DECISION MAKING IN
Ophthalmology

Visit our website at **www.mosby.com**

DECISION MAKING IN
Ophthalmology

W. A. J. van HEUVEN, M.D.
Professor and Herbert F. Mueller Chair of Ophthalmology
The University of Texas Health Science Center at San Antonio
San Antonio, Texas

JOHAN ZWAAN, M.D., PH.D.
Clinical Professor of Ophthalmology
The University of Texas Health Science Center at San Antonio
San Antonio, Texas;
Senior Academic Consultant in Ophthalmology
King Khaled Eye Specialist Hospital
Riyadh, Saudi Arabia

SECOND EDITION

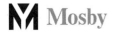 Mosby

A *Harcourt Health Sciences Company*
St. Louis   Philadelphia   London   Sydney   Toronto

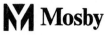
Mosby

A Harcourt Health Sciences Company

Editor: Liz Fathman
Senior Managing Editor: Kathy Falk
Editorial Assistant: Peggy Perel
Project Manager: Patricia Tannian
Senior Production Editor: Anne Salmo
Design Manager: Gail Morey Hudson
Cover Design: Teresa Breckwoldt

SECOND EDITION

Mosby, Inc.
A Harcourt Health Sciences Company
11830 Westline Industrial Drive
St. Louis, Missouri 63146

ISBN 1-55664-454-X

00 01 02 03 04 CL/MV-Y 9 8 7 6 5 4 3 2

CONTRIBUTORS

BRIAN B. BERGER, M.D.

Clinical Professor of Ophthalmology, Department of
  Ophthalmology,
University of Texas Health Science Center,
San Antonio, Texas;
Chief, Department of Ophthalmology
Seton Hospital Network,
Austin, Texas

SUSAN M. BERRY, M.D.

Department of Ophthalmology,
Northeast Methodist Hospital,
San Antonio, Texas

REBECCA J. BROCK, M.D.

Chairman of Ophthalmology, Department of Surgery,
Rose Medical Center
Denver, Colorado

JOHN E. CARTER, M.D.

Associate Professor, Neurology and Ophthalmology,
Department of Medicine-Neurology,
University of Texas Health Science Center,
San Antonio, Texas

CHRISTINE J. CHENG, M.D.

Instructor of Surgery, Department of Surgery,
Division of Plastic and Reconstructive Surgery,
Washington University School of Medicine;
Attending Surgeon, Department of Surgery,
Division of Plastic and Reconstructive Surgery,
Barnes-Jewish Hospital,
St. Louis, Missouri

CONSTANCE L. FRY, M.D.

Clinical Assistant Professor,
Department of Ophthalmology,
Tulane University; Ochsner Clinic,
New Orleans, Louisiana

G. ROBERT HAMPTON, M.D.

Clinical Associate Professor,
Department of Ophthalmology,
SUNY Health Science Center;
Retina Vitreous Surgeons of Central New York,
Syracuse, New York

JOSEPH M. HARRISON, Ph.D.

Associate Professor, Department of Ophthalmology,
The University of Texas Health Science Center at San
  Antonio;
Chief, Visual Function Testing Service,
Department of Ophthalmology, University Hospital
San Antonio, Texas

PETER B. HAY, BA, CRA

Director of Photography,
Retina Vitreous Surgeons of Central New York,
Syracuse, New York

KRISTIN STORY HELD, M.D.

Clinical Associate Professor,
Department of Ophthalmology,
University of Texas Health Science Center at San Antonio,
San Antonio, Texas

DAVID E.E. HOLCK, M.D.

Assistant Professor, Department of Surgery,
Uniformed Services University,
F. Edward Hebert School of Medicine,
Bethesda, Maryland;
Director, Oculoplastics, Orbit & Ocular Oncology Services,
Department of Ophthalmology,
Wilford Hall Medical Center
San Antonio, Texas

MARILYN C. KINCAID, M.D.

Clinical Professor,
Departments of Ophthalmology and Pathology,
St. Louis University School of Medicine,
St. Louis, Missouri

NEIL LALANI, M.D.

Department of Ophthalmology,
University of Texas Health Science Center at San Antonio,
San Antonio, Texas

LORENA LAREZ de MENDIBLE, M.D.

Ophthalmologist, Department of Ophthalmology,
Military Hospital "Dr. Carlos Arvelo" and Clinica El Avila,
Caracas, Venezuela

ANDREW W. LAWTON, M.D.

Little Rock Eye Clinic,
Little Rock, Arkansas

BAILEY L. LEE, M.D.

The Methodist Hospital,
Houston Eye Associates,
Houston, Texas

CHARLES R. LEONE, M.D.

Clinical Professor of Ophthalmology,
Department of Ophthalmology,
University of Texas Health Science Center;
Consultant Staff, Department of Ophthalmology,
St. Luke's Baptist Hospital,
San Antonio, Texas

JEFFREY T. LIEGNER, M.D.

Private Practice—Eye Care Northwest,
Sparta, New Jersey;
Ophthalmologist, Department of Surgery,
Newton Memorial Hospital,
Newton, New Jersey

J. ALBERTO MARTINEZ, M.D.

Clinical Assistant Professor of Ophthalmology,
Georgetown University and George Washington University,
Washington, D.C.;
Department of Ophthalmology,
Georgetown University Hospital/Shady Grove Hospital,
Bethesda, Maryland

LINA M. MAROUF, M.D.

Clinical Associate Professor,
Department of Ophthalmology,
University of Texas Health Science Center,
San Antonio, Texas

MARK McDERMOTT, M.D.

Professor of Ophthalmology,
Kresge Eye Institute, Wayne State University,
Detroit, Michigan

J. KEVIN McKINNEY, M.D., MPH

Ophthalmologist, Glaucoma Specialist,
Eye Health Northwest,
Oregon City, Oregon

MATTHEW B. MILLS, M.D.

Chief, Ophthalmology, Department of Ophthalmology,
Irwin Army Community Hospital,
Fort Riley, Kansas

JAMES L. MIMS III, M.D.

Clinical Professor of Ophthalmology,
Department of Ophthalmology,
University of Texas Health Science Center at San Antonio;
Active Staff, Christus Santa Rosa Children's Hospital,
Baptist Medical Center,
San Antonio, Texas

PETER A. NETLAND, M.D., Ph.D.

Associate Professor, Director Glaucoma Service,
Department of Ophthalmology,
University of Tennessee—Memphis,
Memphis, Tennessee

JOHN D. NG, M.D.

Clinical Faculty, Department of Ophthalmology
University of Texas Health Science Center;
Chief, Oculoplastics and Orbit Service,
Department of Ophthalmology, Service/Department of
   Surgery
Brooke Army Medical Center,
San Antonio, Texas

LANNY ODIN, M.D.

Private Practice, Prairie Eye Center;
Department of Ophthalmology, St. Johns Hospital,
Springfield, Illinois

JOHN M. PARKINSON, M.D.

Clinical Assistant Professor of Ophthalmology,
Department of Ophthalmology,
University of New Mexico School of Medicine,
Albuquerque, New Mexico

KENNETH L. PIEST, M.D.

Clinical Associate Professor,
Departments of Plastic Surgery and Ophthalmology,
University of Texas Health Science Center;
Director, Texas Ophthalmic Plastic Surgery,
San Antonio, Texas

DAVID K. SCALES, M.D.

Assistant Professor of Surgery,
Department of Surgery, Uniformed Services
University of the Health Sciences,
Bethesda, Maryland;
Uveitis Consultant, Department of Ophthalmology,
University of Texas Health Science Center at San Antonio,
San Antonio, Texas

MARTHA P. SCHATZ, M.D.

Clinical Associate Professor of Ophthalmology,
Department of Ophthalmology,
University of Texas Health Science Center at San Antonio;
Neuroophthalmologist, Pediatric Ophthalmologist,
Department of Ophthalmology,
Wilford Hall Medical Center, Lackland AFB,
San Antonio, Texas

FRANK W. SCRIBBICK, M.D.

Clinical Associate Professor,
Department of Ophthalmology,
University of Texas Health Science Center;
Staff Ophthalmologist/Ophthalmic Pathologist,
Brooke Army Medical Center,
San Antonio, Texas

CAMERON K. SHIELDS, M.D.

Ophthalmologist, Department of Surgery,
Virginia Mason Medical Center,
Seattle, Washington

SCOTT D. SMITH, M.D.

Associate Director of Research,
Kind Khaled Eye Specialist Hospital,
Riyadh, Saudi Arabia

TOMY STARCK, M.D.

Assistant Professor, Department of Ophthalmology,
University of Texas Health Science Center at San Antonio;
Assistant Professor, Department of Ophthalmology,
University Hospital,
San Antonio, Texas

ELMER Y. TU, M.D.

Assistant Professor, Department of Ophthalmology,
Director, Refractive Surgery Service,
Illinois Eye and Ear Infirmary,
University of Illinois-Chicago,
Chicago, Illinois

MARTHA WALTON, M.D.

Clinical Associate Professor,
Department of Ophthalmology,
University of Texas Health Science Center at San Antonio;
Active Staff, Department of Ophthalmology,
St. Luke's Baptist Hospital,
San Antonio, Texas

ROY WHITAKER, Jr., M.D.

Department of Surgery,
Moses Cone Health System,
Greensboro, North Carolina

RICHARD W. YEE, M.D.

Clinical Associate Professor,
Department of Ophthalmology and Visual Science,
University of Texas Medical School;
Director of Cornea/External Diseases,
Herman Eye Center, Herman Hospital,
Houston, Texas

ROCKEFELLER S.L. YOUNG, M.D.

Professor,
Department of Ophthalmology and Visual Sciences,
Texas Tech Medical Center,
Lubbock, Texas

To our wives
Constance and **Karen**
for their support.

FOREWORD

My enthusiasm for this book stems from at least two sources. First, I can personally attest that the quality of editors and contributors is first rate. Second, they have taken an already successful book and have gone to the important second edition, which is a testament to the usefulness and quality of the central concept and product.

An additional facet is the discipline needed and exhibited for this task by the authors, Drs. van Heuven and Zwaan. Having known both of them for several decades, their success is not surprising. The value of the decision trees in ophthalmology, as constructed in this book, will likely be more than at first is evident. Our entry with immediate access to Medline and other similar data banks can produce syndrome and disease specificity in surprisingly instant fashions. That disease or syndrome can then be fitted into the decision trees down the several branches, and it is for the user then to climb the branches to look for the more generic testing and results suggested in the tree and the appended text.

Yet another use of this edition will be the amalgamation of practice parameters into the substance of literature searches and decision trees. The final step will be the quality outcomes following treatment.

One can easily imagine how this book may be central to all of the above endeavors. I complement the authors and believe that this second edition will spur a further edition as more branches grow and others are trimmed and yet others are grafted to nonophthalmic branches of medicine, social services, and yes, even payment schedules.

I thank the editors for a work well done.

Robert D. Reinecke, M.D.

Professor of Ophthalmology,
Jefferson Medical College of Thomas Jefferson University

FOREWORD TO THE FIRST EDITION

Drs. van Heuven and Zwaan and their collaborators have undertaken an enormous and difficult task in formalizing the manner in which a skilled practitioner reaches a diagnosis. In the past, this was mainly an intuitive process, but the computer age led naturally to decision trees, decision analysis, decision theory, and related topics. The steps involved in creating a useful decision tree are complicated and have not been previously explored in ophthalmology, to this extent.

I believe this volume emphasizes the reasons why computer programs of differential diagnosis are currently seldom used. Generally, the programs do not indicate the branches of the decision tree being followed, and an enormous amount of time is lost in unrealistic searching. This textbook both demonstrates the problem and solves it in the two decision trees constructed for a patient with loss of vision. The first decision tree is based on either a transient or a persistent loss of vision. The differential diagnosis of persistent visual loss is based mainly on ophthalmoscopic ex-amination. The second decision tree deals with transient visual loss based on the length of time the symptom has been present. Having both decision trees visible in their entirety (and not buried in a computer program) makes the differential diagnosis immediately evident, giving the steps in both the history and the examination that should be considered.

The 130 decision trees presented here contain the differential diagnoses of a wide array of disorders. The volume constitutes a rich ophthalmic resource, for such branched diagrams are exceptionally difficult to prepare. Drs. van Heuven and Zwaan and their co-workers deserve the gratitude and praise of the entire ophthalmic community for indicating the steps by which the skilled practitioner arrives at the final (and correct) diagnosis.

Frank W. Newell, M.D.
Raymond Professor, Emeritus
The University of Chicago

PREFACE

The purpose of *Decision Making in Ophthalmology* is to provide all eye-care providers with algorithms, or "decision trees," that demonstrate logical processes by which clinical problems can be approached. Each decision tree shows how one can proceed methodically either from a symptom or sign to a diagnosis, or from a diagnosis to an appropriate management plan. Each algorithm represents the personal approach of the author to the particular problem. Thus it should not be seen as the only way to solve that problem, but rather as a method favored by the author that has proven to be effective in a clinical setting.

Many of the common signs or symptoms with which patients present to eye-care providers are included. Each algorithm has been intentionally kept simple, yet is detailed enough so that major areas of differential diagnosis are not omitted. Thus the book should be useful for all levels of eye care, whether provided by medical students, residents, optometrists, general practitioners, internists, general ophthalmologists, or even subspecialists in ophthalmology.

Every chapter is best used by observing the tree first. Letters in the tree refer to specific paragraphs in the text, which further explain, add detail, or discuss the rationale of various parts of the tree. The text by itself is not a complete discussion of the problem and may be difficult to understand without reference to the tree. The references are general references about the subject of the tree and are not intended to support any specific statements. Boxes have been placed around invasive procedures and protocols (some drugs) that place the patient at greater risk. Surgical procedures are boxed using capital letters. An index has been provided, which lists symptoms, signs, and some diagnoses and treatments, with the bold reference indicating the main location of their discussion.

Because of the popularity of the first edition, the general outline and organization of the book has not been changed. However, some new chapters have been added to be more complete and other chapters have been deleted or combined. All chapters and their references have been updated with special attention to new therapeutic methods and medications. A new section, entitled "Common Ophthalmic Consultations," has also been added, using the slightly different format of a diagnostic "checklist."

We gratefully acknowledge the help we have received from all of our contributing colleagues, many of them associated with the Department of Ophthalmology at the University of Texas Health Science Center in San Antonio.

W. A. J. van Heuven, M.D.
Johan Zwaan, M.D., Ph.D.

CONTENTS

GENERAL OPHTHALMOLOGY

VISUAL LOSS

W.A.J. van Heuven, M.D.

Vision is the most precious sense, so loss of vision is a serious complaint that requires immediate attention. Untreated and permanent, it changes the patient's life significantly, especially if it is bilateral.

A. If visual loss is spontaneous and without apparent cause (e.g., trauma), the persistence of sudden severe vision loss in one or both eyes may indicate retinal arterial occlusion, a medical emergency. Thus rapid documentation of this condition (vision test, pupil and retina examination), done within 2 hours of the onset of symptoms, may allow early successful emergency treatment, which can consist of ocular massage, paracentesis of the cornea to decrease ocular pressure and increase perfusion, retrobulbar injection of vasodilators, and breathing of CO_2. There is evidence that, after 90 minutes of complete central occlusion of the retinal artery, the retina is permanently damaged and will not recover.

B. *Nontraumatic vitreous hemorrhage* is usually caused by vitreous detachment. The bleeding can originate from vitreous adhesions to vascular structures on the surface of the retina, such as normal disc vessels or neovascularization of any cause, and from retinal vessels when the retina tears. Small vitreous hemorrhages clear rapidly from the visual axis by gravity, so patients may not appreciate the potential danger. Perform a thorough retinal examination in all patients whose eyes have vitreous hemorrhage of any amount to rule out retinal tears and to confirm vitreous detachment. Treat symptomatic horseshoe-shaped retinal tears to prevent retinal detachment. *Vein occlusions* may produce macular edema, which may resolve in weeks or months. Central or branch occlusions of the retinal arterioles are usually embolic and may produce only temporary symptoms when the embolus moves downstream. Treatment is usually directed at making this happen by creating sudden vasodilation. Several *macular disorders* produce transient visual symptoms. Central serous choroidopathy almost resolves completely within 6 weeks to 6 months. Some presumed inflammatory conditions, such as idiopathic stellate neuroretinopathy and acute multifocal punctate pigment epitheliopathy (AMPPE), resolve in a few weeks, as may hemorrhage in some macular degenerations (e.g., age-related or angioid streaks). When these clear, vision may be improved even though the underlying cause persists and will ultimately lead to permanent visual loss. Macular edema caused by a solar burn after eclipse watching or sun gazing often results in surprising recovery of vision. Severe and especially sudden systemic disorders, particularly those causing hypertension (e.g., idiopathic, eclampsial, or severe metabolic imbalance such as acute renal failure), may cause temporary vision loss, usually from macular edema or secondary retinal detachment, until the primary condition is cured.

C. Blunt trauma to the head is less likely to cause visual loss than direct trauma to the eye and orbit but has been known to cause brain injury, especially to the occipital cortex, and contrecoup optic nerve and retinal damage. If optic nerve contusion is suspected, consider high-dose systemic steroids. Direct trauma can take many forms. Blunt injury may cause visual loss by mechanisms ranging from severe lid edema to optic nerve avulsion and includes orbital fractures, ocular hemorrhages, cataracts, and retinal damage. Pupillary examination to elicit an afferent pupillary defect (Marcus Gunn) is helpful in determining damage to the visual pathway. Echography is an easy, cheap, and noninvasive way to rule out a pathologic condition. CT scan and MRI may be helpful, particularly in determining orbital fractures and optic nerve and brain damage. In severe direct trauma, always suspect ocular perforation. Severe hypotony, chemosis, and visual loss are especially suspect. Echography, particularly standardized A-scan, can be helpful. A common ocular perforation is caused by a sliver of steel, usually magnetic, that enters the eye while the patient is hammering on a metal object. Because the sliver is small and thin, it perforates easily through a minute entry wound, which may make it difficult to find. A history of eye injury should thus include detailed questioning about the manner in which the injury occurred. Plain films of the orbit should be routine if any such injury is even remotely suspected. Sharp pointed objects (e.g., darts, pencils, nails) that cause eye injuries, even though they may seem to have perforated the eye anteriorly only, often leave double perforations. Echography can help rule this out.

D. After surgery, visual loss can occur from several obvious ocular complications (e.g., hyphema). However, after ocular or orbital surgery, orbital hemorrhage, optic nerve damage, ocular perforation, and intravascular injection during retrobulbar anesthesia must be considered.

E. Spontaneous "idiopathic" persistent visual loss, when bilateral, most often results from nonocular disease. However, some patients insist that the loss was bilateral when, in fact, the event was unilateral, and the second eye had previously been blinded by another or similar disorder. All cases of visual loss should be considered eye emergencies until the examination indicates otherwise. Of special importance is the severe monocular visual loss in the elderly patient due to temporal (cranial) arteritis. An elevated sedimentation rate helps suggest the diagnosis, at which time systemic steroids should be given immediately to prevent

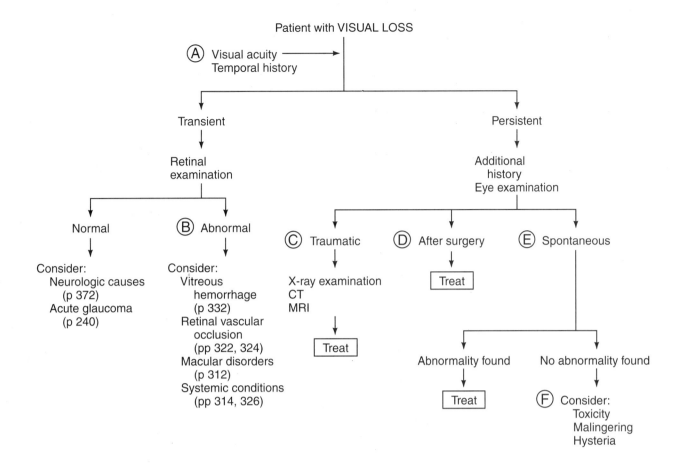

References

Augsburger JI, Magargal LE. Visual prognosis following treatment of acute central retinal artery obstruction. Br J Ophthalmol 1980; 64:913–917.

Deutsch TA, Feller DB. Paton and Goldberg's management of ocular injuries. 2nd ed. Philadelphia: WB Saunders, 1985.

Hayreh SS, Kolder HE, Weingeist TA. Central retinal artery occlusion and retinal tolerance time. Ophthalmology 1980; 87:75–78.

Spoor TC, Hartel WC, Lensink DB, Wilkinson MI. Treatment of traumatic optic neuropathy with corticosteroids. Am J Ophthalmol 1990; 110:665–669.

involvement of the other eye. Biopsy of the temporal artery can confirm the diagnosis later, and results will still be abnormal for several days after steroid treatment has begun.

F. Toxic visual loss is often bilateral and may be caused by quinine methyl alcohol poisoning. The latter, as well as the use of numerous illegal drugs, may be difficult to glean from the patient's history unless specifically elicited.

TRANSIENT VISUAL LOSS

John E. Carter, M.D.
Susan M. Berry, M.D.

The two important factors in the approach to the patient with transient loss of vision are (1) the temporal profile of the transient event and (2) the fundus examination, which is normal in most cases.

A. Patients who experience visual loss when they look to one side usually have an intraorbital mass that compresses or stretches the optic nerve as it moves with rotation of the eye. The examination may be normal, or there may be evidence of a mild optic neuropathy in the form of an afferent pupil defect, color desaturation, or disc edema.

B. Transient obscurations of vision occur in 50% of patients with papilledema secondary to intracranial hypertension. Vision is lost, usually in one eye, just long enough for the patient to be aware of it and blink a few times or rub the eye. The patient is likely to consult a physician only if episodes are frequent or other symptoms are associated with the illness. Any condition resulting in tightly packed nerve fibers as they enter the disc to form the optic nerve may produce similar symptoms.

C. Most patients who experience amaurosis fugax have episodes lasting minutes. Very brief or very prolonged episodes of transient visual loss may be caused by carotid atherosclerotic disease, but the likelihood of carotid occlusive lesions is much smaller. Other factors that identify the patient as having increased risk for cardiovascular disease, including age, hypertension, coronary artery disease, peripheral vascular disease, and family history, must be taken into consideration.

D. The presence of a small area of visual loss or a mild disturbance of vision that progressively increases over 15 minutes or more is highly characteristic of migraine. The patient need not have a headache for this diagnosis to be made. Most patients have some abnormal visual symptoms associated with the episodes, most commonly fortification spectra around an area of scotoma or distortions within the area of visual disturbance resembling heat waves or water running down a glass. Similar abnormal visual disturbances, often accompanied by headache, may occur with cerebral lesions such as arteriovenous malformations or meningiomas, but they do not have the characteristic buildup and resolution. Instead these structural lesions produce symptoms that steadily increase in duration and frequency until they are present daily throughout much of the day.

E. Patients may experience transient monocular visual loss at any age. If the fundus examination is normal, the most helpful indicator of carotid occlusive disease is age. Patients younger than age 40 are unlikely to have carotid disease in the absence of other risk factors. Most cases in these patients are idiopathic, although transient visual loss may occur in association with migraine, Raynaud's phenomenon, diseases causing increased viscosity of the blood, and from cardiogenic embolism.

References

Burde RM, Savino PJ, Trobe ID. Clinical decisions in neuroophthalmology. 2nd ed. St Louis: Mosby, 1992.

Glaser J. Neuro-ophthalmology. 2nd ed. Philadelphia: Lippincott, 1990.

Lee AG, Brazis P. Clinical pathways in neuro-ophthalmology. New York: Thieme, 1998.

Miller NR. Walsh and Hoyt's clinical neuro-ophthalmology. 5th ed. Baltimore: Williams & Wilkins, 1998.

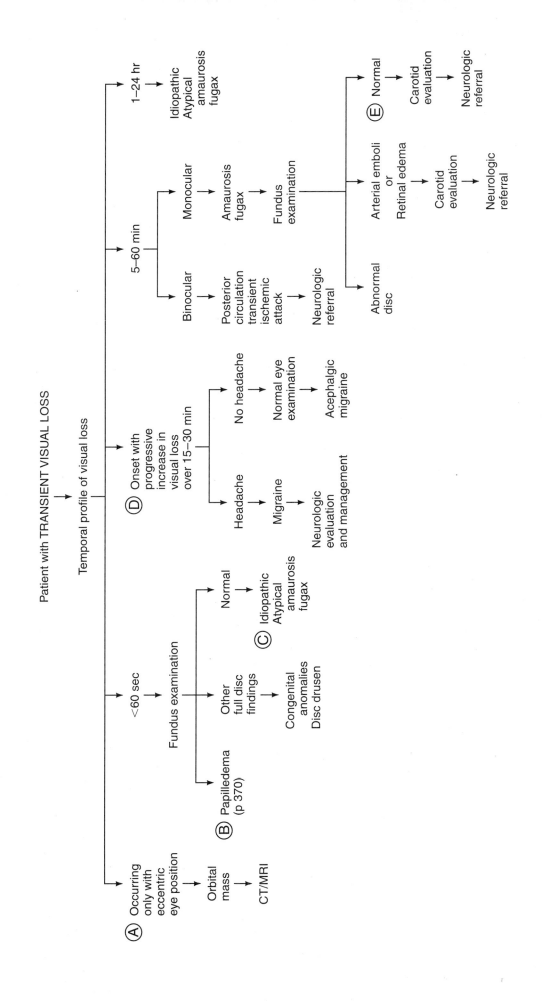

Patient with TRANSIENT VISUAL LOSS

Temporal profile of visual loss

(A) Occurring only with eccentric eye position
→ Orbital mass
→ CT/MRI

< 60 sec
Fundus examination

(B) Papilledema (p 370)

Other full disc findings
→ Congenital anomalies Disc drusen

Normal
→ **(C)** Idiopathic Atypical amaurosis fugax

(D) Onset with progressive increase in visual loss over 15–30 min

Headache
→ Migraine
→ Neurologic evaluation and management

No headache
→ Normal eye examination
→ Acephalgic migraine

5–60 min

Binocular
→ Posterior circulation transient ischemic attack
→ Neurologic referral

Monocular
→ Amaurosis fugax
→ Fundus examination

Abnormal disc

Arterial emboli or Retinal edema
→ Carotid evaluation
→ Neurologic referral

Normal
→ **(E)** Normal
→ Carotid evaluation
→ Neurologic referral

1–24 hr
→ Idiopathic Atypical amaurosis fugax

DISTORTED VISION

W.A.J. van Heuven, M.D.
Bailey L. Lee, M.D.

Distorted vision, or irregularities of lines and figures in the central visual field, is called *metamorphopsia*. Micropsia and macropsia, the two forms of dysmetropsia (seeing abnormal size), are forms of metamorphopsia in which objects appear smaller or larger than they really are.

A. Take a careful history because patients complaining of distorted vision are often nonspecific in describing symptoms. They also often do not know whether the distortion is monocular or binocular or whether it is associated with other symptoms. Testing for distortion, one eye at a time, is easily done using the Amsler grid, which tests the central 20 degrees of vision at reading distance.

B. Some patients use the word *distortion* to describe the perception of blur caused by acquired decreased vision or central scotoma in one eye. Monocular visual acuity and Amsler grid testing elicit these causes. Occasionally, large vitreous floaters, usually from vitreous detachment, may interfere with vision, especially at close range, and mimic monocular distortion. Halos around lights, with or without blurring of vision, may indicate glaucoma. Diplopia or triplopia, whether monocular or binocular, must be investigated initially with a careful examination of muscle balance. Acquired nystagmus requires a thorough neurologic evaluation. Binocular dysmetropsia, although usually retinal in origin, may be cerebral. Cerebral micropsia is more common than macropsia. It may be associated with other neurologic conditions such as migraine, epilepsy, hysteria, schizophrenia, drug intoxication, and focal lesions. These symptoms may be difficult to differentiate from hallucinations. *Palinopsia,* a term meaning visual perseveration, which is the persistence of visual perception after the object has been removed, also requires neurologic evaluation. Visual hallucinations occur from a variety of causes, most of which are not ocular. They represent complex integrative processes and often have little value in topical diagnosis. However, formed hallucinations are often the result of temporal lobe involvement, and unformed ones suggest involvement of the occipital lobe. Many hallucinations are associated with cerebral tumors, although they can be caused by cerebral injury or infection. A complete neurologic evaluation is indicated because different forms of epilepsy, visual field defects, and other neurologic findings may help localize the cause.

C. Micropsia from ocular causes, so-called peripheral metamorphopsia, is often monocular. If binocular, just like binocular macropsia, central metamorphopsia (i.e., resulting from cerebral causes) must be ruled out.

True ocular micropsia is caused by an abnormal separation of the rods and cones, usually in the macular region, which causes fewer retinal receptors to be stimulated by an object than would normally be stimulated by that object. Therefore the brain receives and perceives the object to be smaller. Conditions that separate the retinal receptors, such as stretching or edema of the retina, cause micropsia.

D. True peripheral or retinal macropsia, in contrast to micropsia, is caused by the retinal photoreceptors being closer together than normal. Thus more retinal receptors are stimulated by an object than would normally be stimulated by that object, causing the brain to receive and perceive that the object is larger than actual. Conditions causing shrinkage of the retina, such as retinal scars, are the most common cause of macropsia. If a retinal condition, such as inflammation or trauma, initially causes edema and later causes scarring, macropsia may follow micropsia.

E. Irregular metamorphopsia can result from any condition that causes an irregular distortion of the retina, so the photoreceptors are no longer evenly spaced. Patients perceive straight lines to be crooked and, if the condition involves the fovea, may also have blurred vision. Any condition that causes scarring of the retina or shifting of the retina because of traction may cause metamorphopsia. Patients with impending macular holes or small full-thickness macular holes may also have complaints of metamorphopsia. Like the vitreomacular traction syndrome these may not be obvious unless one performs careful contact lens biomicroscopy.

F. Pars plana vitrectomy and membrane stripping can improve vision and distortion in patients with epiretinal membranes and vitreomacular traction syndrome. Macular holes can be closed with improved vision after vitrectomy and fluid-gas exchange. Because of the high rate of spontaneous resolution of impending macular holes, these are generally observed unless a full-thickness hole develops.

References

Gass JDM. Macular dysfunction caused by vitreous and vitreoretinal interface abnormalities. Stereoscopic atlas of macular diseases: diagnosis and treatment. 4th ed. St Louis: Mosby, 1997.

Miller NR. Walsh and Hoyt's clinical neuro-ophthalmology. 5th ed. Baltimore: Williams & Wilkins, 1998.

Patient with DISTORTED VISION

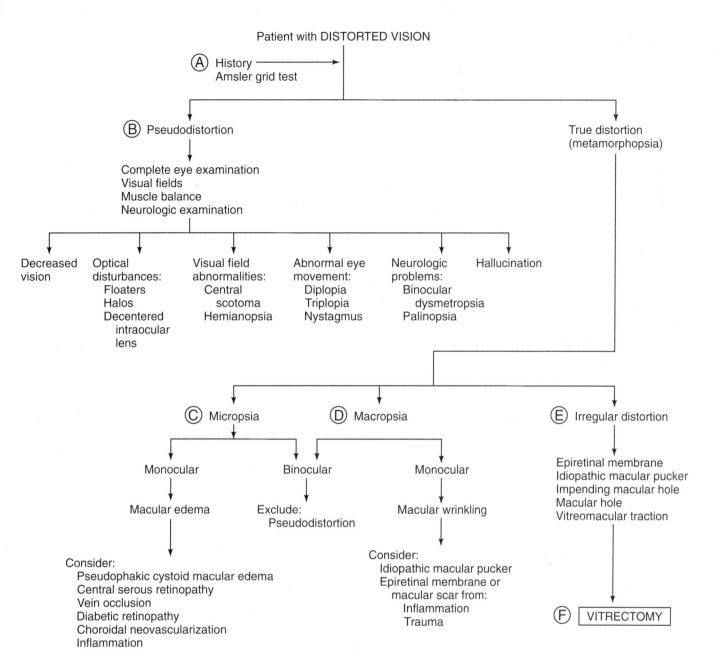

(A) History ⟶
Amsler grid test

(B) Pseudodistortion

True distortion
(metamorphopsia)

Complete eye examination
Visual fields
Muscle balance
Neurologic examination

Decreased
vision

Optical
disturbances:
  Floaters
  Halos
  Decentered
    intraocular
    lens

Visual field
abnormalities:
  Central
    scotoma
  Hemianopsia

Abnormal eye
movement:
  Diplopia
  Triplopia
  Nystagmus

Neurologic
problems:
  Binocular
    dysmetropsia
  Palinopsia

Hallucination

(C) Micropsia

(D) Macropsia

(E) Irregular distortion

Monocular

Binocular

Monocular

Epiretinal membrane
Idiopathic macular pucker
Impending macular hole
Macular hole
Vitreomacular traction

Macular edema

Exclude:
  Pseudodistortion

Macular wrinkling

Consider:
  Pseudophakic cystoid macular edema
  Central serous retinopathy
  Vein occlusion
  Diabetic retinopathy
  Choroidal neovascularization
  Inflammation

Consider:
  Idiopathic macular pucker
  Epiretinal membrane or
    macular scar from:
      Inflammation
      Trauma

(F) VITRECTOMY

POOR COLOR VISION

Rockefeller S.L. Young, Ph.D.
Joseph M. Harrison, Ph.D.

The evaluation of color vision complaints is important primarily because poor color vision may be an early sign of acquired disease or may help differentiate among alternative diagnoses. Occasionally, color vision evaluation is needed in the certification of personnel for occupations that require chromatic discrimination.

A. Color vision problems can be broadly classified as those affecting high-level mental functions involving colors but not the color sense per se and those primarily affecting the color sense. Problems affecting the color sense are manifested by poor color discrimination, abnormal mixtures of primary colors required to match a standard light, disturbances in the color appearance of objects, or the like. Problems affecting high-level mental functions involve the names of colors of familiar objects, the categorization of different colors, topographical memory linked with colors, the attachment of emotion with colors, and so forth.

B. Brain disorders can produce difficulties associated with colors (e.g., color agnosia, anomia, aphasia) without affecting the color sense. Many of the problems are associated with the language aspect of colors, but it is perhaps worth mentioning that visual-verbal or verbal-visual dissociations (i.e., the inability to name the color of shown objects or to correctly point to color-named objects) are not adequate evidence of such problems. Additional information required includes whether color discrimination is normal or whether there is evidence of nonvisual (e.g., verbal-verbal) dissociations, such as the inability to name the color of a named fruit (e.g., banana, apple). Consider neurologic referral.

C. A patient has a defect in the color sense if he or she fails the pseudoisochromatic plates test (e.g., American Optical Hardy-Rand-Rittler, Ishihara, Dvorine, Tokyo Medical College), color arrangement tests (e.g., Farnsworth D-15 and 100-hue, Lanthony Desaturated Panel, Sahlgren saturation test), or color matching tests (e.g., the Nagel, the Neitz, and the Pickford-Nicolson anomaloscopes). Based on the portion of the visible spectrum in which the performance deficits occur, the color vision defects can be further classified as "red-green" (i.e., middle and long wavelength spectrum), "blue" or "blue-yellow" (i.e., short wavelength spectrum), or nonspecific (i.e., the entire spectrum).

D. In the general population, most people with red-green color vision defects have a congenital, stationary, X-linked recessively inherited trait. This trait, present in about 8% of men and 0.42% of women, is generally not considered a health-related problem, but the color vision defect may be important to the patient because it cannot be corrected and may affect early success in school or his or her career plans (e.g., in transportation, military, law enforcement professions). The diagnosis of the inherited color vision trait is supported by a history of a stationary red-green color defect from a young age, the absence of other significant ocular or visual defects (e.g., having good visual acuity), or a family history of color vision problems consistent with X-linked recessive inheritance. Rayleigh matches (the red and green color mixture that appears perceptually identical to a spectral yellow field) provide the definitive data for classifying red-green defects into anomalous trichromacy (i.e., protanomaly and deuteranomaly) or dichromacy (i.e., protanopia and deuteranopia). The Rayleigh matches are made using an anomaloscope.

In the absence of evidence that the red-green defect is stationary, X-linked recessive, and so on, consider the possibility that a red-green defect is secondary to an acquired disorder. The loss of red-green discrimination as demonstrated by pseudoisochromatic plates or color arrangement tests suggests involvement of the central 5 degrees of visual field but, contrary to early clinical correlations, seldom provides information about whether the lesion lies in the optic nerve versus outer retina. However, abnormalities in the Rayleigh matches strongly indicate either a photoreceptor or prereceptoral disturbance.

E. Patients with a "blue" or "blue-yellow" defect typically confuse blues and greens or yellows and violet. Because cases of stationary, inherited, blue-yellow defects are so rarely reported, one would assume, until proven otherwise, that a patient with a blue-yellow defect probably has an acquired problem. The visual pathway for the blue cone signals is thought to be more vulnerable to diseases and ocular insults than the pathway for red or green cone signals. So, a blue-yellow defect may be an indication of early stage disease. In addition to neuronal lesions, a blue-yellow defect may originate from aging changes in the lens of the eye.

F. Nonspecific color vision defects (i.e., significant discrimination losses throughout the entire light spectrum) occur in several distinct clinical entities, all of which fall into the broad classification of "achromatopsia."

G. When nonspecific color discrimination losses are accompanied with normal night vision but poor visual acuity, the cone-mediated vision may be selectively compromised. Progressive cone degeneration and congenital, autosomal recessively inherited, rod monochromacy are among likely diagnoses. Both disorders are associated with poor day-vision function (e.g., visual acuity of 20/200 or worse) and little, if any,

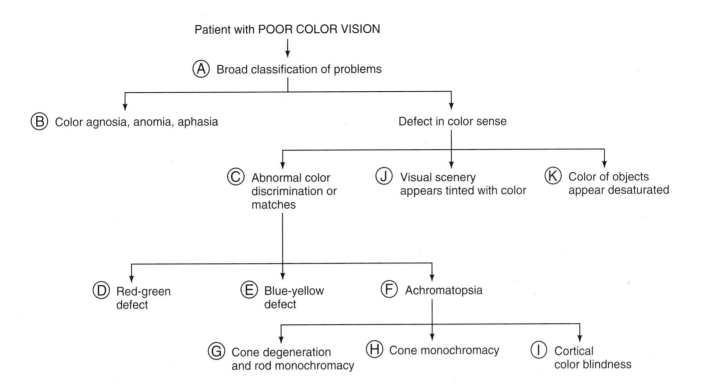

color vision. Rod monochromats also have photophobia and nystagmus, which tend to diminish with age. There is also a rare, X-linked recessive incomplete ("blue-cone") achromatopsia with similar clinical symptoms except for residual blue-yellow color vision and visual acuity as good as 20/60.

H. When nonspecific color discrimination losses are accompanied with normal visual acuity and a history of the disorder from early age, consider cone monochromacy. Cone monochromacy is believed to be a defect of the visual pathway in which chromatic information is not transmitted to the brain despite the presence of cone photoreceptors.

I. When nonspecific color discrimination losses occur after head trauma or vascular cerebral disorder, a probable diagnosis is cortical color blindness. This condition is distinguished from other abnormalities associated with cerebral lesions, such as color agnosia, anomia, or aphasia, in that cortical color blindness involves a loss of the color sense. In the classic cases of cortical color blindness, visual acuity was spared; but the achromatopsia was accompanied by ancillary symptoms such as visual field defects (particularly in the upper quadrant), inability to recognize faces (prosopagnosia), inability to spatially navigate in familiar surroundings (topographical disorientation), or inability to recognize objects (object agnosia).

J. Another clue of an abnormality involving the color sense is the disturbance in color appearance of objects; for example, the patient may report that portions of the visual scenery or the entire visual scenery in one or both eyes appears "tinted" purple, green, blue, red, or yellow (chromatopsia). Depending on the color of the tint, the problem can be classified as erythropsia (red), xanthopsia (yellow), cyanopsia (blue), or chloropsia (green). Chromatopsia almost always suggests an acquired visual defect. It is a symptom reported in association with retinal side effects from drugs and toxic agents. Drugs of particular clinical significance include cardiac glycosides such as digoxin and digitoxin, antimalarial agents such as quinine and chloroquine, and psychotherapeutic drugs such as thioridazine. Chromatopsia may arise optically when substances such as blood or fluorescein collect in front of the retina and alter the wavelength composition of light reaching the photoreceptors. Chromatopsia is also experienced after exposure to high illumination for long periods.

K. Patients may report that the color of an object appears pale, washed-out, or desaturated, another clue of a disturbance of the color sense. Such subjective descriptions are particularly credible when the problem occurs in one eye and the patient is able to appreciate the difference seen by the better eye. The report of color desaturation suggests a loss in the color sense with relatively greater preservation of the luminance sense. Some clinicians believe that the desaturation in the color of red objects is a sensitive indicator of significant macular or optic nerve disease.

References

Grusser OJ, Landis T. The world turns grey: Achromatopsia, colour agnosia and other impairments of colour vision caused by cerebral lesion in visual agnosia and other disturbances of visual perception and cognition. Chap 12. Boca Raton: CRC Press, 1991. This book is volume 12 in the VISION and VISUAL DYSFUNCTION series.

Krastel H, Moreland JD. Colour vision deficiencies in ophthalmic diseases. In: Inherited and acquired colour vision deficiencies. Chap 8. Boca Raton: CRC Press, 1991. This book is volume 7 in the VISION and VISUAL DYSFUNCTION series.

Miller NR. Walsh and Hoyt's Clinical Neuro-ophthalmology. 5th ed. Baltimore: Williams & Wilkins, 1998.

Pokorny J, Smith VC, Verriest G, Pinckers AJLG, eds. Congenital and acquired color vision defects. New York: Grune & Stratton, 1979.

Report of Working Group 41 (Committee on Vision). Procedures for testing color vision. Washington, DC: National Academy Press, 1981.

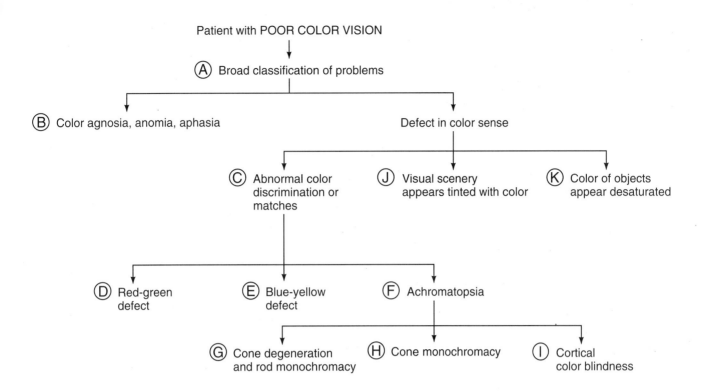

POOR NIGHT VISION

Joseph M. Harrison, Ph.D.
Rockefeller S.L. Young, Ph.D.

A. The patient history for night vision problems is notoriously unreliable. Even in cases of very reduced dark-adapted sensitivity, decreased night vision is often not the patient's complaint. Many complaints of vision problems at night are related to depressed cone rather than rod sensitivity because sufficiently dim ambient illumination is rarely encountered in developed countries.

B. Dark adaptation is tested with a Goldmann-Weekers adaptometer. The pupil is dilated, and the full field of this eye is light adapted for 7 minutes at about 2000 lumens/m² illumination of the interior of the partial sphere used as an adapting field and projection perimeter. The adapting light is turned off, and the test light appears in an area centered at 15 degrees from a dim red fixation spot. At frequent intervals the intensity is decreased and increased to bracket the value that is just visible to the patient. The dark adaptation curve shows the logarithm of the threshold test light intensity as a function of time in the dark after light adaptation (Figure 1). The time of the inflection in the curve separating the cone and rod branches and the threshold in the cone and rod branches are compared with the normal values. Colored test lights can be used to determine relative rod and cone contributions, and the position of the fixation light can be varied to test other parts of the visual field.

C. The electroretinogram (ERG) is the electrical response of the retina produced with flashes of light or other types of visible stimuli. The usual clinical ERG is a mass response arising from the entire retina and can be used to determine rod versus cone and inner versus outer retinal involvement, as well as the lateral extent of the involvement.

D. Localized areas of abnormal retina are usually visible on fundus examination as chorioretinal lesions or pigmentary changes.

E. Chorioretinal abnormality is used to encompass a wide variety of disorders. An important distinction to make is the progressive versus stationary nature of the disease. This is determined by history, but the ERG helps in the diagnosis of type.

F. Fundus findings are an important component of fundus albipunctatus and Oguchi's disease. Both cone and rod adaptation are delayed in fundus albipunctatus, which is associated with slower cone and rod photopigment kinetics. Only rod system adaptation is delayed in Oguchi's disease. Delayed cone-rod break times are also seen in dysfunctions of the retinal pigment epithelium, such as fundus flavimaculatus and dominant drusen. Fundus findings are subtle, if present, in essential congenital stationary night blindness, which can also be distinguished from the two other stationary night-blinding disorders (fundus albipunctatus and Oguchi's disease), which have improved rod sensitivity with prolonged dark adaptation (>180 minutes). Some stationary diseases affect only cone function. In complete achromatopsia or rod monochromatism, there is reduced visual acuity and no cone ERG or cone branch during dark adaptation, but normal rod function exists.

G. Retinitis pigmentosa (RP) and cone-rod degeneration are the two major primary progressive photoreceptor dystrophies associated with decreased night vision. A distinction between the two is that the elevation of the final rod threshold in cone-rod degeneration is usually <100-fold and in rod-cone degeneration >100-fold. Also, in cone-rod degeneration, color vision is affected more than expected on the basis of visual acuity, and photophobia is a more common complaint. Most or all patients with RP have prolonged implicit times for the ERG produced by 30 flashes/sec. The ERG is absent by standard recording techniques in about 70% of patients. The ERG and dark adaptation can be completely normal in central cone dystrophy, which may be detectable only by changes in the fundus, visual acuity, and/or color vision. In some cone degenerations the cone branch of dark adaptation and the cone ERG are absent with a normal rod threshold and ERG. There are also hereditary forms of choroidal atrophy,

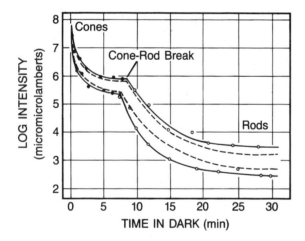

Figure 1 The dark adaptation curve. The area between the dashed lines includes 80% of the data from 110 normal observers. The upper and lower lines represent the upper and lower extremes from this sample. (Adapted from Hecht S, Mandelbaum J. The relation between vitamin A and dark adaptation. JAMA 1939; 112:1911. Copyright 1939, American Medical Association.)

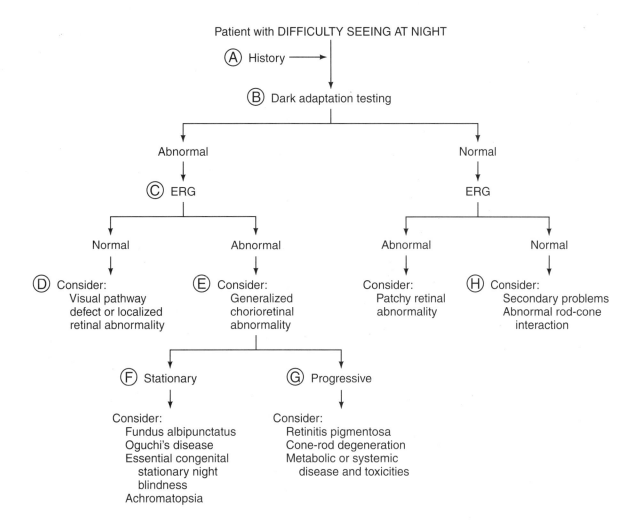

Patient with DIFFICULTY SEEING AT NIGHT

Ⓐ History →

Ⓑ Dark adaptation testing

Abnormal — Normal

Ⓒ ERG — ERG

Abnormal branch (from Ⓒ):
- Normal → Ⓓ Consider: Visual pathway defect or localized retinal abnormality
- Abnormal → Ⓔ Consider: Generalized chorioretinal abnormality

Normal branch:
- Abnormal → Consider: Patchy retinal abnormality
- Normal → Ⓗ Consider: Secondary problems Abnormal rod-cone interaction

From Ⓔ:
- Ⓕ Stationary → Consider: Fundus albipunctatus / Oguchi's disease / Essential congenital stationary night blindness / Achromatopsia
- Ⓖ Progressive → Consider: Retinitis pigmentosa / Cone-rod degeneration / Metabolic or systemic disease and toxicities

such as choroideremia and choroidal sclerosis, which cause a secondary photoreceptor dystrophy and result in poor night vision early in the disease. Avitaminosis is not a common dietary problem in developed countries but may occur secondary to other conditions such as malabsorption syndromes. It can also occur in liver disease and in disorders causing urinary excretion of vitamins. Conditions leading to zinc deficiencies (e.g., alcoholic cirrhosis, chronic pancreatitis) are associated with night vision problems. In addition, a variety of systemic diseases are associated with retinal degenerations affecting night vision: lipid abnormalities (e.g., Bassen-Kornzweig syndrome, or abetalipoproteinemia) resulting in low plasma levels of vitamins A and E, ceroid lipofuscinosis, mucopolysaccharidoses, metabolic disorders such as Refsum's disease (elevated serum phytanic acid) and gyrate atrophy (elevated plasma ornithine), degenerative myopia, and neurologic disease (e.g., Bardet-Biedl, Usher's syndromes). Some forms of occult cancer can also present initially with symptoms of night vision loss. Night vision can be decreased in the later stages of siderosis. Vascular occlusive disease and diabetic retinopathy, luetic retinopathy, panretinal photocoagulation, and phenothiazine, chloroquine, and ethyl alcohol toxicities are also associated with decreased night vision in either the cone or rod branch or both. Glaucoma can cause small losses of dark-adapted sensitivity, which are greater for the rod than cone branch in areas outside of visual field defects. Fundus examination and fluorescein angiography are useful in distinguishing retinal abnormalities.

H. Secondary problems include glare from media opacities; night myopia, which is an inappropriate midpoint accommodation under dark conditions; and miosis from age or drugs. Some patients also show an exaggerated depression of cone sensitivity during the rod branch of dark adaptation detectable with a flickering red stimulus. These patients complain of problems driving at night.

References

Arden CB, Hogg CR. Rod cone interactions and analysis of retinal disease. Br J Ophthalmol 1985; 69:404–415.

Krill AE. Hereditary retinal and choroidal diseases. Vol I. Evaluation. Philadelphia: Harper & Row, 1972:189–226.

Liebowitz HW, Owens DA. Nighttime driving accidents and selective visual degradation. Science 1977; 197:422–423.

Massof RW, Finkelstein D. Two forms of autosomal dominant primary retinitis pigmentosa. Ooc Ophthalmol 1981; 51:289–346.

ISOLATED DIPLOPIA

Susan M. Berry, M.D.
John E. Carter, M.D.

Diplopia most often occurs as an isolated symptom. The presence of other neurologic symptoms indicates more extensive neurologic disease and merits referral for a neurologic evaluation.

A. Monocular diplopia is most commonly caused by some refractive disturbance, including astigmatism or some opacity in the ocular media. The patient may not have realized that there is diplopia when using an eye individually, in which case testing of each eye individually by the clinician may save the patient from an extensive evaluation. Cerebral lesions, usually in the posterior hemisphere, may produce polyopia, but polyopia is usually distinct from the distortion or ghost image seen with ocular disturbances. Patients with cerebral polyopia often see multiple images. This is enhanced when the object is moving; a car passing by may look like a procession of cars. Other visual disturbances, including perseveration of an image in the visual environment (palinopsia) or visual hallucinations, often accompany cerebral polyopia. A homonymous visual field defect is often associated with these phenomena.

B. A comitant strabismus is often benign and may be caused by decompensated congenital phorias or convergency insufficiency.

C. An incomitant strabismus must be classified as neural, myoneural junction, myopathic, or restrictive. Orbital processes causing a restrictive strabismus are usually obvious from the presence of proptosis and abnormal forced ductions. An appropriate lesion is expected on CT or MRI scan of the orbits. Cavernous sinus fistula or thrombosis may mimic orbital disease because of the proptosis and chemosis.

D. The history makes the diagnosis of myasthenia gravis. Ptosis and/or diplopia that varies from hour to hour, day to day, and week to week; that is usually present late in the day; that resolves for a period after a nap; or that had its onset in association with some other illness is likely to be myasthenia gravis. If only ocular muscles are involved, electromyographic studies are unlikely to be positive and cannot be used to exclude the diagnosis. A Tensilon (edrophonium) test is helpful if positive, but in patients with small deviations or with absent symptoms in the office, myasthenia gravis may be difficult to diagnose. A trial of Mestinon (pyridostigmine) for 1–2 weeks may serve better than Tensilon testing in these patients.

E. Diplopia caused by injury to any of the individual ocular motor nerves is most often benign. If the nerve fascicles are involved within the brainstem, the patient is expected to have additional neurologic symptoms or signs. The differential diagnosis for the cause of peripheral third, fourth, and sixth cranial nerve palsies is similar, but the diagnosis of most concern varies with the particular nerve. The third nerve may be injured by a berry aneurysm; surgery before the aneurysm ruptures may be lifesaving, but arteriography has been the only way to rule out an aneurysm definitively. Aneurysmal third nerve palsies involve the pupil in 96% of cases, but the pupil is involved in only 40% of the "vascular" cases attributed to diabetes or hypertension. Pupil sparing suggests a benign cause. Even when the pupil is involved in an older patient or in a patient with diabetes or hypertension, the most likely cause is an ischemic lesion of the nerve simply because this is such a common entity and aneurysmal third nerve palsies are much less common. However, MRI is becoming capable of excluding aneurysm without the morbidity of arteriography. The diagnosis of most concern in the patient with a sixth nerve palsy is neoplasm. Because of its long course along the base of the skull, the sixth nerve is often involved by dural metastases or by nasopharyngeal malignancies eroding through the bone. A CT scan with contrast material demonstrates most such lesions. Benign isolated ocular motor nerve palsies should resolve within 3 months, and pain associated with their onset should resolve within 1–2 weeks. Failure to recover indicates the need for more thorough evaluation and repeat imaging studies.

F. Diplopia associated with an internuclear ophthalmoplegia (INO) or with skew deviation indicates intrinsic brainstem disease and requires a neurologic evaluation. Skew deviation is diagnosed when the patient complains of an acquired vertical diplopia that is not caused by orbital disease or myasthenia and that on examination cannot be attributed to a dysfunction of the third or fourth nerve. The vertical strabismus may be comitant or incomitant, and 50% of patients with a skew deviation also have an INO.

G. Although patients with progressive supranuclear palsy, chronic progressive external ophthalmoplegia (CPEO), and Fisher's variant of acute postinfectious polyradiculitis (ataxia, ophthalmoplegia, and depressed reflexes) have strabismus, many do not complain of diplopia. These entities are characterized by weakness in most

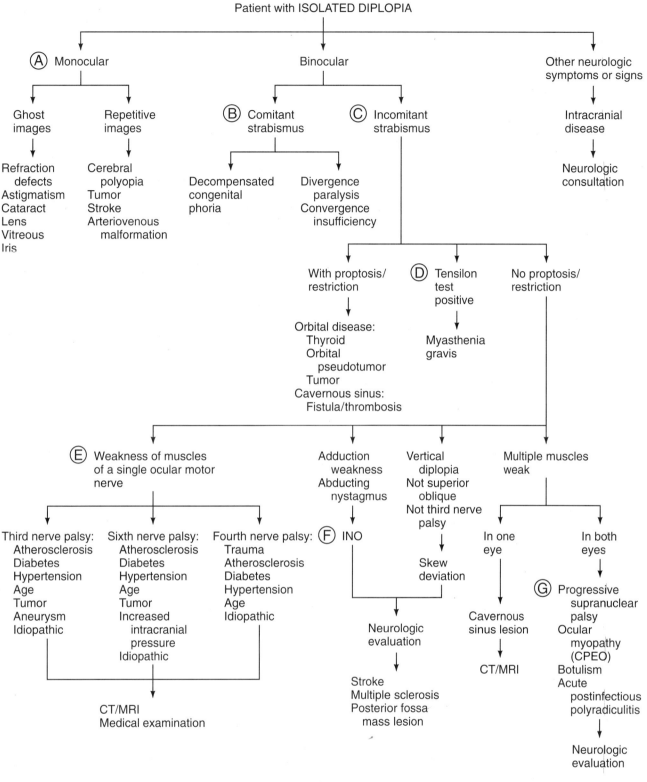

Patient with ISOLATED DIPLOPIA

(A) Monocular

Ghost images
- Refraction defects
- Astigmatism
- Cataract
- Lens
- Vitreous
- Iris

Repetitive images
- Cerebral polyopia
- Tumor
- Stroke
- Arteriovenous malformation

Binocular

(B) Comitant strabismus
- Decompensated congenital phoria
- Divergence paralysis
- Convergence insufficiency

(C) Incomitant strabismus

With proptosis/restriction
- Orbital disease:
  - Thyroid
  - Orbital pseudotumor
  - Tumor
- Cavernous sinus:
  - Fistula/thrombosis

(D) Tensilon test positive
- Myasthenia gravis

No proptosis/restriction

Other neurologic symptoms or signs
- Intracranial disease
- Neurologic consultation

(E) Weakness of muscles of a single ocular motor nerve

Third nerve palsy:
- Atherosclerosis
- Diabetes
- Hypertension
- Age
- Tumor
- Aneurysm
- Idiopathic

Sixth nerve palsy:
- Atherosclerosis
- Diabetes
- Hypertension
- Age
- Tumor
- Increased intracranial pressure
- Idiopathic

Fourth nerve palsy:
- Trauma
- Atherosclerosis
- Diabetes
- Hypertension
- Age
- Idiopathic

CT/MRI
Medical examination

Adduction weakness
Abducting nystagmus

(F) INO
- Neurologic evaluation
  - Stroke
  - Multiple sclerosis
  - Posterior fossa mass lesion

Vertical diplopia
Not superior oblique
Not third nerve palsy
- Skew deviation

Multiple muscles weak

In one eye
- Cavernous sinus lesion
- CT/MRI

In both eyes
- **(G)** Progressive supranuclear palsy
- Ocular myopathy (CPEO)
- Botulism
- Acute postinfectious polyradiculitis
- Neurologic evaluation

References

extraocular muscles in both eyes. Progressive supranuclear palsy usually has additional abnormalities in the form of involuntary eye movements such as square wave jerks and neurologic signs of parkinsonism.

Burde RM, Savino PJ, Trobe JD. Clinical decisions in neuro-ophthalmology. 2nd ed. St Louis: Mosby, 1992:224–288.

Glaser JS. Neuro-ophthalmology. 2nd ed. Philadelphia: Lippincott, 1990.

Miller NR. Walsh and Hoyt's clinical neuro-ophthalmology. 5th ed. Baltimore: Williams & Wilkins, 1998.

PHOTOPHOBIA

Jeffrey T. Liegner, M.D.

Photophobia is abnormal intolerance to light, which is difficult to quantitate but may be a helpful symptom in diagnosing ocular disease.

A. The history is helpful to determine onset. However, if the history is vague, suspect nontraumatic ocular disease.

B. Oculocutaneous (autosomal recessive) and ocular (X-linked) albinism have iris transillumination defects, fundus hypopigmentation, and macular hypoplasia. Aniridia, an underdevelopment of the iris, also shows macular aplasia, nystagmus, lens opacities, late corneal pannus, and glaucoma. Of patients with aniridia, 30% develop Wilms' tumor. Infants with photophobia, which may be apparent only from excessive tearing or oculodigital gouging, may have congenital glaucoma. Corneal clouding, buphthalmos, and optic nerve cupping can occur quickly.

C. Achromatopsia is a congenital, autosomal-recessive condition with absent or poor cone function, poor vision, nystagmus, color blindness, and a normal fundus appearance. These patients avoid lights to keep their rods dark-adapted for improved vision. Cone dystrophy has similar symptoms but often with a bull's eye appearance of the macula. The advanced stage of cone dystrophy can have the same retinal appearance as retinitis pigmentosa. Electrophysiologic studies (e.g., electroretinography, visual evoked response, dark adaptation) are important for early diagnosis and differentiation of these entities.

D. A photophobic response to direct versus consensual illumination is helpful in distinguishing corneal or conjunctival abnormalities from intraocular disease. With surface problems, direct illumination of the affected eye produces a more pronounced photophobic response than does contralateral testing. Photophobia produced with contralateral illumination indicates iritis. In addition, relief of photophobia with a topical anesthetic confirms surface irritation. Fluorescein staining may point to an abrasion or foreign body.

E. Patients with photophobia need a complete eye examination, including peripheral retinal examination, to rule out other consequences of trauma such as lens injury, optic nerve injury, and retinal edema, tears, or detachment.

F. Prophylactic topical antibiotics and a tight patch for 24 hours to prevent lid motion facilitate corneal healing. Cycloplegia reduces ciliary spasm and consensual photophobia. Reevaluation after the patch is removed is important to exclude infections, a persistent epithelial corneal defect, or improper healing.

G. Numerous drugs can produce photophobia: anticonvulsants (mephenytoin, methsuximide, paramethadione, trimethadione, valproic acid), antineoplastic agents (cytarabine, fludarabine, procarbazine, vindesine), topical medications (belladonna-like products, dexamethasone, vidarabine), as well as clofibrate, oral retinoids, ketoconazole, phenothiazines, some κ-blockers, and nalidixic acid.

H. Corneal inflammatory conditions produce photophobia from irritated corneal nerves. This may be diagnostically reduced with topical anesthetics. However, because topical anesthetics retard wound healing, incite corneal inflammation, and obscure worsening symptoms, they should never be prescribed as treatment. Anterior uveitis (iridocyclitis) may be symptomatic 12–24 hours before aqueous cell and flare are detectable. A history of uveitis or photophobia or clinical evidence of old inflammation in the anterior segment may suffice for early treatment decisions.

I. Papillitis presents with disc edema and hyperemia, hemorrhage, venous sheathing, and fine vitreous opacities, which can result from inflammation, infiltration, or vascular disorders. Posterior scleritis has characteristic deep orbital pain with exudative retinal detachment, optic nerve edema, cystoid macular edema, simulated subretinal tumor, and annular choroidal detachments. Diagnostic ultrasonography is helpful in defining thickening of the sclera and choroid, as well as the associated choroidal and retinal detachments.

J. Color desaturation with an afferent pupillary defect may be sufficient to diagnose retrobulbar optic neuritis. If photophobia is combined with meningeal or cerebral signs, consider emergency referral to a neurologist. If photophobia is accompanied by sudden severe headache, consider subarachnoid hemorrhage from a ruptured congenital aneurysm or arteriovenous malformation. Photophobia could also be a prominent part of migraine in all its various manifestations. When photophobia is associated with trigeminal neuralgia, there may be focal skin hypersensitivity to touch, as well as excessive corneal sensitivity. Pseudophotophobia represents the subjective hypersensitivity to light that does not exceed the clinician's definition of photophobia. This is seen occasionally in lightly pigmented eyes but may also occur in psychiatric disorders, in adolescent behavior, and for secondary gain.

References

Drug Evaluation Monographs. Micromedex, Inc. (Computerized Clinical Information System). vol. 68, 1991.

Nussenblatt RB, Palestine AG. Uveitis: Fundamentals and clinical practice. Chicago: Year Book, 1989.

Ryan S, ed. Retina. St Louis: Mosby, 1989.

Smolin G, Thoft RA, eds. The cornea. In: Scientific foundations and clinical practice. Boston: Little, Brown, 1987.

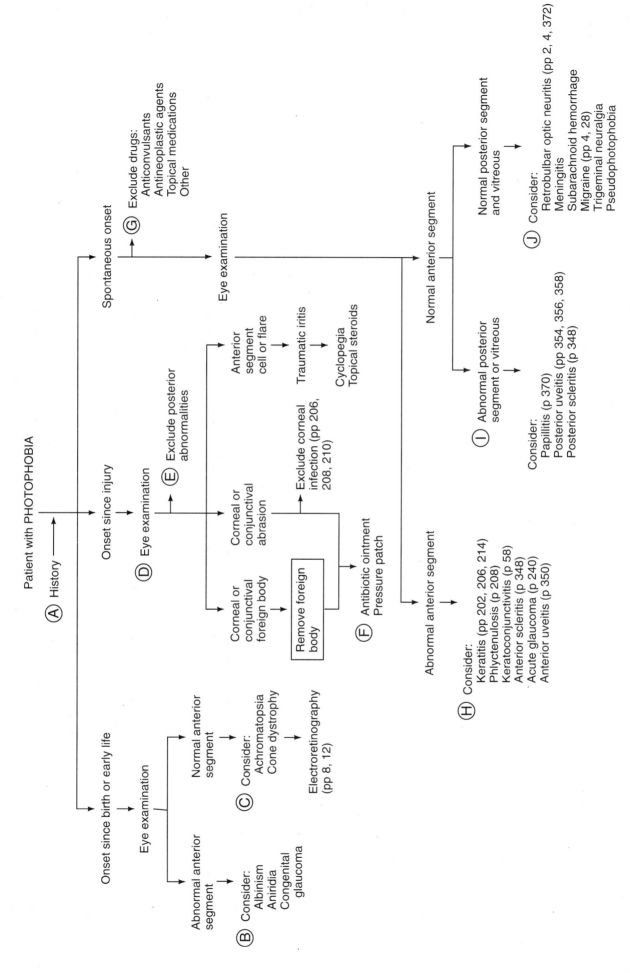

Patient with PHOTOPHOBIA

(A) History

Onset since birth or early life

Eye examination

Abnormal anterior segment

(B) Consider:
Albinism
Aniridia
Congenital glaucoma

Normal anterior segment

(C) Consider:
Achromatopsia
Cone dystrophy

Electroretinography (pp 8, 12)

Onset since injury

(D) Eye examination

(E) Exclude posterior abnormalities

Corneal or conjunctival foreign body

Remove foreign body

Corneal or conjunctival abrasion

Exclude corneal infection (pp 206, 208, 210)

(F) Antibiotic ointment
Pressure patch

Anterior segment cell or flare

Traumatic iritis

Cyclopegia
Topical steroids

Abnormal anterior segment

(H) Consider:
Keratitis (pp 202, 206, 214)
Phlyctenulosis (p 208)
Keratoconjunctivitis (p 58)
Anterior scleritis (p 348)
Acute glaucoma (p 240)
Anterior uveitis (p 350)

Spontaneous onset

(G) Exclude drugs:
Anticonvulsants
Antineoplastic agents
Topical medications
Other

Eye examination

Normal anterior segment

Abnormal posterior segment or vitreous

(I) Consider:
Papillitis (p 370)
Posterior uveitis (pp 354, 356, 358)
Posterior scleritis (p 348)

Normal posterior segment and vitreous

(J) Consider:
Retrobulbar optic neuritis (pp 2, 4, 372)
Meningitis
Subarachnoid hemorrhage
Migraine (pp 4, 28)
Trigeminal neuralgia
Pseudophotophobia

17

FLASHES AND FLOATERS

W.A.J. van Heuven, M.D.
Bailey L. Lee, M.D.

A common chief complaint, particularly in adults, is "seeing flashes or floaters." These symptoms usually stem from ocular sources. The flashes of light indicate mechanical stimulation of the retina and arc best seen in the dark or with the eyes closed, when the flashes do not compete with ambient light. When the retina is mechanically stimulated, a message is transmitted to the brain, which the brain presumes to be light because the stimulus originated in the retina. Firm massage of the globe can produce such retinal stimulation with resultant flashes. Floaters, which are usually caused by opacities in the ocular media that cause shadows to be cast on the retina, are best seen in bright light or against a bright background. Floaters caused by opacities near the retina appear small and distinct, whereas those farther forward are larger and blurrier. Floaters move with eye movement and, depending on the tissue in which they are embedded, either follow the eye movements precisely, overshoot the eye movements, or move with gravity.

A. A history is important to determine whether flashes are true entoptic flashes or pseudoflashes. True flashes are better seen in the dark and are usually vertical and temporal. Some patients complain of the flashes only at night.

B. When flashes occur mostly in or around bright lights, the patient may really be complaining of glare, halos, or photophobia. Glare is usually caused by media opacities, varying from cataracts to intraocular lenses to contact lenses or dirty and scratched spectacles. Although halos can be caused by any opacities in the ocular media, a common cause is corneal edema from increased intraocular pressure. In fact, when eliciting a history of glaucoma, ask for the symptom of halo or rainbow vision. Many drugs that affect the corneal epithelium can also produce halos. Photophobia, abnormal intolerance to bright light, may be caused by glare. However, photophobia in children, in whom media opacities are less common, warrants consideration of congenital disorders such as cone dystrophy, albinism, or achromatopsia. Numerous systemic drugs can also cause photophobia. Hysteria and malingering are also more common than generally appreciated. As with all entoptic phenomena, cerebral causes such as migraine headaches and their variants must be considered, and a careful history and neurologic examination may be indicated (p 28).

C. True flashes, with or without floaters, indicate retinal stimulation, which is most often caused by traction on the retina. The most common form of retinal traction is vitreous traction, in which the vitreous gel, at a point of firm vitreoretinal adhesion, pulls the retina forward. This problem can be caused by congenital abnormalities, such as congenital retinal traction tufts and congenital meridional folds at the ora serrata. Vitreous traction can also be acquired when the vitreous gel, which tends to liquefy with increasing age, collapses forward and produces sudden traction on the retina at the posterior edge of the vitreous base. Vitreous traction can also occur in "secondary" vitreous detachment, in which a slow shrinkage of the vitreous gel, caused by inflammation or chronic vascular leakage, causes slowly progressive traction on those retinal structures to which the vitreous is firmly attached, such as the disc, major retinal vessels, and areas of abnormal retinal vascular lesions, such as neovascularization and vascular tumors (von Hippel). Retinal traction can also occur tangentially to the retina from preretinal fibrosis, which occurs in spontaneous idiopathic macular pucker and in proliferative vitreoretinopathy. The latter most often results from proliferation of retinal pigment epithelial cells, which have migrated through a retinal hole into the vitreous cavity and settled on the retina. Intraretinal traction can also occur after chorioretinal injuries with resultant scars, which shrink with time. A complete retinal examination, using indirect ophthalmoscopy and scleral depression, usually permits diagnosis of the source of flashes and floaters caused by retinal traction.

D. In addition to vitreoretinal traction, other retinal pathologic conditions can also lead to symptoms of photopsias. These include inflammatory disorders such as multiple evanescent white dot syndrome (MEWDS), acute zonal occult outer retinopathy (AZOOR), birdshot retinochoroidopathy, and punctate inner choroidopathy (PIC). Also patients with decreased central vision from choroidal neovascularization can have symptoms of flashing lights or even formed hallucinations (Charles Bonnet syndrome).

E. Acute and sudden symptoms of flashes and floaters usually indicate vitreous detachment. Patients may call the office for an appointment, and the determination of whether the patient should be seen immediately must often be made during the telephone conversation. Thus it is wise, particularly in a retina practice, to instruct the secretaries to ask whether the floaters are fewer or more than a dozen. If the floaters are few, it is often safe to assume that a benign vitreous detachment has occurred, in which the floaters represent the opacities on the posterior vitreous surface, where the vitreous was previously attached to the disc. If the floaters are numerous, particularly if they are described as a "cloud," "spider web," or "curtain," assume that there has been a vitreous hemorrhage, which may mean that there is now a retinal tear. Other common causes of vitreous hemorrhage are vitreous detachment without retinal tear, in which the hemorrhage originates at the disc, and vitreous traction on neovascularization of the retina as a result of diabetic retinopathy, retinal vein occlusion, or other ischemic retinopathies. Ocular trauma can also produce vitreous hemorrhage.

F. Acute, or rhegmatogenous, vitreous detachment is a sudden collapse of the vitreous gel caused by a sudden outpouring of central liquefied vitreous through one of the posterior holes in the vitreous cortex overlying the disc and macula. The vitreous gel usually retracts forward with the central liquefied vitreous moving through the posterior vitreous hole into the space between the vitreous surface and the retina. The separation of vitreous from the retina stops anteriorly at the posterior edge of the vitreous base, which represents the strongest adhesion between vitreous and retina. The sudden cessation of the vitreous detachment at the vitreous base creates traction on the retina at that location and may tear the retina. When that occurs, there is usually bleeding, causing many floaters. If no retinal tear occurs, the floaters represent small pieces of glial tissue on the posterior surface of the vitreous, where it separated from the optic disc. Always examine the fellow eye for vitreous detachment. If it is not present, advise the patient that symptoms of floaters in the fellow eye should again prompt a visit to the ophthalmologist.

G. Progressively worsening floaters, although they could represent rebleeding from neovascularization of the retina, often indicate uveitis, particularly peripheral uveitis (pars planitis). Also consider reticulum cell sarcoma.

H. If the vitreous appears liquefied or is detached, vitreous biopsy can be done easily with a needle through the pars plana. If the vitreous is solid and not detached,

it is safer to do a partial vitrectomy to avoid causing vitreous traction on the retina during the biopsy. Specimens should be cultured and stained for cytologic examination. Fungi may need special stains (e.g., silver).

I. Vitreous floaters that are chronic and stable and move precisely with eye movement are common, particularly in myopic patients. They represent opacities in the posterior vitreous near the retina and are of no clinical significance. They may remain constant for decades.

J. Vitreous opacities that overshoot (i.e., move more than the eye movement and then return to the visual axis) indicate vitreous opacities on the posterior surface of a detached vitreous gel. No matter how long the symptoms have been present, examine the fellow eye for vitreous detachment. If it is not present, advise the patient of the significance of new floaters in the fellow eye.

References

Brown GC, Murphy RP. Visual symptoms associated with choroidal neovascularization: Photopsias and the Charles Bonnet syndrome. Arch Ophthalmol 1992; 110:1251–1256.

Eisner G. Biomicroscopy of the peripheral fundus. New York: Springer-Verlag, 1973.

Gass JDM. Acute zonal occult outer retinopathy. J Clin Neuro-Ophthalmol 1993; 13:79–97.

Jampol LM, Sieving PA, Pugh D, et al. Multiple evanescent white dot syndrome. I. Clinical findings. Arch Ophthalmol 1984; 102:671–674.

Schepens CL. Retinal detachment and allied diseases. Philadelphia: WB Saunders, 1983.

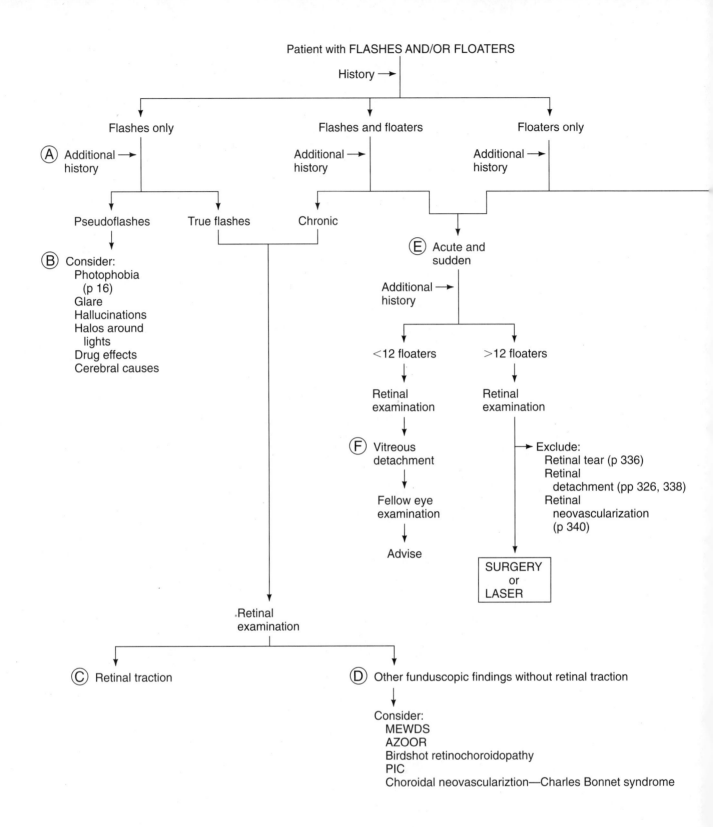

Patient with FLASHES AND/OR FLOATERS

History →

Flashes only

Ⓐ Additional →
history

Flashes and floaters

Additional →
history

Floaters only

Additional →
history

Pseudoflashes

True flashes

Chronic

Ⓑ Consider:
  Photophobia
    (p 16)
  Glare
  Hallucinations
  Halos around
    lights
  Drug effects
  Cerebral causes

Ⓔ Acute and
  sudden

Additional →
history

<12 floaters

>12 floaters

Retinal
examination

Retinal
examination

Ⓕ Vitreous
  detachment

Fellow eye
examination

Advise

Exclude:
  Retinal tear (p 336)
  Retinal
    detachment (pp 326, 338)
  Retinal
    neovascularization
    (p 340)

SURGERY
or
LASER

.Retinal
examination

Ⓒ Retinal traction

Ⓓ Other funduscopic findings without retinal traction

Consider:
  MEWDS
  AZOOR
  Birdshot retinochoroidopathy
  PIC
  Choroidal neovasculariztion—Charles Bonnet syndrome

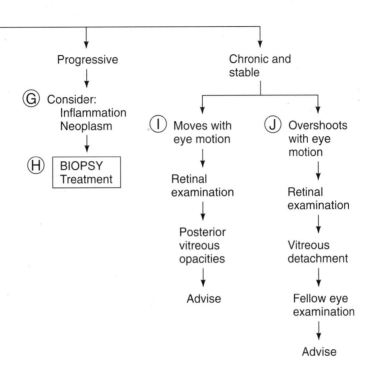

Progressive

Chronic and stable

(G) Consider:
Inflammation
Neoplasm

(H) BIOPSY
Treatment

(I) Moves with
eye motion

Retinal
examination

Posterior
vitreous
opacities

Advise

(J) Overshoots
with eye
motion

Retinal
examination

Vitreous
detachment

Fellow eye
examination

Advise

ACQUIRED INCREASING MYOPIA

Johan Zwaan, M.D., Ph.D.

Four factors determine the ocular refractive state: the optical power of the cornea, the optical power of the lens, the distance between these two (i.e., anterior chamber depth), and axial length. Accommodation for near vision and scleral resistance versus intraocular pressure (IOP) play a role in the genesis of myopia, and both genetic and environmental influences are suspected.

Myopia is the most common ocular anomaly seen in developed countries. Most affected individuals have so-called simple myopia. In the United States 15%–25% of the population has or will have this type of myopia. In most people the refractive error becomes manifest between the ages of 7 and 13 and worsens, becoming reasonably stable around age 17. A much smaller group, almost all college students, becomes myopic in early adulthood.

Second, a large group of syndromes and inherited diseases are commonly associated with myopia. Examples are Marfan's, Ehlers-Danlos, Stickler's, Down's, fetal alcohol syndromes and retinitis pigmentosa. The diagnosis of these diseases obviously does not depend on the finding of myopia.

In a third group of patients myopia is a major presenting sign. These are discussed in this chapter. It is useful to divide these patients by age and to consider the anatomic structures involved in the genesis of myopia (i.e. cornea, lens, ciliary body [muscle], and vitreous size [axial length]).

A. Up to age 3 years corneal power and lens power are adjusted to correlate with different increases of axial length. The result is that >95% of eyes end up with a refraction close to emmetropia (between +4.00 and −4.00 diopters of refractive error). The regulatory factors involved are only poorly understood.

B. Megalocornea is associated with myopia because the cornea is steeper than normal. It is inherited and all three patterns of Mendelian inheritance have been reported. It is usually an isolated condition but can be associated with juvenile glaucoma or ectopia lentis.

C. Ectopia lentis can cause significant myopia as a result of tilting of the lens. In some types (Marfan's syndrome, autosomal-recessive ectopia lentis et pupillae) the axial length is also increased. Fluctuation of the refraction is common, related to shifts in lens position, and the patient may indeed go all the way from high myopia to high hyperopia if the lens dislocates completely and disappears out of the visual axis.

D. Posterior lentiglobus is an axial deformation of the posterior aspect of the lens. It results in high myopia through the center of the lens, although the periphery can be emmetropic.

E. An enlarging corneal diameter and an axial length increasing beyond the expected normal growth in an infant should alert one to the possible presence of con-

genital glaucoma, even in the absence of clearly abnormal IOP. Other signs usually present are an enlarging optic cup and corneal edema.

F. Even mild cicatricial retinopathy of prematurity, expressed as retinal pigmentation and dragging of retinal vessels and macula, is almost always associated with myopia. It is less well known that prematurity per se is a risk factor for the development of severe myopia.

G. Both animal experiments and findings in patients with capillary hemangiomas, severe ptosis, plexiform neurofibroma, or patching have demonstrated that, in addition to causing severe amblyopia, prolonged eyelid closure may cause myopia as a result of an increase in axial eye length.

H. A severely blurred image on the fovea during infancy not only is amblyopiogenic but can also cause myopia. Typical causes are a cloudy cornea resulting from birth trauma, a cataract, or a vitreous hemorrhage.

I. Congenital hereditary endothelial dystrophy (CHED), an autosomal-recessive disease leading to diffuse corneal clouding, is always associated with myopia. It is differentiated from congenital glaucoma because the IOP is normal or close to normal, the cornea is greatly thickened, and its diameter does not increase.

J. A vitreous hemorrhage related to birth can cause high myopia. It is often not recognized because retinal examinations are not done routinely on all newborns. Because of the dense structure of the infant vitreous, such a hemorrhage clears only slowly and its amblyopiogenic influence may be present for months.

K. A syndrome has been reported in which monocular presence of significant myelination of retinal nerve fibers is combined with high myopia, fairly intractable amblyopia, and strabismus. The pathogenesis is not understood.

L. Inability to obtain a clear endpoint on retinoscopy should lead to slit-lamp examination. Central thinning of the cornea and irregular mires and rings seen with keratometry, keratoscopy, or corneal topographical determinations, confirm the presence of keratoconus, which usually manifests itself at puberty.

M. Fluctuating distance vision is often the presenting sign for previously undiagnosed diabetes. The fluctuations are presumably caused by changes in lens hydration, related to the variations in osmotic effects of swings in blood glucose. Ask patients about other signs and symptoms, such as weight loss, polydipsia, and polyuria. A simple dipstick test can confirm glucosuria, which should lead to immediate referral to the internist or endocrinologist.

N. Episodes of blurred and double vision, associated with headaches or eye pain, may be caused by a spasm of the near reflex. Examination should reveal convergence of the eyes and miosis during the attacks. The problem is most often seen in female adolescents and is self-limited, although it may recur for several years. The attacks can be incapacitating and may last several hours. Although underlying abnormalities are rare and the problem is almost always functional, neurologic and neuroophthalmologic examinations are recommended. Treatment consists of cycloplegics and binocular glasses, although paradoxically, miotics have also been used with success, presumably by reducing the central drive.

O. Pilocarpine is notorious for inducing disturbing, if transient, myopia in young people. Other miotics, sometimes used in the treatment of accommodative esotropia (echothiophate; isoflurophate), can also cause myopia.

Many drugs may occasionally lead to myopia, presumably because of induced edema of the ciliary body. In cases of unexplained recently acquired myopia, it is worthwhile to question the patient about medication use.

P. In elderly patients, gradually increasing myopia is almost always the result of lens changes. These changes may be subtle, but eventually it becomes clear that a nuclear cataract is developing.

References

Curtin BJ. The myopias: Basic science and clinical management. Philadelphia: Harper & Row, 1985.

Dagi LR, Chrousos GA, Cogan DG. Spasm of the near reflex associated with organic disease. Am J Ophthalmol 1987; 103:582–585.

Goldberg MF. Clinical manifestations of ectopia lentis et pupillae in 16 patients. Ophthalmology 1988; 95:1080–1088.

Rosner M, Belkin M. Intelligence, education, and myopia in males. Arch Ophthalmol 1987; 105:1508–1511.

Straatsma BR, Foos RY, Heckenlively JR, Taylor GN. Myelinated retinal nerve fibers. Am J Ophthalmol 1981; 91:25–38.

Weale RA. Corneal shape and astigmatism: With a note on myopia. Br J Ophthalmol 1988; 72:696–699.

Working Group on Myopia Prevalence and Progression. Myopia: Prevalence and progression. Washington DC: National Academy Press, 1989.

Patient with ACQUIRED INCREASING MYOPIA

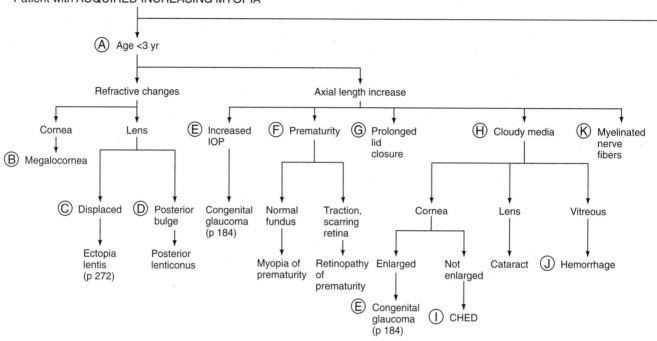

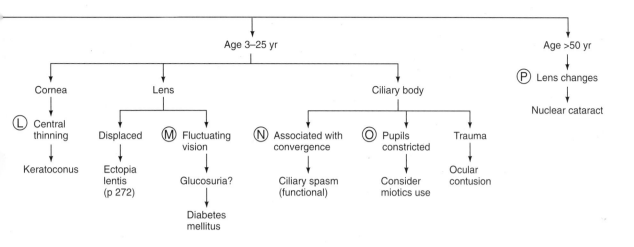

Age 3–25 yr

Cornea

Ⓛ Central
thinning

Keratoconus

Lens

Displaced

Ectopia
lentis
(p 272)

Ⓜ Fluctuating
vision

Glucosuria?

Diabetes
mellitus

Ciliary body

Ⓝ Associated with
convergence

Ciliary spasm
(functional)

Ⓞ Pupils
constricted

Consider
miotics use

Trauma

Ocular
contusion

Age >50 yr

Ⓟ Lens changes

Nuclear cataract

ACQUIRED HYPEROPIA

W.A.J. van Heuven, M.D.

Hyperopia is the optical condition in which an infinitely distant object is focused behind the retina. Eyes with hyperopia tend to be smaller and shorter. As a consequence, the optical system needs to converge light more than in a myopic (larger and longer) eye if light is to be focused on the retina. One could say that the optical system of a hyperopic eye is not strong enough and therefore needs to be given additional power (+ lenses) to bring distant objects in focus. Because eyes are capable of accommodation until late adulthood, hyperopia can be easily overcome for many years and may not be diagnosed until adulthood. Early in life, the additional accommodation required for reading and other near tasks can also be easily performed. As patients get older, accommodation capabilities decrease. Emmetropic eyes (neither hyperopic nor myopic) usually lose enough accommodative capability by age 40 that the 3 diopters of accommodation required for reading vision are no longer available from accommodation alone. Such patients report difficulty with near vision, and reading glasses should be prescribed. Patients with hyperopia, because of their need to accommodate for their hyperopia as well as for near tasks, may get symptoms of presbyopia (old eye) earlier and may require reading glasses during their thirties and bifocals (reading as well as distance correction) by their forties.

A. In any evaluation of acquired hyperopia, the history should elicit whether this affects both near and far vision equally. In presbyopia, near vision is affected selectively. Testing for normal pupillary reactions is important to rule out interference with accommodation as the cause of hyperopic symptoms. Cycloplegic refraction should be done to uncover latent hyperopia.

B. In the absence of surgical or nonsurgical trauma and after accommodative problems have been ruled out, perform a thorough ocular, orbital, and systemic examination to rule out ocular reasons for acquired hyperopia. Any condition that elevates the retina without compromising its function is tantamount to shortening of the optic pathway, which can manifest as hyperopia. Thus central serous choroidopathy and retinal detachment secondary to intraocular tumors or posterior ocular inflammation, in which retinal edema does not occur quickly, should be considered. Orbital lesions that press the posterior ocular wall anteriorly may have the same effect. Systemic conditions, which can cause macular edema, produce hyperopia initially. However, later, the edematous retina also produces blurred vision.

C. A common form of acquired loss of accommodation is caused by the inadvertent rubbing of atropine-like substances into the eye, which often occurs in medical personnel. Anticholinergic agents used in the management of gastrointestinal disorders, respiratory disorders, hyperactive carotid sinus, Parkinson's disease, or dysmenorrhea can also cause accommodative paresis. Similar effects can be caused by ergotamine (often used to produce illicit abortion) and penicillamine.

D. Once drugs are ruled out as a cause, consider severe, generalized debilitating illnesses that can cause a dynamic insufficiency of accommodation, usually in asthenic individuals. Consider food poisoning, especially botulism. Neurologic causes, from lesions of the parasympathetic nuclei in the midbrain, may be caused by encephalitis or a tumor of the pineal body.

E. Operations that remove the lens produce hyperopia and a loss of accommodation. In addition, operations or trauma that cause corneal flattening change the optics of the eye in a hyperopic direction.

F. Injuries that contuse or tear the iris or ciliary body may produce paresis of accommodation, simulating acquired hyperopia. Scarring of the cornea can flatten the corneal surface, changing the refractive power of the eye toward hyperopia, as does lens subluxation in a posterior direction. Retinal edema or ocular compression from retrobulbar hemorrhage or orbital fractures also effectively shortens the optical pathway to produce acquired hyperopia.

References

Duane TD. Clinical ophthalmology. Philadelphia: Harper & Row, 1985.

Fraunfelder FT. Drug-induced ocular side effects and drug interactions. 3rd ed. Philadelphia: Lea & Febiger, 1989.

Miller NR. Walsh & Hoyt's clinical neuro-ophthalmology. 5th ed. Baltimore: Williams & Wilkins, 1998.

Patient with ACQUIRED HYPEROPIA

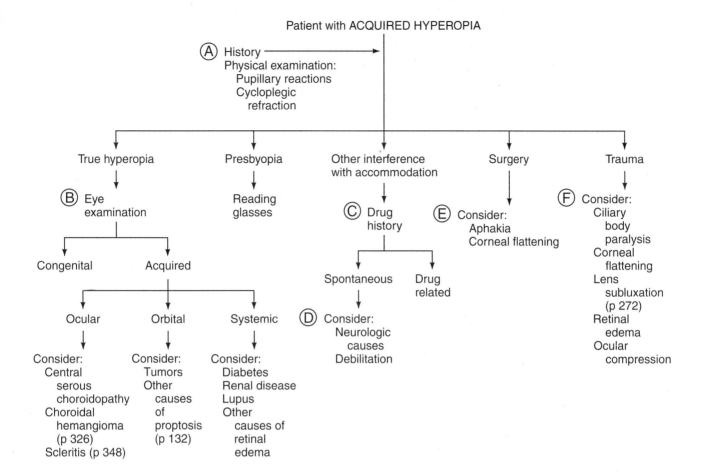

(A) History
Physical examination:
   Pupillary reactions
   Cycloplegic
    refraction

True hyperopia

Presbyopia

Other interference
with accommodation

Surgery

Trauma

(B) Eye
   examination

Reading
glasses

(C) Drug
   history

(E) Consider:
   Aphakia
   Corneal flattening

(F) Consider:
   Ciliary
    body
    paralysis
   Corneal
    flattening
   Lens
    subluxation
    (p 272)
   Retinal
    edema
   Ocular
    compression

Congenital

Acquired

Spontaneous

Drug
related

Ocular

Orbital

Systemic

(D) Consider:
   Neurologic
    causes
   Debilitation

Consider:
   Central
    serous
    choroidopathy
   Choroidal
    hemangioma
    (p 326)
   Scleritis (p 348)

Consider:
   Tumors
   Other
    causes
    of
    proptosis
    (p 132)

Consider:
   Diabetes
   Renal disease
   Lupus
   Other
    causes of
    retinal
    edema

HEADACHE

Johan Zwaan, M.D., Ph.D.

One of the most common reasons for referral of a patient to the ophthalmologist is the complaint of headache, even though an ocular cause for headache is uncommon. Eye findings may be important and sometimes essential in the diagnosis of the type of headache. Muscular or tension headaches are by far the most common, followed by migraines. Other causes for headaches are much less common.

The diagnosis of headaches relies to a large extent on the history, which should be taken in great detail. Of particular importance are the length of the headache symptoms, its frequency and duration, location, associated symptoms such as nausea, exacerbating and relieving features, possible triggers, and family history. The results of various examinations are useful for specific types of headaches but are generally less informative than the history. However, because patients present in the belief that their headache is caused by an eye problem, a full eye examination is necessary.

In some headaches (e.g., subarachnoid hemorrhage, temporal arteritis, bacterial meningitis), a rapid and accurate diagnosis is essential to avoid permanent harm to the patient.

A. Patients report that the headache caused by a subarachnoid hemorrhage is the worst pain they have ever experienced. The pain reaches maximum intensity in a few minutes or less ("thunderclap"). A milder forewarning "sentinel" headache may occur before the severe attack. In a few patients the headache is less severe and less acute. The diagnosis is missed in up to 25% of patients, half of whom will have bleeding again within 2 weeks, with an increased mortality rate.

B. An early CT scan done within 72 hours is highly diagnostic with a sensitivity of up to 95%. If the CT is normal, a lumbar puncture (LP) will show blood in the CSF and, starting a few hours after the onset, xanthochromia. To avoid possible brain herniation, an LP should not be done if the CT is abnormal. If CT is unavailable, performing an LP is controversial.

C. Chronic sinusitis is rarely the cause of a headache. Acute sinusitis, associated with an upper respiratory tract infection, gives a dull, constant ache, which increases when the patient bends over. Pressing on the area over the paranasal sinuses is uncomfortable. The diagnosis is confirmed by x-ray film or CT scan.

D. Most patients with headache and fever have an acute systemic illness and the headache will resolve when the temperature comes down. In meningitis the headache increases in severity over hours to days. It often radiates to the neck and back and is somewhat relieved by lying flat. Altered consciousness and vomiting are common. Nuchal rigidity is highly typical. An LP is essential for the diagnosis.

E. Acute encephalitis overlaps in its symptoms with meningitis because the meninges are usually involved in any inflammation of the brain. However, altered state of consciousness and mental status, seizures, and focal neurologic signs are more severe than in meningitis.

F. The role of chronic hypertension in the causation of headache is controversial. Most authors now believe that it is not a factor. Acute, severe (diastolic pressure >130 mm Hg) hypertension, on the other hand, can cause headache and is common when the blood pressure elevation is acute. Papilledema and retinopathy may be present.

G. An epidural hematoma is the result of arterial bleeding after a temporal or parietal skull fracture. Patients usually lose consciousness immediately after the trauma. They then regain it and a headache begins to develop. The headache increases over a few hours, and vomiting, seizures, and focal signs occur. Loss of consciousness and often death follow. This typical scenario is not always followed, and some patients never regain consciousness after the trauma.

H. Subdural hematomas are caused by rupture of the bridging veins of dura and arachnoid. Trauma is the most common cause. In the acute form most patients are comatose after the injury. In subacute and chronic cases minor trauma is common, but in one third of patients such a history is absent. Older patients, epileptics, alcoholics, and patients with coagulation disorders are prone to subdural hematomas developing. The headache is severe and may last days to weeks. Tapping on the head increases the pain.

I. Headache is never the only symptom of a migraine. In fact, migraine can be present without a headache. To be classified as migraineurs, patients should have at least five attacks lasting 4–72 hours. The headache should have two or more of the following characteristics: unilateral, throbbing, moderate to severe, and aggravated by movement. It should be accompanied by at least one of the following three: nausea, photophobia, or phonophobia.

J. The term *common migraine* has been replaced by *migraine without aura*. Migraine without aura is considerably more common than that with aura.

K. Patients with migraine with aura, previously called classical migraine, often have a prodromal stage of fluid retention, changes in energy level and appetite, and a decrease in mental alertness as much as a day before the onset of the headache. The aura occurs within 1 hour before the headache and starts with scintillating scotomata consisting of jagged, often colored lines, which begin in the periphery of the visual field and gradually move centrally. Quadrantanopsia or hemianopsia may develop. Other sensory auras, such as paresthesias, are uncommon. The aura resolves in less than 60 minutes. Rarely, the deficits become permanent because of cerebral infarction. The headache follows the aura or occasionally coincides with it.

L. In complicated migraine the headache is accompanied by focal neurologic deficits such as hemiplegia. Loss of consciousness may occur. The neurologic dysfunctions tend to outlast the headache.

M. A positive family history is common in migraine patients. Familial hemiplegic migraine shows autosomal-dominant inheritance and a responsible gene has been localized on chromosome 19p13.1. It encodes a protein subunit of one of the cellular calcium channels.

N. Basilar migraine is rare. The headache is preceded or accompanied by bilateral occipital lobe dysfunction (visual field abnormalities), brainstem abnormalities (diplopia), and/or cerebellar dysfunction (dysarthria, ataxia). Other cranial nerve signs may be present. This syndrome is usually seen in children. It is thought to result from disturbed blood flow in the vertebrobasilar arterial system.

O. Cluster headaches are uncommon and affect primarily adult men. The pain is severe and lasts only a few minutes. Attacks are frequent during a period of days to weeks and then disappear for prolonged periods, only to recur later. Alcohol is a known trigger. The conjunctiva is injected on the affected side and the nose is congested. A mild Horner's syndrome may be present. The cause is unknown.

P. The attacks of trigeminal neuralgia last only a few seconds but are very painful. They occur within the distribution of the second and third division of the trigeminal nerve and are repeated at a high frequency, often for weeks on end. Touching of the face or lips will trigger the attack. In most patients no cause is found. The condition can be so disabling that some patients become suicidal.

Q. Acute hydrocephalus, as seen when a ventriculoperitoneal shunt malfunctions, or when a tumor, such as the subependymal astrocytomas of tuberous sclerosis, blocks the CSF flow, produces severe headache. Papilledema and later optic atrophy are usually the result. Other visual disturbances include cranial sixth nerve palsies and even concomitant esotropia.

R. In pseudotumor cerebri, papilledema is usually the sign leading to the diagnosis. The headache is initially relatively mild and may be present for weeks before the diagnosis is made. A CT scan is normal, but the ventricles may appear smaller than average. The opening pressure found by LP is elevated to up to 450 mm H_2O. Visual disturbances are frequent (i.e., cranial sixth nerve palsies with resulting diplopia, slightly blurred vision, enlarged blind spots, and constricted peripheral visual fields).

S. Intracranial hypotension (pressure <90 mm H_2O) may be caused by a CSF leak, usually after an LP is performed. A traumatic dura tear or an avulsed nerve root and systemic dehydration may also lower the CSF pressure.

T. Tension-type headaches, previously called muscular contraction or tension headaches, are the most common headaches. They cause a steady pressurelike pain that may last for days. The headache is precipitated or exacerbated by stress. The patient has no nausea, photophobia, or aura. The headache is generalized with frequent occipital or neck pain.

U. Temporomandibular joint disease (TMJ), usually malocclusion, may lead to preauricular pain associated with chewing. Most patients develop facial pain and headache.

V. Temporal arteritis or giant cell arteritis needs to be diagnosed and treated promptly to avoid severe visual loss. This disease strikes older people and is diagnosed by the tenderness of the temporal artery, elevated sedimentation rate, and temporal artery biopsy. The patient often has a history of malaise, anorexia, mild fever and aches, and anemia. In half of the patients this granulomatous arteritis is associated with polymyalgia rheumatica. If the disease is suspected, start treatment with high-dose steroids immediately, even before the results of the biopsy are known, to prevent progression of visual deficits. Once ischemic optic neuropathy has started, it may progress with startling rapidity.

W. Although "eye strain" is a popular explanation by the lay public for all types of headaches, particularly tension-type, this opinion is usually wrong. If the headache is related to a refractive error or muscle imbalance, it will be absent in the morning and appear and then increase with use of the eyes.

References

Ducros A, Denier C, Joutel A, et al. Recurrence of the T666M calcium channel CAGNAlA gene mutation in familial hemiplegic migraine with progressive cerebellar ataxia. Am J Hum Genet 1999; 64:89–98.

Frishberg BM. The utility of neuroimaging in the evaluation of headache in patients with normal neurological examinations. Neurology 1994; 44:1191–1197.

Goadsby PJ, Olesen J. Diagnosis and management of migraine. Br J Med 1996; 312:1279–1283.

Rassmussen BK. Epidemiology of headache. Cephalalgia 1995; 15:45–68.

Weir B. Headaches from aneurysms. Cephalalgia 1994; 14:79–87.

Ziegler DK, Schwertfeger TL, Murrow RW. Headache. Clin Neurol 1996; 2:1–56.

Patient presenting with HEADACHE

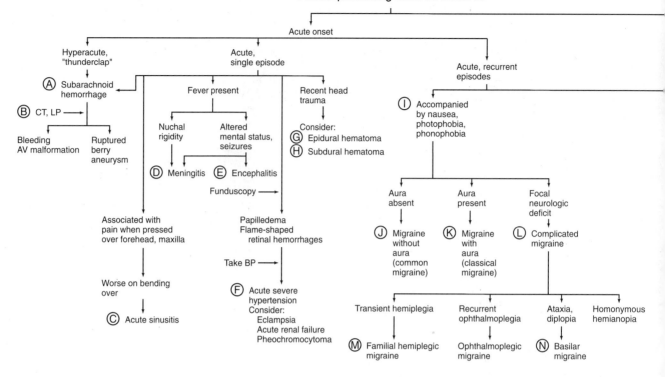

Acute onset

Hyperacute, "thunderclap"

Ⓐ Subarachnoid hemorrhage

Ⓑ CT, LP →

Bleeding AV malformation

Ruptured berry aneurysm

Acute, single episode

Fever present

Nuchal rigidity

Altered mental status, seizures

Ⓓ Meningitis

Ⓔ Encephalitis

Funduscopy →

Associated with pain when pressed over forehead, maxilla

Worse on bending over

Ⓒ Acute sinusitis

Recent head trauma

Consider:
Ⓖ Epidural hematoma
Ⓗ Subdural hematoma

Papilledema Flame-shaped retinal hemorrhages

Take BP →

Ⓕ Acute severe hypertension
Consider:
Eclampsia
Acute renal failure
Pheochromocytoma

Acute, recurrent episodes

Ⓘ Accompanied by nausea, photophobia, phonophobia

Aura absent

Aura present

Focal neurologic deficit

Ⓙ Migraine without aura (common migraine)

Ⓚ Migraine with aura (classical migraine)

Ⓛ Complicated migraine

Transient hemiplegia

Recurrent ophthalmoplegia

Ataxia, diplopia

Homonymous hemianopia

Ⓜ Familial hemiplegic migraine

Ophthalmoplegic migraine

Ⓝ Basilar migraine

30

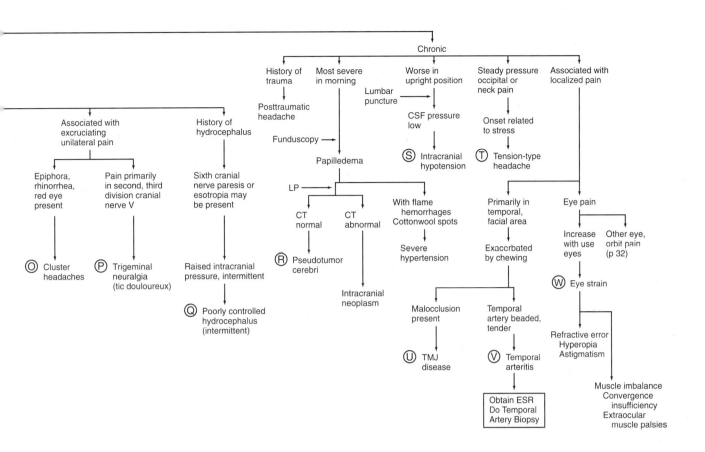

Chronic

History of trauma

Posttraumatic headache

Most severe in morning

Funduscopy →

Papilledema

LP →

CT normal

Ⓡ Pseudotumor cerebri

CT abnormal

Intracranial neoplasm

Worse in upright position

Lumbar puncture →

CSF pressure low

Ⓢ Intracranial hypotension

Steady pressure occipital or neck pain

Onset related to stress

Ⓣ Tension-type headache

Associated with localized pain

With flame hemorrhages Cottonwool spots

Severe hypertension

Primarily in temporal, facial area

Exacerbated by chewing

Malocclusion present

Ⓤ TMJ disease

Temporal artery beaded, tender

Ⓥ Temporal arteritis

Obtain ESR
Do Temporal
Artery Biopsy

Eye pain

Increase with use eyes

Ⓦ Eye strain

Other eye, orbit pain (p 32)

Refractive error
Hyperopia
Astigmatism

Muscle imbalance
Convergence
 insufficiency
Extraocular
 muscle palsies

Associated with excruciating unilateral pain

Epiphora, rhinorrhea, red eye present

Ⓞ Cluster headaches

Pain primarily in second, third division cranial nerve V

Ⓟ Trigeminal neuralgia (tic douloureux)

History of hydrocephalus

Sixth cranial nerve paresis or esotropia may be present

Raised intracranial pressure, intermittent

Ⓠ Poorly controlled hydrocephalus (intermittent)

EYE PAIN

Tomy Starck, M.D.
Lorena Larez de Mendible, M.D.

A. The diagnosis of ocular pain covers a broad spectrum of ophthalmic and nonophthalmic entities and may be a sign of a more serious underlying disease process. A thorough clinical history, including detailed review of systems, adds to the complete physical examination.

B. Ocular pain without redness most likely does not involve the ocular surface, with the exception of Thygeson's punctate keratopathy. Multiple small corneal epithelial and subepithelial areas of staining with fluorescein dye usually highlight the diagnosis. Hypotony secondary to end-stage ocular diseases (phthisis bulbi) may be accompanied by chronic dull pain.

C. Patients with orbital pain and a history of trauma may reveal old orbital wall fractures on CT scan, especially of the lesser wing of the sphenoid.

D. Homer's syndrome should be considered in patients with ocular pain associated with anisocoria, ptosis, and anhidrosis. Although unlikely, microvascular causes, such as diabetes mellitus, may occasionally induce ophthalmoplegias with pain and anisocoria. Pain, with or without visual loss on ocular movement, suggests optic neuritis and requires careful evaluation of the visual pathways.

E. Headache is believed to be a common related symptom of refractive errors, although in reality the association is uncommon. Several migraine syndromes may also prove to be causes of ocular-related pain (p 28). Systemic debilitating symptoms, such as loss of weight, loss of appetite, and scalp tenderness, may indicate an arteritis.

F. Limitation of ocular motility secondary to nerve involvement, called *ophthalmoplegia*, may be associated with pain. The differential diagnosis should include migraine syndromes, orbital inflammatory disease, contiguous sinusitis, tumors of the parasellar area, and superior orbital-cavernous sinus syndrome caused by vascular anomalies, tumors, or infection.

G. Pain, diffuse conjunctival injection, hazy cornea, high intraocular pressure (IOP), mid-dilated pupil, the absence of an advanced cataract, and iris bombé make the diagnosis of simple angle-closure glaucoma. Gonioscopy confirms the diagnosis.

H. In the case of an advanced cataract with the findings in section J, phacomorphic glaucoma is the diagnosis, and immediate lens extraction is indicated.

I. After a thorough ocular examination reveals only a red eye with severe pain but no obvious ocular disease, further studies are indicated, including orbital ultrasonography, CT, or MRI. Also consider posterior scleritis, orbital myositis, or pseudotumor.

J. Painful infiltrates of the cornea (with and without epithelial defects) can be a diagnostic dilemma. An infective corneal ulcer must be differentiated from a sterile ulcer by scraping the lesion for Gram stain and cultures. Bacterial, fungal, and viral ulcers with infiltrates must be treated specifically. Sterile corneal infiltrates are caused by immune responses in the cornea to a specific toxin or antigen and respond well to steroids.

K. Fluorescein staining of the cornea is usually associated with a diffusely red eye and some pain. The differential diagnosis of the corneal staining includes corneal abrasion, foreign body, keratitis sicca, herpes simplex keratitis, keratoconjunctivitis, corneal ulcers, corneal dystrophies, and degenerations.

L. Lid abnormalities that may cause exposure or mechanical abrasion of the cornea are trichiasis, ectropion, entropion, lagophthalmos, lid coloboma, and scarring of the lids that leaves the globe exposed.

M. In the red eye with pain and ciliary injection the presence of a hypopyon (layer of white cells in the anterior chamber) helps narrow the diagnosis. Considerations are endophthalmitis, Behçet's syndrome, malignancy (retinoblastoma, leukemia, lymphoma), and severe anterior uveitis.

N. Hyphema (a layer of red cells in the anterior chamber) after trauma makes the diagnosis in a painful red eye simple. In contrast, spontaneous hyphema, especially in children, should raise suspicion of juvenile xanthogranuloma (JXG) or child abuse. In adults, consider neovascularization and tumors.

O. If thorough examination reveals only anterior inflammation, the differential diagnosis is HLA-B27–positive disease (Reiter's syndrome, ankylosing spondylitis, inflammatory bowel disease, psoriasis), Behçet's syndrome, or idiopathic iritis, the last one being the most common.

P. The painful red eye with anterior chamber inflammation may also exhibit posterior chamber inflammation in the form of vitreitis, retinitis, vasculitis, or infective endophthalmitis. Consider life-threatening systemic diseases such as syphilis, tuberculosis, sarcoidosis, and AIDS.

REFERENCES

Albert D, Jacobiec F. Atlas of clinical ophthalmology. Philadelphia: Saunders, 1996.

Basic and Clinical Science Course. Sections 3, 4, and 7. San Francisco: American Academy of Ophthalmology, 1998.

Cullom D, Chang B. Wills Eye Hospital: Office and emergency room diagnosis and treatment of eye disease. Philadelphia: Lippincott, 1993.

Duane T, Jaeger E. Clinical ophthalmology. Vol 2. Philadelphia: Lippincott, 1988.

Tomsak RL. Handbook of treatment in neuro-ophthalmology. Washington: Butterworth-Heinemann, 1997.

Patient with OCULAR PAIN

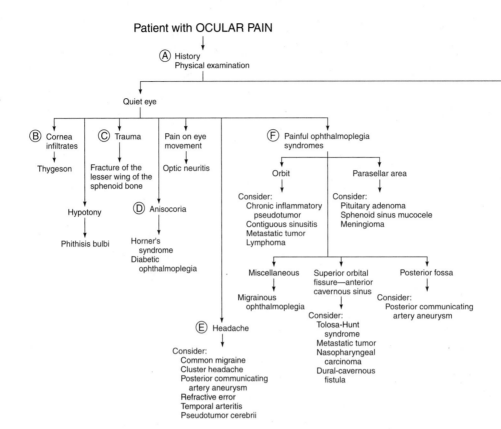

(A) History
Physical examination

Quiet eye

(B) Cornea
infiltrates

Thygeson

Hypotony

Phithisis bulbi

(C) Trauma

Fracture of the
lesser wing of the
sphenoid bone

(D) Anisocoria

Horner's
syndrome
Diabetic
ophthalmoplegia

Pain on eye
movement

Optic neuritis

(E) Headache

Consider:
  Common migraine
  Cluster headache
  Posterior communicating
    artery aneurysm
  Refractive error
  Temporal arteritis
  Pseudotumor cerebrii

(F) Painful ophthalmoplegia
syndromes

Orbit

Consider:
  Chronic inflammatory
    pseudotumor
  Contiguous sinusitis
  Metastatic tumor
  Lymphoma

Parasellar area

Consider:
  Pituitary adenoma
  Sphenoid sinus mucocele
  Meningioma

Miscellaneous

Migrainous
ophthalmoplegia

Superior orbital
fissure—anterior
cavernous sinus

Consider:
  Tolosa-Hunt
    syndrome
  Metastatic tumor
  Nasopharyngeal
    carcinoma
  Dural-cavernous
    fistula

Posterior fossa

Consider:
  Posterior communicating
    artery aneurysm

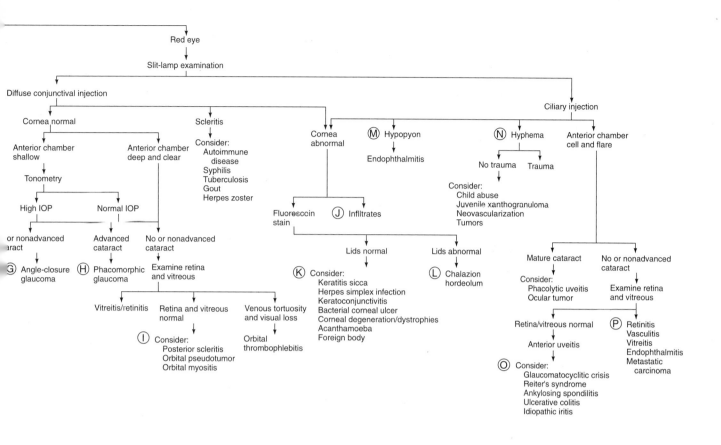

Red eye
↓
Slit-lamp examination

Diffuse conjunctival injection

Cornea normal

Anterior chamber shallow

Tonometry

High IOP | Normal IOP

Ⓖ or nonadvanced cataract

Ⓖ Angle-closure glaucoma

Anterior chamber deep and clear

Ⓗ Advanced cataract

Ⓗ Phacomorphic glaucoma

No or nonadvanced cataract

Examine retina and vitreous

Vitreitis/retinitis

Retina and vitreous normal

Ⓘ Consider:
Posterior scleritis
Orbital pseudotumor
Orbital myositis

Venous tortuosity and visual loss

Orbital thrombophlebitis

Scleritis

Consider:
Autoimmune disease
Syphilis
Tuberculosis
Gout
Herpes zoster

Cornea abnormal

Fluorescein stain

Ⓙ Infiltrates

Lids normal

Ⓚ Consider:
Keratitis sicca
Herpes simplex infection
Keratoconjunctivitis
Bacterial corneal ulcer
Corneal degeneration/dystrophies
Acanthamoeba
Foreign body

Lids abnormal

Ⓛ Chalazion hordeolum

Ⓜ Hypopyon
↓
Endophthalmitis

Ciliary injection

Ⓝ Hyphema

No trauma | Trauma

Consider:
Child abuse
Juvenile xanthogranuloma
Neovascularization
Tumors

Anterior chamber cell and flare

Mature cataract

Consider:
Phacolytic uveitis
Ocular tumor

Retina/vitreous normal

Anterior uveitis

Ⓞ Consider:
Glaucomatocyclitic crisis
Reiter's syndrome
Ankylosing spondilitis
Ulcerative colitis
Idiopathic iritis

No or nonadvanced cataract

Examine retina and vitreous

Ⓟ Retinitis
Vasculitis
Vitreitis
Endophthalmitis
Metastatic carcinoma

RED EYE

Tomy Starck, M.D.
Lorena Larez de Mendible, M.D.

The differential diagnosis of the red eye encompasses a wide range of ophthalmic conditions, many of which are discussed in detail in other chapters.

A. One of the more helpful differentiating symptoms of the red eye, obtained from the history and physical examination, is pain. In general, the nonpainful red eye denotes a less serious, non–vision-threatening cause. A painful red eye is often a more serious problem.

B. Slit-lamp examination, by which more than 90% of the red eye can be diagnosed, is most helpful. However, more than one disease process may be taking place, so perform a complete eye examination.

C. A nonpainful red eye with diffuse conjunctival injection may be caused by abnormalities of the lids. Debris and bacterial growth found in blepharitis and meibomitis can spill over into the conjunctiva. Ocular rosacea, a skin disease involving facial erythema and telangiectasias, is often associated with dysfunction of the meibomian glands. Trichiasis (ingrowth of eyelashes) may cause mechanical irritation. Malpositions of the eyelid may cause exposure. Molluscum contagiosum lesions on the lid margin usually result in a follicular conjunctivitis.

D. Diffuse nonpainful conjunctival injection in the absence of lid abnormalities may be caused by conjunctivitis. The distinction between follicular and papillary conjunctivitis is helpful to determine treatment. Follicles are best seen in the inferior conjunctival cul-de-sac and appear as smooth elevations with vessels surrounding but not within each follicle. Papillae can be small or "giant" and present a mosaic-like pattern. Each papilla has a central fibrovascular core. Papillary conjunctival injection is a nonspecific inflammatory response.

E. Rarely, a nonpainful diffusely red eye harbors a malignancy of the ciliary body, retina, or choroid. The differential diagnosis of the tumor depends on the patient's age. Retinoblastoma leads in the pediatric age group, and melanoma leads in adults.

F. Generalized dilated episcleral vessels, with or without conjunctival injection, should raise suspicion of vascular anomalies such as carotid-cavernous fistula or low-grade flow dural-carotid shunts. Focal dilated episcleral vessels may signal an underlying intraocular malignancy ("sentinel vessels").

G. Nonpainful focal lesions of the conjunctiva may become irritated and inflamed. Pinguecula and pterygium are easily diagnosed. Atypical inflamed lesions may need to be excised to rule out malignancy. Localized nonpainful "redness" of the conjunctiva usually represents episcleritis, which includes episcleral vascular injection, or a subconjunctival hemorrhage, which is a localized collection of blood beneath the conjunctiva with normal conjunctival vessels. Both conditions are benign, but occasionally, the first may require the use of topical nonsteroidal drugs. Recurrent subconjunctival hemorrhage without trauma warrants a hematologic work-up.

H. Proptosis, conjunctival injection, and pain are highly suggestive of inflammatory orbital disease (orbital pseudotumor). When pain is absent, consider thyroid ophthalmopathy in the differential diagnosis.

I. Pain, diffuse conjunctival injection, high intraocular pressure (IOP), mid-dilated pupil, the absence of an advanced cataract, and iris bombé make the diagnosis of simple angle-closure glaucoma. Gonioscopy confirms the diagnosis.

J. In the case of an advanced cataract with the findings in section M, phacomorphic glaucoma is the diagnosis, and immediate lens extraction is indicated.

K. If a thorough ocular examination reveals only a red eye with severe pain but no obvious ocular disease, further studies are indicated, including orbital ultrasonography, CT, or MRI. Consider posterior scleritis, orbital myositis, or pseudotumor.

L. Pain, diffuse conjunctival injection, and scleral edema (scleritis) require a systemic work-up based on a thorough review of systems to rule out both generalized immune diseases as well as infectious causes.

M. Fluorescein staining of the cornea is usually associated with a diffusely red eye and some pain. The differential diagnosis of the corneal staining includes corneal abrasion, foreign body, keratitis sicca, herpes simplex keratitis, keratoconjunctivitis, corneal ulcers, corneal dystrophies, and degenerations.

N. Lid abnormalities that may cause exposure or mechanical abrasion of the cornea are trichiasis, ectropion, entropion, lagophthalmos, and scarring of the lids that leaves the globe exposed.

O. Painful infiltrates of the cornea (with and without epithelial defects) can be a diagnostic dilemma. An infective corneal ulcer must be differentiated from a sterile ulcer by scraping the lesion for Gram stain and cultures. Bacterial, fungal, and viral ulcers with infiltrates must be treated specifically. Sterile corneal infiltrates are caused by immune responses in the cornea to a specific toxin or antigen and usually respond well to steroids.

P. With ciliary injection, anterior chamber cell and flare and hypermature cataract, phacolytic uveitis (and possibly glaucoma) is the diagnosis. Diagnostic echography should be done to rule out a hidden malignancy of the posterior segment.

Q. If a thorough examination reveals only anterior inflammation, the differential diagnosis is HLA-B27–positive disease (Reiter's syndrome, ankylosing spondylitis, inflammatory bowel disease, psoriasis), Behçet's syndrome, or idiopathic iritis, the last one being the most common.

R. The painful red eye with anterior chamber inflammation may also exhibit posterior chamber inflammation in the form of vitreitis, retinitis, vasculitis, or infective endophthalmitis. Consider life-threatening systemic diseases such as syphilis, tuberculosis, sarcoidosis, and AIDS.

S. In the red eye with pain and ciliary injection the presence of a hypopyon (layer of white cells in the anterior chamber) helps narrow the diagnosis. Considerations are endophthalmitis, Behçet's syndrome, malignancy (retinoblastoma, leukemia, lymphoma), and severe anterior uveitis.

T. Hyphema (a layer of red cell in the anterior chamber) after trauma makes the diagnosis of a painful red eye simple. In contrast, spontaneous hyphema, especially in children, should raise suspicion of juvenile xanthogranuloma (JXG) or child abuse. In adults, consider neovascularization and tumors.

REFERENCES

Albert D, Jacobiec F. Atlas of clinical ophthalmology. Philadelphia: Saunders, 1996.

Basic and Clinical Science Course. Sections 3, 4, and 7. San Francisco: American Academy of Ophthalmology, 1998.

Cullom D, Chang B. Wills Eye Hospital: Office and emergency room diagnosis and treatment of eye disease. Philadelphia: Lippincott, 1993.

Duane T, Jaeger E. Clinical ophthalmology. Vol 2. Philadelphia: Lippincott, 1988.

Hampton F. Ocular differential diagnosis. Baltimore: Williams & Wilkins, 1997.

Newell FW. Ophthalmology: Principles and concepts. St Louis: Mosby, 1992.

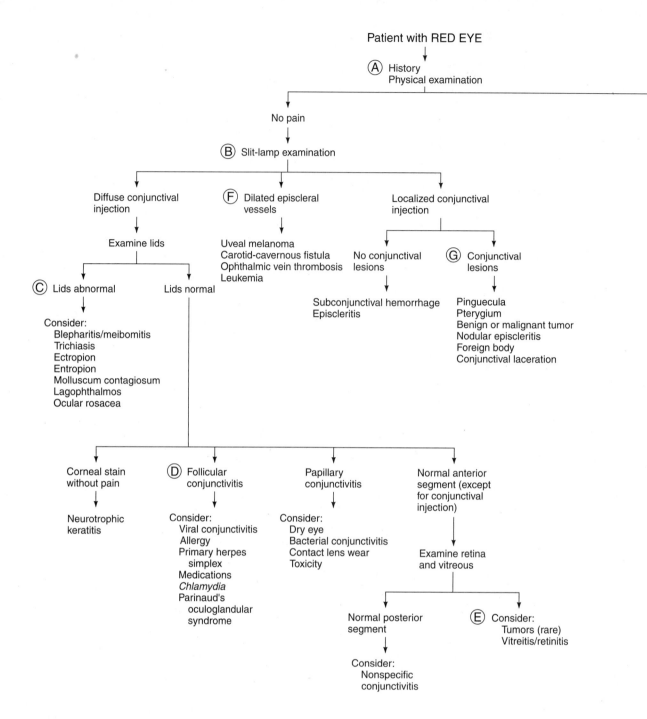

Patient with RED EYE

Ⓐ History
Physical examination

No pain

Ⓑ Slit-lamp examination

Diffuse conjunctival injection

Ⓕ Dilated episcleral vessels

Localized conjunctival injection

Examine lids

Uveal melanoma
Carotid-cavernous fistula
Ophthalmic vein thrombosis
Leukemia

No conjunctival lesions

Ⓖ Conjunctival lesions

Ⓒ Lids abnormal

Lids normal

Subconjunctival hemorrhage
Episcleritis

Pinguecula
Pterygium
Benign or malignant tumor
Nodular episcleritis
Foreign body
Conjunctival laceration

Consider:
    Blepharitis/meibomitis
    Trichiasis
    Ectropion
    Entropion
    Molluscum contagiosum
    Lagophthalmos
    Ocular rosacea

Corneal stain without pain

Ⓓ Follicular conjunctivitis

Papillary conjunctivitis

Normal anterior segment (except for conjunctival injection)

Neurotrophic keratitis

Consider:
    Viral conjunctivitis
    Allergy
    Primary herpes simplex
    Medications
    Chlamydia
    Parinaud's oculoglandular syndrome

Consider:
    Dry eye
    Bacterial conjunctivitis
    Contact lens wear
    Toxicity

Examine retina and vitreous

Normal posterior segment

Ⓔ Consider:
    Tumors (rare)
    Vitreitis/retinitis

Consider:
    Nonspecific conjunctivitis

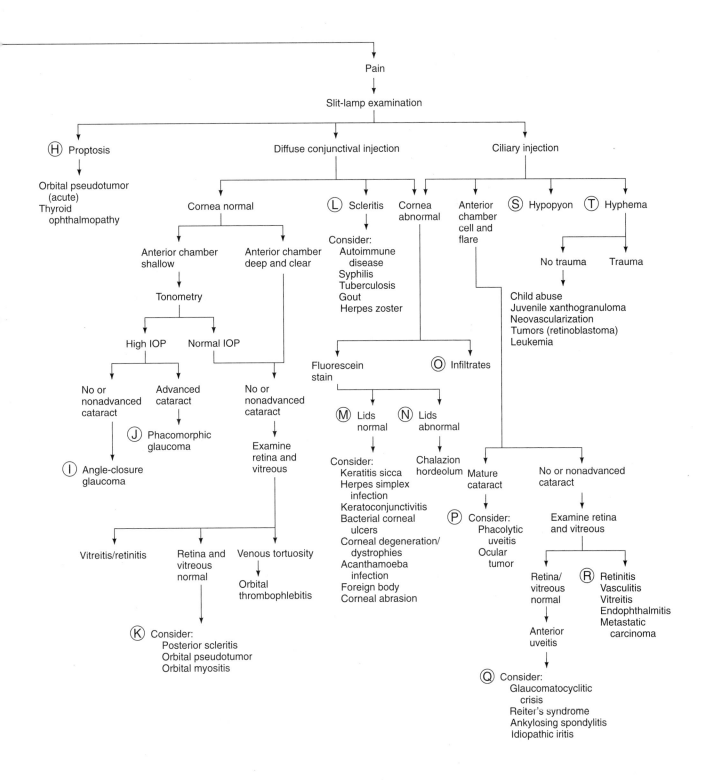

Pain

Slit-lamp examination

(H) Proptosis

Orbital pseudotumor
(acute)
Thyroid
ophthalmopathy

Diffuse conjunctival injection

Ciliary injection

Cornea normal

(L) Scleritis

Cornea
abnormal

Anterior
chamber
cell and
flare

(S) Hypopyon (T) Hyphema

Anterior chamber
shallow

Anterior chamber
deep and clear

Consider:
  Autoimmune
    disease
  Syphilis
  Tuberculosis
  Gout
  Herpes zoster

No trauma   Trauma

Tonometry

Child abuse
Juvenile xanthogranuloma
Neovascularization
Tumors (retinoblastoma)
Leukemia

High IOP   Normal IOP

No or
nonadvanced
cataract

Advanced
cataract

No or
nonadvanced
cataract

Fluorescein
stain

(O) Infiltrates

(J) Phacomorphic
     glaucoma

Examine
retina and
vitreous

(M) Lids
     normal

(N) Lids
     abnormal

(I) Angle-closure
    glaucoma

Consider:
  Keratitis sicca
  Herpes simplex
    infection
  Keratoconjunctivitis
  Bacterial corneal
    ulcers
  Corneal degeneration/
    dystrophies
  Acanthamoeba
    infection
  Foreign body
  Corneal abrasion

Chalazion
hordeolum Mature
           cataract

No or nonadvanced
cataract

Vitreitis/retinitis

Retina and
vitreous
normal

Venous tortuosity

Orbital
thrombophlebitis

(P) Consider:
     Phacolytic
     uveitis
     Ocular
     tumor

Examine retina
and vitreous

Retina/
vitreous
normal

(R) Retinitis
     Vasculitis
     Vitreitis
     Endophthalmitis
     Metastatic
       carcinoma

(K) Consider:
     Posterior scleritis
     Orbital pseudotumor
     Orbital myositis

Anterior
uveitis

(Q) Consider:
     Glaucomatocyclitic
       crisis
     Reiter's syndrome
     Ankylosing spondylitis
     Idiopathic iritis

ITCHY EYE

Kristin Story Held, M.D.

Itching is a common symptom of many ocular external diseases, including viral conjunctivitis, blepharitis, dry eye syndrome, and allergic blepharoconjunctivitis. It is just one of many other more significant symptoms in conjunctivitis, blepharitis, and dry eye syndrome, but it is the primary and overwhelming complaint in allergic blepharoconjunctivitis. Intense itching is the most common and significant symptom of ocular allergic disease. Nonallergic causes can usually be ruled out after the initial history and physical examination.

A. After making the diagnosis of allergic blepharoconjunctivitis, collect additional historical information. The types of allergic blepharoconjunctivitis include contact blepharoconjunctivitis, drug hypersensitivity reactions, giant papillary conjunctivitis, vernal keratoconjunctivitis, atopic keratoconjunctivitis, and hay fever conjunctivitis. Elucidation of the patient's history and the clinical setting in which the itchy eye developed will lead to a highly accurate diagnosis. Key questions must be asked of every patient: What is the primary symptom? Is there a history of atopic disease, hay fever, asthma, or eczema? Has there been exposure to specific environmental agents or topical preparations (e.g., eye drops, cosmetics)? Does the patient wear contact lenses, or has he or she had ocular surgery? Associated signs include red eyes, swollen lids, tearing, rhinorrhea, stringy discharge, chemosis, and papillary hypertrophy. Evert the lids to evaluate the superior tarsal conjunctiva.

B. Allergic contact blepharoconjunctivitis develops acutely, usually within 48 hours after contact with the offending agent. The patient is reexposed to a topical ophthalmic preparation to which he or she has been previously sensitized. A delayed (type IV) T-lymphocyte–mediated hypersensitivity reaction occurs. Neomycin sulfate is the most common offending ocular preparation. Other agents include chloramphenicol, antazoline phosphate, atropine sulfate, idoxuridine thimerosal, chlorhexidine, facial soaps, perfumes, and cosmetics. The eyes and surrounding skin become acutely erythematous and edematous, and intense itching develops, accompanied by a characteristic eczematoid dermatitis of the eyelid skin. Symptoms resolve upon removal of the causative agent. Supportive measures provide symptomatic relief.

C. Anaphylactoid reactions to topical preparations are rapid in onset and characterized by lid edema and conjunctival erythema and chemosis. Anaphylactoid reactions are type I (IgE-mediated) hypersensitivity reactions. These rarely occur, but the main offending agents are topical penicillin, sulfacetamide, bacitracin, and topical anesthetics.

D. Long-term use of topical preparations such as gentami-

ALLERGY DROPS

Over-the-counter
Naphazoline hydrochloride/pheniramine maleate eye drops (OcuHist, Opcon-A, Naphcon-A)
Naphazoline hydrochloride/antazoline phosphate eye drops (Vasocon-A)
H₁ antihistamines
Levocabastine hydrochloride ophthalmic suspension (Livostin)
H₁ antihistamines plus mast-cell stabilizer
Olopatadine hydrochloride ophthalmic solution (Patanol)
Mast-cell stabilizer
Cromolyn sodium ophthalmic solution (Crolom, Opticrom)
Mast-cell stabilizer plus eosinophil suppressor
Lodoxamide tromethamine ophthalmic solution (Alomide)
NSAID
Ketorolac tromethamine ophthalmic solution (Acular)
Steroids
Loteprednol etabonate ophthalmic suspension (Alrex 0.2%, Lotemax 0.5%)
Rimexolone ophthalmic suspension (Vexol)
Fluorometholone (FML, Fluor-Op, Eflone, Flarex)

cin, idoxuridine, pilocarpine, and echothiophate iodide may result in a cytotoxic (type II) reaction. The reaction is slow to develop and often follows use of a drug for weeks, months, or even years. A conjunctival follicular response is usually present, and significant conjunctival scarring can develop.

E. Giant papillary conjunctivitis occurs in otherwise healthy persons who wear contact lenses or an ocular prosthesis or who have monofilament nylon or another foreign body on the ocular surface. No history of atopic disease is associated. Eversion of the upper lid reveals the characteristic giant papillae. Definitive treatment is removal of the foreign body.

F. Vernal keratoconjunctivitis typically occurs in young males in the second decade of life. Symptoms peak in the spring and fall. The condition is worse in warm climates. Ocular symptoms are severe, but there are no associated systemic symptoms. There is a patient or family history of atopic disease. The classic sign is papillary hypertrophy of the superior tarsal conjunctiva and limbus. Trantas' dots and shield ulcers may be seen. Abundant eosinophils and free eosinophilic granules are seen on conjunctival scrapings. No granules and fewer eosinophils are seen with atopic and hay fever keratoconjunctivitis. Because vernal keratoconjunctivitis tends to be self-limited, the goal of treatment is palliation.

G. Atopic dermatitis is familial and begins in childhood. From 10% to 20% of the population is atopic, and 25%–40% of these patients have ocular involvement, which usually appears in the teens. The eye signs are accompanied by characteristic skin lesions on the face, trunk, and flexor surfaces of the arms and legs. Atopic dermatitis is neither seasonal nor exacerbated by warm climates. Atopic keratoconjunctivitis is characterized by recurrent inflammation of the lids and conjunctiva. The inferior fornix and palpebral conjunctiva are predominately involved. Serious potentially blinding consequences may occur in relation to the corneal complications. One must take great care to recognize and treat associated acne rosacea, herpetic disease, and keratitis sicca. Systemic antihistamines and strict environmental controls are important in successful management.

H. Hay fever conjunctivitis is characterized by hyperemic chemotic, baggy conjunctiva accompanied by allergic rhinitis, mild asthma, and/or sinusitis. Many allergens may cause this reaction. If pollens are the cause, the symptoms may vary with season and geographic location. If molds, house dust, or dander is the allergen, no seasonal variation exists. Conjunctival scrapings stained with Giemsa stain show eosinophils. The mainstay of treatment is removing the offending agent; treatment is otherwise supportive.

References

Colby K, Dohlman C. Vernal keratoconjunctivitis. In: Jakobiec FA, Adamis AP, Pineda RA, eds. International ophthalmology clinics—Noninfectious inflammatory disorders of the eye and adnexa. Boston: Little, Brown, 1996; 36:15–20.

Friedlaender MH. Management of ocular allergy. Ann Allerg Asthma Immunol 1995; 75:212–224.

Power WJ, Tugal-Tutkun I, Foster CS. Long-term follow-up of patients with atopic keratoconjunctivitis. Ophthalmology 1998; 105.4:637–642.

Titi MJ. A critical look at ocular allergy drugs. Am Fam Physician 1996; 53:2637–2642.

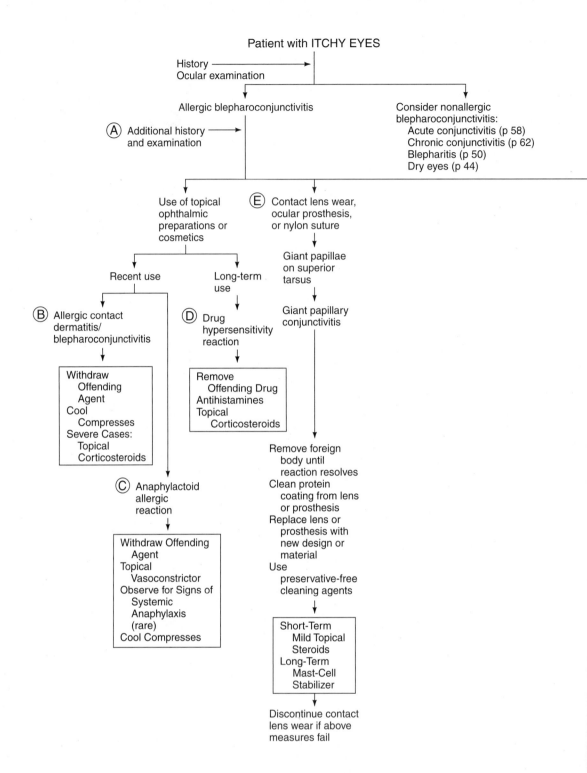

Patient with ITCHY EYES

History ⎯⎯⎯⎯⎯⎯
Ocular examination

Allergic blepharoconjunctivitis

Ⓐ Additional history ⎯⎯⎯→
and examination

Consider nonallergic
blepharoconjunctivitis:
    Acute conjunctivitis (p 58)
    Chronic conjunctivitis (p 62)
    Blepharitis (p 50)
    Dry eyes (p 44)

Use of topical
ophthalmic
preparations or
cosmetics

Ⓔ Contact lens wear,
ocular prosthesis,
or nylon suture

Giant papillae
on superior
tarsus

Giant papillary
conjunctivitis

Recent use

Long-term
use

Ⓑ Allergic contact
dermatitis/
blepharoconjunctivitis

Ⓓ Drug
hypersensitivity
reaction

Withdraw
    Offending
    Agent
Cool
    Compresses
Severe Cases:
    Topical
    Corticosteroids

Remove
    Offending Drug
Antihistamines
Topical
    Corticosteroids

Ⓒ Anaphylactoid
allergic
reaction

Remove foreign
    body until
    reaction resolves
Clean protein
    coating from lens
    or prosthesis
Replace lens or
    prosthesis with
    new design or
    material
Use
    preservative-free
    cleaning agents

Withdraw Offending
    Agent
Topical
    Vasoconstrictor
Observe for Signs of
    Systemic
    Anaphylaxis
    (rare)
Cool Compresses

Short-Term
    Mild Topical
    Steroids
Long-Term
    Mast-Cell
    Stabilizer

Discontinue contact
lens wear if above
measures fail

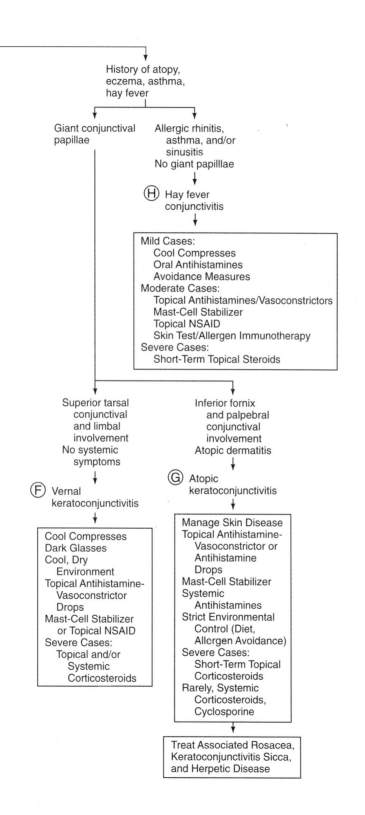

History of atopy,
eczema, asthma,
hay fever

Giant conjunctival
papillae

Allergic rhinitis,
asthma, and/or
sinusitis
No giant papilllae

(H) Hay fever
conjunctivitis

Mild Cases:
    Cool Compresses
    Oral Antihistamines
    Avoidance Measures
Moderate Cases:
    Topical Antihistamines/Vasoconstrictors
    Mast-Cell Stabilizer
    Topical NSAID
    Skin Test/Allergen Immunotherapy
Severe Cases:
    Short-Term Topical Steroids

Superior tarsal
conjunctival
and limbal
involvement
No systemic
symptoms

Inferior fornix
and palpebral
conjunctival
involvement
Atopic dermatitis

(F) Vernal
keratoconjunctivitis

(G) Atopic
keratoconjunctivitis

Cool Compresses
Dark Glasses
Cool, Dry
    Environment
Topical Antihistamine-
    Vasoconstrictor
    Drops
Mast-Cell Stabilizer
    or Topical NSAID
Severe Cases:
    Topical and/or
    Systemic
    Corticosteroids

Manage Skin Disease
Topical Antihistamine-
    Vasoconstrictor or
    Antihistamine
    Drops
Mast-Cell Stabilizer
Systemic
    Antihistamines
Strict Environmental
    Control (Diet,
    Allergen Avoidance)
Severe Cases:
    Short-Term Topical
    Corticosteroids
    Rarely, Systemic
    Corticosteroids,
    Cyclosporine

Treat Associated Rosacea,
Keratoconjunctivitis Sicca,
and Herpetic Disease

DRY EYE

Kristin Story Held, M.D.

Dry eye affects millions of people worldwide and is a common problem leading patients to the ophthalmologist's office. There are many causes of dry eye, which results ultimately from abnormalities of the tear film and/or ocular surface. The tear film is composed of three layers: (1) the outermost lipid layer, derived from the meibomian glands; (2) the largest layer, the aqueous layer, derived from the main and accessory lacrimal glands; and (3) the mucin layer, derived from the goblet cells. Abnormalities of the meibomian glands, lacrimal glands, or conjunctiva, which contains the goblet cells, obviously result in a defective tear film mechanism, as does any abnormality of the ocular surface (i.e., the cornea, eyelids, conjunctiva). An accurate diagnosis is important in determining appropriate treatment and resolving patients' complaints. A thorough history and physical examination are essential in making a proper diagnosis. Laboratory evaluation and histologic studies provide further information supporting the diagnosis.

A. The symptoms are variable and range from burning and foreign body sensation to severe pain and irritation out of proportion to clinical signs. Symptoms are often exacerbated by smoke, wind, or prolonged use of the eyes. Paradoxical tearing may be present. One may complain of ropy mucus, vision that fluctuates with blinking, and photophobia.

B. The patient history may often disclose the cause of the dry eye. Most types of dry eye are more common in women, and postmenopausal women are more likely to have aqueous tear deficiencies than premenopausal women. Many commonly prescribed medications, systemic and topical, can affect the tear film and should be eliminated when possible. Ask about specific systemic complaints that might suggest an underlying systemic disorder associated with dry eyes, particularly the autoimmune collagen vascular disorders and lymphoma. Dry eyes have been associated with certain dermatologic diseases as well. Congenital conditions associated with lacrimal hyposecretion include lacrimal gland hypoplasia, familial dysautonomia, and multiple endocrine neoplasia. Acquired conditions include rheumatoid arthritis, systemic lupus erythematosus, polyarteritis nodosa, lymphoma, thrombocytopenia purpura, hypergammaglobulinemia, Hashimoto's thyroiditis, sarcoidosis, graft-versus-host disease, and viral dacryoadenitis. Conjunctival or lip biopsy may be useful in diagnosing Sjögren's syndrome. Irradiation, chemical burns, or mechanical trauma to the lacrimal gland produces hyposecretion as well. A history of factors leading to vitamin A deficiency must be elicited because this is a common cause of dry eye worldwide, and rapid improvement in the ocular surface abnormalities occurs with systemic vitamin A therapy.

C. Perform a thorough evaluation of the lid structure and function, including observation of the blink mecha-

nism and Bell's phenomenon. Lid abnormalities such as ectropion, entropion, trichiasis, and margin irregularity must be detected so that surgical repair can be undertaken. Rule out nocturnal lagophthalmos, Bell's palsy, and thyroid disease. Assess the integrity of the fifth and seventh cranial nerves.

D. The inferior marginal tear strip is observed initially. Normally, the height of the tear meniscus should be at least 1 mm and convex. A small, scanty tear strip suggests deficient tear volume. Debris in the tear film may indicate an inadequate tear volume in addition to blepharitis.

E. The conjunctival examination may indicate the underlying cause of the dry eyes such as ocular cicatricial pemphigoid, trachoma, chemical burn, or Stevens-Johnson syndrome. Conjunctival biopsy is useful in the diagnosis of ocular pemphigoid. Severe cases may require systemic and topical immunosuppressive therapy. Conjunctival impression cytologic examination may be useful in evaluating the epithelium for squamous metaplasia and the presence of goblet cells.

F. Proper use of dye tests is of ultimate importance in diagnosing the dry eye. A fluorescein strip is moistened with a drop of preservative-free saline solution and gently touched to the inferior tear meniscus. The amount of fluorescence is an indirect measure of the aqueous tear volume. Observe the cornea for areas of punctate stain. Fluorescein stains areas that are devoid of epithelium as the water-soluble dye penetrates into the underlying corneal stroma. The tear breakup time, which indicates the stability of the tear film, is then recorded. It is the time between a blink and the appearance of a corneal dry spot. Normally it should be >10 seconds. Tear breakup time is often abnormal (<10 seconds) in all types of dry eye conditions. The tear breakup time may help in assessing the efficacy of treatment; that is, a positive therapeutic effect would be indicated by an increased tear breakup time. If corneal drying repeatedly appears in the same area, suspect and treat a localized corneal abnormality. Rose bengal is a vital dye that stains devitalized epithelial cells rather than areas of actual epithelial cell loss. It is common to see rose bengal staining in the interpalpebral zone of exposure in keratoconjunctivitis sicca. Rose bengal stains this region in many cases in which fluorescein would show no defect.

G. Schirmer's test is performed to measure tear secretion. Place a standardized strip (Whatman's 41 filter paper, 5 mm wide) in the lateral third of the lower eyelid for 5 minutes. The test is first performed without anesthesia to indicate the reflex or maximum amount of lacrimal gland secretion. Wetting of less than 15 mm at 5 minutes is abnormal. When performed after the instillation of topical anesthesia, the test measures the minimum or basal tear secretion. The normal value is >10 mm at 5 minutes.

H. The tear film osmolality, lysozyme level, and lactoferrin level are three laboratory tests that measure lacrimal gland function and may be useful in diagnosing dry eye. Tear film osmolality is increased (>312 mOsm/kg) in patients with keratoconjunctivitis sicca, whereas lysozyme and lactoferrin levels are decreased in tears of patients with decreased lacrimal gland secretion. Kits are available to perform these tests.

I. After establishing the diagnosis of dry eye by a thorough patient history and complete systematic clinical examination, initiate treatment in a logical, stepwise fashion. First, address the underlying cause of the dry eye. Lid abnormalities may be surgically corrected, blepharitis and meibomitis shows are treated, and associated inflammation is controlled. Refer patients with underlying systemic conditions for further medical consultation, and control the associated inflammation and immune processes by local and systemic immunosuppression as needed. Next, address localized conjunctival and corneal abnormalities. Modify systemic medications. The mainstay of dry eye treatment is artificial tear replacement. Treatment with preserved artificial tears with strict adherence to a schedule of four times daily is used on a conscientious basis in mild cases. Lubricating ointment may be added at bedtime. Patching with the lubrication may be helpful if nocturnal lagophthalmos is present. Niteye, a "dry eye bandage," is now available in the form of a plastic eye shield that acts as a moisture chamber for use when resting. Once the need for artificial tears exceeds four times daily, preservative-free drops must be used and in some cases may be used every 15–60 minutes. Celluvisc (carboxymethylcellulose sodium 1% lubricant),

Occucoat PF (hydroxypropyl methylcellulose), and sodium hyaluronate (dilute Healon) may afford decreased frequency of administration because of their increased viscosity. Lacriserts, sustained-release tear inserts, are available but difficult for many patients to insert. Patients should decrease external factors that increase the evaporation of the tear film or exacerbate symptoms. In cases of excess mucous strands, 10% acetylcysteine may be effective. As a rule, wearing soft contact lenses should be avoided, particularly if the tear breakup time is <10 seconds; however, on a short-term basis they may be useful in resolving persistent epithelial defects or filamentary keratopathy. If symptoms and signs of ocular surface injury persist, perform temporary punctal occlusion using absorbable collagen plugs or nonabsorbable silicone plugs. If occlusion of all four puncta affords clinical improvement and the patient tolerates this well, proceed with permanent punctal occlusion using thermal cautery, laser, or radiodiathermy. In severe cases refractory to all preceding measures, perform lateral tarsorrhaphy. Consider topical cyclosporine in severe cases. Patient reassurance is extremely important. The efficacy of therapy may be assessed by following the tear breakup time and the staining pattern with rose bengal, but the most important gauge is the patient's symptoms.

References

Arffa, RC, ed. Grayson's diseases of the cornea. 4th ed. St Louis: Mosby, 1997: 355.

deLuise VP. Management of dry eyes. In: Focal points: Clinical modules for ophthalmologists. San Francisco: American Academy of Ophthalmology, 1985.

Nelson ID. Dry eye syndrome—Current diagnosis and management. In: Schachat AP, ed. Current practice in ophthalmology. St Louis: Mosby, 1992: 49.

Smolin G, Friedlaender M, eds. International Ophthalmology Clinics—Dry eye. Vol 34.1. Boston: Little, Brown, 1994.

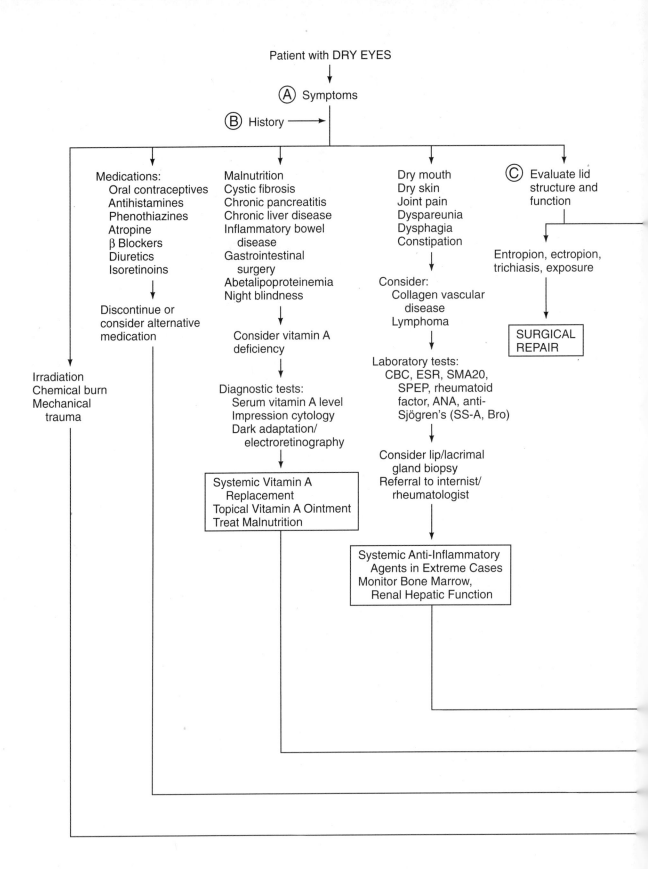

Patient with DRY EYES

Ⓐ Symptoms

Ⓑ History

Medications:
  Oral contraceptives
  Antihistamines
  Phenothiazines
  Atropine
  β Blockers
  Diuretics
  Isoretinoins

Discontinue or
consider alternative
medication

Irradiation
Chemical burn
Mechanical
  trauma

Malnutrition
Cystic fibrosis
Chronic pancreatitis
Chronic liver disease
Inflammatory bowel
  disease
Gastrointestinal
  surgery
Abetalipoproteinemia
Night blindness

Consider vitamin A
deficiency

Diagnostic tests:
  Serum vitamin A level
  Impression cytology
  Dark adaptation/
    electroretinography

Systemic Vitamin A
  Replacement
Topical Vitamin A Ointment
Treat Malnutrition

Dry mouth
Dry skin
Joint pain
Dyspareunia
Dysphagia
Constipation

Consider:
  Collagen vascular
    disease
  Lymphoma

Laboratory tests:
  CBC, ESR, SMA20,
  SPEP, rheumatoid
  factor, ANA, anti-
  Sjögren's (SS-A, Bro)

Consider lip/lacrimal
  gland biopsy
Referral to internist/
  rheumatologist

Systemic Anti-Inflammatory
  Agents in Extreme Cases
Monitor Bone Marrow,
  Renal Hepatic Function

Ⓒ Evaluate lid
structure and
function

Entropion, ectropion,
trichiasis, exposure

SURGICAL
REPAIR

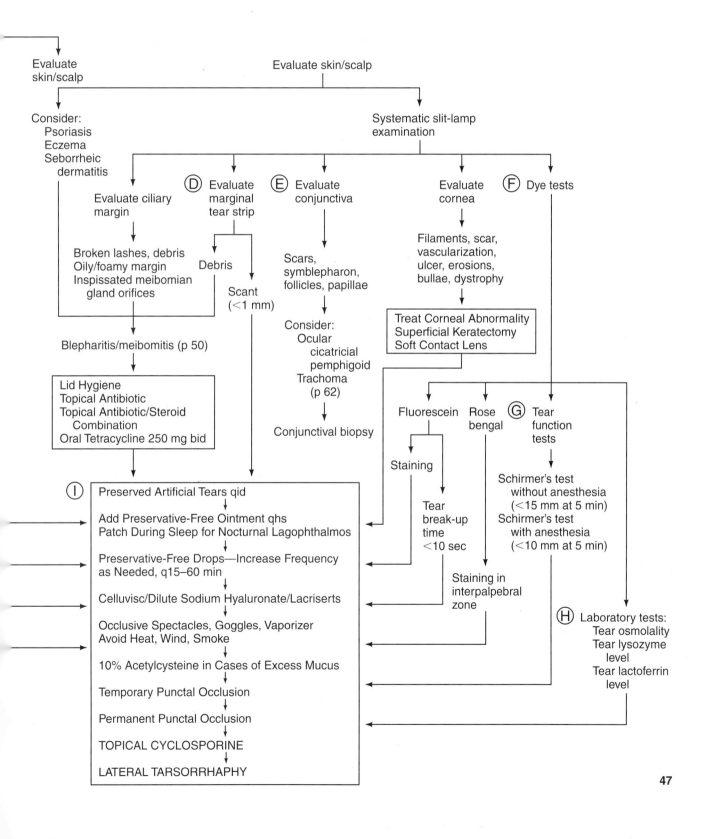

Evaluate
skin/scalp

Evaluate skin/scalp

Consider:
  Psoriasis
  Eczema
  Seborrheic
    dermatitis

Systematic slit-lamp
examination

Evaluate ciliary
margin

ⒹEvaluate
marginal
tear strip

ⒺEvaluate
conjunctiva

Evaluate
cornea

ⒻDye tests

Broken lashes, debris
Oily/foamy margin
Inspissated meibomian
  gland orifices

Debris

Scant
(<1 mm)

Scars,
symblepharon,
follicles, papillae

Filaments, scar,
vascularization,
ulcer, erosions,
bullae, dystrophy

Blepharitis/meibomitis (p 50)

Consider:
  Ocular
    cicatricial
    pemphigoid
  Trachoma
    (p 62)

Treat Corneal Abnormality
Superficial Keratectomy
Soft Contact Lens

Lid Hygiene
Topical Antibiotic
Topical Antibiotic/Steroid
  Combination
Oral Tetracycline 250 mg bid

Conjunctival biopsy

Fluorescein

Rose
bengal

ⒼTear
function
tests

Staining

Schirmer's test
  without anesthesia
  (<15 mm at 5 min)
Schirmer's test
  with anesthesia
  (<10 mm at 5 min)

ⒾPreserved Artificial Tears qid

Add Preservative-Free Ointment qhs
Patch During Sleep for Nocturnal Lagophthalmos

Preservative-Free Drops—Increase Frequency
as Needed, q15–60 min

Celluvisc/Dilute Sodium Hyaluronate/Lacriserts

Occlusive Spectacles, Goggles, Vaporizer
Avoid Heat, Wind, Smoke

10% Acetylcysteine in Cases of Excess Mucus

Temporary Punctal Occlusion

Permanent Punctal Occlusion

TOPICAL CYCLOSPORINE

LATERAL TARSORRHAPHY

Tear
break-up
time
<10 sec

Staining in
interpalpebral
zone

ⒽLaboratory tests:
  Tear osmolality
  Tear lysozyme
    level
  Tear lactoferrin
    level

EPIPHORA

Kenneth L. Piest, M.D.
Martha A. Walton, M.D.

A. Tearing may result from reflex lacrimation, which may be caused by ocular surface irritation. It can also result from other entities that stimulate the ophthalmic division of the fifth cranial nerve, as in iritis or glaucoma.

B. Congenital nasolacrimal duct obstruction is a common disorder, occurring in up to 30% of newborns.

C. The basal tear secretion (BTS) is assessed by anesthetizing the conjunctiva and ocular surface with a topical agent and then measuring tear production. If the BTS is low, the quantity of tears required to keep the cornea moist is insufficient. This condition stimulates the reflex arc of the fifth and seventh cranial nerves, producing excessive reflex secretion. The lacrimal drainage system cannot handle the sporadic increase in volume, and overflow tearing (pseudoepiphora) occurs. Topical ocular lubrication is required to prevent stimulation of the reflex arc.

D. Dye disappearance testing (DDT) is one of the most useful tests of lacrimal outflow. A moistened fluorescein strip or 2% solution is placed in the conjunctival fornices. Clearance of the dye over 5 minutes is observed. Retention of dye after this period is abnormal and suggests obstruction. Further testing is necessary to determine the condition responsible for the obstruction.

E. The primary dye test (Jones I), like the DDT, is a functional test investigating lacrimal outflow under normal physiologic conditions. However, it gives an abnormal result in approximately one third of normal patients and is often performed improperly. The test consists of attempting to recover fluorescein dye from the inferior meatus by passing a cotton-tipped wire probe beneath the inferior turbinate. A wire is used because of the close approximation of the turbinate to the wall of the nose. A cotton-tip applicator is too large to enter this space. Attempts at dye recovery are also often accompanied by anesthetizing and shrinking of the mucosa to provide comfort and better visualization. This procedure may mask the true pathologic condition in patients in whom hypertrophy and impaction of the turbinate are compressing the opening of the nasolacrimal duct.

F. In selected patients diagnostic testing may provide additional information. Scintigraphy can be used to evaluate the physiologic flow of tears and therefore is a functional test. Structural information can be provided by dacryocystography. Newer digital subtraction imaging can provide detailed images and is useful when a mass, diverticulum, or stenosis is suspected.

G. The secondary dye test (irrigation) is performed after an abnormal DDT and a primary dye test. It differentiates partial from complete obstructions and provides an estimate of the site of the block. Clear saline solution is used. If irrigation fails to transmit fluid into the nose, a total obstruction is present. If irrigation produces dye-containing fluid from the nose, dye was able to enter the lacrimal sac under physiologic conditions but could not pass down the duct.

H. A pump mechanism is responsible for the excretion of tears. A normal-functioning orbicularis muscle is a prerequisite. With eyelid closure, the heads of the pretarsal orbicularis compress the ampulla and shorten the canaliculi, while the preseptal fibers expand the sac. This action creates negative pressure and draws fluid into the sac from the ampulla and canaliculi. When the eye opens, the muscles relax. The resilience of the lacrimal sac fascia collapses the sac and forces tears from the sac into the duct. Disorders that affect this pumping mechanism, such as seventh cranial nerve palsy or lower lid laxity, can produce tearing.

References

Bueger DG, Schaefer AJ, Campbell CB, Flanagan JC. Acquired lacrimal disorders. In: Smith BC, Della Rocca RC, Nesi FA, Lisman RD, eds. Ophthalmic plastic and reconstructive surgery. St Louis: Mosby, 1988: 661.

Katowitz JA, Kropp TM. Congenital abnormalities of the lacrimal drainage system. In: Hornblass A, ed. Oculoplastic, orbital and reconstructive surgery. Vol 2. Baltimore: Williams & Wilkins, 1990: 1397.

Leone CR. The management of pediatric lacrimal problems. Ophthalmic Plast Reconstr Surg 1989; 1:34–39.

Patrinely JR, Anderson RL. A review of lacrimal drainage surgery. Ophthalmic Plast Reconstr Surg 1986; 2:97–102.

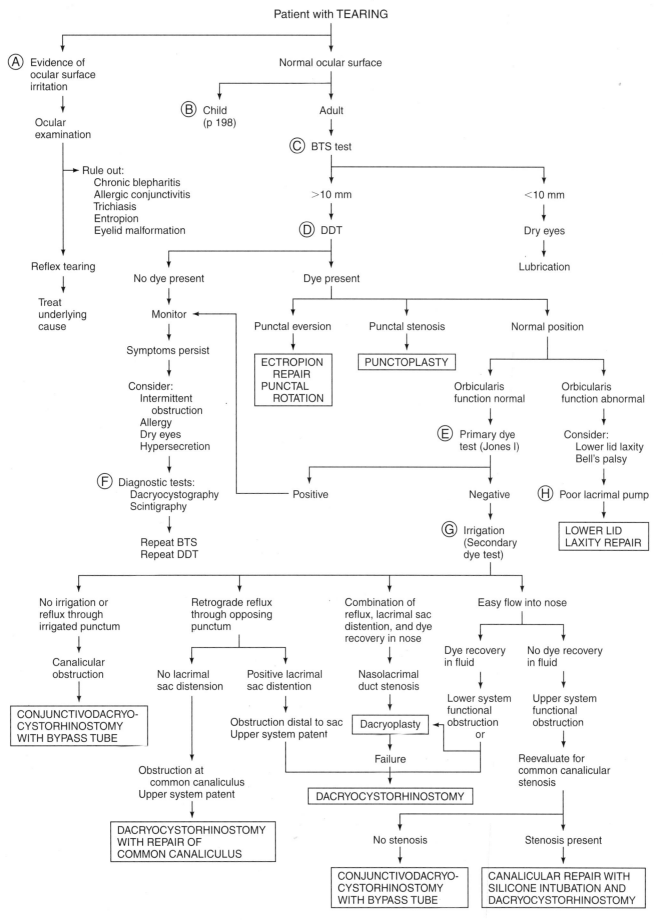

Patient with TEARING

(A) Evidence of ocular surface irritation

Ocular examination

Rule out:
Chronic blepharitis
Allergic conjunctivitis
Trichiasis
Entropion
Eyelid malformation

Reflex tearing

Treat underlying cause

Normal ocular surface

(B) Child (p 198)

Adult

(C) BTS test

>10 mm

(D) DDT

<10 mm

Dry eyes

Lubrication

No dye present

Monitor

Symptoms persist

Consider:
Intermittent obstruction
Allergy
Dry eyes
Hypersecretion

(F) Diagnostic tests:
Dacryocystography
Scintigraphy

Repeat BTS
Repeat DDT

Dye present

Punctal eversion

ECTROPION REPAIR PUNCTAL ROTATION

Punctal stenosis

PUNCTOPLASTY

Normal position

Orbicularis function normal

(E) Primary dye test (Jones I)

Positive

Negative

(G) Irrigation (Secondary dye test)

Orbicularis function abnormal

Consider:
Lower lid laxity
Bell's palsy

(H) Poor lacrimal pump

LOWER LID LAXITY REPAIR

No irrigation or reflux through irrigated punctum

Canalicular obstruction

CONJUNCTIVODACRYO-CYSTORHINOSTOMY WITH BYPASS TUBE

Retrograde reflux through opposing punctum

No lacrimal sac distension

Positive lacrimal sac distension

Obstruction distal to sac Upper system patent

Obstruction at common canaliculus Upper system patent

DACRYOCYSTORHINOSTOMY WITH REPAIR OF COMMON CANALICULUS

Combination of reflux, lacrimal sac distention, and dye recovery in nose

Nasolacrimal duct stenosis

Dacryoplasty

Failure

DACRYOCYSTORHINOSTOMY

No stenosis

CONJUNCTIVODACRYO-CYSTORHINOSTOMY WITH BYPASS TUBE

Easy flow into nose

Dye recovery in fluid

Lower system functional obstruction or

No dye recovery in fluid

Upper system functional obstruction

Reevaluate for common canalicular stenosis

Stenosis present

CANALICULAR REPAIR WITH SILICONE INTUBATION AND DACRYOCYSTORHINOSTOMY

BLEPHARITIS

Kristin Story Held, M.D.

Blepharitis is chronic inflammation of the eyelids secondary to a broad spectrum of infectious and noninfectious causes. Patients with acne rosacea, seborrheic dermatitis, atopic disease, and Down's syndrome have a greater than normal predisposition for blepharitis. Accurate diagnosis requires a complete patient history and thorough clinical examination. Once the appropriate diagnosis has been established, proper therapy can be implemented.

A. Patients often complain of burning, irritation, foreign body sensation, itching, and mattering of the eyes particularly upon awakening. The course is usually chronic, with varying degrees of waxing and waning. Associated dermatologic conditions may be present and helpful in establishing the diagnosis.

B. Staphylococcal blepharoconjunctivitis is by far the most common cause of infectious blepharitis and probably the most common chronic infection of the external eye. It occurs in a younger population (mean age, 42 years), and 80% of patients are female. The symptoms are generally shorter in duration, more severe, and maximally waxing and waning in nature. The classic clinical sign is the collarette. Other signs are poliosis, madarosis, misdirected lashes, erythema, ulcerated lid margins, and hordeolum. Of patients, 15% exhibit bulbar and tarsal conjunctival changes. Recent studies have shown that a large percentage of lid cultures from these patients are positive for *Staphylococcus aureus* and *S. epidermidis*. A keratitis may develop secondary to the toxic effects of the organism. Punctate epithelial erosions develop over the inferior third of the cornea. Marginal catarrhal infiltrates may occur secondary to the bacterial antigen and host-antibody interaction, most often at the 8- and 10- and 2- and 4-o'clock positions. Secondary infections of these lesions may lead to an infectious corneal ulcer. Finally, phlyctenulosis may develop as a result of cell-mediated immunity. In most cases the diagnosis is based on clinical evidence of infection, and cultures are not routinely done because most staphylococcal species are sensitive to bacitracin, erythromycin, and the aminoglycosides. Cultures with sensitivity testing of the lid margins may be useful in patients who have keratitis, marginal infiltrates, or phlyctenules or who have recalcitrant symptoms. The goal of treatment for staphylococcal blepharitis is to cure it. To achieve this goal, treatment must be implemented aggressively for a prolonged initial period before tapering of the regimen is begun. Of these patients, 50% have associated keratoconjunctivitis sicca, which must be treated concurrently.

C. Seborrheic blepharitis occurs in an older age group (mean age, 50 years). The course is more chronic with minimal waxing and waning of symptoms that last longer. The classic clinical sign is scurf, which is oily, greasy debris on the lid margin. The lids are less inflamed than with staphylococcal blepharitis or meibo-

mianitis. Most patients have associated seborrheic dermatitis and may benefit by dermatologic consultation. Associated keratitis may be present. Many have concurrent keratoconjunctivitis sicca. The goal of treatment is to control and prevent complications. Topical antibiotics are unnecessary.

D. Patients may exhibit signs of both seborrheic and staphylococcal blepharoconjunctivitis. Most have underlying seborrheic dermatitis, and 35% have associated keratoconjunctivitis sicca. The course is that of chronic seborrheic blepharitis intermittently exacerbated by the staphylococcal component. Clinical findings include both collarettes on the lashes and oily, greasy crusting of the anterior eyelid. Almost all of these patients have positive lid cultures for *S. epidermidis,* and more than 80% are positive for *S. aureus.* Treatment is aimed at control of clinical signs and symptoms and requires a long-term commitment to compliance by the patient and diligent attention by the ophthalmologist.

E. Patients with primary meibomitis exhibit more inflammation than those with seborrheic blepharitis. The anterior lamellae are minimally involved with scurf; however, the meibomian glands are diffusely inflamed and inspissated with retained, thick secretions that are not easily expressed. These patients are predisposed to chalazia. Of patients, 63% have associated rosacea. Many have punctate epithelial erosions and stain with rose bengal in the interpalpebral zone. Systemic tetracycline is indicated; it is believed to alter the nature of the oily secretions.

F. Patients who have seborrheic blepharitis associated with meibomitis have more exacerbations than those with pure seborrheic blepharitis. They may complain of severe burning in the morning. The meibomian glands are engorged with retained secretions, and the tear film is foamy, especially laterally.

G. Successful treatment requires accurate diagnosis based on thorough patient history and clinical examination. Pure staphylococcal blepharoconjunctivitis may be cured with aggressive long-term lid hygiene and topical antibiotics. The other types of blepharitis are difficult or impossible to eradicate. The goals of treatment are to improve the patient's symptoms and signs, stabilize the course with decreased exacerbations, prevent complications, and preserve vision. This requires a great deal of commitment by the patient and the treating physician. The foundation of treatment is consistent lid hygiene that (1) removes eyelid debris and (2) restores normal flow of the meibomian secretions. Topical antibiotics are used in all patients except those with purely seborrheic blepharitis. Oral tetracycline is used in all patients with primary meibomitis, particularly in association with rosacea, and in refractory

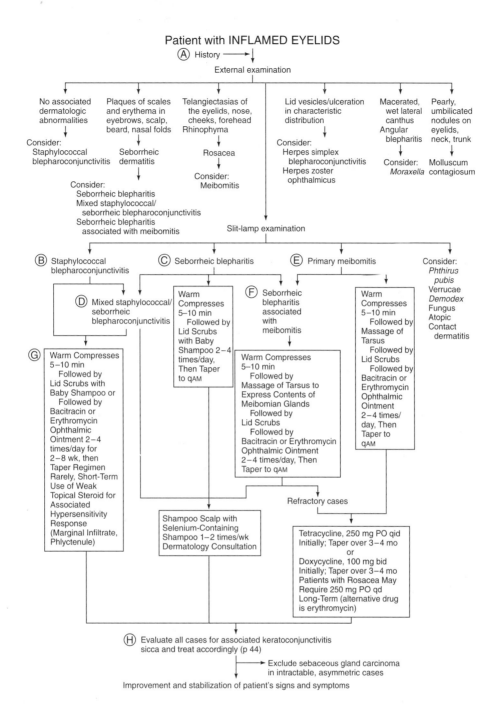

Patient with INFLAMED EYELIDS

(A) History → External examination

No associated dermatologic abnormalities
↓
Consider:
Staphylococcal blepharoconjunctivitis

Plaques of scales and erythema in eyebrows, scalp, beard, nasal folds
↓
Seborrheic dermatitis
↓
Consider:
Seborrheic blepharitis
Mixed staphylococcal/ seborrheic blepharoconjunctivitis
Seborrheic blepharitis associated with meibomitis

Telangiectasias of the eyelids, nose, cheeks, forehead Rhinophyma
↓
Rosacea
↓
Consider:
Meibomitis

Lid vesicles/ulceration in characteristic distribution
↓
Consider:
Herpes simplex blepharoconjunctivitis
Herpes zoster ophthalmicus

Macerated, wet lateral canthus Angular blepharitis
↓
Consider:
Moraxella

Pearly, umbilicated nodules on eyelids, neck, trunk
↓
Molluscum contagiosum

Slit-lamp examination

(B) Staphylococcal blepharoconjunctivitis

(C) Seborrheic blepharitis

(E) Primary meibomitis

Consider:
Phthirus pubis
Verrucae
Demodex
Fungus
Atopic
Contact dermatitis

(D) Mixed staphylococcal/ seborrheic blepharoconjunctivitis

(F) Seborrheic blepharitis associated with meibomitis

Warm Compresses 5–10 min
Followed by Lid Scrubs with Baby Shampoo 2–4 times/day, Then Taper to qAM

Warm Compresses 5–10 min
Followed by Massage of Tarsus
Followed by Lid Scrubs
Followed by Bacitracin or Erythromycin Ophthalmic Ointment 2–4 times/day, Then Taper to qAM

(G) Warm Compresses 5–10 min
Followed by Lid Scrubs with Baby Shampoo or
Followed by Bacitracin or Erythromycin Ophthalmic Ointment 2–4 times/day for 2–8 wk, then Taper Regimen Rarely, Short-Term Use of Weak Topical Steroid for Associated Hypersensitivity Response (Marginal Infiltrate, Phlyctenule)

Warm Compresses 5–10 min
Followed by Massage of Tarsus to Express Contents of Meibomian Glands
Followed by Lid Scrubs
Followed by Bacitracin or Erythromycin Ophthalmic Ointment 2–4 times/day, Then Taper to qAM

Shampoo Scalp with Selenium-Containing Shampoo 1–2 times/wk Dermatology Consultation

Refractory cases

Tetracycline, 250 mg PO qid Initially; Taper over 3–4 mo
or
Doxycycline, 100 mg bid Initially; Taper over 3–4 mo
Patients with Rosacea May Require 250 mg PO qd Long-Term (alternative drug is erythromycin)

(H) Evaluate all cases for associated keratoconjunctivitis sicca and treat accordingly (p 44)
→ Exclude sebaceous gland carcinoma in intractable, asymmetric cases

Improvement and stabilization of patient's signs and symptoms

cases of seborrheic blepharitis associated with meibomitis. Initially, aggressive treatment is required and then tapered. The morning is the most important time for lid hygiene because it targets organisms and debris that have accumulated overnight. Short courses of mild topical steroids may be used to treat staphylococcal hypersensitivity reactions. Furthermore, associated dermatologic conditions and underlying keratoconjunctivitis sicca must be managed.

H. Because 25%–60% of patients with chronic blepharitis have concurrent keratoconjunctivitis sicca, all patients with blepharitis must be evaluated for dry eye and treated accordingly.

References

Arffa RC, ed. Grayson's diseases of the cornea. 4th ed. St Louis: Mosby, 1997: 339.

Brown DD, McCulley JP. Staphylococcal and mixed staphylococcal/seborrheic blepharoconjunctivitis. In: Fraunfelder FT, Roy FH, eds. Current ocular therapy. 3rd ed. Philadelphia: WB Saunders, 1990: 525.

Halsted M, McCulley JP. Seborrheic blepharitis. In: Fraunfelder FT, Roy FH, eds. Current ocular therapy. 3rd ed. Philadelphia: WB Saunders, 1990: 522.

McCulley JP. Meibomitis. In: Kaufman HE, Barron BA, McDonald MB, Waitman SR, eds. The cornea. New York: Churchill Livingstone, 1988: 125.

NONPIGMENTED LESION OF THE EYELID

Marilyn C. Kincaid, M.D.
Andrew W. Lawton, M.D.

A.   Cystic dermoids contain skin appendages, such as hair shafts, differentiating them from epidermal inclusion cysts. They usually grow slowly and are located in the region of the lacrimal fossa, superotemporal to the globe. Occasionally, trauma results in cyst rupture, yielding an intense inflammatory response that mimics orbital cellulitis. When this diagnosis is suspected and excision contemplated, a CT scan is crucial to determine the extent of the lesion because they sometimes extend into the deep orbit.

B.   The pilomatrixoma, also called *calcifying epithelioma of Malherbe,* is a benign lesion of hair-shaft origin. It tends to necrose and calcify at its center and may mimic an epidermal inclusion cyst. Treatment is total excision.

C.   Sebaceous carcinoma is an aggressive tumor with high morbidity and mortality rates. It can mimic a chalazion and must be considered in the differential of recurrent chalazion, especially in the elderly. It can also mimic a unilateral blepharitis or conjunctivitis. The diagnosis should be suspected when the latter do not respond to topical medication. Tissue diagnosis and appropriate surgical intervention are mandatory under these circumstances.

D.   Capillary hemangiomas are hamartomas and are not malignant. They generally resolve spontaneously. However, depending on location, they may cause amblyopia either by corneal distortion with resultant astigmatism or by eyelid ptosis with pupillary occlusion. In such circumstances, intralesional corticosteroid injection may hasten resolution.

E.   Basal cell carcinomas grow slowly and almost never metastasize. Morbidity results from local extension. The most dangerous variant is morpheaform because the spread is subcutaneous, with accompanying fibrous proliferation that mimics scar tissue. Frozen section-controlled excision may be necessary to ensure complete removal.

F.   Molluscum contagiosum is a pox viral infection that historically has been seen most commonly in children. However, it is also associated with HIV infection and can be considered a sexually transmitted disease.

G.   Keratoacanthomas grow extremely rapidly and can attain a large size in weeks to months. They regress spontaneously but may erode surrounding tissues, including bone, with significant scarring and damage before doing so. Histologically, they may appear worrisome, but they are benign. However, for accurate histologic diagnosis, the entire lesion must be removed because otherwise they may be confused with a well-differentiated squamous cell carcinoma.

H.   Squamous cell carcinoma in this location is relatively slow growing and is unlikely to metastasize. The prognosis is excellent if recognized early and excised completely. Frozen section control of surgical margins to ensure complete excision of the tumor is strongly recommended.

References

Deans RM, Harris GJ, Kivlin JD. Surgical dissection of capillary hemangiomas. Arch Ophthalmol 1992; 110:1743–1747.

Depot MJ, Jakobiec FA, Dodick JM, Iwamoto T. Bilateral and extensive xanthelasma palpebrarum in a young man. Ophthalmology 1984; 91:522–527.

Doxanas MT, Iliff WJ, Iliff NT, Green WR. Squamous cell carcinoma of the eyelids. Ophthalmology 1987; 94:38–51.

Glatt HJ, Olson JJ, Putterman AM. Conventional frozen sections in periocular basal-cell carcinoma: A review of 236 cases. Ophthalmic Surg 1992; 23:6–9.

Kass LG, Hornblass A. Sebaceous carcinoma of the ocular adnexa. Surv Ophthalmol 1989; 33:477–490.

Lane CM, Ehrlich WW, Wright JE. Orbital dermoid cyst. Eye 1987; 1:504–511.

Robinson MR, Udell IJ, Garber PF, et al. Molluscum contagiosum of the eyelids in patients with acquired immune deficiency syndrome. Ophthalmology 1992; 99:1745–1747.

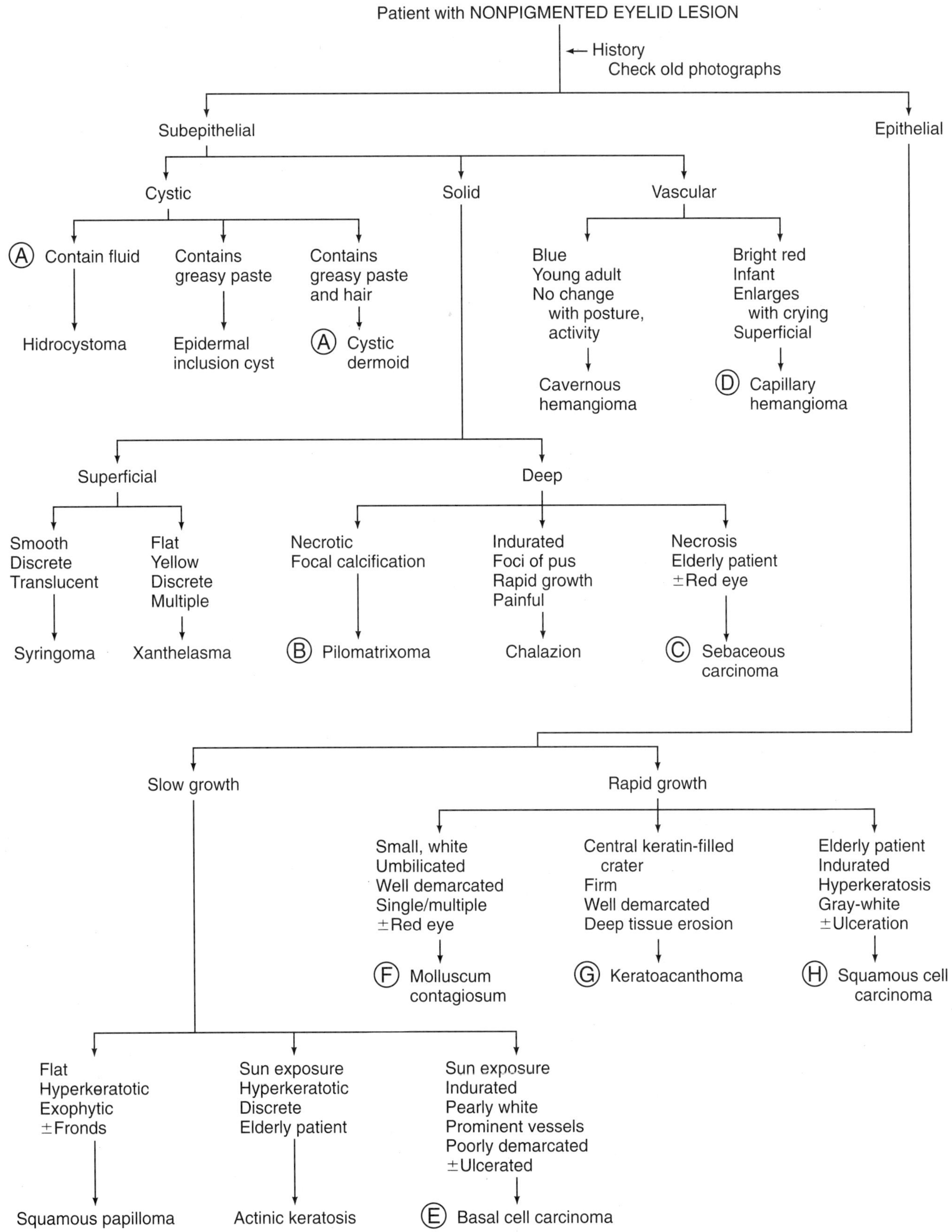

Patient with NONPIGMENTED EYELID LESION

← History
  Check old photographs

Subepithelial

Cystic

Ⓐ Contain fluid → Hidrocystoma

Contains greasy paste → Epidermal inclusion cyst

Contains greasy paste and hair → Ⓐ Cystic dermoid

Solid

Vascular

Blue
Young adult
No change with posture, activity
→ Cavernous hemangioma

Bright red
Infant
Enlarges with crying
Superficial
→ Ⓓ Capillary hemangioma

Superficial

Smooth
Discrete
Translucent
→ Syringoma

Flat
Yellow
Discrete
Multiple
→ Xanthelasma

Deep

Necrotic
Focal calcification
→ Ⓑ Pilomatrixoma

Indurated
Foci of pus
Rapid growth
Painful
→ Chalazion

Necrosis
Elderly patient
±Red eye
→ Ⓒ Sebaceous carcinoma

Epithelial

Slow growth

Rapid growth

Small, white
Umbilicated
Well demarcated
Single/multiple
±Red eye
→ Ⓕ Molluscum contagiosum

Central keratin-filled crater
Firm
Well demarcated
Deep tissue erosion
→ Ⓖ Keratoacanthoma

Elderly patient
Indurated
Hyperkeratosis
Gray-white
±Ulceration
→ Ⓗ Squamous cell carcinoma

Flat
Hyperkeratotic
Exophytic
±Fronds
→ Squamous papilloma

Sun exposure
Hyperkeratotic
Discrete
Elderly patient
→ Actinic keratosis

Sun exposure
Indurated
Pearly white
Prominent vessels
Poorly demarcated
±Ulcerated
→ Ⓔ Basal cell carcinoma

PIGMENTED LESION OF THE EYELID

Marilyn C. Kincaid, M.D.
Andrew W. Lawton, M.D.

A. Nevus of Ota is characterized by a large blue nevus of the eyelid (see section B), scleral pigmentation, and increased numbers of uveal melanocytes. Affected patients are at higher risk for developing uveal and intracranial melanoma and must be carefully evaluated. Cranial CT scanning allows earlier diagnosis and a better prognosis.

B. A blue nevus results from proliferation of darkly pigmented, spindle-shaped melanocytic cells deep within the dermis. Diffraction of light waves by the skin fibroblasts results in a blue rather than a brown appearance. Blue nevi, like other melanocytic nevi, are benign and can be excised for cosmetic reasons.

C. Melanocytic nevi only rarely undergo malignant transformation. The chief reason for excision is cosmetic.

D. Pigmented basal cell carcinomas occur because benign melanocytes become passively entrapped in the proliferating mass of epithelial cells. Pigmentation in a basal cell carcinoma does not alter prognosis but may mislead the clinician into an incorrect diagnosis.

E. Malignant melanomas of the eyelid skin are very rare. They can arise from a pre-existing nevus, from lentigo maligna (melanoma in situ), or apparently de novo. A new pigmented nodule demands prompt evaluation because the depth of invasion is strongly associated with the prognosis. The entire lesion is excised with frozen section control of the margins.

F. An older term for lentigo maligna is *Hutchinson's freckle.* Lentigo maligna is really melanoma in situ, a flat lesion composed of atypical melanocytes. Generally, they grow slowly, but development of nodules (the vertical growth phase) indicates invasive melanoma and demands prompt evaluation and excision.

References

Garner A, Koornneef L, Levene A, Collin JRO. Malignant melanoma of the eyelid skin: Histopathology and behaviour. Br J Ophthalmol 1985; 69:180–186.

Grossniklaus HE, McLean IW. Cutaneous melanoma of the eyelid: Clinicopathologic features. Ophthalmology 1991; 98:1867–1873.

Hartmann LC, Oliver CF, Winkelman RK, et al. Blue nevus and nevus of Ota associated with dural melanoma. Cancer 1989; 64:182–186.

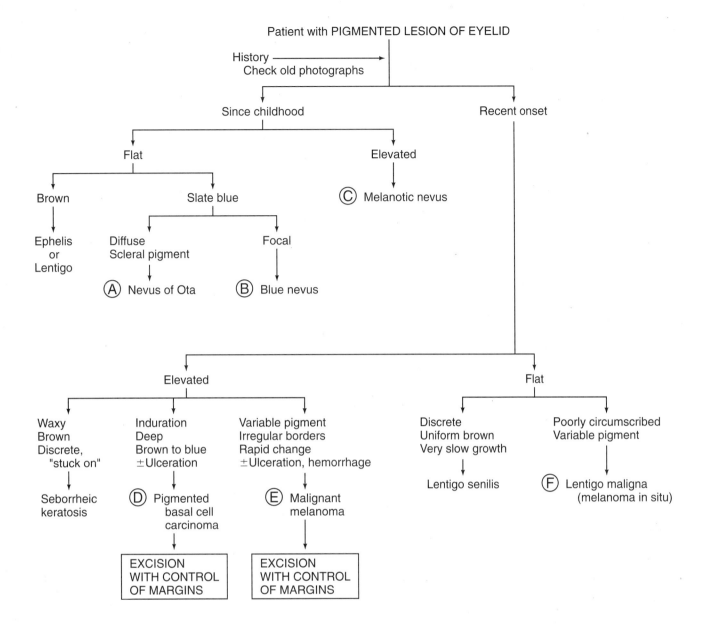

Patient with PIGMENTED LESION OF EYELID

History
Check old photographs

Since childhood

Recent onset

Flat

Elevated

Brown

Slate blue

Ⓒ Melanotic nevus

Ephelis
or
Lentigo

Diffuse
Scleral pigment

Focal

Ⓐ Nevus of Ota

Ⓑ Blue nevus

Elevated

Flat

Waxy
Brown
Discrete,
"stuck on"

Induration
Deep
Brown to blue
±Ulceration

Variable pigment
Irregular borders
Rapid change
±Ulceration, hemorrhage

Discrete
Uniform brown
Very slow growth

Poorly circumscribed
Variable pigment

Seborrheic
keratosis

Ⓓ Pigmented
basal cell
carcinoma

Ⓔ Malignant
melanoma

Lentigo senilis

Ⓕ Lentigo maligna
(melanoma in situ)

EXCISION
WITH CONTROL
OF MARGINS

EXCISION
WITH CONTROL
OF MARGINS

LESION OF THE CONJUNCTIVA

Marilyn C. Kincaid, M.D.
Andrew W. Lawton, M.D.

Conjunctival lesions are extremely common. A complete history and physical examination are mandatory. Often, excisional biopsy will also help establish the diagnosis.

A. Interpalpebral melanin deposition in the bulbar conjunctiva is extremely common in darker-skinned individuals. The combination of presence since childhood without subsequent change implies benign racial pigmentation.

B. Conjunctival nevi typically occur in the interpalpebral bulbar conjunctiva. They grow slowly but may become more prominent during puberty or young adulthood. Histologically, epithelial cysts are virtually always present, although they may be subtle clinically. Alternatively, they may be the predominant feature. Rarely, conjunctival nevi become malignant, necessitating regular follow-up examinations. Excision may be indicated for cosmesis.

C. Solid dermoids contain hair shafts. Other types of epibulbar choristomas generally do not have hair but may have a variety of ectodermal or mesodermal elements. Excision must be approached with care because these lesions may extend into the interior of the eye. Also, epibulbar dermoids (usually bilateral) are features of Goldenhar's syndrome, which may include renal and vertebral malformations, as well as preauricular skin tags.

D. Benign intraepithelial dyskeratosis is an uncommon autosomal-dominant condition originally traced to a kindred in North Carolina, although more recent patients do not belong to this group. Despite a possibly worrisome clinical appearance, this lesion is not malignant.

E. Bitot spots are areas of keratinization associated with vitamin A deficiency. In developed countries, vitamin A deficiency is rare except in individuals who have undergone extensive small bowel resection.

F. Squamous papillomas result from proliferation of conjunctival epithelium with associated fibrovascular stroma. They are usually found at the lid margin, caruncle, or limbus. Their occurrence in young individuals distinguishes them from the lesions of conjunctival intraepithelial neoplasia. They are probably caused by a virus.

G. Conjunctival intraepithelial neoplasia ranges from mild dysplasia to frank carcinoma in situ. Even lesions that are histologically more benign can lead to invasive squamous cell carcinoma if not attended to. These lesions are best completely excised with freezing of the surgical base, ideally at the first surgical procedure.

Margins should be examined by frozen section methods to ensure completeness of the excision. Recurrences are nearly always histologically more malignant.

H. The conjunctival lesions of sarcoidosis are the ideal site for histologic confirmation of the diagnosis because there is virtually no morbidity of a biopsy at this site. However, the yield of blind biopsies is low.

I. Localized subconjunctival amyloid deposition is rare but distinctive. The deposits can be removed surgically and generally do not recur.

J. The "salmon patch" is virtually pathognomonic for conjunctival lymphoma. Evaluate the patient for more widespread local or systemic disease. Consider a biopsy of the salmon patch, with fresh tissue submitted for flow cytometric analysis. The area may require irradiation to induce regression.

K. Recently acquired melanosis in an older person should prompt mapping biopsies because atypical changes in primary acquired melanosis cannot be diagnosed clinically. If excisional surgery is indicated, treat the excision base with cryotherapy to help prevent recurrence.

L. Conjunctival malignant melanoma may arise from acquired melanosis, from a pre-existing nevus, or de novo. Once the melanoma has invaded, there is a significant risk of metastasis and mortality. Complete excision with cryotherapy and a complete metastatic work-up are indicated.

References

Elsas FJ, Green WR. Epibulbar tumors in childhood. Am J Ophthalmol 1975; 79:1001–1007.

Folberg R, Jakobiec FA, Bernardino VB, Iwamoto T. Benign conjunctival melanocytic lesions: Clinicopathologic features. Ophthalmology 1989; 96:436–461.

Grossniklaus HE, Green WR, Luckenbach M, Chan CC. Conjunctival lesions in adults: A clinical and histopathologic review. Cornea 1987; 2:78–116.

Kiratli H, Shields CL, Shields JA, DePotter P. Metastatic tumors to the conjunctiva: Report of 10 cases. Br J Ophthalmol 1996; 80:5–8.

Lee GA, Hirst LW. Ocular surface squamous neoplasia. Surv Ophthalmol 1995; 39:429–450.

Mansour AM, Barber JC, Reinecke RD, Wang FM. Ocular choristomas. Surv Ophthalmol 1989; 33:339–358.

McDonnell, Carpenter JE, Jacobs P, et al. Conjunctival melanocytic lesions in children. Ophthalmology 1989; 96:986–993.

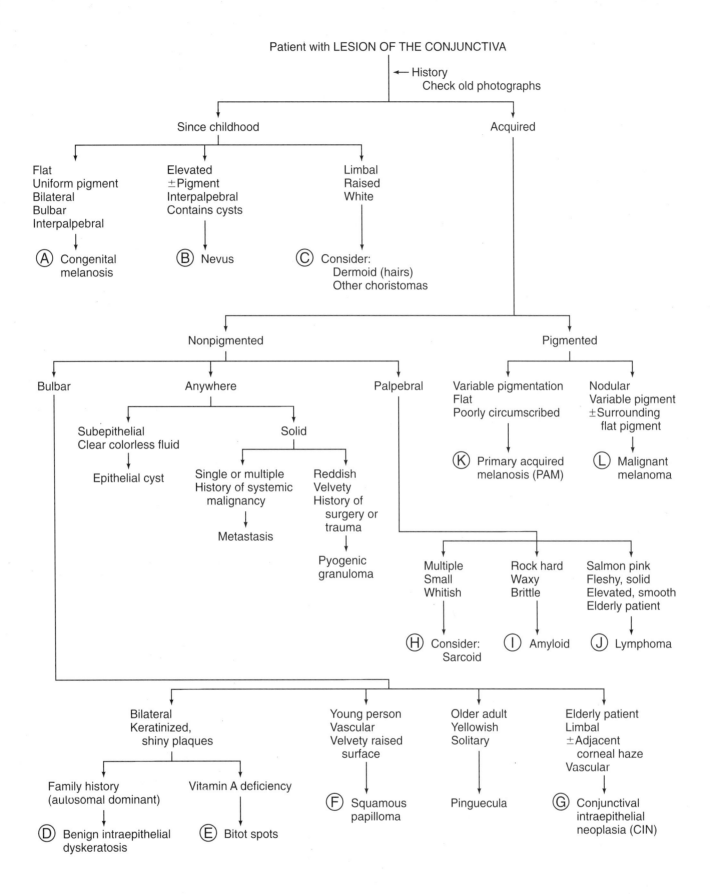

Patient with LESION OF THE CONJUNCTIVA

← History
Check old photographs

Since childhood

Flat
Uniform pigment
Bilateral
Bulbar
Interpalpebral

Ⓐ Congenital
melanosis

Elevated
±Pigment
Interpalpebral
Contains cysts

Ⓑ Nevus

Limbal
Raised
White

Ⓒ Consider:
Dermoid (hairs)
Other choristomas

Acquired

Nonpigmented

Bulbar

Anywhere

Subepithelial
Clear colorless fluid

Epithelial cyst

Solid

Single or multiple
History of systemic
malignancy

Metastasis

Reddish
Velvety
History of
surgery or
trauma

Pyogenic
granuloma

Palpebral

Multiple
Small
Whitish

Ⓗ Consider:
Sarcoid

Rock hard
Waxy
Brittle

Ⓘ Amyloid

Salmon pink
Fleshy, solid
Elevated, smooth
Elderly patient

Ⓙ Lymphoma

Pigmented

Variable pigmentation
Flat
Poorly circumscribed

Ⓚ Primary acquired
melanosis (PAM)

Nodular
Variable pigment
±Surrounding
flat pigment

Ⓛ Malignant
melanoma

Bilateral
Keratinized,
shiny plaques

Family history
(autosomal dominant)

Ⓓ Benign intraepithelial
dyskeratosis

Vitamin A deficiency

Ⓔ Bitot spots

Young person
Vascular
Velvety raised
surface

Ⓕ Squamous
papilloma

Older adult
Yellowish
Solitary

Pinguecula

Elderly patient
Limbal
±Adjacent
corneal haze
Vascular

Ⓖ Conjunctival
intraepithelial
neoplasia (CIN)

ACUTE CONJUNCTIVITIS

Kristin Story Held, M.D.

Conjunctivitis implies an inflammatory process of the conjunctival ocular surface. Certain characteristic clinical features may allow determination of an accurate clinical diagnosis (type of exudate, conjunctival response, preauricular adenopathy, and associated symptoms or signs).

A. Acute conjunctivitis is present <4 weeks, is abrupt in onset, and is usually unilateral at first with involvement of the second eye occurring within 1 week. History should include the patient's age, allergies, medications, exposure to irritants, and ocular, genitourinary, and respiratory symptoms. A history of contagion is common. Patients often complain of red eye with discharge, eyelids sticking on awakening, and burning or foreign body sensation. Vision is near normal, as are pupillary response, intraocular pressure, and funduscopic examination.

B. Inflammation of the conjunctiva can produce only a few clinical signs. A papillary response is nonspecific, resulting from any type of inflammation. Papillae occur in the tarsal conjunctiva and contain a central vessel that branches on the surface in a spokelike pattern readily evident on biomicroscopic examination. Numerous small papillae give the conjunctiva a red velvety appearance characteristic of bacterial conjunctivitis.

C. Hyperacute purulent conjunctivitis suggests infection with *Neisseria gonorrhoeae,* a highly virulent bacterium that can penetrate an intact corneal epithelium. There is rapid progression of a highly purulent conjunctivitis with lid edema, conjunctival hyperemia, and limbal chemosis to corneal perforation and blindness. This is the only bacterial conjunctivitis that commonly produces preauricular adenopathy. *Neisseria meningitidis* is less common but can produce septicemia and meningitis. Prompt laboratory evaluation and institution of specific treatment are mandatory. Smears for Gram and Giemsa stains should be taken from conjunctival scrapings rather than the exudate. Gram stain shows gram-negative intracellular diplococci in an overwhelming acute inflammatory response (polymorphonuclear lymphocytes [PMLs]). Cultures are obtained on blood and chocolate agar (37° C, 10% CO_2). Carbohydrate fermentation studies should be obtained to differentiate *N. gonorrhoeae* from *N. meningitidis.* The patient with suspected gonococcal conjunctivitis is admitted for systemic parenteral full-dose antibiotics according to current recommendations of the Centers for Disease Control and Prevention. IV aqueous penicillin C, 10 million U/day for 5 days, is recommended for penicillin-sensitive gonorrhea. Ceftriaxone, 1 g IM daily for 5 days, is desirable for penicillinase-producing strains and ease of administration. Tetracycline or erythromycin, 500 mg PO four times per day,

is given for at least 1 week because of the high rate of associated chlamydial infections. Topical bacitracin may be administered but is of secondary importance. The copious discharge should resolve within the first 24–48 hours, and the lid edema and hyperemia clear within 7–14 days.

D. Bacterial conjunctivitis is the most common type of infectious conjunctivitis. Historically, clinical diagnosis is made on the basis of a specific constellation of signs and symptoms; that is, the presence of a mucopurulent discharge, the absence of conjunctival follicles, and the absence of preauricular adenopathy. In adults the most common organisms isolated are *Streptococcus pneumoniae, Staphylococcus aureus,* and *Staphylococcus epidermidis.* In children the chief organisms are *Haemophilus influenzae, S. pneumoniae,* and *S. aureus. S. pneumoniae* is classically seen in cooler, temperate climates, whereas *H. aegyptius* is seen in warmer, southern climates. Bacterial conjunctivitis predominates over viral in the winter and spring. Most cases of bacterial conjunctivitis are self-limited, but appropriate antibiotics can shorten the course from 10–14 days to 1–3 days. Exceptions are *Moraxella lacunata* and *S. aureus,* which may result in chronic follicular conjunctivitis and chronic blepharoconjunctivitis, respectively. Initial treatment consists of broad-spectrum topical antibiotic solution or ointment (e.g., sulfacetamide drops or ointment four times daily, bacitracin ointment four times daily, or erythromycin ointment four times daily, for 5–10 days). Therapy is adjusted according to culture and sensitivity in refractory cases.

E. Because bacterial conjunctivitis is sufficiently identifiable on clinical grounds, self-limited and benign in nature, and highly responsive to empiric treatment, extensive laboratory evaluation is usually not needed. If the diagnosis is unclear or if the conjunctivitis is refractory to initial empiric treatment, perform a laboratory evaluation. Discontinue antibiotic treatment for 24 hours before obtaining specimens. Investigate all conjunctivitis in children. Obtain conjunctival scrapings for Gram and Giemsa stains. PMLs may be seen with Giemsa stain. Bacteria may be seen with Gram stain with a high level of specificity. Routine culture and sensitivity are obtained on blood and chocolate agar. Gram stain characteristics may allow presumptive diagnosis of the pathogen until culture and sensitivity results are available to guide selection of the specific topical antibiotics. Numerous preparations are available in the United States. Sulfacetamide covers *Staphylococcus, Pneumococcus, Haemophilus,* and *Moraxella* and is inexpensive and relatively nontoxic. Agents containing neomycin are broad spectrum, but there is a high incidence of sensitivity to neomycin.

Chloramphenicol is broad spectrum and especially useful for *Haemophilus* and *Moraxella,* but a small risk of aplastic anemia exists, although no adverse systemic effects have been seen with short-term use. Aminoglycosides are broad spectrum but are associated with a significant incidence of local hypersensitivity and toxicity. Furthermore, they are unreliable for *Pneumococcus* and other *Streptococcus* species and cause emergence of resistant strains. Fluoroquinolones are broad spectrum and highly effective but are more expensive. Topical therapy is preferred because it circumvents the toxic systemic side effects of many agents and allows the use of highly effective bactericidal agents such as neomycin and bacitracin. Exceptions are *Neisseria, Chlamydia,* and *Haemophilus influenzae* type B in children (risk of septicemia, meningitis, orbital cellulitis, and endogenous endophthalmitis), which require systemic treatment.

F. Giant papillae suggest a narrower differential diagnosis. They have a cobblestone appearance and are >1 mm. They are more common in allergic and chronic conjunctivitis.

G. A pseudomembrane or membrane forms in certain inflammatory conditions as proteinaceous fluid and fibrin coagulate on the conjunctival surface. Pseudomembranes are easily removed without bleeding. Membranes are more firmly adherent and bleed when stripped from the conjunctival surface.

H. The follicle is a focal lymphoid hyperplasia, which appears as a gray or white round structure with small vessels arising at its border and encircling it. A follicular response is a more specific clinical sign. Follicles are seen in most cases of viral conjunctivitis and all cases of chlamydial conjunctivitis except neonatal. Only trachoma produces a more severe follicular response in the upper tarsal conjunctiva than in the inferior fornix.

I. The clinical complex of a watery discharge, conjunctival follicles, and preauricular adenopathy suggests viral or chlamydial disease. Viral conjunctivitis occurs in all age groups. Epidemics are common. Adenoviruses are responsible for the most frequent epidemics in the United States. Viral conjunctivitis predominates over bacterial in the summer. Because viral isolation techniques are expensive and of low yield, they are not routinely used. A morphologic diagnosis may be possible if the patient has associated corneal changes or systemic symptoms. However, if performed early in appropriately selected patients, viral isolation techniques may be helpful. The laboratory should be informed of a presumed diagnosis so that the appropriate cell line in which to inoculate the specimen may be selected. Cultures may also be taken from the pharynx and nares. Giemsa-stained conjunctival smears show predominantly lymphocytes or may show multinucleated giant cells. A Pap smear may show intranuclear inclusions. Immunofluorescent antibody techniques are available for diagnosing herpes simplex, herpes zoster, adenovirus and *Chlamydia.*

J. Characteristic periorbital vesicles or pustules associated with a follicular, sometimes membranous, conjunctivitis and a palpable preauricular node are seen in primary herpes simplex blepharoconjunctivitis, which most often affects young children. The conjunctivitis caused by herpes simplex is self-limited but may be followed by the classic dendritic keratitis; therefore topical antiviral agents for both the skin and eye are advocated. Trifluridine 1% solution or vidarabine 3% ointment are given five times daily for 7–10 days until the conjunctivitis has resolved. Topical acyclovir ointment or topical antibiotic ointment may be applied to the skin lesions in conjunction with warm soaks three times a day. Cool compresses may provide symptomatic relief. Examine the patient every 2–3 days for the development of keratitis. Use oral acyclovir in primary cases of herpetic disease with eyelid involvement.

K. Pharyngoconjunctival fever (PCF) is typically caused by adenovirus with serotypes 3 and 7. The clinical complex of pharyngitis, fever, and follicular conjunctivitis help identify this diagnosis. Epidemics are often associated with public swimming pools in the summer.

L. Epidemic keratoconjunctivitis (EKC) is caused by adenovirus with serotypes 8 and 19. The clinical syndrome consists of preauricular lymphadenopathy, follicular conjunctivitis, pharyngitis, and characteristic subepithelial infiltrates that develop 5–12 days after the initial symptoms.

M. Viral conjunctivitis is usually self-limited and has a low morbidity rate, requiring no treatment. Antiviral agents are ineffective. Cool compresses provide symptomatic relief, as do artificial tears. Vasoconstricting antihistamine drops (naphazoline, pheniramine) may be given for itching. Inform the patient that the condition might worsen before it improves, and advise him or her to perform meticulous handwashing and to avoid direct contact with others. Health care personnel should refrain from direct patient contact for 14 days after the onset of symptoms.

References

Arffa RC. Grayson's diseases of the cornea. St Louis: Mosby, 1997: 107.

Dawson CR, Sheppard JD. Follicular conjunctivitis. In: Duane TD, ed. Clinical ophthalmology. Vol 4. Philadelphia: Harper & Row, 1990.

Fitch CP, Rapoza PA, Owens S, et al. Epidemiology and diagnosis of acute conjunctivitis at an inner-city hospital. Ophthalmology 1989; 96:1215–1220.

Friedlaender MH. A review of the causes and treatment of bacterial and allergic conjunctivitis. Clin Ther 1995; 17:800.

Mannis MJ. Bacterial conjunctivitis. In: Duane TD, ed. Clinical ophthalmology. Vol 4. Philadelphia: Harper & Row, 1990.

McDonnell PJ, Green WR. Conjunctivitis. In: Mandell GL, Douglas RG Jr, Bennett JE, eds. Principles and practice of infectious diseases. 3rd ed. Vol 1. New York: Churchill Livingstone, 1990: 975.

Patient with ACUTE CONJUNCTIVITIS

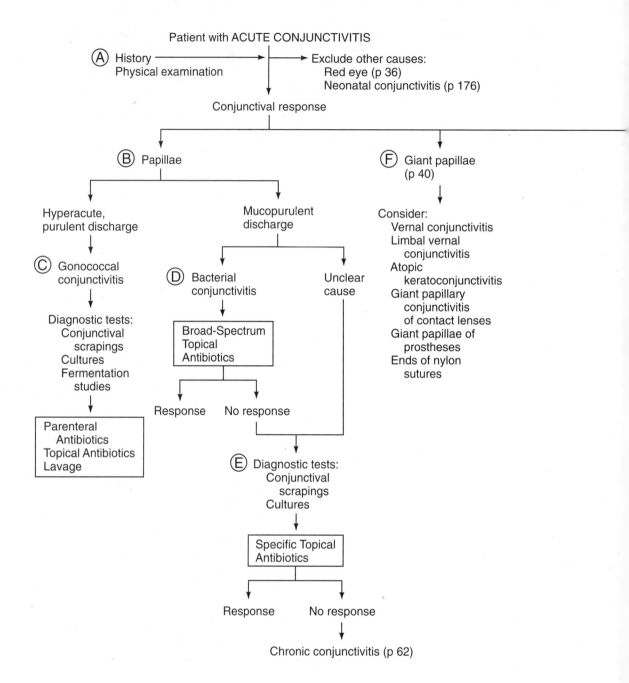

(A) History ──────────────► Exclude other causes:
    Physical examination   Red eye (p 36)
                                      Neonatal conjunctivitis (p 176)

Conjunctival response

(B) Papillae

Hyperacute,   Mucopurulent
purulent discharge   discharge

(C) Gonococcal   (D) Bacterial   Unclear
    conjunctivitis   conjunctivitis   cause

Diagnostic tests: Broad-Spectrum
  Conjunctival   Topical
    scrapings   Antibiotics
  Cultures
  Fermentation
    studies   Response   No response

Parenteral
  Antibiotics
Topical Antibiotics
Lavage

(E) Diagnostic tests:
      Conjunctival
        scrapings
      Cultures

    Specific Topical
    Antibiotics

  Response   No response

  Chronic conjunctivitis (p 62)

(F) Giant papillae
    (p 40)

Consider:
  Vernal conjunctivitis
  Limbal vernal
    conjunctivitis
  Atopic
    keratoconjunctivitis
  Giant papillary
    conjunctivitis
    of contact lenses
  Giant papillae of
    prostheses
  Ends of nylon
    sutures

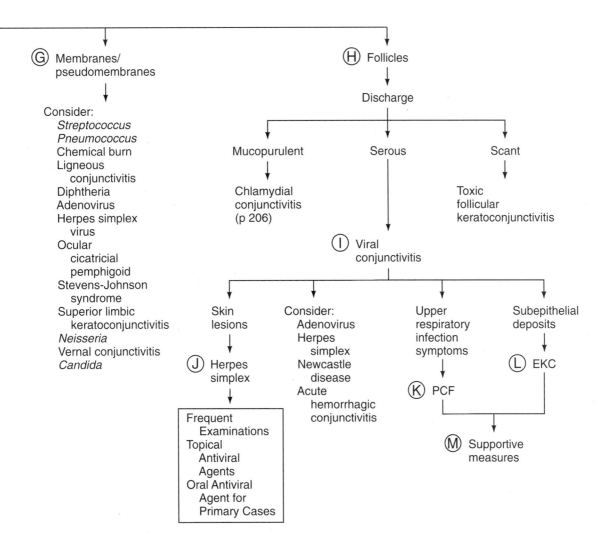

G Membranes/
pseudomembranes

Consider:
   Streptococcus
   Pneumococcus
   Chemical burn
   Ligneous
     conjunctivitis
   Diphtheria
   Adenovirus
   Herpes simplex
     virus
   Ocular
     cicatricial
     pemphigoid
   Stevens-Johnson
     syndrome
   Superior limbic
     keratoconjunctivitis
   Neisseria
   Vernal conjunctivitis
   Candida

H Follicles

Discharge

Mucopurulent | Serous | Scant

Chlamydial
conjunctivitis
(p 206)

Toxic
follicular
keratoconjunctivitis

I Viral
conjunctivitis

Skin
lesions

Consider:
   Adenovirus
   Herpes
     simplex
   Newcastle
     disease
   Acute
     hemorrhagic
     conjunctivitis

Upper
respiratory
infection
symptoms

Subepithelial
deposits

J Herpes
simplex

L EKC

K PCF

Frequent
   Examinations
Topical
   Antiviral
   Agents
Oral Antiviral
   Agent for
   Primary Cases

M Supportive
measures

CHRONIC CONJUNCTIVITIS

Kristin Story Held, M.D.

Chronic conjunctivitis is inflammation of the conjunctiva that persists >2–4 weeks. There are many causes of chronic conjunctivitis, and effective treatment is available to alleviate the signs and symptoms of most types. Accurate identification of the specific cause of chronic conjunctivitis is the key to successful management. The symptoms are variable, and clinical signs may seem equally nonspecific. A systematic approach to the investigation of chronic conjunctivitis, including detailed history, thorough examination, and specific diagnostic tests, affords the most accurate diagnosis and treatment.

A. A detailed patient history provides important clues in the diagnosis of chronic conjunctivitis. Explore any history of exposure. Chronic adenoviral conjunctivitis is a clinical diagnosis, and laboratory tests are often of little help. Likewise, a history of asthma, allergy, atopy, or exposure to a specific allergen suggests one type of allergic blepharoconjunctivitis; itching is the predominant complaint in these patients. Associated systemic symptoms may suggest a specific diagnosis such as the fever and malaise associated with Parinaud's oculoglandular conjunctivitis or the genitourinary symptoms associated with chlamydial disease. Finally, inquire about all topical preparations used, including cosmetics, contact lens solutions, and contact lenses.

B. A thorough systemic examination is essential and includes external inspection and examination of associated lymphadenopathy, dermatologic conditions, and local adnexal eye disease, including examination for lagophthalmos and poor Bell's phenomenon. Slit-lamp examination should evaluate the characteristics of the conjunctival reaction, discharge, presence of foreign bodies or irritants, adequacy of tearing, and presence of keratopathy.

C. Parinaud's oculoglandular conjunctivitis is a syndrome characterized by a unilateral granulomatous lesion of the conjunctiva surrounded by follicles and large visible preauricular or submandibular lymph nodes on the same side. Fever, malaise, and rash may be present. Several microorganisms may produce this syndrome, most commonly the bacillus of cat-scratch fever. More than two thirds of these patients have been scratched by a cat 1–2 weeks before the onset of symptoms. Other common causes are tularemia, sporotrichosis, tuberculosis, and other mycobacteria; syphilis; coccidioidomycosis; and less commonly, leukemia, lymphoma, mumps, mononucleosis, fungi, and sarcoidosis. Perform a diagnostic laboratory evaluation when the cause is unclear because treatment is directed at the specific causative agent.

D. *Moraxella lacunata,* large square gram-negative diplobacillus, produces a chronic angular blepharoconjunctivitis characterized by conjunctival injection and maceration of the inner and outer canthal angles. It can produce a chronic follicular conjunctivitis and keratitis. Culture and cytologic examination help establish this diagnosis. *M. lacunata* is readily cultured on blood and chocolate agar. *Moraxella* responds well to topical sulfacetamide, tetracycline, or erythromycin. Culture and sensitivity help guide treatment.

E. Molluscum contagiosum, a skin disease caused by a poxvirus, is characterized by multiple dome-shaped umbilicated nodules on the eyelid or lid margin. The virus causes a toxic reaction, which results in a chronic follicular conjunctivitis and keratitis that can progress to a trachoma-like picture. Recognition of the typical molluscum lesions, which may be inconspicuous or hidden by the lashes, is crucial. Treatment involves simple excision, incision and curettage, cryotherapy, or electrocautery of the lesions.

F. *Chlamydia* is an extremely common cause of chronic eye infection, specifically trachoma, adult inclusion conjunctivitis, and neonatal inclusion conjunctivitis. Trachoma is the most common cause of preventable blindness or decreased vision in the world, affecting about 500 million people. It is a chronic follicular conjunctivitis that results in conjunctival and corneal scarring. The cicatricial phase of the disease causes conjunctival and lid deformation that ultimately leads to the blinding complications of corneal ulceration and opacification. Trachoma occurs primarily in Third World countries in association with poverty and poor sanitation. The presence of two of the following signs suggests the diagnosis of trachoma: (1) lymphoid follicles on the upper tarsal conjunctiva, (2) typical conjunctival scarring, (3) vascular pannus, and (4) limbal follicles or their sequela, Herbert's pits. Cytologic examination of Giemsa-stained conjunctival smears to look for chlamydial inclusions is helpful. Direct fluorescent monoclonal antibody staining of conjunctival smears and McCoy cell culture for *C. trachomatis* are available as well.

G. Because many causes exist for chronic conjunctivitis, laboratory evaluation is required for diagnosis. Obtain conjunctival smears for cytologic evaluation with Gram and Giemsa stains. This is rapid and cost-effective. Gram stain reveals bacterial pathogens, and Giemsa stain reveals cellular morphology. Bacterial infections are characterized by polymorphonuclear cells. Viral infections are characterized by lymphocytes. A mixed response is seen in chlamydial infection. Intraepithelial cytoplasmic inclusions are diagnostic of chlamydial infections; however, inclusions can be seen more readily in acute than in chronic chlamydial infection. Eosinophils suggest allergic eye disease. Cytologic examination may also reveal dysplasia or keratinization of the ocular surface. Bacterial culture is useful, particularly in partially treated or resistant cases. Cultures are taken after the patient has stopped taking antibiotics for 24–72 hours. Sensitivity results are particularly useful in guiding therapy. Blood and chocolate agar should be used. The rate of isolation in the chronic phase of an infection is often lower than during the acute phase, especially for viruses (e.g., adenovirus). Viral cultures are not particularly helpful in chronic conjunctivitis. McCoy cell culture is the standard for the laboratory-confirmed diagnosis of chlamydial conjunctivitis. Direct monoclonal antibody staining of conjunctival smears has been reported to have a sensitivity of 100%, specificity of 94%, and positive and negative predictive values of 94% and 100%, respectively. However, the diagnostic tests are not perfect and sexually active patients with follicular conjunctivitis should be considered to have chlamydial disease until proven otherwise. Therapeutic trials of tetracycline or erythromycin are important diagnostic and therapeutic steps in selected patients. In refractory cases, conjunctival biopsy is useful for detection of other potentially treatable causes, such as pemphigoid or malignancy (e.g., sebaceous gland carcinoma).

H. Chlamydial organisms are responsible for trachoma and adult inclusion conjunctivitis. Adult inclusion conjunctivitis usually occurs in sexually active adults, 15–30 years of age, who have acquired a new sexual partner within the past 2 months. It presents as an acute follicular conjunctivitis with mucopurulent discharge and has a chronic course. Keratitis may be a prominent feature later in the disease. Reiter's syndrome has been reported in association with adult inclusion conjunctivitis. Nonspecific urethritis in men and chronic vaginal discharge in women are common. More than 4 million Americans acquire genital chlamydial infection each year, and 1 in 300 of these patients gets inclusion conjunctivitis. Treat all sexual partners simultaneously to prevent reinfection. Refer patients for evaluation for other venereal infections such as gonorrhea and syphilis.

I. *C. trachomatis* is the most common cause of chronic follicular conjunctivitis. Topical antibiotics are relatively ineffective. Adequate treatment requires systemic administration of tetracycline or doxycycline for 3 weeks. Tetracycline should not be administered to children <7 years of age or to pregnant or lactating women. In patients who are intolerant of tetracycline, use oral erythromycin. Administer erythromycin, tetracycline, or sulfacetamide ointment as an adjunct. Treat sexual partners concurrently, and refer the patient for genitourinary examination.

References

Dawson CR, Sheppard JD. Follicular conjunctivitis. In: Duane TD, ed. Clinical ophthalmology. Vol 4. Philadelphia: Harper & Row, 1990.

Huang MC, Dreyer B. Parinaud's oculoglandular conjunctivitis and cat-scratch disease. In: Jakobiec FA, Lucarelli MJ, eds. International Ophthalmology Clinics—Ocular adnexal infections. Vol 36.3. Boston: Little, Brown, 1996: 29.

Mannis MJ. Bacterial conjunctivitis. In: Duane TD, ed. Clinical ophthalmology. Vol 4. Philadelphia: Harper & Row, 1990.

Rapoza PA, Quinn TC, Terry AC, et al. A systematic approach to the diagnosis and treatment of chronic conjunctivitis. Am J Ophthalmol 1990; 109:138–142.

Patient with CHRONIC CONJUNCTIVITIS

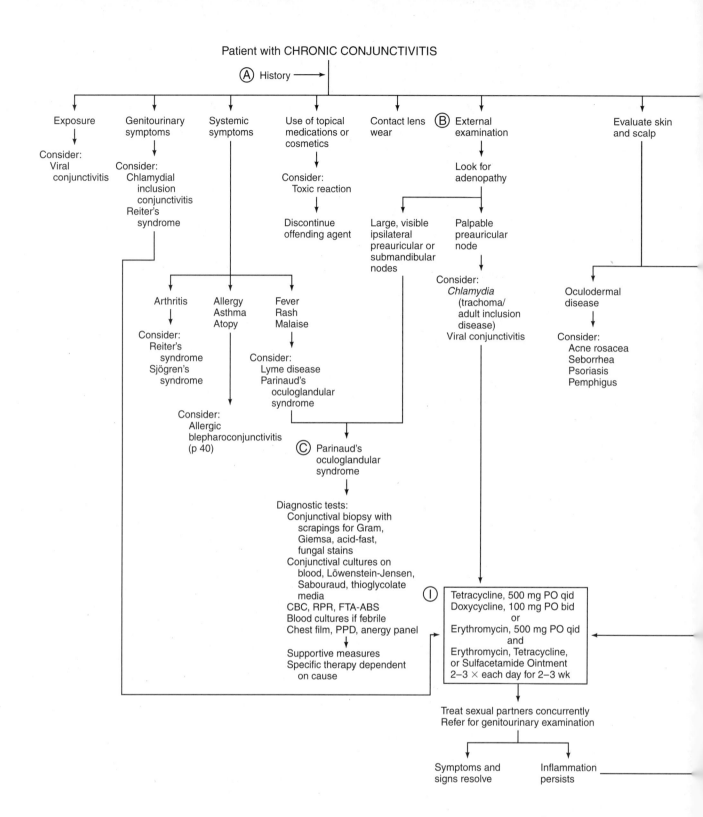

(A) History ⟶

| Exposure | Genitourinary symptoms | Systemic symptoms | Use of topical medications or cosmetics | Contact lens wear | (B) External examination | Evaluate skin and scalp |

Consider:
Viral conjunctivitis

Consider:
Chlamydial inclusion conjunctivitis
Reiter's syndrome

Consider:
Toxic reaction

Discontinue offending agent

Look for adenopathy

Large, visible ipsilateral preauricular or submandibular nodes

Palpable preauricular node

Consider:
Chlamydia (trachoma/adult inclusion disease)
Viral conjunctivitis

Oculodermal disease

Consider:
Acne rosacea
Seborrhea
Psoriasis
Pemphigus

Arthritis

Consider:
Reiter's syndrome
Sjögren's syndrome

Allergy
Asthma
Atopy

Fever
Rash
Malaise

Consider:
Lyme disease
Parinaud's oculoglandular syndrome

Consider:
Allergic blepharoconjunctivitis (p 40)

(C) Parinaud's oculoglandular syndrome

Diagnostic tests:
Conjunctival biopsy with scrapings for Gram, Giemsa, acid-fast, fungal stains
Conjunctival cultures on blood, Löwenstein-Jensen, Sabouraud, thioglycolate media
CBC, RPR, FTA-ABS
Blood cultures if febrile
Chest film, PPD, anergy panel

Supportive measures
Specific therapy dependent on cause

(I) Tetracycline, 500 mg PO qid
Doxycycline, 100 mg PO bid
or
Erythromycin, 500 mg PO qid
and
Erythromycin, Tetracycline, or Sulfacetamide Ointment
2–3 × each day for 2–3 wk

Treat sexual partners concurrently
Refer for genitourinary examination

Symptoms and signs resolve

Inflammation persists

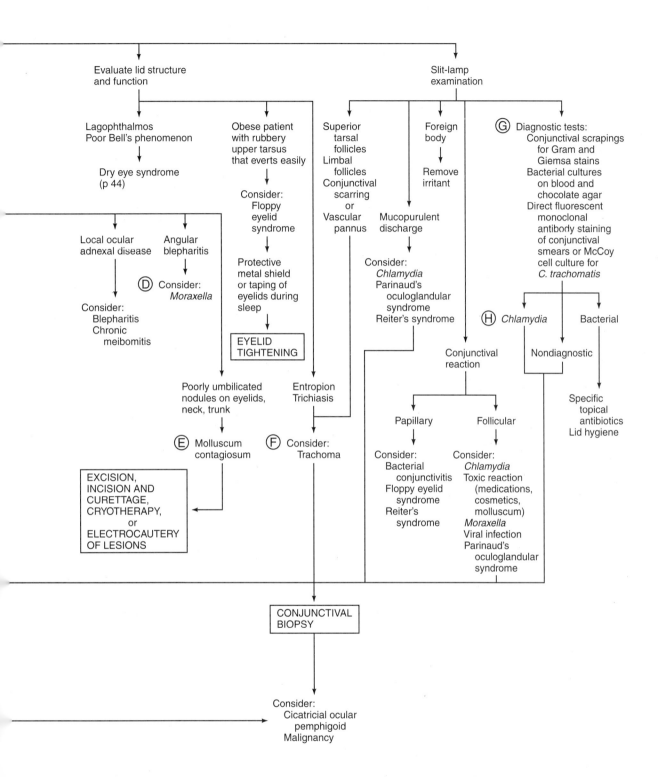

Evaluate lid structure
and function

Slit-lamp
examination

Lagophthalmos
Poor Bell's phenomenon

Obese patient
with rubbery
upper tarsus
that everts easily

Superior
tarsal
follicles
Limbal
follicles
Conjunctival
scarring
or
Vascular
pannus

Foreign
body

Ⓖ Diagnostic tests:
Conjunctival scrapings
for Gram and
Giemsa stains
Bacterial cultures
on blood and
chocolate agar
Direct fluorescent
monoclonal
antibody staining
of conjunctival
smears or McCoy
cell culture for
C. trachomatis

Dry eye syndrome
(p 44)

Remove
irritant

Consider:
Floppy
eyelid
syndrome

Mucopurulent
discharge

Local ocular
adnexal disease

Angular
blepharitis

Consider:
Chlamydia
Parinaud's
oculoglandular
syndrome
Reiter's syndrome

Ⓗ *Chlamydia*

Bacterial

Ⓓ Consider:
Moraxella

Protective
metal shield
or taping of
eyelids during
sleep

Nondiagnostic

Consider:
Blepharitis
Chronic
meibomitis

Conjunctival
reaction

Specific
topical
antibiotics
Lid hygiene

EYELID
TIGHTENING

Poorly umbilicated
nodules on eyelids,
neck, trunk

Entropion
Trichiasis

Papillary

Follicular

Ⓔ Molluscum
contagiosum

Ⓕ Consider:
Trachoma

Consider:
Bacterial
conjunctivitis
Floppy eyelid
syndrome
Reiter's
syndrome

Consider:
Chlamydia
Toxic reaction
(medications,
cosmetics,
molluscum)
Moraxella
Viral infection
Parinaud's
oculoglandular
syndrome

EXCISION,
INCISION AND
CURETTAGE,
CRYOTHERAPY,
or
ELECTROCAUTERY
OF LESIONS

CONJUNCTIVAL
BIOPSY

Consider:
Cicatricial ocular
pemphigoid
Malignancy

SUBCONJUNCTIVAL HEMORRHAGE

W.A.J. van Heuven, M.D.

Blood under the ocular conjunctiva should be differentiated from other conditions that cause redness, such as inflammation. Slit-lamp examination shows its precise location under the conjunctiva. The most common fresh appearance is a bright red patch with a relatively normal surrounding, which can show enlargement and thinning with gravity during the first few days. Because no inflammation is present, the conjunctival vessels around the patch are normal and not dilated. If the hemorrhage is thick, it may present as a dark red, almost black elevation. With time and blood breakdown, it may become green or yellow, like a bruise, and usually disappears within 2 weeks.

A. Subconjunctival hemorrhage most commonly is idiopathic and spontaneous in a healthy adult. The patient often wakes up with the condition, possibly caused by eye rubbing during sleep. It becomes more common with increasing age and increased capillary fragility, arteriosclerosis, and hypertension. In young patients without a history of trauma or infection, rule out systemic causes, particularly hematologic or hepatic diseases, diabetes, lupus erythematosus, parasites, and vitamin C deficiency.

B. Several febrile systemic infections, including meningococcal septicemia, scarlet fever, typhoid fever and cholera, rickettsia (typhus), parasites (malaria), and viruses (influenza, smallpox, measles, yellow fever, sandfly fever), can be the cause.

C. Many drugs and chemicals, including not only those that can cause blood dyscrasias or act as "blood thinners" but also various antibiotics, contraceptives, steroids, and vitamins A and D, have been associated with subconjunctival hemorrhage.

D. Many drugs and chemicals may cause hemorrhage directly or cause irritation, leading to eye rubbing, which produces the hemorrhage.

E. Subconjunctival hemorrhage after direct ocular trauma should lead one to question whether there is an ocular perforation, often underneath the blood, which would require surgical repair. If the conjunctiva appears intact, vision is good, pupillary responses are normal, the intraocular pressure (IOP) is normal, the media are clear, and the rest of the eye examination is normal, it is usually safe to assume that the eye is not perforated. However, there may be hyphema or vitreous hemorrhage, which prevents visualization of the fundus. Ultrasound examination is then indicated, as well as x-ray studies in cases of possible retained foreign bodies or suspected fractures. Particularly grave prognostic signs, which suggest perforation, are an afferent pupillary defect (Marcus Gunn) or a retinal detachment discovered by ultrasonography. Intraocular air or foreign bodies prove perforation. Very low IOP also suggests perforation, although moderately low IOP may simply mean ciliary body contusion. Occasionally, perforated eyes have normal or even high pressures.

F. Subconjunctival hemorrhage has been reported as a result of emboli from long bone fractures, chest compression, cardiac angiography, open-heart surgery, and other "remote" operations.

G. Blood under the conjunctiva is a normal sequela of ocular surgery, even if no conjunctival incision is made, as in transconjunctival cryotherapy. Because the surgery has made the conjunctival vessels more fragile, the bleeding may actually increase during the first few days after the operation.

H. The occurrence of a subconjunctival hemorrhage in an eye that has undergone a scleral buckling procedure indicates a buckle infection unless proven otherwise, even if the operation occurred years before. Usually, there is focal tenderness somewhere over the buckle. Even without this sign, it is wise to treat the patient with broad-spectrum systemic antibiotics for at least 10 days. Even if the hemorrhage and the tenderness clear, they may recur. Most buckle infections eventually require surgery to remove all implants and permanent sutures.

I. With the modern exercise craze, subconjunctival hemorrhages are now more often seen in young, healthy persons, especially after weight lifting and gravity inversion maneuvers. Severe coughing, sneezing, or wind instrument blowing may also be causes.

References

Fraunfelder FT. Drug induced ocular side effects and drug interactions. 3rd ed. Philadelphia: Lea & Febiger, 1989.

Friberg TR, Weinreb RN. Ocular manifestations of gravity inversion. JAMA 1985; 253:1755–1757.

Russell SR, Olson KR, Folk JC. Predictors of scleral rupture and the role of vitrectomy in severe ocular blunt trauma. Am Ophthalmol 1988; 105:253.

Patient with SUBCONJUNCTIVAL HEMORRHAGE

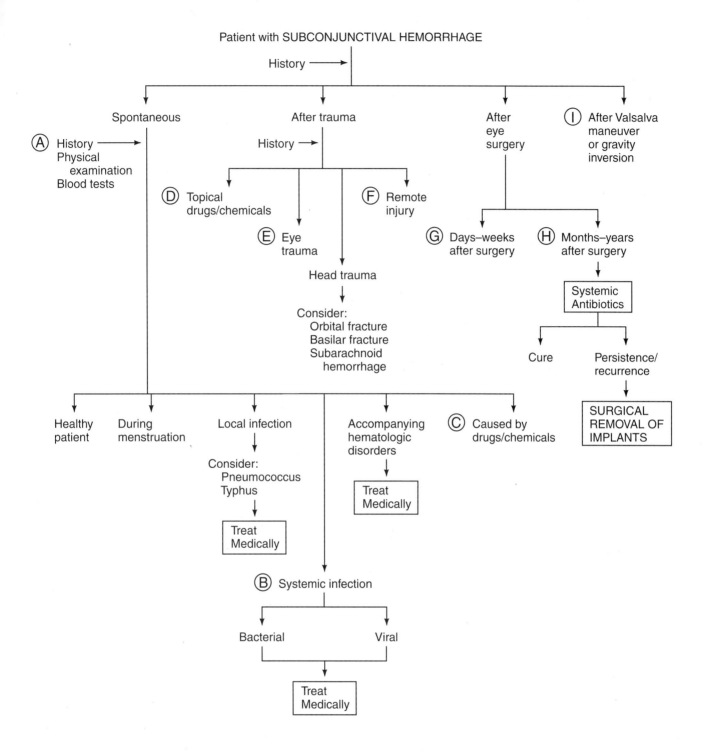

History →

Spontaneous

(A) History →
Physical
examination
Blood tests

After trauma

History →

(D) Topical
drugs/chemicals

(E) Eye
trauma

(F) Remote
injury

Head trauma

Consider:
  Orbital fracture
  Basilar fracture
  Subarachnoid
    hemorrhage

After
eye
surgery

(I) After Valsalva
maneuver
or gravity
inversion

(G) Days–weeks
after surgery

(H) Months–years
after surgery

Systemic
Antibiotics

Cure

Persistence/
recurrence

SURGICAL
REMOVAL OF
IMPLANTS

Healthy
patient

During
menstruation

Local infection

Consider:
  Pneumococcus
  Typhus

Treat
Medically

Accompanying
hematologic
disorders

Treat
Medically

(C) Caused by
drugs/chemicals

(B) Systemic infection

Bacterial

Viral

Treat
Medically

PIGMENT ALTERATIONS OF THE IRIS

Marilyn C. Kincaid, M.D.
Andrew W. Lawton, M.D.

A. Brushfield spots are often an isolated finding, unrelated to any other condition. However, clinically, they are associated with Down's syndrome, in which case other stigmata of trisomy 21 will be evident.

B. Oculocutaneous albinism is generally a straightforward diagnosis. In ocular albinism the skin and hair may appear normally pigmented. However, examination of family members may show that the patient has less pigmentation than typical for that family. Skin biopsy or hair bulb analysis may help provide the diagnosis.

C. Bilateral heterochromia, or bilateral variable pigmentation of the iris, can be a solitary defect or can be associated with Hirschsprung's disease (aganglionic megacolon), Waardenburg's syndrome (deafness, white forelock), or other pigmentary changes of the skin and hair (piebaldism).

D. Melanosis oculi and nevus of Ota have been associated with increased risk of uveal, orbital, and intracranial melanoma. Consider MRI or CT scans to evaluate for these tumors.

E. Iris atrophy can result from the trauma of cataract surgery or from ongoing rubbing of the intraocular lens against the iris. Usually, the lens can be left in place, but occasionally, the uveitis-glaucoma-hyphema syndrome results from continued iris irritation, inflammation, and prostaglandin release. In such cases the lens must be removed.

F. Anterior segment necrosis occurs when extraocular muscle surgery interrupts the blood supply from the anterior ciliary arteries. Less commonly, it can be seen after an episode of shock or other cause of hypoperfusion.

G. In herpes zoster infections the iris atrophy results from intraocular inflammation. This is particularly likely if the tip of the nose is involved in the cutaneous process because the nasociliary nerve also supplies the iris.

H. The inflammation of Fuchs' heterochromic iridocyclitis causes iris depigmentation on the involved side. However, if the atrophy is sufficiently severe, the affected iris may actually appear darker because of the exposed iris pigment epithelium. These patients may develop cataract and glaucoma.

I. Glaucomatocyclitic crisis is characterized by recurrent bouts of elevated intraocular pressure with corneal edema and anterior uveitis that last hours to weeks. There is relatively little pain, and the angle typically remains open. The iris becomes hypopigmented on the affected side. Mild miotics are used to treat the glaucoma. The ultimate prognosis is good, with retention of the full visual field.

J. Leukemic infiltration can cause a unilateral or bilateral darkening of the iris and can be the first manifestation of the initial diagnosis or of relapse. Systemic treatment of the leukemia typically causes the iris color to return to normal.

K. The clinical history of trauma can be misleadingly trivial or absent. Be particularly suspicious if the patient has been engaged in an activity likely to produce a ferrous foreign body. It is essential to remove the foreign body to prevent further deterioration in ocular function.

L. Early recognition of iridocorneal endothelial syndrome is crucial because these patients are prone to develop glaucoma and corneal decompensation.

References

Britt JM, Karr DJ, Kalina RE. Leukemic iris infiltration in recurrent acute lymphocytic leukemia. Arch Ophthalmol 1991; 109:1456–1457.

Diesenhouse MC, Palay DA, Newman NJ, et al. Acquired heterochromia with Horner syndrome in two adults. Ophthalmology 1992; 99:1815–1817.

Gartner S, Henkind P. Neovascularization of the iris (rubeosis iridis). Surv Ophthalmol 1978; 22:291–312.

Harding SP. Natural history of herpes zoster ophthalmicus: Predictors of postherpetic neuralgia and ocular involvement. Br J Ophthalmol 1987; 71:353–358.

Lewen RM. Ocula albinism. Arch Ophthalmol 1988; 106:120–121.

Liang JC, Juarez CP, Goldberg MF. Bilateral bicolored irides with Hirschsprung's disease. Arch Ophthalmol 1983; 101:69–73.

Perry HD, Yanoff M, Scheie HG. Rubeosis in Fuchs heterochromic iridocyclitis. Arch Ophthalmol 1975; 93:337–339.

Singh AD, De Potter P, Fijal BA, et al. Lifetime prevalence of uveal melanoma in white patients with oculo(dermal) melanocytosis. Ophthalmology 1998; 105:195–198.

Thompson WS, Curtin VT. Congenital bilateral heterochromia of the choroid and iris. Arch Ophthalmol 1994; 112:1247–1248.

Wilson MC, Shields MB. A comparison of the clinical variations of the iridocorneal endothelial syndrome. Arch Ophthalmol 1989; 107:1465–1468.

Patient with PIGMENT ALTERATIONS OF THE IRIS

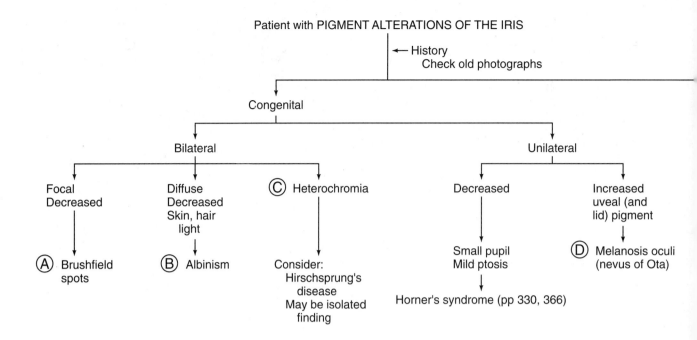

←— History
Check old photographs

Congenital

Bilateral

Focal
Decreased

Ⓐ Brushfield
spots

Diffuse
Decreased
Skin, hair
light

Ⓑ Albinism

Ⓒ Heterochromia

Consider:
Hirschsprung's
disease
May be isolated
finding

Unilateral

Decreased

Small pupil
Mild ptosis

Horner's syndrome (pp 330, 366)

Increased
uveal (and
lid) pigment

Ⓓ Melanosis oculi
(nevus of Ota)

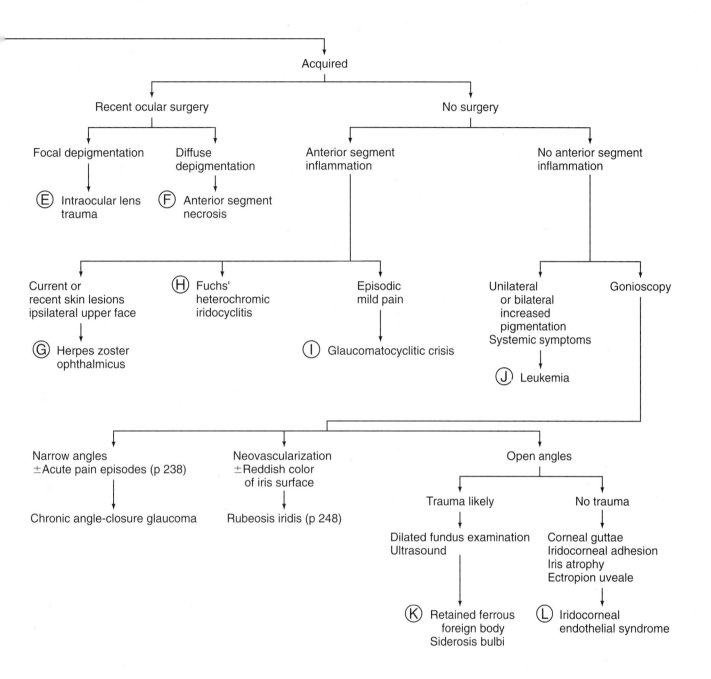

Acquired

Recent ocular surgery

Focal depigmentation

Ⓔ Intraocular lens trauma

Diffuse depigmentation

Ⓕ Anterior segment necrosis

Current or recent skin lesions ipsilateral upper face

Ⓖ Herpes zoster ophthalmicus

Ⓗ Fuchs' heterochromic iridocyclitis

No surgery

Anterior segment inflammation

Episodic mild pain

Ⓘ Glaucomatocyclitic crisis

No anterior segment inflammation

Unilateral or bilateral increased pigmentation Systemic symptoms

Ⓙ Leukemia

Gonioscopy

Narrow angles ±Acute pain episodes (p 238)

Chronic angle-closure glaucoma

Neovascularization ±Reddish color of iris surface

Rubeosis iridis (p 248)

Open angles

Trauma likely

Dilated fundus examination Ultrasound

Ⓚ Retained ferrous foreign body Siderosis bulbi

No trauma

Corneal guttae Iridocorneal adhesion Iris atrophy Ectropion uveale

Ⓛ Iridocorneal endothelial syndrome

INCREASED TRANSILLUMINATION OF THE IRIS

Johan Zwaan, M.D., Ph.D.

Transillumination of the iris indicates reduced melanin pigment in the double layer of pigmented iris epithelium that covers the posterior aspect of the iris. It may result from the absence or decrease of melanin within the cells, or there may be defects within the cell layers. The latter can be the result of congenital anomalies, trauma, or disease.

A. When there is a significant lack of pigment, the defects can be seen by transscleral transillumination with a bright light, such as a muscle light. In general, careful slit-lamp examination in a darkened room is essential to evaluate more subtle defects. In patients with dark rides the defects may be particularly difficult to see because pigment in the iris stroma blocks the light.

B. In oculocutaneous albinism the eyes, as well as the skin and hairs, show a significant lack of pigment. In tyrosinase-negative type 1 (OCA 1), melanin is completely missing. The lashes and hair are white, and transillumination of the iris is complete. Vision is significantly reduced because of foveal hypoplasia and lack of fundus pigment. Nystagmus is found. In tyrosinase-positive OCA 2, some pigment accumulates over time and the hair and lashes are yellowish. Vision is reduced less than in OCA 1. At least 10 different genetic types of OCA exist. Their discussion is beyond the scope of this chapter.

C. Patients with ocular albinism also have reduced vision, foveal hypoplasia, and nystagmus. Expression can be varied even within one family. Although skin changes are not obvious, electron microscopy has shown that abnormalities of pigmentation are present, primarily macromelanosomes. Four different types of ocular albinism exist.

D. Loss of pigment from the iris epithelium in pigment dispersion syndrome occurs primarily in a spokelike midperipheral pattern. It is caused by rubbing of the posterior leaflet of the iris epithelium against the lenticular zonules, associated with a concave iris plateau and a deep anterior chamber. It is found primarily in young adults with myopia and affects males more than females. The dislodged pigment granules are deposited in the trabecular meshwork and are visible with gonioscopy as a dense band of pigment. This may interfere with aqueous drainage and lead to glaucoma. Pigment also is deposited on the corneal endothelium in a vertical band, Krukenberg's spindle, and on other anterior segment structures.

E. The deposition of flaky white material on the anterior surface of the lens is the hallmark of pseudoexfoliation. The material also may be found on the zonules, the drainage angle, the corneal endothelium, ciliary processes, and anterior vitreous face. Pigment accumulation in the drainage angle is less pronounced than in pigment dispersion. The pigment is derived from the iris epithelium at the pupillary ruff as evidenced by scattered peripupillary transillumination defects. This pattern of pigment loss is not pathognomonic for pseudoexfoliation because it can also occur with aging.

F. Trauma, manipulation of the iris during surgery, and inflammation can lead to loss of pigment, usually in a patchy fashion. A careful history and slit-lamp examination will usually lead to the proper diagnosis.

G. Fuchs' heterochromic iridocyclitis is a unilateral anterior uveitis that affects young adults. It manifests as progressive heterochromia; a painless decrease of vision may occur. The anterior chamber reaction is low grade with small keratic precipitates and no posterior synechiae. Cataracts may develop. Atrophy of the iris pigment epithelium is patchy.

H. Abnormal shapes of the pupil (dyscoria), corectopia, and holes in the iris (pseudopolycoria) can result from hypoplasia of the iris stroma. The hypoplasia may be congenital, as in Axenfeld-Rieger's syndrome, or acquired, as in iridocorneal endothelial (ICE) syndrome. In both cases it can be progressive.

I. Axenfeld's anomaly usually shows autosomal-dominant inheritance. It is characterized by posterior embryotoxon and bridges of iris tissue crossing the anterior chamber angle and inserting at Schwalbe's line. It is often associated with glaucoma. This may be congenital or develop later, necessitating monitoring of the intraocular pressure (IOP) throughout life. In Rieger's anomaly the iris stroma is hypoplastic, in addition to the abnormalities found in Axenfeld's anomaly. Both anomalies are termed syndromes if systemic abnormalities are present. Because both may be found within the same family, they are now considered variable manifestations of the same gene defect and the syndrome or anomaly is labeled Axenfeld-Rieger's. The syndrome has been mapped to two different gene loci: 4q25 and 13q14. Autosomal-dominant iris hypoplasia and iridogoniodysgenesis with systemic features also map to the first locus.

J. ICE syndrome includes progressive essential iris atrophy, Chandler's syndrome, and the iris-nevus, or Cogan-Reese, syndrome. It is almost always unilateral. Glaucoma is combined with corneal endothelial abnormalities, anterior synechiae, iris atrophy leading to pseudopolycoria, and iris nodules. The three subtypes show different degrees of these manifestations of the same disease.

K. Ectopia lentis et pupillae is an autosomal-recessive anomaly. The lens dislocation is in the opposite direction from the displacement of the pupil. The iris shows transillumination defects. Axial myopia is the rule.

References

Brooks AMV, Gillies WE. The presentation and prognosis of glaucoma in pseudoexfoliation of the lens capsule. Ophthalmology 1988; 95:271–274.

Farrar SM, Shields MB, Miller KN, Stoup CN. Risk factors for the development and severity of glaucoma in the pigment dispersion syndrome. Am J Ophthalmol 1989; 108:223–227.

Goldberg MF. Clinical manifestations of ectopia lentis et pupillae in 16 patients. Ophthalmology 1988; 95:1080–1087.

Jones N. Fuchs' heterochromic uveitis: An update. Surv Ophthalmol 1993; 37:253–272.

King RA, Hearing VJ, Creel D, Qetting WS. Albinism. In: Scriver CR, Beaudet AL, Sly WS, Valle D, eds. The metabolic and molecular basis of inherited disease. New York: McGraw-Hill 1995: 4353–4390.

Semina EV, Reiter R, Leysens NJ, et al. Cloning and characterization of a novel bicoid-related homeobox transcription factor, RIEG, involved in Rieger syndrome. Nature Genet 1996; 14:392–399.

Wilson MC, Shields MB. A comparison of the clinical variations of the iridocorneal endothelial syndrome. Arch Ophthalmol 1989; 107:1465–1468.

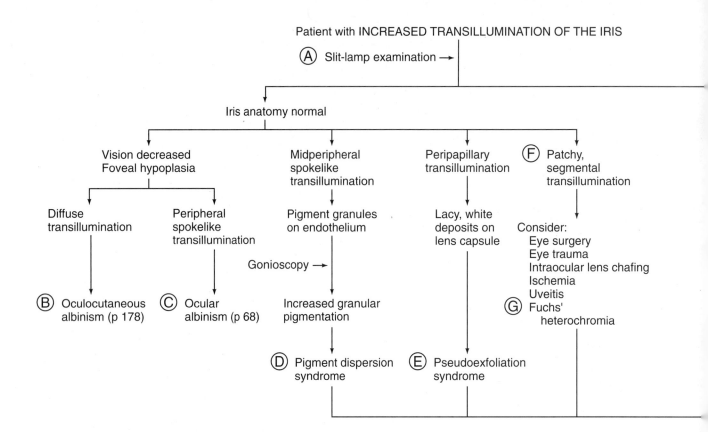

Patient with INCREASED TRANSILLUMINATION OF THE IRIS

(A) Slit-lamp examination →

Iris anatomy normal

Vision decreased
Foveal hypoplasia

Midperipheral
spokelike
transillumination

Peripapillary
transillumination

(F) Patchy,
segmental
transillumination

Diffuse
transillumination

Peripheral
spokelike
transillumination

Pigment granules
on endothelium

Lacy, white
deposits on
lens capsule

Consider:
Eye surgery
Eye trauma
Intraocular lens chafing
Ischemia
Uveitis
(G) Fuchs'
heterochromia

Gonioscopy →

(B) Oculocutaneous
albinism (p 178)

(C) Ocular
albinism (p 68)

Increased granular
pigmentation

(D) Pigment dispersion
syndrome

(E) Pseudoexfoliation
syndrome

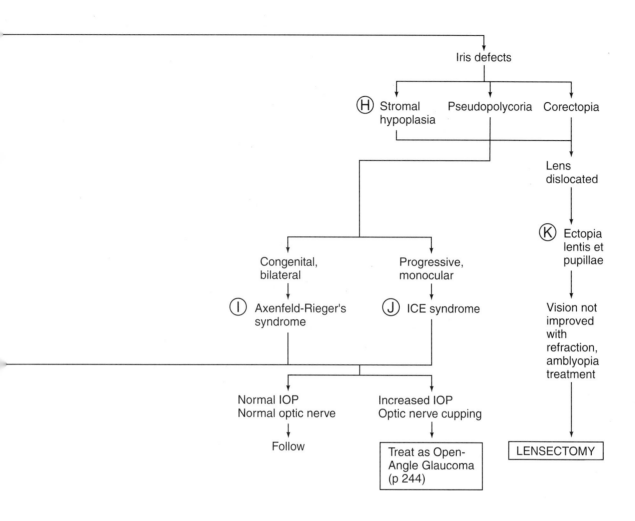

Iris defects

Ⓗ Stromal hypoplasia   Pseudopolycoria   Corectopia

Lens dislocated

Ⓚ Ectopia lentis et pupillae

Congenital, bilateral

Progressive, monocular

Ⓘ Axenfeld-Rieger's syndrome

Ⓙ ICE syndrome

Vision not improved with refraction, amblyopia treatment

Normal IOP
Normal optic nerve

Increased IOP
Optic nerve cupping

Follow

Treat as Open-Angle Glaucoma (p 244)

LENSECTOMY

TUMOR OF THE IRIS

Marilyn C. Kincaid, M.D.
Andrew W. Lawton, M.D.

A. The hallmark of neurofibromatosis is the Lisch nodule, a discrete, pigmented stromal mass that appears toward the end of the first decade of life. These masses are generally bilateral and multiple. They have no prognostic significance. Patients with neurofibromatosis may also have schwannomas and neurofibromas of the iris. The earlier that patients with neurofibromatosis can be identified, the more likely it is that possibly life-threatening neoplasms such as pheochromocytoma and acoustic neuroma can be found and treated.

B. Epithelial implantation cysts are the cyst form of epithelial ingrowth. Such cysts must be removed in toto; if ruptured, they may become an open downgrowth, which can be difficult to treat.

C. Sarcoidosis is a systemic granulomatous disease of unknown cause. It has a propensity for the iris, resulting in iridocyclitis and discrete nodules. The nodules tend to be vascular and multiple. Those at the pupil margin are called *Koeppe nodules,* and those at the periphery are called *Busacca nodules.* Systemic evaluation for sarcoid, including angiotensin-converting enzyme levels, chest radiograph, and biopsy of skin or conjunctival lesions, is indicated. Corticosteroid therapy may be indicated.

D. Juvenile xanthogranuloma is a true neoplasm that continues to grow if untreated, with significant consequences if located on the iris. These lesions are very sensitive to corticosteroids and irradiation; attempt these treatments before resorting to iridocyclectomy.

E. Iris melanomas have a low malignant potential, probably because of their minute size. However, in rare instances they can metastasize and kill. Follow patients for growth of the lesion before contemplating any surgery. Rarely, melanocytomas may grow and simulate melanomas. Sometimes, fine-needle aspiration of the anterior chamber with cytologic analysis of the fluid can help establish the diagnosis. Undertake gonioscopy to assess angle involvement and evaluation for a ciliary body component before doing a sector iridectomy for iris melanoma.

F. Metastatic lesions of the iris are much rarer than those of the choroid. Fine-needle aspiration of the anterior chamber with cytologic analysis of the fluid can help establish a primary site. These patients generally have widespread disease and a poor prognosis. Treatment is directed toward the underlying disease. External beam irradiation to help shrink the iris lesions can be instituted if appropriate.

References

Brown D, Boniuk M, Font RL. Diffuse malignant melanoma of the iris with metastases. Surv Ophthalmol 1990; 34:357–364.

Huson S, Jones D, Beck JL. Ophthalmic manifestations of neurofibromatosis. Br J Ophthalmol 1987; 71:235–238.

Offret H, Saraux H. Adenoma of the iris pigment epithelium. Arch Ophthalmol 1980; 98:875–883.

Shields JA. Primary cysts of the iris. Trans Am Ophthalmol Soc 1981; 79:771–809.

Shields JA, Shields CL, Kiratli H, De Potter P. Metastatic tumors to the iris in 40 patients. Am J Ophthalmol 1995; 119:422–430.

Tracy KW, Letson RD, Summers CG. Subconjunctival steroid in the management of uveal juvenile xanthogranuloma: A case report. J Pediatr Ophthalmol Strabismus 1990; 27:26–28.

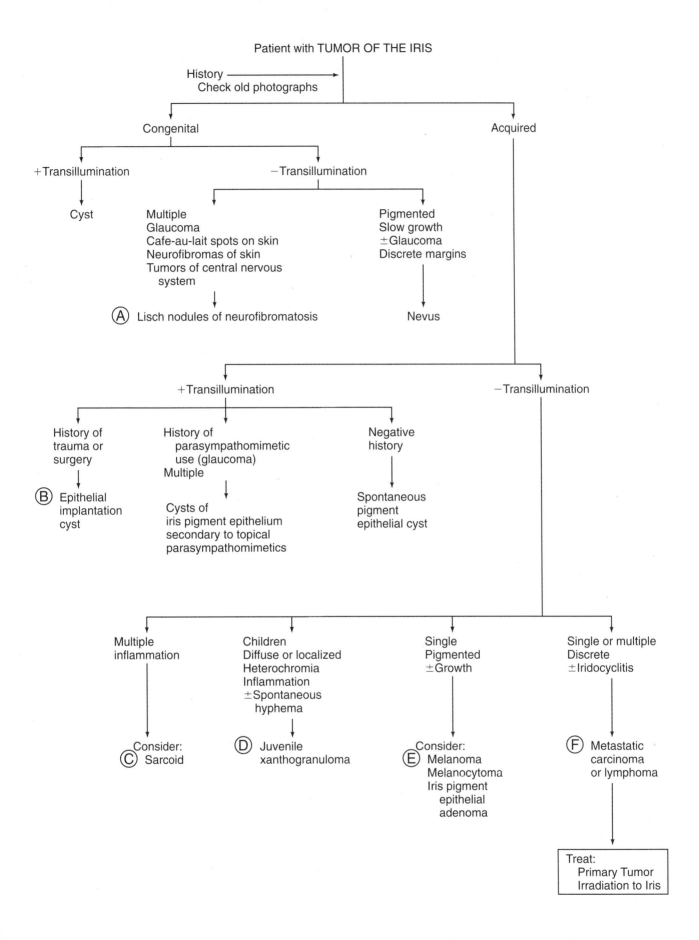

Patient with TUMOR OF THE IRIS

History
Check old photographs

Congenital

+Transillumination

Cyst

−Transillumination

Multiple
Glaucoma
Cafe-au-lait spots on skin
Neurofibromas of skin
Tumors of central nervous
  system

(A) Lisch nodules of neurofibromatosis

Pigmented
Slow growth
±Glaucoma
Discrete margins

Nevus

Acquired

+Transillumination

History of
trauma or
surgery

(B) Epithelial
implantation
cyst

History of
parasympathomimetic
use (glaucoma)
Multiple

Cysts of
iris pigment epithelium
secondary to topical
parasympathomimetics

Negative
history

Spontaneous
pigment
epithelial cyst

−Transillumination

Multiple
inflammation

Consider:
(C) Sarcoid

Children
Diffuse or localized
Heterochromia
Inflammation
±Spontaneous
  hyphema

(D) Juvenile
xanthogranuloma

Single
Pigmented
±Growth

Consider:
(E) Melanoma
Melanocytoma
Iris pigment
epithelial
adenoma

Single or multiple
Discrete
±Iridocyclitis

(F) Metastatic
carcinoma
or lymphoma

Treat:
Primary Tumor
Irradiation to Iris

HYPHEMA

W.A.J. van Heuven, M.D.

Hyphema, the presence of blood in the anterior chamber of the eye, occurs most commonly after trauma. Bleeding can arise from the iris or ciliary body when a tear of these tissues occurs at the time of contusion and ocular deformation. During a blow to the front of the eye, the anteroposterior dimension of the globe suddenly decreases, causing a compensatory increase in the anterior equatorial circumference of the globe. Structures such as the iris root, the ciliary body, and the peripheral retina, which are attached circumferentially to the ocular wall, may disinsert, producing dialysis of the iris root, tears in the ciliary body, and dialysis of the retina at the ora serrata. In addition, the anteroposterior compression can cause contusion injury to the lens and the retina. Thus, after a hyphema clears, a thorough ocular examination, with special attention to anterior peripheral structures, must be done. Partial or complete iridodialysis may be accompanied by injury to the trabecular meshwork, causing late glaucoma, even many years after the injury. Cyclodialysis may produce low intraocular pressure (IOP), resulting in choroidal detachments and macular edema. Retinal dialysis may lead to late retinal detachment unless treated with cryotherapy or photocoagulation. Commotio retinae (Berlin's edema) is retinal edema resulting from a contusion. It appears as a grayness of the retina often confined to the macula. It may be accompanied by retinal or preretinal hemorrhages and choroidal rupture. In many cases the condition clears without permanent damage, but it may be associated with severe visual loss and chorioretinal scarring. Occasionally, it may result in retinal hole formation.

A. Because many patients with hyphema are children or young adults, a precise history may be difficult to obtain. Always suspect ocular perforation, especially in a patient with a history of using a sharp, pointed object or hammering metal. When the eye ruptures from blunt trauma alone, it tends to do so at normally weak places in the sclera near the limbus or under the muscle insertions. Radiologic and echographic examinations are indicated when posterior ocular injury is suspected or when the eye examination shows severe limitation of motion to suggest orbital fracture. Severe chemosis, "reverse" Marcus Gunn afferent pupillary defect, and severe visual loss are especially ominous signs that indicate trauma beyond the simple hyphema.

B. Although many hyphemas can be seen grossly, hyphema can best be detected using slit-lamp examination because even small hyphemas become obvious. The recommended treatment is rest (hard to achieve in a child) and hospital admission with sedation, sometimes with bilateral patching. Avoid bilateral patching if it excites the patient more. The use of dilating or constricting drops is controversial, and there is no evidence that either is of definite benefit. The use of IV aminocaproic acid (Amicar) to stop bleeding and to prevent rebleeding is also still controversial but is becoming more accepted. Amicar acts by competitive inhibition of the conversion of plasminogen into plasmin and has a direct antiplasmin effect. It is used at a dosage of 100 mg/kg every 4 hours, with a maximum of 30 g/day orally for 5 days. Do not use Amicar in hyphemas occupying more than 70% of the anterior chamber because the clot may persist longer. Because rebleeding often occurs on the fourth or fifth day after injury, hospitalization should continue for 5 days. If rebleeding occurs, the same treatment can be repeated, unless a 100% hyphema occurs, resulting in increased IOP. This combination can lead to blood staining of the cornea and optic nerve damage, which can be prevented with surgical evacuation of the hyphema.

C. Most hyphemas, including total hyphemas, should be treated medically for the first 4 days, unless microscopic corneal blood staining occurs or the IOP rises to >50 mm Hg and is unresponsive to all medical management. Hyphemas >50% and lasting more than 5 days and hyphemas in patients with sickle cell disease or trait who have an IOP >35 mm Hg should also be surgically evacuated. There is some controversy relative to the length of time that any given pressure elevation can be observed before surgery is indicated.

D. Although most hyphemas are traumatic and occur in children, some diseases of childhood can produce hyphema and must be ruled out because of their medical significance. The most important of these is retinoblastoma, which can rarely present as a hyphema. Retinoblastoma can be ruled out with ophthalmic ultrasonography, which should be done in all hyphemas in any case to rule out ocular ruptures, vitreous hemorrhages, inflammatory conditions, other tumors, retinoschisis, and retinopathy of prematurity. Hyphemas can also result from vascular tumors of the iris, particularly juvenile xanthogranuloma, which is a disease of children <3 years. Usually, the ocular involvement is monocular and not associated with skin lesions. Iris xanthogranulomas may respond to topical steroids and mydriatics. Otherwise, surgical excision or radiation therapy may be used.

E. Systemic conditions that cause bleeding may rarely cause hyphema. Usually, however, the hyphema is secondary to ocular ischemia, which has caused iris or angle neovascularization. A type of hyphema observed with increasing frequency follows a vitrectomy for diabetic vitreous hemorrhage, in which case rebleeding into the vitreous cavity, once the vitreous barrier has been removed, spreads into the anterior chamber.

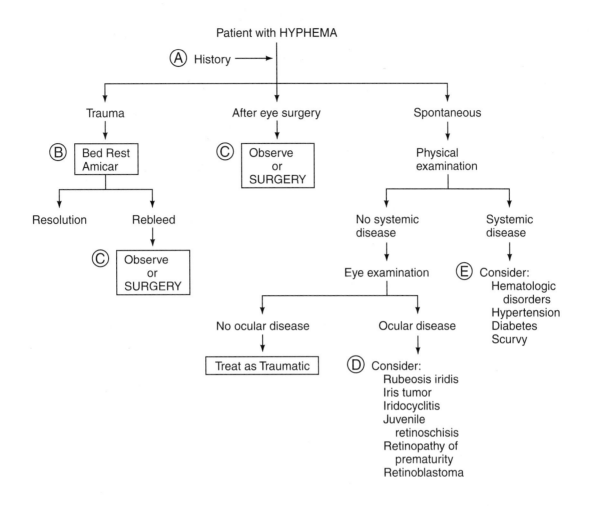

References

Deutsch TA, Fellar AB. Paton and Goldberg's management of ocular injuries. Philadelphia: WB Saunders, 1988.

Gottsch JD. Hyphema: Diagnosis and management. Retina 1990; 10:S65–S71.

Kearns P. Traumatic hyphaema: A retrospective study of 314 cases. Br Ophthalmol 1991; 75:137–141.

Tasman W, Jaeger EA. Duane's clinical ophthalmology. Philadelphia: JB Lippincott, 1998.

HYPOPYON

Bailey L. Lee, M.D.

A *hypopyon* is an accumulation of inflammatory cells in the anterior chamber. It is a nonspecific reaction resulting from intraocular inflammation with many causes. A complete history and physical examination are important in narrowing the differential diagnosis.

A. Patients typically have symptoms of pain, tearing, photophobia, and decreased vision when there is significant anterior chamber reaction to result in a hypopyon. Others signs on examination include injection; keratic precipitates, which can be of the granulomatous or nongranulomatous type; cell and flare in the anterior chamber; elevated intraocular pressure; and lens opacity. Patients with microbial keratitis may have an epithelial defect and a stromal infiltrate. A history is important to determine whether there is an associated systemic disease with the hypopyon or if it is primarily a manifestation of an ocular disease.

B. A pseudohypopyon can be an accumulation of tumor cells or khaki-colored cells of ghost cell glaucoma following intraocular hemorrhage; it can mimic a true hypopyon. A diagnostic paracentesis may be helpful when the diagnosis is in doubt.

C. In a patient with a history of contact lens wear, consider microbial keratitis; in cases that appear to be sterile, also consider a tight-fitting contact lens. After any ophthalmic procedure, including laser treatment in either the anterior or posterior segment, there can be postoperative inflammation. After intraocular surgery, one should always be concerned of postoperative endophthalmitis, but sterile causes can result from severe postoperative inflammation or a reaction to retained lens fragments after cataract surgery. HIV-positive patients with a drug history of rifabutin use can develop a sterile hypopyon. In this case treat with topical corticosteroids.

D. Exogenous endophthalmitis is an ocular emergency that requires immediate attention and should always be suspected in patients after intraocular surgery or in the setting of penetrating ocular trauma. The benefit of early vitrectomy and intravitreal antibiotic injection in postoperative endopthalmitis after cataract surgery with vision worse than hand motions has been demonstrated in the Endophthalmitis Vitrectomy Study (EVS). The EVS also showed the lack of benefit of systemic IV antibiotics. However, these results do not necessarily apply to cases of postoperative endophthalmitis after trabeculectomy or in traumatic endophthalmitis. In the latter case, *Bacillus* species endophthalmitis can develop into a fulminant infection with poor visual outcome.

E. The most common cause of endogenous endophthalmitis is infection of a fungal species, but bacterial species can also be involved. A history of immunosuppression and an indwelling catheter are risk factors, along with a history of IV drug abuse (IVDA). Treatment can involve both systemic and local intravitreal antifungal therapy. Severe cases may require vitrectomy.

References

Ayliffe W, Foster CS, Marcoux P, et al. Relapsing acute myeloid leukemia manifesting as hypopyon uveitis. Am J Ophthalmol 1995; 119:361–364.

Colvard DR, Roberston DM, O'Duffy JD. The ocular manifestations of Behcet's disease. Arch Ophthalmol 1997; 95:1813–1817.

Endophthalmitis Vitrectomy Study Group. Results of the Endophthalmitis Vitrectomy Study. A randomized trial of immediate vitrectomy and of intravenous antibiotics for the treatment of postoperative bacterial endopthalmitis. Arch Ophthalmol 1995; 113:1479–1496.

Saran BR, Maguire AM, Nichols C, et al. Hypopyon ueveitis in patients with acquired immunodeficiency syndrome treated for systemic *Mycobacterium avium* complex infection with rifabutin. Arch Ophthalmol 1994; 112:1159–1165.

Shields JA, Shields CL, Eagle RC, Blair CJ. Spontaneous pseudohypopyon secondary to diffuse infiltrating retinoblastoma. Arch Ophthalmol 1988, 106:1301–1302.

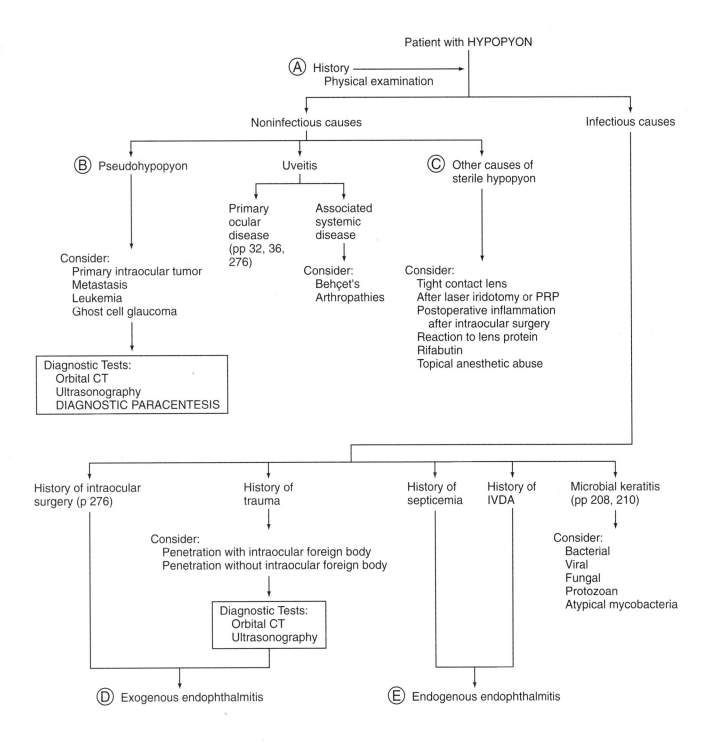

Patient with HYPOPYON

(A) History ⎯⎯⎯⎯⎯⎯
Physical examination

Noninfectious causes   Infectious causes

(B) Pseudohypopyon   Uveitis   (C) Other causes of
                                                                      sterile hypopyon

                              Primary   Associated
                              ocular   systemic
                              disease   disease
                              (pp 32, 36,
                              276)   Consider:
                                             Behçet's
                                             Arthropathies

Consider: Consider:
   Primary intraocular tumor   Tight contact lens
   Metastasis   After laser iridotomy or PRP
   Leukemia   Postoperative inflammation
   Ghost cell glaucoma   after intraocular surgery
                                                                  Reaction to lens protein
                                                                  Rifabutin
                                                                  Topical anesthetic abuse
┌─────────────────────────────┐
│ Diagnostic Tests: │
│   Orbital CT   │
│   Ultrasonography   │
│   DIAGNOSTIC PARACENTESIS   │
└─────────────────────────────┘

History of intraocular   History of   History of   History of   Microbial keratitis
surgery (p 276)   trauma   septicemia   IVDA   (pp 208, 210)

                     Consider: Consider:
                        Penetration with intraocular foreign body   Bacterial
                        Penetration without intraocular foreign body   Viral
                                                                                Fungal
                              ┌─────────────────────────┐   Protozoan
                              │ Diagnostic Tests: │   Atypical mycobacteria
                              │   Orbital CT   │
                              │   Ultrasonography   │
                              └─────────────────────────┘

(D) Exogenous endophthalmitis   (E) Endogenous endophthalmitis

MICROPHTHALMOS

Johan Zwaan, M.D., Ph.D.

Microphthalmos is defined as an eye that is congenitally smaller than the norm. This means an axial length of <21 mm in an adult or <16 mm in a newborn. The anomaly consists of a group of diverse disorders, which is classified as simple (no other ocular anomalies) or complex (combination with other eye anomalies, cataract, or vitreoretinal disease). The complex category is further divided in colobomatous and noncolobomatous.

A. When a patient or parent reports that an eye appears smaller than normal, true microphthalmos may be present or the eye may have microcornea. A microcornea has a horizontal diameter of <10 mm in the adult or <9 mm in an infant. Although usually occurring in combination, microphthalmos can be present with a normal-sized cornea and vice versa. Narrowing of the lid fissure may cause the eye to look smaller than it is.

B. The blepharophimosis syndrome is characterized by shortening of the horizontal lid fissure, ptosis, telecanthus, and epicanthus inversus. There are two types with autosomal inheritance, in one of which the affected women are infertile. It may also occur sporadically and is often secondary to anophthalmos or extreme microphthalmos, in which orbital and eyelid growth are reduced.

C. Ptosis may give the impression that the eye on the involved side is small, particularly when the ptosis is one-sided or asymmetric (p 116).

D. Several intrauterine infections can affect eye size. Infections with the rubella virus in the first trimester cause infection of the embryo in 50% of cases. In the rubella syndrome microphthalmos may be combined with cataracts and pigmentary "salt-and-pepper" retinopathy. The retinopathy usually does not reduce vision significantly. Glaucoma and keratitis are less common. Systemic problems include congenital heart defects, sensorineural deafness, and growth and mental retardation.

E. The offspring of women who become infected with toxoplasmosis in the first trimester have the most severe manifestations of the disease. Although infections later in pregnancy may give minimal or no abnormalities, some neonates who have initially negative examinations may later develop the syndrome. Microphthalmos is always accompanied in this syndrome by chorioretinitis, which is the most common expression of the syndrome. Other findings include intracranial calcifications, hydrocephalus, microcephalus, seizures, and jaundice. The intracranial abnormalities may cause blindness more often than the chorioretinitis, which will reduce vision, particularly when the macular area is involved, but not abolish it.

F. CMV infects up to 2.3% of newborns, making it the most common intrauterine infection. However, less than one fifth of the infected babies develop congenital anomalies. Microphthalmos is relatively mild. Chorioretinitis, which causes less pigmented scars than toxoplasmosis, and optic atrophy develop in 6% of the fetuses of women having a primary CMV infection during pregnancy. Microcephalus, hydrocephalus, cerebral calcifications that are typically located periventricularly, and cerebral atrophy may be present. Less common eye manifestations are cataract, glaucoma, and keratitis.

G. All of the anterior segment dysgenesis syndromes, as well as aniridia, may be associated with microcornea.

H. Nuclear cataracts often are found together with microcornea. This combination may be autosomal dominant. The microcornea and small anterior chamber make lensectomy or lens aspiration more difficult.

I. Anterior persistent hyperplastic primary vitreous (PHPV) is characterized by persistence of the hyaloid vasculature. A fibrovascular membrane covers the posterior surface of the lens and sometimes invades the lens. It is connected to the optic disc or less commonly to retinal vessels by a stalk containing the hyaloid artery. Contraction of the membrane pulls the ciliary processes under the lens, resulting in a highly characteristic pigmented fringe behind the lens periphery. This same contraction moves the lens-iris diaphragm forward, narrowing the anterior chamber angle and eventually leading to angle-closure glaucoma, which is difficult to treat. Most cases are sporadic and involve only one eye, although bilateral and familial PHPV have been reported. Visual outcome after surgery is often surprisingly good and depends partially on the extent of retinal involvement and on the patient's age at surgery. In less severe cases the fibrovascular membrane is limited to a peripheral sector of the lens and the vascular stalk inserts into the peripheral retina.

J. Chronic uveitis or hypotony may lead to atrophy of the eye. The eye shrinks and the contents become disorganized. This is called *phthisis bulbi*. Tumors may be present in such an eye and need to be excluded. In young children retinoblastoma can occur, whereas in adults uveal melanomas may be present.

K. Posterior PHPV is also called *congenital retinal fold*. There is a fold of retina and condensed vitreous running from the disc to the periphery, sometimes up to the ora serrata. Abnormal blood vessels are seen within the fold, presumably remnants of anastomoses between hyaloid and retinal vasculature. The eye is microphthalmic, and there is no cataract, unlike in anterior PHPV. Because of macular involvement the vision is usually poor and esotropia and nystagmus may result.

L. Patients with Hallermann-Streiff's syndrome have a birdlike face with hypotrichosis, dental abnormalities, and short stature. The eyes are severely microphthalmic, with small corneae and cataracts, which often reabsorb spontaneously. The inheritance pattern is unclear.

M. Colobomas are the most common cause of microphthalmos. They may be isolated or part of a syndrome with systemic abnormalities. The inheritance is autosomal dominant with variable expression, although recessive inheritance has been reported. Many cases are sporadic. Vision is always reduced because the chorioretinal colobomas have to be large for the eye to become microphthalmic.

N. In Lenz's syndrome microphthalmia is combined with vertebral, dental, and urogenital anomalies and with heart defects. Inheritance is X-linked.

O. CHARGE syndrome stands for coloboma, heart defects, choanal atresia, retarded growth, genital anomalies, and ear anomalies. It usually is sporadic, although rare familial occurrences have been reported.

P. A variety of chromosomal anomalies may be associated with colobomatous microphthalmia. Common syndromes are Patau's syndrome (trisomy 13), cat-eye syndrome (trisomy or tetrasomy 22pter), Wolf-Hirschhorn's syndrome (4p−), and triploidy. There are numerous other rare associations.

Q. The main characteristics of Patau's syndrome are colobomas, cleft lip and palate, and polydactyly. The colobomas are extensive and involve the iris, ciliary body, retina/choroid, and optic disc. The eye is usually microphthalmic, although not always. The retina is dysplastic, and cartilage develops in the eye. Almost all organ systems can be involved. Severe cardiac and CNS anomalies limit life expectancy. Only 5% of the infants survive beyond age 3 years.

R. Various reports indicate that 50%–80% of patients with simple microphthalmos have a systemic disease such as fetal alcohol syndrome, fetal exposure to other toxins (vitamin A, thalidomide, warfarin) or to maternal diabetes mellitus, fetal infections (rubella and others), or a large variety of inherited syndromes.

S. Nanophthalmos is a rare form of microphthalmos in which the eye is proportionally smaller in all directions. The axial length is 16.0–18.5 mm and the eye is very hyperopic (≥10 diopters). The lens is large relative to eye size, and the cornea is small. This causes the iris to bow forward, resulting in a very shallow anterior chamber and a narrow chamber angle. Angle-closure glaucoma often follows. The sclera is thicker than usual, impeding venous outflow through the vortex veins. This causes uveal effusions and choroidal detachments spontaneously, but in particular during and after intraocular surgery. The detachments also contribute to angle-closure glaucoma.

References

Fowler KB, Stagno S, Pass RE, et al. The outcome of congenital cytomegalovirus infection in relation to maternal antibody status. N Engl J Med 1992; 326:693–703.

Koppe JG, Loewer-Sieger DH, Roever-Bonnet H. Results of 20-year follow-up of congenital toxoplasmosis. Lancet 1986; i:254–256.

Mullaney PB, Karcioglu ZA, Al-Mesfer SA, Abboud EB. Presentation of retinoblastoma as phthisis bulbi. Eye 1997; 11:403–408.

Pollard Z. Treatment of persistent hyperplastic primary vitreous. J Pediatr Ophthalmol Strabismus 1985; 22:180–183.

Warburg M. Classification of microphthalmos and coloboma. J Med Genet 1993; 30:664–669.

Weiss AH, Kouseff BG, Ross EA, Longbottom J. Complex microphthalmos. Arch Ophthalmol 1989; 107:1619–1624.

Weiss AH, Kouseff BG, Ross EA, Longbottom J. Simple microphthalmos. Arch Ophthalmol 1989; 107:1625–1630.

Wright KW, Christensen LE, Noguchi BA. Results of late surgery for presumed congenital cataracts. Am J Ophthalmol 1992; 114:409–415.

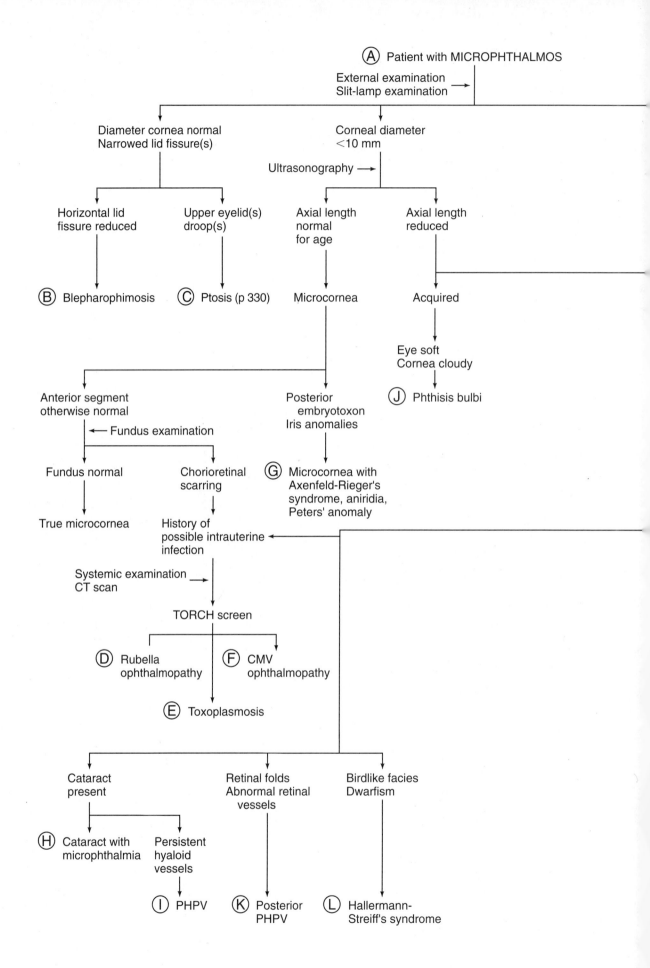

A. Patient with MICROPHTHALMOS

External examination
Slit-lamp examination →

Diameter cornea normal
Narrowed lid fissure(s)

Corneal diameter
<10 mm

Ultrasonography →

Horizontal lid
fissure reduced

Upper eyelid(s)
droop(s)

Axial length
normal
for age

Axial length
reduced

B. Blepharophimosis

C. Ptosis (p 330)

Microcornea

Acquired

Eye soft
Cornea cloudy

J. Phthisis bulbi

Anterior segment
otherwise normal

← Fundus examination

Posterior
embryotoxon
Iris anomalies

Fundus normal

Chorioretinal
scarring

G. Microcornea with
Axenfeld-Rieger's
syndrome, aniridia,
Peters' anomaly

True microcornea

History of
possible intrauterine ←
infection

Systemic examination →
CT scan

TORCH screen

D. Rubella
ophthalmopathy

F. CMV
ophthalmopathy

E. Toxoplasmosis

Cataract
present

Retinal folds
Abnormal retinal
vessels

Birdlike facies
Dwarfism

H. Cataract with
microphthalmia

Persistent
hyaloid
vessels

I. PHPV

K. Posterior
PHPV

L. Hallermann-
Streiff's syndrome

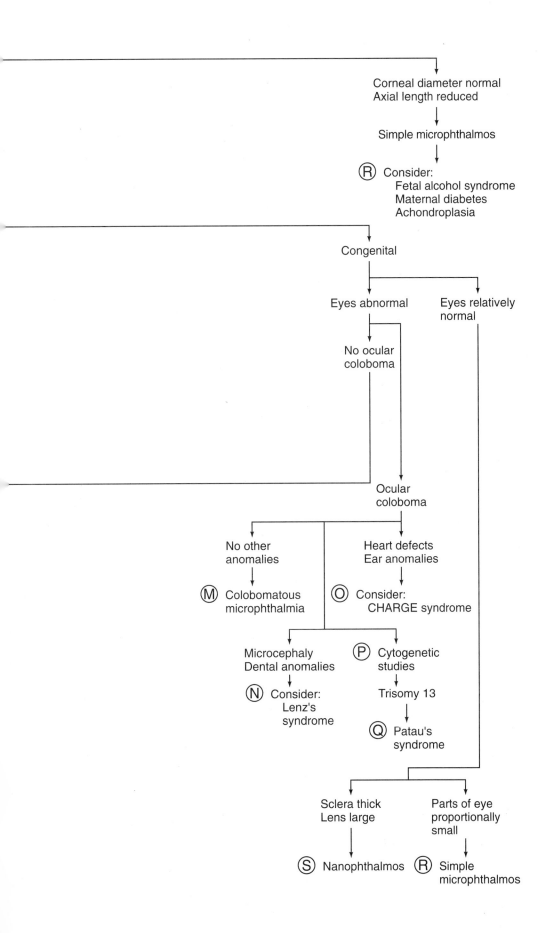

Corneal diameter normal
Axial length reduced

Simple microphthalmos

Ⓡ Consider:
Fetal alcohol syndrome
Maternal diabetes
Achondroplasia

Congenital

Eyes abnormal

Eyes relatively
normal

No ocular
coloboma

Ocular
coloboma

No other
anomalies

Heart defects
Ear anomalies

Ⓜ Colobomatous
microphthalmia

Ⓞ Consider:
CHARGE syndrome

Microcephaly
Dental anomalies

Ⓟ Cytogenetic
studies

Ⓝ Consider:
Lenz's
syndrome

Trisomy 13

Ⓠ Patau's
syndrome

Sclera thick
Lens large

Parts of eye
proportionally
small

Ⓢ Nanophthalmos

Ⓡ Simple
microphthalmos

MACROPHTHALMOS

Johan Zwaan, M.D., Ph.D.

An eye that is larger than the norm expected for a patient's age is called *macrophthalmos.* The size of the normal eye changes dramatically during the first few years of life. Axial length averages 16–17 mm at term. Because of the very rapid postnatal growth phase it gains 3.5–4 mm in the next 18 months. Growth slows down to 1.1 mm from age 2–5 years and even more from age 5–13 years (1.3 mm). After age 13, growth is negligible. The average axial length from this time on is 23 mm.

A. Certain conditions give the appearance of macrophthalmos even when the ocular size is normal. The corneal diameter may be increased or the eye may be more prominent than usual because of exophthalmos or retraction of the eyelids. Measurement of the diameter of the cornea by slit-lamp examination or with calipers and of the ocular axial length by ultrasonography may be necessary to differentiate megalocornea and anterior megalophthalmos from true macrophthalmos. The normal cornea has a horizontal diameter of 9.5–10 mm at birth. At 1 year of age it has grown to 11.5–12.0 mm and at age 3 years and beyond the diameter is 12.5 mm. If the cornea is adult size at birth (12.5 mm) or 13.0 mm at age 2 years and beyond, it is considered enlarged and called *megalocornea.*

B. When the eye is proptotic because of thyroid orbitopathy (p 132), or another orbital pathologic condition, when the orbits are shallow as seen in craniofacial anomalies such as Apert's or Crouzon's syndrome, or in eyelid retraction, patients or parents often believe that the globe is enlarged. Standard clinical examination is usually adequate to lay this idea to rest.

C. Euryblepharon is a congenital abnormality of the eyelids. The lateral canthus is displaced downward and outward and the lower eyelid downward. The palpebral fissure is enlarged. This may give the erroneous impression that the eye is larger than normal. The abnormality may be autosomal dominant. It is sometimes seen in Down's syndrome and in craniofacial anomalies.

D. In myopia the cornea usually is normal in diameter. Refraction or cycloplegic retinoscopy will give the diagnosis.

E. Keratoglobus is a congenital or acquired anomaly of the cornea. The corneal stroma is thinned in the midperiphery, leading to a bulging out of the cornea in a globular configuration. It may be inherited (X-linked) or occur in association with blue sclerae. In Down's and Rubinstein-Taybi's syndromes it may occur acutely as a form of hydrops.

F. Congenital glaucoma is present at birth; infantile glaucoma occurs in the first 1–2 years of life. Because the sclera and cornea are more elastic at these ages, increased ocular pressure causes expansion of the globe. If the pressure is not controlled, the eye will become significantly enlarged, leading to buphthalmos.

G. Mucopolysaccharidoses cause clouding of the cornea and rarely enlargement of the cornea. Rule out secondary glaucoma caused by thickening of the cornea and consequent anterior chamber angle narrowing and/or the accumulation of metabolites in the trabecular meshwork.

H. If congenital or infantile glaucoma is controlled early enough by surgical or medical means, the corneal diameter may still be within normal limits. If the control is borderline or poor, elongation of the eye may continue. Monitoring of the axial length is a useful way to assess control.

I. Marfan's syndrome is autosomal dominant. It is caused by mutations of the fibrillin gene on chromosome 1 Sq 21.1. In addition to the systemic findings of cardiac and skeletal anomalies, ocular abnormalities are present. It is the most common cause for ectopia lentis. Cataracts may form, and high myopia and retinal detachments are common. Rarely, enlargement of the entire anterior segment is present (anterior megalophthalmos). Expression may vary from family to family because of the different mutations of the gene.

J. In (anterior) megalophthalmos the ciliary ring and the lens-iris diaphragm are enlarged as well as the cornea. Iridodonesis, iris transillumination, lens dislocation and high myopia/astigmatism can result. This may be an isolated condition, but it has been found in association with Apert's syndrome, Marfan's syndrome, and mucolipidosis type 2.

K. Simple megalocornea is an X-linked disorder, although other inheritance patterns have been reported. The cornea is clear, and thickness and endothelial cell density are normal. The diameter may be as large as 18 mm. It is differentiated from congenital glaucoma because the cornea is clear and intraocular pressure (IOP) is normal, as is the optic nerve.

L. Megalocornea may be associated with a variety of systemic disorders, such as Alport's syndrome, craniofacial anomalies, Marfan's syndrome, facial hemihypertrophy, mucolipidosis type 2, and Down's syndrome.

References

Curtin BJ. The myopias: Basic science and clinical management. Philadelphia: Harper & Row, 1985.

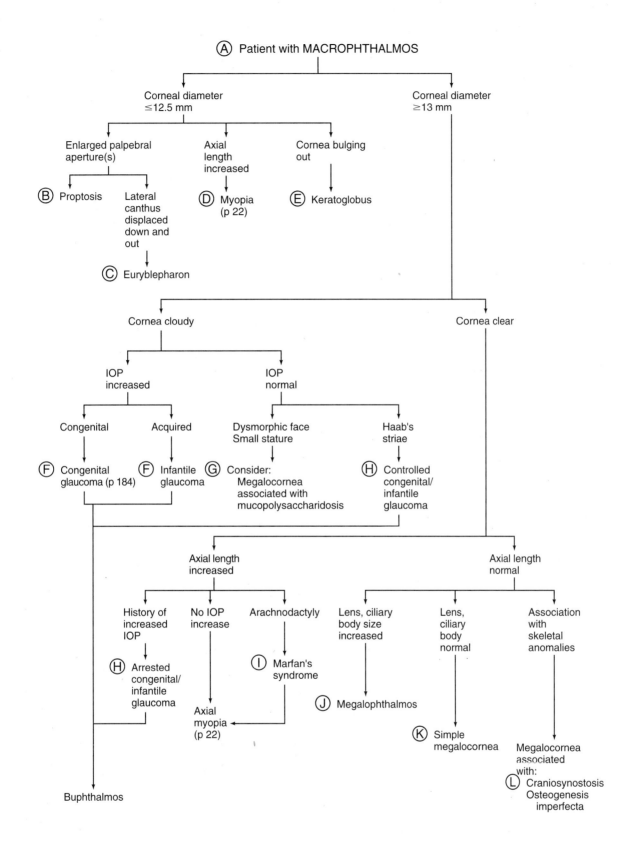

Egbert JB, Kushner BJ. Excessive loss of hyperopia. A presenting sign of juvenile aphakic glaucoma. Arch Ophthalmol 1990; 108:1257–1259.

Hoskins HD, Shaffer RN, Hetherington J. Anatomical classification of developmental glaucomas. Arch Ophthalmol 1984; 102:1331–1334.

Mackey DA, Buttery RG, Wise GM, Denton MJ. Description of X-linked megalocornea with identification of the gene locus. Arch Ophthalmol 1991; 109:829–833.

Maumenee I. The Marfan syndrome is caused by a point mutation in the fibrillin gene. Arch Ophthalmol 1992; 110:472–473.

PAINFUL ORBITAL SWELLING

Charles R. Leone, M.D.

Painful orbital swelling can result from inflammation, infection, or tumor. The most common cause is inflammatory and, excluding Graves' disease, is usually an idiopathic condition called *orbital inflammatory disease* (OID).

A. Examination of the patient includes a complete eye examination with emphasis on visual acuity, extraocular muscle movement (EOM), exophthalmometer readings, and palpation for any mass, particularly in the lacrimal gland fossa area. Obtain a CT scan to gain information about the orbit itself, its bony contours, and the condition of the paranasal sinuses. If a specific mass is detected, standardized A-scan ultrasonography can determine its tissue consistency. An A-scan is also the most precise technique for measuring extraocular muscles (enlarged in Graves' disease) or the thickness of the optic nerve. Consider MRI to delineate any process in the apex of the orbit because bone is not imaged and thus does not interfere with the orbital image. Also, the apex of the orbit is beyond echographic reach.

B. Orbital cellulitis is usually associated with an ethmoiditis and possible medial orbital infiltrate. This can be seen clearly on a CT scan. It is fairly common in children, who present with pain, fever, and toxicity. This may have been preceded by an upper respiratory tract infection. The eye findings are proptosis, restricted EOMs, and possibly decreased vision. The common pathogens are *Haemophilus influenzae, Streptococcus,* and *Staphylococcus,* and there may be an abscess formation within the orbit. It is important to obtain ENT and pediatric consultations to use a team approach in treating this emergency situation. Institute IV antibiotics as soon as possible, and monitor vision. If no improvement occurs within 24 hours, consider surgery consisting of sinus drainage and/or direct orbital drainage, if there is an abscess.

C. If there is noticeable improvement, continue IV antibiotics for several more days, followed by oral antibiotics for a total of 10–14 days.

D. If the sinuses are clear and an orbital infiltrate is present, consider OID, especially in middle-aged women. However, all patient groups are affected. The typical clinical features include the abrupt onset of unilateral painful orbital swelling associated with chemosis, conjunctival hyperemia, limited gaze, and sometimes a palpable mass. Occasionally, these can be associated with an underlying systemic disease such as sarcoidosis or rheumatoid arthritis. One of the extraocular muscles can be affected and would show a localized infiltrative process, usually involving the entire muscle from insertion to origin, producing a clinical paresis. In sarcoidosis the lacrimal gland is often involved and presents as a swollen, tender mass in the superior temporal quadrant. Most cases of OID respond to oral steroids (prednisone, 40–60 mg/day). Once control is achieved, tapering the daily dose by 2.5–10 mg/wk usually provides control until the condition resolves. If oral steroids are not effective, give IV dexamethasone, 4 mg every 6 hours. Once control is achieved, oral steroids can then be reinstituted.

E. If there is not a resolution of the process or the mass, consider biopsy. If inflammatory tissue is found at the time of biopsy, intralesional triamcinolone, 20–40 mg, can be injected.

F. If control is not achieved with intralesional steroid therapy, consider radiation therapy, 1000–3000 cGy. If this is unsuccessful, consider chemotherapy. Even then it is usually necessary to continue steroids until improvement starts.

G. If a neoplasm is found in the biopsy, the diagnostic possibilities include lymphoma or adenocystic carcinoma of the lacrimal gland. Other painful neoplasms are squamous cell carcinoma and metastatic lesions. One cause of pain with the carcinomas is perineural invasion of the fifth nerve. Lymphoma and metastatic lesions require further systemic work-up, followed by chemotherapy, radiation therapy, or both. When taking a biopsy of lymphoid or metastatic lesions, obtain enough tissue for cell marker studies and receptor cell assays. Adenocystic carcinoma and squamous cell carcinoma are usually treated with exenteration with or without radiation therapy.

References

Jakobiec FA, Iwamoto T, Knowles DM. Ocular adnexal lymphoid tumors: Correlative ultrastructural and immunological marker studies. Arch Ophthalmol 1982; 100:84–98.

Leone CR, Lloyd WC. Treatment protocol for orbital inflammatory disease. Ophthalmology 1985; 92:1325–1331.

Weiss A, Friendly D, Eglin K, et al. Bacterial periorbital and orbital cellulitis in childhood. Ophthalmology 1983; 90:195–203.

Wright JE, Stewart WB, Krohel GB. Clinical presentation in the management of lacrimal gland tumors. Br J Ophthalmol 1979; 63:600–606.

Patient with PAIN AND SWELLING AROUND THE EYE

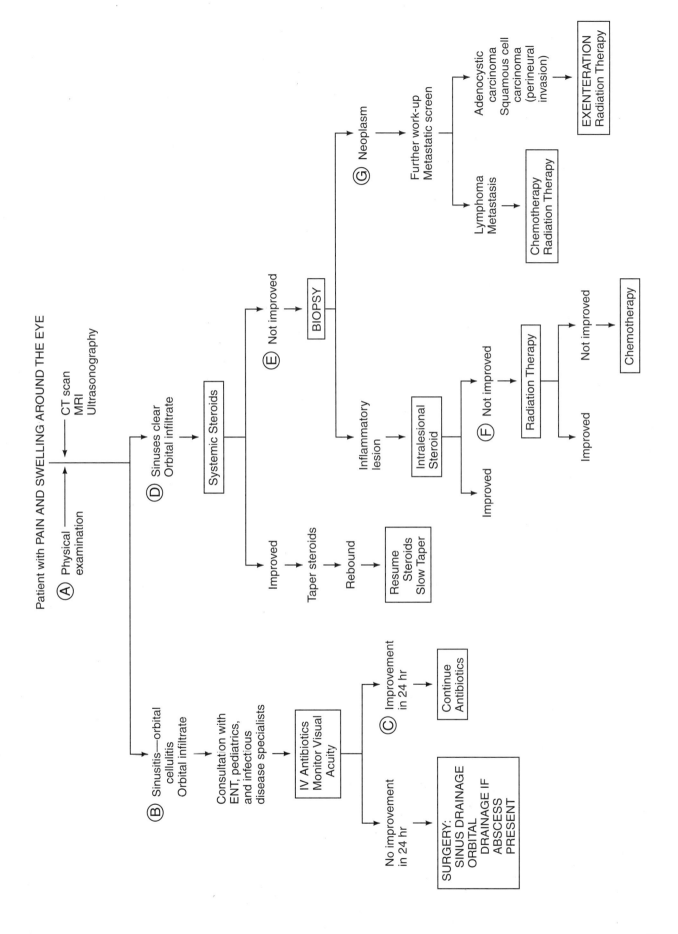

A — Physical examination

CT scan
MRI
Ultrasonography

B — Sinusitis—orbital cellulitis
Orbital infiltrate

Consultation with ENT, pediatrics, and infectious disease specialists

IV Antibiotics
Monitor Visual Acuity

No improvement in 24 hr

SURGERY:
SINUS DRAINAGE
ORBITAL DRAINAGE IF ABSCESS PRESENT

C — Improvement in 24 hr

Continue Antibiotics

D — Sinuses clear
Orbital infiltrate

Systemic Steroids

Improved

Taper steroids

Rebound

Resume Steroids Slow Taper

E — Not improved

BIOPSY

Inflammatory lesion

Intralesional Steroid

Improved

F — Not improved

Radiation Therapy

Improved

Not improved

Chemotherapy

G — Neoplasm

Further work-up
Metastatic screen

Lymphoma
Metastasis

Chemotherapy
Radiation Therapy

Adenocystic carcinoma
Squamous cell carcinoma (perineural invasion)

EXENTERATION
Radiation Therapy

89

EYE TRAUMA

Johan Zwaan, M.D., Ph.D.

The initial evaluation of a patient with eye trauma should be as complete as possible because decisions about diagnostic and treatment options hinge on it. At the same time, the evaluation should not worsen the ocular condition. A careful history is extremely important in directing the required therapeutic interventions. Emergency situations should be recognized and treated immediately, with the remainder of the examination being postponed if necessary. If the patient is cognizant, a visual acuity should be obtained for prognostic and legal reasons.

A. If the initial evaluation reveals any life-threatening conditions, the treatment of those takes precedence over the treatment of any eye injury.

B. If no light perception is present in a severely traumatized eye and enucleation is contemplated, it may be preferable to do a primary repair, repeat the visual acuity measures, obtain a visually evoked response (VER), and possibly get a second opinion. As long as the enucleation is done within 2 weeks after the initial injury, the rare complication of sympathetic ophthalmia can be avoided. Consider primary enucleation if a second general anesthesia puts the patient at risk.

C. An afferent pupillary defect (APD) implies dysfunction of the optic nerve or the retina. Whether dense media opacities, such as a vitreous hemorrhage, can cause an APD in the absence of optic nerve or retina damage is still being debated.

D. After a blunt injury the pupil first reacts with spastic miosis. Then, the spasm relaxes and traumatic mydriasis sets in.

E. Stretching at the iris root, usually by blunt trauma, may damage the circular iris blood vessels and cause a hyphema. The iris root can be torn off, leading to iris dialysis. Other sequelae are angle recession and rarely a cyclodialysis cleft. Initial treatment of any of these abnormalities is generally conservative, with definitive surgical repair postponed until the swelling has subsided.

F. Minimal sphincter rupture merely causes mild anisocoria with the sphincter function remaining intact. Severe trauma may lead to a dilated, nonreactive pupil. If the rupture is localized, a teardrop or sector deformity can result. A teardrop-shaped pupil may also result from prolapse, and if one is found, the presence of an open globe should be excluded.

G. Asymmetry of the pupil does not necessarily indicate trauma to the eye per se. A variety of neurologic insults may be the cause, some of which may indicate intracranial injury. If photographs dating to before the accident are available, they are useful in excluding pre-existing conditions. Pharmacologic causes for pupillary asymmetry may be obtained from the history.

H. If there is overt prolapse of the iris or the pupil is eccentric or peaked, corneal or scleral integrity may have been compromised and an open globe may be present. Defer further examination of the eye until an examination under anesthesia can be performed.

I. A ruptured lens leads to liberation of lens material into the anterior chamber, where it may induce phacoanaphylactic uveitis or phakolytic glaucoma. Lens removal (usually by aspiration) at the time of primary repair is indicated. A fibrinoid anterior chamber reaction can be prominent, particularly in children, and can mimic the release of lens proteins. It should be differentiated from lens rupture. Hydration of the lens through the capsular rupture can cause lens swelling and lead to pupillary block. The decision to remove a traumatic cataract or dislocated lens at the time of initial repair depends on visual acuity, the presence of other eye problems (e.g., hyphema, lens swelling), and other potential complications of the cataract (e.g., pupillary block). In many cases primary removal is not necessary, and a secondary procedure can be contemplated under more controlled conditions. Implantation of a posterior chamber intraocular lens in the capsular bag, if possible, or in the sulcus as part of the primary repair is becoming more common. Vitreous loss is common during removal of a traumatic cataract or dislocated lens and must be prepared for.

J. A conjunctival laceration or foreign body, a subconjunctival hemorrhage, conjunctival chemosis, a shallow anterior chamber in the absence of a corneal laceration, and a soft eye should lead to the suspicion of a scleral laceration. Shotgun pellet and other injuries to the eyelids may appear small and inconsequential externally, but they may have penetrated the globe through the eyelid. A high index of suspicion is necessary to avoid overlooking scleral lacerations. Ultrasonography (through the eyelids) and CT scanning are useful auxiliary tools. If any doubt exists about a possible scleral laceration, careful surgical exploration is mandatory.

K. Even the smallest pressure on an open globe can lead to extrusion of ocular contents. If an open globe is diagnosed or even suspected, manipulation may lead to increased damage and should therefore be avoided. Cover the eye with a shield for protection. If deemed necessary, give antibiotics intravenously rather than topically to avoid introduction of high and potentially toxic concentrations into the eye. When the patient is taken to the operating room, use general anesthesia rather than local anesthesia so that anesthetic solution is not injected into the eye. Once the patient has been anesthetized, muscle contractions are relaxed and the risk for squeezing ocular contents out of the eye lessens.

L. If possible, perform indirect ophthalmoscopy early so that continued hemorrhage does not blur the image. Avoid scleral depression until an open globe has been excluded. The pupil needs to be dilated for the examination, and this should be recorded clearly on the chart to avoid confusion with neurologic reasons for a dilated pupil.

M. If the vasculature is compromised with the optic nerve avulsion, which is usually the case, the disc and retina will be edematous. Blood may be present on the disc. A hole or crater may be seen at the level of the disc where the nerve was torn.

N. In central retinal artery occlusion (CRAO), vision is lost within seconds, usually because of embolization of the artery. Thrombosis, vasculitis, spasm, and dissecting aneurysm can also cause CRAO. There is an afferent pupillary defect, and the retina is pale and edematous with a cherry-red macula. Treatment within 60 minutes after onset may restore vision. The treatment aims at dislodging the embolus to a more peripheral arteriole by increasing arterial diameter (by carbogen inhalation) or reducing intraocular pressure (paracentesis, massage, IV acetazolamide).

O. Optic nerve injuries of any type are relatively uncommon. Compression of the nerve may result from dis-placed bone fragments of the sphenoid or, more commonly, from edema or hemorrhage. Imaging studies, in particular CT scanning, are essential in reaching the proper diagnosis.

P. Treatment of optic nerve injuries is controversial. IV steroids are helpful if given early.

Q. Consider decompression of the compressed optic nerve if IV steroids do not improve the clinical condition.

R. A chemical burn, especially an alkali burn, is an ophthalmic emergency. Start treatment by lavage immediately, even before the exact nature of the burn is known.

References

Alfaro DV, Liggett PE, eds. Vitreoretinal surgery of the injured eye. Philadelphia: Lippincott, Williams & Wilkins, 1998.

Kuhn F, Morris R, Witherspoon D, et al. A standardized classification of ocular trauma. Ophthalmology 1996; 103: 240–243.

Kylstra JA, Lamkin JC, Runyan DK. Clinical predictors of scleral rupture after blunt ocular trauma. Am J Ophthalmol 1993; 115:530–535.

MacCumber MW. Management of ocular injuries and emergencies. Philadelphia: Lippincott-Raven, 1998.

Shingleton BJ, Hersh PS, Kenyon KR. Eye trauma. St Louis: Mosby, 1991.

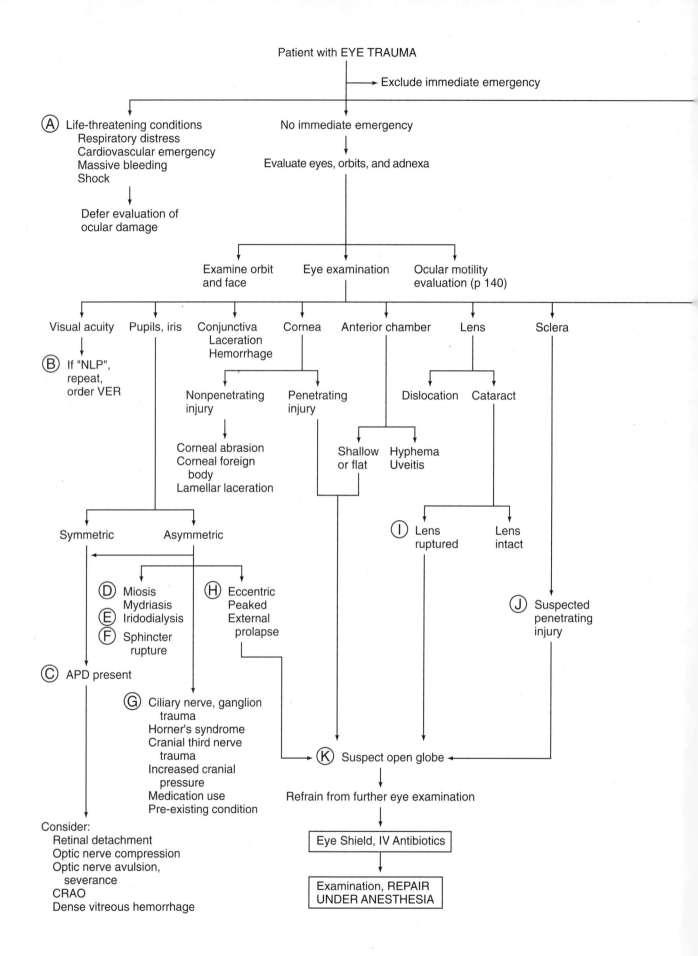

Patient with EYE TRAUMA

→ Exclude immediate emergency

Ⓐ Life-threatening conditions
Respiratory distress
Cardiovascular emergency
Massive bleeding
Shock

↓

Defer evaluation of
ocular damage

No immediate emergency

Evaluate eyes, orbits, and adnexa

Examine orbit
and face

Eye examination

Ocular motility
evaluation (p 140)

Visual acuity

Pupils, iris

Conjunctiva
Laceration
Hemorrhage

Cornea

Anterior chamber

Lens

Sclera

Ⓑ If "NLP",
repeat,
order VER

Nonpenetrating
injury

Penetrating
injury

Dislocation

Cataract

Corneal abrasion
Corneal foreign
body
Lamellar laceration

Shallow
or flat

Hyphema
Uveitis

Symmetric

Asymmetric

Ⓘ Lens
ruptured

Lens
intact

Ⓓ Miosis
Mydriasis
Ⓔ Iridodialysis
Ⓕ Sphincter
rupture

Ⓗ Eccentric
Peaked
External
prolapse

Ⓙ Suspected
penetrating
injury

Ⓒ APD present

Ⓖ Ciliary nerve, ganglion
trauma
Horner's syndrome
Cranial third nerve
trauma
Increased cranial
pressure
Medication use
Pre-existing condition

Ⓚ Suspect open globe ←

Refrain from further eye examination

Consider:
Retinal detachment
Optic nerve compression
Optic nerve avulsion,
severance
CRAO
Dense vitreous hemorrhage

Eye Shield, IV Antibiotics

Examination, REPAIR
UNDER ANESTHESIA

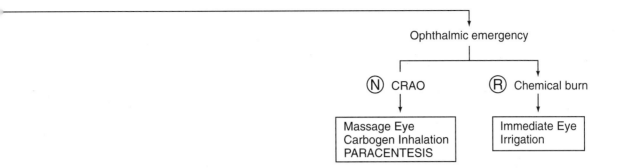

Ophthalmic emergency

Ⓝ CRAO

Ⓡ Chemical burn

Massage Eye
Carbogen Inhalation
PARACENTESIS

Immediate Eye
Irrigation

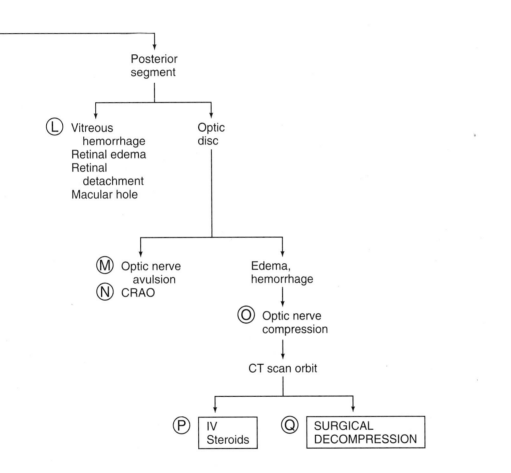

Posterior
segment

Ⓛ Vitreous
  hemorrhage
Retinal edema
Retinal
  detachment
Macular hole

Optic
disc

Ⓜ Optic nerve
  avulsion
Ⓝ CRAO

Edema,
hemorrhage

Ⓞ Optic nerve
  compression

CT scan orbit

Ⓟ IV
  Steroids

Ⓠ SURGICAL
  DECOMPRESSION

INTRAOCULAR CALCIUM DENSITY

Marilyn C. Kincaid, M.D.
Andrew W. Lawton, M.D.

A. Penetrating injuries of the globe, particularly when hidden by intact conjunctiva, often result in relatively minor patient complaints despite the presence of a retained intraocular foreign body. When a CT scan indicates fracture of the orbital bones, check the image of the globe for the possibility of an intraocular bone fragment.

B. Traumatic cataracts often develop calcification over time, especially when the original injury occurred in childhood. The location of the calcification on CT or ultrasound scan along with a clinically evident opaque lens helps make the diagnosis.

C. *Phthisis bulbi* is shrinkage and disorganization of the globe. Often, it is hypotonous as well, although later this may be less evident because of fibrosis and ossification. The shrunken globe also takes on a "squared-off" appearance because of the remodeling action of the rectus muscles. The intraocular calcification may develop into true ossification with fatty or hematopoietic marrow. Eyes with opaque media may develop occult intraocular neoplasms and should be evaluated with ultrasound or CT scan.

D. Massive gliosis of the retina describes a posterior segment mass composed of proliferating glial cells disorganizing and replacing the retina. The dilated blood vessels within the mass often develop calcification in their walls, and the mass itself may develop focal or diffuse calcification. This is a benign condition, requiring no surgical intervention.

E. Most retinoblastomas demonstrate small, diffuse foci of calcification on CT or ultrasound. Histologically, these calcific foci are found in areas of focal necrosis. Although calcification is characteristic of retinoblastoma, its absence does not rule it out.

F. Optic nerve head drusen can simulate papilledema, but CT or ultrasound readily discloses the drusen.

G. Episcleral osseous choristomas are typically found in the interpalpebral region and are completely benign. The confirmation of dense calcification can allay the family's fears.

H. Choroidal osteomas are classically found in the choroid posteriorly in women. The cause is obscure. They are elevated and yellowish and can simulate a melanoma or metastatic tumor. However, the presence of dense calcification confirms the diagnosis of osteoma.

I. Scleral plaques anterior to the rectus muscles, especially the horizontal recti, are common in older persons. No therapy is indicated.

References

Atta HR. Imaging of the optic nerve with standardized echography. Eye 1988; 2:358–366.

Henke V, Philip W, Naumann GO. Intraocular ossification in clinically unsuspected malignant melanoma of the uva in phthisis bulbi. Klin Monatsbl Augenheilkd 1986; 1989: 243–246.

Mansour AM, Barber JC, Reinecke RD, Wang FM. Ocular choristomas. Surv Ophthalmol 1989; 33:339–358.

Shields CL, Shields JA, Augsburger JJ. Choroidal osteoma. Surv Ophthalmol 1988; 33:17–27.

INTRAOCULAR CALCIUM DENSITY Detected during Imaging Studies

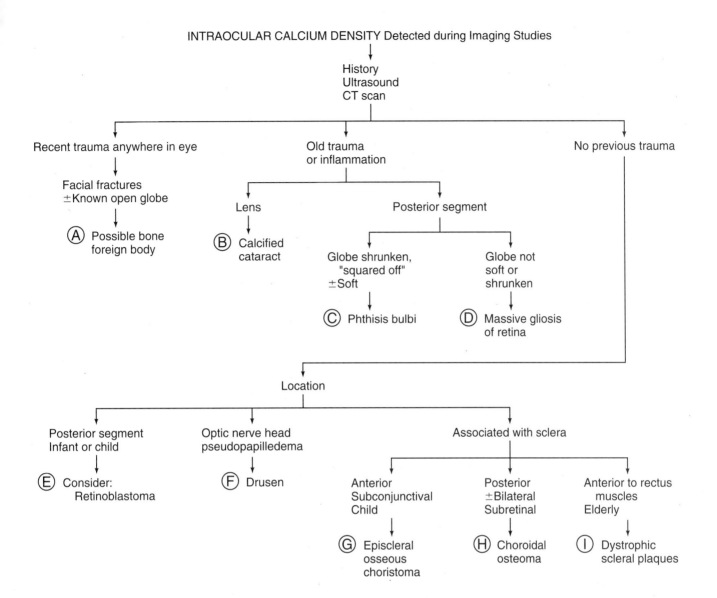

COMMON OPHTHALMIC CONSULTATIONS

DIABETES MELLITUS

W.A.J. van Heuven, M.D.

Checklist for Patients with Diabetes Mellitus

History

A. Date of diagnosis and insulin dependence
B. Type of vision disturbance (e.g., floaters, intermittent)
C. Diplopia
D. Pain
E. Dialysis
F. Hypertensive medications

General Physical Examination

G. Blood pressure
H. Weight
I. Carotid auscultation

Eye Examination

TEST	SIGN OR SYMPTOM
J. Best corrected vision	Vision improveable
K. Pupil examination	Reactive pupil
L. Muscle function	Diplopia
M. Test corneal sensitivity	Decreased sensitivity
N. Slit-lamp examination of iris, undilated	Rubeosis iridis
O. Gonioscopy	Rubeosis of angle
P. Indirect ophthalmoscopy, dilated	High-risk characteristics
Q. Direct ophthalmoscopy, dilated	Neovascularization of disc
R. Slit-lamp with precorneal lens examination, dilated	Macular edema
S. Photography and fluorescein angiography	Macular leakage

A. Type 1 diabetes, so-called insulin-dependent diabetes, usually starts before the age of 30 and is caused by an autoimmune destruction of pancreatic β cells. Eye disease of any type is usually not present for at least 5 years. Type 2 diabetes, so-called non–insulin-dependent diabetes, is caused by insulin resistance and represents most diabetic patients. It usually occurs later in life and has a strong genetic disposition. Diabetic eye changes, particularly retinopathy, are often present at the time of diagnosis.

B. The two most common visual symptoms of diabetes are blurring of vision and "floaters." Intermittent blurring is caused by fluctuations in blood sugar, which affect the hydration of the lens, which in turn affects the refractive state of the eye. The blurring is often present each day at the same time and is often related to food intake. Intermittent blurring may occasionally lead to the diagnosis of diabetes. Constant blurring of vision usually results from other causes, such as cataract or diabetic macular edema. Floaters in the visual field may represent vitreous hemorrhage in advanced diabetic retinopathy. In a known diabetic patient, vitreous floaters are highly significant and may indicate bleeding from proliferative diabetic retinopathy, meeting the criteria for laser treatment. Quick referral to an ophthalmologist is desirable so that laser treatment can be performed before the vitreous hemorrhage becomes too dense.

C. Diplopia may be caused by a mononeuropathy of cranial nerve III, IV, or VI. Third nerve palsy is the most common, and the eye is directed down and out. Ptosis of the eyelid may preclude diplopia. The pupillary reaction is usually normal, distinguishing this diabetic nerve palsy from more serious intracranial lesions. Mononeuropathy results from microinfarction of nerves that innervate ocular muscles. Complete recovery usually occurs within 9 months.

D. Eye pain is unusual in diabetes, except when corneal erosion is present or when acute glaucoma from neovascularization of the iris (rubeosis iridis) is present.

E. The history of dialysis should lead one to suspect advanced retinal disease. Dialysis often requires the use of heparin, which may promote bleeding from neovascular retinal vessels, causing vitreous hemorrhage and visual loss. Communication with the dialysis unit is important so that the use of heparin can be minimized.

F. Be aware of the systemic medications of the patient, especially antihypertensive drugs. Communication between the ophthalmologist and internist is important to ensure that blood pressure is kept well controlled.

G. Ophthalmologists should take blood pressure readings of all patients with diabetes and other systemic vascular disease. A higher-than-normal blood pressure reading should be reported to the referring physician because the combination of diabetes and uncontrolled hypertension causes rapid microvascular disease progression.

H. Most type 2 diabetic patients are obese, which is associated with hypertriglyceridemia and a reduction in high-density lipoprotein (HDL) cholesterol, both of which represent cardiovascular risk factors. Exercise and weight loss can be effective cures. Exercise, which is difficult for obese persons, becomes even more difficult if the patient is visually handicapped. The ophthalmologist can be helpful in recommending weight loss and exercise as part of a regimen that will decelerate the progression of microvascular disease.

I. Perform auscultation of the neck because obstructions of the carotid circulation increase the ischemia to the eyes, which can further increase neovascularization of the retina or iris. Occasionally, patients with minimal diabetic retinopathy may have iris neovascularization and secondary glaucoma (rubeotic glaucoma) not caused by diabetes but rather caused by obstruction of the carotid circulation.

J. A best corrected vision is important because periodic blurring from refractive changes related to hydration of the lens when blood sugar fluctuates needs to be differentiated from macular edema.

K. In a patient with mononeuropathy, the reactivity of the pupil will usually be intact and will be important to differentiate the cause of the nerve palsy from more serious intracranial causes.

L. Test extraocular movements to rule out mononeuropathies.

M. Diabetic patients often have decreased corneal sensitivity, so physicians should have a high index of suspicion when a diabetic patient complains of eye tearing, with or without pain, because a corneal abrasion, infection, or ulcer may be present.

N. Undilated pupillary examination is important to rule out the presence of rubeosis of the iris, a result of ocular ischemia. If present, the cause of the ischemia must be determined, whether diabetic or carotid. If the cause can be eliminated, possibly through carotid surgery, the rubeosis may regress. Otherwise, perform laser panretinal photocoagulation in the eye with rubeosis iridis.

O. Perform gonioscopy in all diabetic patients before dilation, at least once yearly, to rule out neovascularization of the anterior chamber angle, which may be present with or without rubeosis of the pupillary margin.

P. Do indirect ophthalmoscopy through a dilated pupil at every office visit to classify the degree of retinopathy present. High-risk factors, which would indicate that panretinal laser photocoagulation should be done, include the presence of neovascularization in the retina, neovascularization of the disc, and vitreous hemorrhage.

Q. Do direct ophthalmoscopy through a dilated pupil to rule out neovascularization of the disc.

R. Perform a slit-lamp examination of the lens and of the macula, using a precorneal examination lens, at every visit. Cataracts are more common in diabetic patients and may need to be removed surgically, not only because the patient may benefit visually but also because cataract removal will enhance the ability to diagnose retinal disease and treat when indicated. Macular examination will help diagnose macular edema, which, if clinically significant, should be treated with laser photocoagulation.

S. Perform standard retina photography of at least three areas (disc, macula, peripheral quadrant) once yearly to monitor the progression of details of the retinopathy so that early intervention can be done. Fluorescein angiography may be needed to differentiate neovascularization from normal vessels and to delineate specific leaks causing macular edema so that laser treatment can be adequately planned.

References

DeFronzo RA, van Heuven WAJ. Diabetic retinopathy. In: DeFronzo RF, ed. Current therapy of diabetes mellitus. St Louis: Mosby, 1998: 154–159.

The Diabetic Retinopathy Study Research Group. Report no. 8: Photocoagulation treatment of proliferative diabetic retinopathy: Clinical applications of diabetic retinopathy study (DRS) findings. Ophthalmology 1981; 88:583–600.

Early Treatment Diabetic Retinopathy Study Research Group. Photocoagulation for diabetic macular edema: ETDRS Report no. 1. Arch Ophthalmol 1985; 103:1796–1806.

Jacobson DM. Pupil involvement in patients with diabetes-associated oculomotor nerve palsy. Arch Ophthalmol 1998; 116:723–727.

ARTHRITIS

Marilyn C. Kincaid, M.D.

Checklist for Patients with Arthritis

Eye Examination

TEST	SIGN OR SYMPTOM
A. Best corrected vision	Vision improveable
B. Eyelid inspection	Skin lesions, lid edema
C. Conjunctival inspection	Injection, papillary reaction
D. Scleral inspection	Scleritis, episcleritis
E. Corneal inspection	Dry eyes, marginal ulcer
F. Intraocular pressure	May be elevated
G. Pupils	Irregular pupils, nonreactive pupils
H. Muscle function	Brown syndrome
I. Iris	Iritis, iridocyclitis
J. Gonioscopy	Peripheral anterior synechiae
K. Lens	Cataract, posterior synechiae
L. Ophthalmoscopy	Retinal ischemia, vasculitis
M. Optic nerve	Optic atrophy, optic neuritis
N. Visual fields	Glaucomatous, optic neuropathic, or CNS field changes

The term *arthritis* refers collectively to more than 100 different disorders, many of which affect the eyes. Indeed, patients often do not realize that their "joint disease" is really a systemic disease affecting many organs and systems, and thus they may not think to connect ocular symptoms with their arthritis. Typically, an internist, pediatrician, or rheumatologist will already have made the diagnosis and have the patient under care. However, occasionally, ocular manifestations may be the first evidence of rheumatic disease.

The ophthalmologist should be aware of the various ocular manifestations of rheumatic disease because some are potentially devastating to the eye and to vision. Moreover, certain drugs, such as systemic corticosteroids, antimalarials, and gold, used in the treatment of the various rheumatic diseases themselves have ocular effects.

A. Visual acuity may be normal but is often reduced because of intraocular inflammation, macular edema, optic neuropathy, corneal haze, or cataract.

B. Patients with rheumatoid arthritis (RA) may have rheumatoid nodules in the eyelids, as in the skin elsewhere. These are subcutaneous nodules of variable size that histologically are necrotizing granulomas. Systemic lupus erythematosus (SLE) causes a photosensitivity reaction. Discoid skin lesions can occur in systemic lupus also; these lesions consist of keratin plugs and surrounding superficial edema. Skin biopsy discloses immunoglobulins and complement at the dermal-epidermal junction. The typical "butterfly" malar rash may extend to involve the lids. The upper lids may show a horizontal band of telangiectatic vessels just above the lash line. Scleroderma, a fibrosing disease of skin and of viscera, can cause firmness and immobility of the eyelids, although this alteration does not usually cause exposure keratopathy.

C. The conjunctiva may be injected. Patients with gout often have chronically dusky-red eyes, involving both palpebral and bulbar conjunctiva. The precise cause is uncertain. In one series, 58% of patients with Reiter's syndrome had ocular manifestations, most often papillary conjunctivitis with a mucopurulent discharge. The conjunctivitis can also be follicular. It tends to resolve spontaneously without sequelae; symblepharon formation is unusual. Patients with RA who are taking gold, either orally or parentally, may develop gold deposits in the conjunctiva and cornea. These deposits are minute, gold to violaceous flecks in both the cornea and conjunctiva. They are not visually disabling and are not an indication to discontinue gold therapy.

D. Episcleritis and scleritis are also manifestations of rheumatic disease. Several different types exist; four varieties are seen in RA alone. Nodular episcleritis is comparable to rheumatoid nodules in the skin or elsewhere. A yellowish nodule is present on the sclera with surrounding deep vessel injection. Although painful, nodular scleritis is self-limited and does not imply ocular disease elsewhere. It is generally treated with topical steroid drops. Necrotizing scleritis is more serious. An area of the sclera shows blanching, consistent with a focal vascular closure. This phenomenon may herald vasculitis elsewhere in the body. Also, the necrotic sclera may thin and perforate. Scleromalacia perforans typically is bilateral and painless and occurs in older women with long-standing RA. Contrary to the implication of its name, the sclera only seldom perforates, but it does thin, baring the underlying uvea and allowing it to prolapse. Brawny scleritis is a massive granulomatous inflammation of the sclera, with considerable scleral thickening. The cornea can become involved as well. Brawny scleritis is usually unilateral. The deep episcleral vessels can be distinguished from more superficial vessels by placing a drop of 10% phenylephrine on the conjunctiva; conjunctival vessels will blanch, whereas deep episcleral vessels will not.

E. Keratoconjunctivitis sicca is probably the most common ocular complication of the rheumatic diseases. The patient may not complain of dry eye per se, but rather of sandiness, grittiness, or foreign body sensation. It can be isolated but is usually part of Sjögren's syndrome, an inflammatory reaction to lacrimal and salivary glands. Schirmer's test and rose Bengal staining are helpful tests. The latter gives a characteristic staining reaction lateral and medial to the cornea, staining surface cells that are devoid of mucin. Sjögren's syndrome can be primary or secondary. The secondary syndrome consists of either keratoconjunctivitis sicca or xerostomia associated with rheumatoid disease. It may progress to systemic lymphoma, although this is less likely with the secondary form. The cornea may develop melting in RA, usually in a peripheral location. This marginal furrow can extend to form a complete ring ulcer. There is little pain with this; the initial manifestation can be alterations in visual acuity consistent with alteration in corneal curvature. Keratoconjunctivitis sicca may predispose to corneal melting; however, the precise cause of the melting is uncertain. It can proceed to descemetocele formation and perforation; secondary infection may also occur. Patients with chronic anterior uveitis may develop band keratopathy. This is particularly common in patients with juvenile rheumatoid arthritis (JRA). Patients with gout rarely have corneal crystals that are possibly urate.

F. Intraocular pressure may be elevated by several mechanisms. Uveitis itself can cause glaucoma. The trabecular meshwork can be directly affected by granulomas. Inflammatory debris can also collect in the trabecular meshwork. Posterior synechiae and iris bombé may cause pressure elevation, as can peripheral anterior synechiae. Open-angle glaucoma can also occur on the basis of long-term steroid use in steroid-sensitive patients.

G. The pupils may be irregular because of posterior synechiae. As seen in anterior uveitis from any cause, the pupils may be relatively miotic and poorly reactive.

H. The superior oblique tendon has a synovial sheath and thus can, on rare occasions, be involved by RA. The result is a Brown's syndrome type of restricted movement of the superior oblique muscle.

I. Anterior uveitis is no more common in most of the rheumatic diseases than in the general population. However, it often occurs in disorders such as ankylosing spondylitis and Reiter's syndrome. In such diseases it presents as a typical uveitis with circumlimbal injection, pain, and cell and flare. The HLA antigen B27 is strongly associated; it is positive in ≥50% of patients with anterior uveitis (normal, <8%); in turn, about 1% of patients who are B27 positive have uveitis. An insidious variant occurs in JRA. The eye is deceptively quiet and painless, yet slip-lamp biomicroscopy discloses considerable cell and flare. Affected children tend to be girls ≤10 years old, with antinuclear antigen (ANA)-positive pauciarticular disease, although other forms of JRA (polyarticular, systemic; ANA-negative) may show ocular involvement less often. These children may have considerable ocular damage with a high risk of blindness if the uveitis is not detected and appropriately treated. Because there are no obvious signs or symptoms, such patients should be screened every 6 months.

J. Peripheral anterior synechiae, sequelae from long-term uveitis, may be evident.

K. Anterior uveitis can cause nuclear sclerosis, which can be quite dense. Corticosteroids can lead to posterior subcapsular cataracts. Cataract extraction may be necessary not only for visual rehabilitation but also to monitor retinal changes. Posterior synechiae can result from chronic anterior uveitis.

L. Retinal vasculitis is most often seen in SLE, polyarteritis nodosa, and scleroderma, and it often correlates well with the level of systemic disease activity and CNS involvement. Changes similar to those of hypertension, including cotton-wool spots and retinal hemorrhages, are often seen. Other findings include venous tortuosity, serous retinal detachment, optic atrophy, and microaneurysms. Less commonly, severe retinal vasoocclusive disease, including branch and central artery occlusion, can occur, associated with a poor visual prognosis. Depo-steroids, systemic steroids, or even immunosuppressive agents may be necessary to control the process. Posterior scleritis may give rise to a serous sensory retinal detachment, as can lupus choroidopathy. A case of optic nerve head neovascularization without retinal ischemia in ANA-positive pauciarticular JRA has been reported. Patients with polymyalgia rheumatica have a higher-than-average risk of temporal arteritis. Retinal findings include cotton-wool spots and central or branch arterial occlusion. Patients with gout may have a higher-than-expected incidence of asteroid hyalosis.

Patients receiving antimalarial treatment (chloroquine and analogs) may develop a bull's eye maculopathy, which is dose dependent.

M. Various types of optic neuropathy, including optic neuritis and optic atrophy, have rarely been reported in SLE. The cause appears to be vasoocclusion of the small vessels in the optic nerve. Optic neuropathy often correlates with CNS involvement. Visual outcome is variable.

N. Visual fields can show changes secondary to glaucoma or evidence of optic neuropathy. In SLE, there can be retrochiasmal field defects from CNS involvement.

References

Boone MI, Moore TL, Cruz OA. Screening for uveitis in juvenile rheumatoid arthritis. J Pediatr Ophthalmol Strabismus 1998; 34:41–43.

Chumbley LC. Rheumatologic disorders. In: Ophthalmology in internal medicine. Philadelphia: WB Saunders, 1981: 103–143.

Jabs DA, Miller NR, Newman SA, et al. Optic neuropathy in systemic lupus erythematosus. Arch Ophthalmol 1986; 104:564–568.

Lee DA, Barker SM, Su WPD, et al. The clinical diagnosis of Reiter's syndrome: Ophthalmic and nonophthalmic aspects. Ophthalmology 1986; 93:350–356.

HIV-POSITIVE PATIENT

Bailey L. Lee, M.D.

Checklist for Patients with HIV

History

A. Date of diagnosis
B. Opportunistic infections and malignancies
C. Type of visual symptoms
D. Medication history (e.g., antiretroviral therapy, protease inhibitors, anti-CMV medications)
E. Laboratory studies (e.g., CD4 count, viral load, renal function, CBC, head imaging studies)

Eye Examination

TEST	SIGN OR SYMPTOM
F. Best corrected visual acuity	Vision improvable
G. External examination	Lid lesions, proptosis
H. Pupillary examination	Afferent pupillary defect
I. Muscle function	Diplopia, limited motility
J. Visual field	Visual field defect
K. Intraocular pressure (IOP)	Decreased IOP
L. Slit-lamp examination of the anterior segment	Conjunctival lesions, corneal findings, inflammation
M. Slit-lamp examination of vitreous	Inflammation
N. Indirect ophthalmoscopy/slit-lamp biomicroscopy	Retinal lesions, disc edema, macular edema

A. The median time from exposure to HIV to the development of AIDS is approximately 11 years. Thus the longer the duration of HIV, the more likely one will develop the opportunistic infection and malignancies associated with AIDS.

B. AIDS patients are susceptible to opportunistic infections and occult malignancies that may have ocular manifestations. These include CMV, *Pneumocystic carinii, Mycobacterium avium* complex (MAC), cryptococcosis, tuberculosis, microsporidiosis, toxoplasmosis, candidiasis, Kaposi's sarcoma, and lymphoma. Remember syphilis as a cause of ocular inflammation.

C. Visual complaints depend on the site of the pathologic condition. It can range from blurred or decreased vision, foreign body sensation, photophobia, diplopia, and headache to flashes or floaters.

D. Patients with HIV typically take several medications. These can include a combination of antiviral and protease inhibitors for the HIV, also known as highly active antiretroviral therapy (HAART), and medications prophylaxis of opportunistic infections. Some medications may have ocular side effects. HAART may boost the immune system and cause ocular inflammation in patients with a history of CMV retinitis. Rifabutin, used in the prophylaxis for MAC, can lead to hypopyon uveitis, and treatment of CMV with cidofovir can cause uveitis and hypotony.

E. Laboratory studies can be helpful in following the immune status. CD4 counts <50 cells/mm^3 put patients at higher risk of developing CMV retinitis. Viral load is the newer parameter used to follow the immune status. These patients may have low blood counts or impaired renal function, which should be considered before choosing an anti-CMV medication. Head imaging studies are important to rule out orbital and intracranial abnormalities.

F. Complaints of decreased vision may simply be caused by a refractive error. When the vision cannot be corrected, the cause needs to be identified.

G. External examination may reveal proptosis caused by orbital inflammation or mass effect. Lid lesions such as Kaposi's sarcoma, *Molluscum contagiosum,* and herpes zoster ophthalmicus may be present.

H. Causes of an afferent pupillary defect include optic nerve disorders caused by infections such as CMV papillitis, syphilitic optic neuritis, and cryptococcal meningitis, or infiltrative disorders such as lymphoma. Also, a CMV retinal detachment can lead to an afferent pupillary defect.

I. Deceased motility may be caused by cranial nerve palsies from infections (e.g., cryptococcal meningitis) or infiltration (e.g. lymphoma). Orbital inflammation or masses can also restrict ocular movement.

J. Visual field abnormalities may be caused by retinal, optic nerve, or intracranial pathologic conditions. To exclude the possibility of intracranial causes, obtain a head imaging study.

K. The intraocular pressure (IOP) may be decreased or increased with intraocular inflammation. Cidofovir has been associated with hypotony. A retinal detachment can also cause decreased IOP.

L. Conjunctival findings include Kaposi's sarcoma. Corneal findings include infectious causes such as herpes simplex, herpes zoster, and microsporidiosis. An anterior chamber reaction may be present if there is vitreous reaction.

M. In the initial descriptions of CMV retinitis in AIDS patients, there was little vitreous reaction, presumably because of the significant immune suppression. However, this is not true today in view of HAART medications. Also consider *Toxoplasmosis,* acute retinal necrosis, and syphilis as causes of retinitis associated with vitreous reaction.

N. HIV retinopathy, a retinal microvasculopathy, is the most common retinal finding in AIDS patients, whereas CMV retinitis is the most common opportunistic ocular infection in AIDS patients. Counsel patients about the symptoms of retinal detachment and follow them closely for reactivation once the initial diagnosis is made. Serial photography is helpful. Progressive outer retinal necrosis, a variant of acute retinal necrosis occurring in the immunocompromised host, can be difficult to treat and may respond to antiviral therapy. Other infectious causes of retinochoroiditis include *Toxoplasmosis,* syphilis, *Pneumocystis carinii,* cryptococcus, and *Nocardia.* Also, if these patients have an indwelling catheter, there is the risk of endogenous endophthalmitis. There have been recent reports of HIV causing anterior and posterior uveitis as well as chronic multifocal retinal infiltrates that respond to antiretroviral therapy. Disc edema may be caused by an infection or an intracranial mass. There

have been reports of cystoid macular edema and serous macular exudation in patients with CMV retinitis.

References

Davis JL, Taskintuna I, Freeman WR, et al. Iritis and hypotony after treatment with intravenous cidofovir for cytomegalovirus retinitis. Arch Ophthalmol 1997; 115:733–737.

Graham K, Pinnolis M. AIDS and the posterior segment. Int Ophthalmol Clin 1998; 38:265–280.

Kupperman BD, Petty JG, Richman DD, et al. Correlation between CD4+ counts and prevalence of cytomegalovirus retinitis and human immunodeficiency virus-related noninfectious retinal vasculopathy in patients with acquired immunodeficiency syndrome. Am J Ophthalmol 1993; 115:575–582.

Ryan-Graham MA, Durand M, Pavan-Langston D. AIDS and the anterior segment. Int Ophthalmol Clin 1998; 38:241–263.

Zegans ME, Walton RC, Holland GN, et al. Transient vitreous inflammatory reactions associated with combination antiretroviral therapy in patients with AIDS and cytomegalovirus retinitis. Am J Ophthalmol 1998; 125:292–300.

SARCOIDOSIS

Marilyn C. Kincaid, M.D.

Checklist for Patients with Sarcoidosis

Eye Examination

TEST	SIGN OR SYMPTOM
A. Best corrected vision	Generally normal
B. Eyelid inspection	"Millet seed" skin lesions
C. Conjunctiva inspection	Whitish nodules
D. Sclera and episclera	Scleritis, episcleritis
E. Pupils	Irregular pupils, nonreactive pupils
F. Intraocular pressure	May be elevated
G. Muscle function	Pain on movement, diplopia, palsy
H. Cornea	Keratic precipitates, keratitis sicca
I. Iris	Nodules
J. Gonioscopy	Nodules, peripheral anterior synechiae
K. Lens	Cataract
L. Ophthalmoscopy	Choroidal, retinal, optic nerve, vitreal involvement
M. Optic nerve	Papilledema, neuritis, atrophy
N. Orbit	Lacrimal gland fullness
O. Visual fields	Changes consistent with glaucoma or optic neuropathy

Sarcoidosis is a multisystem disease of unknown cause. Virtually any organ can be involved by this noncaseating granulomatous disease.

The classic patient with sarcoid is a young, African-American woman. However, sarcoid does occur in white patients, in older individuals, and in men. Ocular involvement occurs in about 25% of patients and is more common in African-American patients with sarcoid (31% versus 8% in one series).

Sarcoid is primarily a diagnosis of exclusion because there is no specific test. The cause is unknown. A positive gallium scan and elevated angiotensin-converting enzyme (ACE) level help establish the diagnosis, along with the finding of hilar lymphadenopathy on chest radiography. However, hilar lymphadenopathy is not always present. The chest x-ray film may be normal, or there may be pulmonary fibrosis with or without lymphadenopathy. Gallium citrate tends to localize where T lymphocytes collect; thus the gallium scan tends to be more sensitive than chest x-ray study and tends to correlate better with disease activity. The lacrimal gland may also take up gallium. Although this test is sensitive, it is not specific for sarcoid. Other causes of granulomatous disease, especially tuberculosis, must be ruled out.

The ophthalmologist is in a position to make the diagnosis of sarcoid, both through recognition of the clinical findings and also by biopsy of periorbital skin, conjunctiva, or lacrimal gland, all easily accessible tissues. Patients may be referred to the ophthalmologist for such a biopsy. About 25% of all patients with sarcoid have ocular involvement, with or without symptoms. Ocular signs of sarcoid can precede pulmonary involvement, sometimes by years. Also, the course of the ocular disease does not necessarily parallel the systemic disease. Optimal management for preservation of sight and of life requires cooperation between the ophthalmologist and primary physician.

A. Visual acuity in sarcoid may be decreased as a result of variety of factors, including anterior segment inflammation, secondary glaucoma, cataract, and chorioretinal involvement. Cystoid macular edema is common with posterior uveitis. Vision may also be decreased from optic nerve and CNS involvement.

B. The eyelid, like skin elsewhere, may have small "millet seed" nodules. Other lesions include larger granulomata, which may be ulcerated.

C. Conjunctival lesions resemble those of the skin; small, yellow-white, round "millet seed" lesions that are primarily located in the fornix. These lesions are accessible and easy to biopsy. There can also be a nonspecific follicula conjunctival reaction. Random biopsy of these follicles, or even of apparently normal conjunctiva, is positive for sarcoid in up to 50% of patients with sarcoid. Because other diseases can cause granulomatous inflammation of the conjunctiva, special stains for fungi and acid-fast bacilli, and careful examination for foreign material, should be done.

D. Nodular episcleritis occurs in sarcoid. There is injection of the deep vessels overlying the sclera in the area of a scleral nodule. Histologically, these nodules are granulomas.

E. Pupils may be irregular or adherent to the lens because of granulomatous iritis. As with other causes of iritis, the pupil may react only sluggishly and there can be associated pain with photophobia.

F. Intraocular pressure may be elevated by several mechanisms. The uveitis itself can cause glaucoma. The trabecular meshwork can be directly affected by granulomas. Posterior synechiae and iris bombé may cause pressure elevation, as can peripheral anterior synechiae. Glaucoma can also occur on the basis of long-term steroid use in steroid-sensitive patients. Patients tend to have a poor response to antiglaucoma medications and surgery.

G. The cranial nerves can be affected in sarcoidosis; the most commonly involved is the facial nerve (cranial nerve VII), manifest as facial palsy. Extraocular muscle involvement is rare but has been proven by biopsy.

Signs and symptoms include diplopia and pain on movement.

H. The classic keratic precipitates are large, gray-yellow, greasy-appearing deposits on the posterior surface of the cornea, commonly called *mutton fat*. Histologically, these have been shown to consist of small granulomas, often with pigment. Patients with sarcoid may have a dry eye, secondary to lacrimal gland involvement. the corneal surface may therefore show small punctate erosions. Band keratopathy may occur because of the systemic hypercalcemia that often accompanies this disease.

I. Koeppe's and Busacca's nodules may be present on the iris surface at the pupil or within the stroma, respectively. These are whitish, solid nodules that histologically are foci of granulomatous inflammation. Typically, they are associated with active anterior uveitis. The anterior chamber reaction typically shows considerable cell and flare.

J. Gonioscopy may show nodules of ciliary body and peripheral iris that are not visible by ordinary slit-lamp biomicroscopy. Peripheral anterior synechiae, sequelae from long-term uveitis, may also be evident.

K. Long-term sarcoidosis and uveitis may cause cataracts. The lens may also become cataractous as a result of steroid therapy.

L. The retina shows inflammatory changes that are characteristic but not diagnostic of sarcoid. Similar changes may be seen in other diseases associated with granulomatous choroiditis. The retinal vasculature may show patchy or diffuse periphlebitis with hemorrhages. Dalen-Fuchs' nodules are small granulomata beneath the retinal pigment epithelium; they appear as yellow-white subretinal infultrates. Larger choroidal granulomata may occur, appearing as yellow subretinal elevated masses with irregular borders. They may cause a secondary serous retinal detachment. Granulomata may also be present within the retina or in the vitreous. The latter give a "string of pearls" appearance. Another unusual but classic finding is the "tache de bougie" or candle-wax drippings. These are discrete, small, pale perivascular chorioretinal infiltrates, present in about one third of all patients with biopsy-confirmed sarcoid. They can resemble the lesions of birdshot choroidopathy or multifocal choroiditis.

Cystoid macular edema can be the result of retinitis or uveitis, and is one cause of visual loss.

Neovascularization of the optic nerve head and of peripheral retina is unusual but has been reported in sarcoid. Secondary vitreous hemorrhage may occur. Treatment with corticosteroids, without photocoagulation, has been effective.

M. Of the cranial nerves, the optic nerve is second only to the facial nerve in sarcoid involvement. Although unusual, optic nerve involvement can be manifest without retinal lesions. Disc edema, granulomata of the optic nerve head, papillitis, optic atrophy, and retrobulbar optic neuritis are all possible manifestations. Optociliary shunt vessels are seen rarely with granulomatous inflammation of the optic nerve.

N. The lacrimal glands are involved in sarcoid in up to 6% of patients, and this is often bilateral. The lateral aspect of the upper lids shows a classic fullness, and there can be a secondary keratoconjunctivitis sicca. The palpebral lobe of the lacrimal gland can often be prolapsed forward and is easily biopsied; however, care must be taken to avoid severing the lacrimal gland duct. Apart from the lacrimal gland, orbital involvement is rare.

O. Visual fields can show any of the changes of glaucoma, evidence of optic neuropathy, or enlarged blind spot. Sarcoid can involve the pituitary region, and thus it is an important non-neoplastic cause of chiasmal visual field defects.

References

Chumbley LC. Sarcoidosis. In: Chumbley LC, ed. Ophthalmology in internal medicine. Philadelphia: WB Saunders, 1981:231–238.

Cornblath WT, Elner V, Rolfe M. Extraocular muscle involvement in sarcoidosis. Ophthalmology 1993; 100:501–505.

Galetta S, Schatz NJ, Glaser JS. Acute sarcoid optic neuropathy with spontaneous recovery. J Clin Neuro-ophthalmol 1989; 9:27–32.

Jabs DA, Johns CJ. Ocular involvement in chronic sarcoidosis. Am J Ophthalmol 1986; 102:297–301.

Karcioglu ZA, Brear R. Conjunctival biopsy in sarcoidosis. Am J Ophthalmol 1985; 99:68–73.

Vrabec TR, Augsburger JJ, Fischer DH, et al. Taches de bougie. Ophthalmology 1995; 102:1712–1721.

Weinreb RN, Lipson BK, Ryder MI, Freeman W. Diagnostic testing in ophthalmic sarcoidosis. Semin Ophthalmol 1987; 2:257–272.

HEAD AND FACIAL TRAUMA

David E.E. Holck, M.D.
John D. Ng, M.D.

Checklist for Patients with Head and Facial Trauma

TEST	SIGN OR SYMPTOM
A. History and symptomatology	Directs the examination
B. Visual acuity	Ocular, orbital or optic nerve damage
C. Afferent pupillary defect	Optic nerve damage
D. Intraocular pressure	± elevated in field of gaze antagonistic to entrapped muscle
E. External examination	Canthal dystopia, bony and soft tissue misalignment
F. Exophthalmometry	Swelling versus retrobulbar hemorrhage
G. Palpation	Bony step-offs, bony mobility, crepitus, malocclusion
H. Extraocular motility	Strabismus, paralytic and restrictive
I. Forced ductions and force generations	Strabismus, paralytic or restrictive, paretic myopathy
J. Visual fields and color vision testing	Optic nerve pathology
K. Eye examination	Anterior segment pathology, transmitted orbital pathology
L. Imaging studies	Bony orbital pathology, soft tissue pathology

Ophthalmologists are often the first specialists to evaluate patients with head and facial trauma. Many others are not comfortable evaluating ophthalmic injuries, which are commonly seen in these types of trauma. Early and proper ophthalmic evaluation will help prioritize which injuries should be addressed first and which ancillary studies are needed. Ophthalmic evaluation will be different in unconscious and conscious patients and should be accomplished only after the patient is medically stable for examination.

A. Although the history and symptoms may be nonspecific, certain complaints may assist in focusing the examination. Visual loss from blunt trauma may suggest optic neuropathy. Binocular diplopia in specific fields of gaze may indicate restrictive strabismus from orbital fractures or extraocular muscle contusions or a muscle paralysis. Significant pain while looking in extreme gazes may suggest extraocular muscle impingement and ischemia. Associated trismus or malocclusion may be associated with a trimalar or Le Fort fractures. Par-

esthesias in the distribution of specific sensory nerves may also pinpoint a specific site of injury.

B. Visual acuity is often an unreliable indicator. Often, patients will not have their glasses when they are evaluated. Lack of patient cooperation and associated injuries may preclude an accurate measurement of visual acuity. Certainly, unconscious or intubated patients will be unresponsive.

C. Pupillary evaluation for reactivity and evidence of an afferent pupillary defect (Marcus Gunn pupil) will give useful information until the patient is able to cooperate fully to determine the presence or absence of traumatic optic neuropathy (TON). If traumatic mydriasis or anterior segment trauma is observed in one eye, the presence of a "reverse" afferent pupillary defect may suggest TON.

D. Intraocular pressures (IOPs) may vary greatly. With elevated pressures, hemorrhagic chemosis, and facial fractures, a retrobulbar hemorrhage must be ruled out. In medial wall or inferior wall blowout fractures, extraocular muscle entrapment may be seen. In these instances, IOP may be elevated when the patient attempts to look in the opposite direction from the entrapped muscle.

E. External examination of the traumatized patient is often rewarding. In the periocular areas, in addition to ecchymosis and soft tissue swelling, malposition of the canthal angles may suggest soft tissue disruption or bony orbital wall fractures. Lateral canthal tendon displacement may suggest a trimalar of Le Fort 3 fracture. Similarly, medial canthal displacement may suggest an underlying Le Fort type 2, 3, or naso-orbital-ethmoid (NOE) fracture. Telescoping nasal fractures may demonstrate a characteristic nasal bridge depression. Associated observations of epistaxis or a CSF leak may also point to a fracture in the cribriform plate. Soft tissue telecanthus further suggests traumatic bony expansion or detachment of the anterior and posterior crura of the medial canthal tendon. Also, medial canthal trauma may involve the lacrimal drainage system. Early treatment of canalicular trauma is superior to delayed treatment. Hemorrhagic chemosis should lead one to suspect a ruptured globe, which requires surgical exploration and takes precedence over any associated facial or soft tissue pathologic condition.

F. Gross proptosis suggests a retrobulbar hemorrhage, especially with orbital fractures and a tense orbit. Exophthalmometry can differentiate true proptosis from soft tissue swelling. With lateral orbital wall trauma, exophthalmometers that fix to the frontal and maxillary bones should be used. If not available, looking over the patient's head from behind can give an approximation of proptosis.

G. Gentle palpation of swollen tissues may demonstrate additional pathologic conditions. Soft tissue crepitus suggests fractures along the perinasal sinuses, especially medially. Bony "step-offs" may be palpable along the orbital walls and laterally along the zygoma. Trimalar fractures and Le Fort 1, 2, and 3 fractures may also be associated with malocclusion. Mobility of the maxillary alveolar ridge associated with vertical facial lengthening may demonstrate a Le Fort 1 fracture. Evidence of an NOE fracture, with a depressed nasal and midface contour, and a step-off along the inferior rim suggests a Le Fort 2 fracture. Lateral orbital rim defects with malocclusion and vertical lengthening of the midface suggest Le Fort 3 fractures.

H. Extraocular motility measurements may demonstrate a restrictive or paralytic strabismus. In blow-out fractures of the orbital floor or medial wall, the inferior or medial rectus muscles may be entrapped. This would result in limitations of gaze in the opposite functional field of the affected muscle. Paretic muscles would result in motility limitations in the field of action of the affected muscle.

I. Forced ductions and differential IOPs are helpful to determine which muscles are entrapped, whereas force generations determine the paretic muscle. Following these tests, binocular diplopic visual fields are helpful in following patients with marginal findings to determine which are surgical candidates and which should be observed.

J. Visual field and color vision testing will help determine any additional optic nerve pathologic condition. These tests can be reliably conducted only in a cooperative, stable patient.

K. Anterior segment examination and dilated fundus evaluation are critical to determine the extent of the pathologic condition and visual sequelae after head and facial trauma. Evidence of globe rupture takes priority over associated orbital fractures or soft tissue lacerations. Carotid-cavernous fistulas may be seen. Anterior segment findings of pulsatile proptosis, arterialization of conjunctival vessels, chemosis, and elevated IOP may help make this diagnosis. In addition, evidence of an anterior segment or retinal pathologic condition may limit the overall visual potential.

L. After initial patient examination, associated studies may be indicated. Orbital and head CT scanning is the most useful ancillary test to determine the full extent of

bony and some soft tissue pathology. Thin axial sections of 1- to 1.5-mm cuts should be requested. Direct coronal views are more desirable than reconstructed coronal views. Caution should be taken to avoid MRI while it is unknown whether metallic foreign bodies are in critical anatomic locations. Also, in the acute setting, a bony pathologic condition is better visualized using standard CT scanning modalities. Occasionally, if evidence of an arteriovenous fistula is present by clinical evaluation and initial imaging studies, arteriography may be necessary. After metallic foreign bodies have been ruled out, MRI scanning may allow better evaluation of soft tissues, especially the optic nerve. Orbital and ocular ultrasound may also provide useful information in the acute setting and are good and economic adjuncts to CT and MRI scanning. External photography is invaluable when multiple observers are evaluating the patient or when the patient is being followed over time.

Once the patient's airway, breathing, and circulation are stabilized, most ophthalmic and associated head and facial pathologic conditions do not require emergency care. One exception is a retrobulbar hemorrhage causing central retinal artery occlusion. In this instance a canthotomy and cantholysis must be performed in the emergency room to relieve the elevated orbital pressure. If it is inadequate, surgical orbital decompression by an orbital surgeon should be done. Another exception is a ruptured globe, which requires surgical repair as soon as possible. Consultation by neurosurgery is indicated if CSF leaks are suspected or abnormalities in neuroimaging are seen (orbital roof fractures, air, blood, or contusions in the CNS). In addition, otorhinolaryngology (ENT) and oromaxillofacial (OMS) specialists should be consulted for midface trauma that is outside the scope of the treating ophthalmologist.

References

Deutsch TA, Feller DB, eds. Paton and Goldberg's management of ocular injuries. 2nd ed. Philadelphia: WB Saunders, 1985.

Dortzbach RK, ed. Ophthalmic plastic surgery: Prevention and management of complications. New York: Raven 1994.

Dutton JJ. Atlas of ophthalmic surgery. Vol. 2: Oculoplastic, lacrimal, and orbital surgery. St Louis: Mosby, 1992.

Homblass A, Hanig, CJ, eds. Oculoplastic, orbital and reconstructive surgery. Baltimore: Williams & Wilkins, 1990.

McCord CD, Tanenbaum M, Nunery WR, eds. Oculoplastic surgery. 3rd ed. New York: Raven 1995.

Shingleton BJ, Hersh PS, Kenyon KR, eds. Eye trauma. St Louis: Mosby, 1991.

THYROID ORBITOPATHY

Johan Zwaan, M.D., Ph.D.

Checklist for Patient with Thyroid Eye Disease

TEST	SIGN OR SYMPTOM
A. Visual acuity	Uncommonly reduced
B. Inspect eyelids	Lid lag, retraction; fullness
C. Inspect conjunctiva	Chemosis, injection over muscle insertions
D. Exophthalmometry	Proptosis; if not axial, exclude other causes
E. Pupillary reactions	Afferent pupillary defect
F. Motility examination, forced ductions test	Diplopia, restrictive hypotropia and estropia, positive forced duction
G. Slit-lamp examination cornea	Punctate staining, tearfilm deficiencies
H. Intraocular pressure measurement in primary and upgaze	Increase of at least 6 mm Hg in upgaze
I. Ophthalmoscopy	Swollen or pale disc
J. Visual fields test	Central or cecocentral scotoma with inferior altitudinal or nerve fiber bundle defect

Patients with suspected or proven thyroid orbitopathy are commonly referred for ocular evaluation to assist in the diagnosis of the disease or to assess and treat its complications. Graves' disease is the most common thyroid disorder associated with orbitopathy, but other thyroid abnormalities, such as Hashimoto's thyroiditis, can also result in orbitopathy. Of Graves' patients, 40% develop overt thyroid orbitopathy, but subclinical orbit changes are present in almost all patients. Generally, the orbitopathy becomes detectable within 18 months after diagnosis of thyroid disease. However, the onset of the orbitopathy is unpredictable and may occur before or many years after Graves' disease is diagnosed. It progresses slowly and stabilizes after several months or even many years, resolving eventually.

Initial complaints may be nonspecific, such as eye irritation, fullness of the eyelids, and tearing. The correct diagnosis of thyroid orbitopathy may not be made until the symptoms become more pronounced.

All signs and symptoms of thyroid orbitopathy are related to an immune-mediated inflammation of the soft tissues and muscles of the orbit. Acute inflammation is accompanied by edema and deposition of glycosaminoglycans. Fibroblasts produce hyaluronic acid and collagen, eventually causing a fibrosis of the orbital tissues.

Classification of disease stages is not very helpful because signs and symptoms vary among patients and do not follow an orderly progression. Patients are referred for consultation because (1) they have clear thyroid orbitopathy; (2) they have proptosis; (3) they have thyroid disease, but ocular manifestations are absent or minimal; (4) they have a condition often associated with thyroid disease (myasthenia gravis or other autoimmune disorders, e.g., superior limbic keratitis). For all of these patients the following parts of the eye examination are of particular importance.

A. Visual acuity decrease is not a reliable indicator. Exposure keratitis is often limited to the inferior cornea, not interfering with the visual axis until late in the disease. Ophthalmopathy is uncommon, and of the affected patients, one fifth have entirely normal vision.

B. External examination of the eyelids may yield the first indications of thyroid orbitopathy. Mild eyelid edema can be an early sign of dysthyroid eye disease. The eyelids may show lid lag (easiest tested by having the patient perform fairly fast vertical pursuit eye movements) or retraction of upper or lower lid. Early retraction may be mistaken for ptosis of the opposite eye. Lagophthalmos may cause exposure keratitis. There are numerous eponymous signs describing eyelid abnormalities, which are related to eyelid retraction. For the upper lid this may be caused by adrenergic overaction of Mueller's muscle or by fibrosis of the levator palpebrae. Similarly, fibrosis of the retractor of the lower lid or of the capsulopalpebral fascia may lead to lower lid retraction.

C. The conjunctiva may show conjunctival chemosis and infection early in the disease, particularly over the extraocular muscle insertions. Blood vessels in these areas may be dilated and tortuous.

D. Proptosis is the result of inflammation in the orbital connective tissue, edema, impaired venous drainage, and accumulation of glycosaminoglycans, particularly in the connective tissues of the extraocular muscles and the orbital fat. The displacement of the eye is axial, and proptosis in other directions necessitates excluding other causes. The proptosis is usually bilateral but often asymmetric. Unilateral proptosis is uncommon but does not exclude thyroid orbitopathy.

E. An afferent pupillary defect indicates optic neuropathy.

F. Diplopia is caused by extraocular muscle fibrosis, which results in limitations of eye movements and abnormal eye positions. In extreme cases the eye may be "frozen." The inferior rectus muscle is most commonly involved, followed by the medial rectus. Thus the diplopia is usually vertical and may have an uncrossed horizontal component. Forced-duction tests are positive for elevation and abduction of the eye. Restrictive fibrosis of the superior rectus and lateral rectus muscle is uncommon. Ultrasonography is very sensitive in detecting muscle enlargement even in early stages, when no overt eye findings are present. CT is useful. The lendinous insertions are not involved in thyroid orbitopathy, which differentiates the disease from myositis. Thyroid disease is the most common cause for adult-onset strabismus and should be excluded in all such patients.

G. Exposure keratitis may result from proptosis, eyelid retraction, or lagophthalmos. In addition, the lacrimal gland's tear production may be reduced or the tears may be abnormal. Perform fluorescein staining of the cornea and tear film testing at each visit. Ulceration and even perforation of the cornea may occur in extreme cases, but they are uncommon.

H. Later in the disease, intraocular pressure increases in upward gaze because of restriction of the inferior rectus muscle. This also happens to an extent in normal eyes, and the pressure rise should be at least 6 mm Hg to be meaningful. The absence of this phenomenon does not exclude thyroid disease.

I. Optic neuropathy occurs in only 5% of patients with thyroid orbitopathy but is a potentially severe complication. Vision loss can range from none (in about one fifth of the patients) to total blindness. An afferent pupillary defect is seen in one third of the patients, a swollen or pale disc in about half. Pattern reversal visually evoked potentials and color testing, particularly when done with the Farnsworth-Munsell 100-hue test, can detect early optic neuropathy. Visual field defects are common. The optic neuropathy is caused by compression of the optic nerve at the right orbital apex by swollen extraocular muscles. It may occur without significant proptosis.

J. Visual field defects consist of central or cecocentral scotomas. They are often combined with inferior fiber bundle defects, which sometimes are misdiagnosed as being caused by glaucoma. Inferior altitudinal defects or generalized constriction may be found.

References

Fries PD. Thyroid dysfunction: Managing the ocular complications of Graves' disease. Geriatrics 1992; 47:58.

Nugent RA, Belkin RI, Niegel JM, et al. Graves' orbitopathy: Correlation of computed tomography and clinical findings. Radiology 1990; 177:675.

Panzo GJ, Tomsak RL. A retrospective review of 26 cases of dysthyroid optic neuropathy. Am J Ophthalmol 1983; 96:190.

Shammas HJ, Minckler DS, Ogden C. Ultrasound in early orbitopathy. Arch Ophthalmol 1980; 98:277.

Spierer A, Eisenstein Z. The role of increased intraocular pressure on upgaze in the assessment of Graves' ophthalmopathy. Ophthalmology 1991; 98:1491.

Tallstedt L, Lundell G, Torring O, et al. Occurrence of ophthalmopathy after treatment for Graves' hyperthyroidism. N Engl J Med 1992; 326:1733.

OCULOPLASTICS

EYELID EDEMA

Kenneth L. Piest, M.D.

The eyelid easily accumulates fluid as a result of the laxity and extensibility of the subcutaneous tissue. Edema is not a diagnosis but a symptom of many pathologic conditions of both local and systemic origins. It is helpful to differentiate inflammatory from noninflammatory edema. In either case in the acute phase, the skin is tense and smooth. As resolution occurs, fine wrinkling of the skin develops. This can be an important sign in determining whether the condition is improving.

A. One of the first steps should be to determine whether ocular involvement is present. Inflammatory conditions of the conjunctiva or globe can affect the lids. Proptosis or motility disturbances indicate orbital involvement.

B. Many infectious processes often appear as unilateral edema. A localized mass below the medial canthal tendon suggests dacryocystitis. Tenderness above the tendon suggests sinusitis as a possible cause. Rarer entities include Chagas' disease, filariasis, onchocerciasis, and cat-scratch disease.

C. Most viral infections are self-limited. In severe cases involving herpetic infections, acyclovir is sometimes recommended. Consultation with an infectious disease specialist can be helpful.

D. Age, rate of progression, and location are important considerations. Rhabdomyosarcomas, the most common primary orbital malignancy in childhood, may mimic an inflammatory process. Carcinoma of the sebaceous gland may resemble an inflammatory process, particularly chalazion and blepharoconjunctivitis.

E. The eyelid is the most common site involved in ocular allergy. The extreme thinness of the lid skin makes the lid particularly susceptible to allergic inflammation. The allergic response may be caused by local agents such as contact dermatitis, sunlight, or insect bites or may be part of a generalized reaction such as urticaria or drug reactions. Involvement may range from mild erythema of the lid margin to diffuse lid and facial involvement.

F. Lymphomatous lesions, be it a pseudotumor or malignant process, may present bilaterally. Imaging is often necessary to determine the extent of involvement and the area to undergo biopsy. Immunologic surface markers can help in the diagnosis and treatment plans.

G. Generalized infectious diseases of a bacterial, viral, or parasitic nature may produce a toxic or allergic type of edema. Similarly, erysipelas and serum sickness also produce lid swelling.

H. Tumors may be mistaken for an edematous lid. Examples include hemangiomas, lymphangiomas, neurofibromas, and lymphocytic tumors. Close examination and history may provide a diagnosis. If a mass of uncertain origin is present, consider a biopsy.

I. Fluid retention in cardiovascular, renal, and endocrine abnormalities may produce lid edema. Edema of the lid is also common in pregnancy and the premenstrual period. Angioneurotic edema is a chronic condition of vasomotor origin of uncertain cause that affects the subcutaneous tissue. The attacks, lasting days to weeks, may be cyclic or irregular. A history of atopic disease, allergies, or endocrine abnormality is often discovered.

J. Blepharochalasis is a condition of unknown cause. It may appear at any time from infancy to adulthood but is most commonly seen between 10 and 18 years of age. Recurrent attacks of transient, painless lid edema that occur over time produce permanent tissue changes. Rare unilateral cases have been reported.

K. Trauma can produce hemorrhage and edema in the lids. Fractures of the skull can also produce hemorrhage into the lid area, especially in basilar skull fractures in which extravasated blood seeps along the floor of the orbit and into the lids.

L. Any local cause that impedes lymphatic drainage from the lid area can produce edematous changes. Scarring secondary to trauma or surgery may impair drainage, especially in the temporal region. Malignant disease, skin disease, or irradiation can also impede lymphatic outflow.

References

Duke-Elder S, MacFaul PA. System of ophthalmology. Vol. 13. Part 1: The ocular adnexa: Diseases of the eyelids. St Louis: Mosby, 1974: 11–23.

Font RL. Eyelids and lacrimal drainage system. In: Spencer WH, ed. Ophthalmic pathology: An atlas and textbook. 3rd ed. Philadelphia: WB Saunders, 1986: 2141–2312.

Orentreich DS, Orentreich N. Dermatology of the eyelids. In: Smith BC, Nesi FA, Lisman RD, Levine MR, eds. Ophthalmic, plastic, and reconstructive surgery. St Louis: Mosby, 1998: 485–530.

Roy FH. Ocular differential diagnosis. 5th ed. Philadelphia: Lea & Febiger, 1993.

Starr MB. Infectious and hypersensitivity of the eyelids. In: Smith BC, Nesi FA, Lisman RD, Levine MR, eds. Ophthalmic, plastic, and reconstructive surgery. St Louis: Mosby, 1998: 531–556.

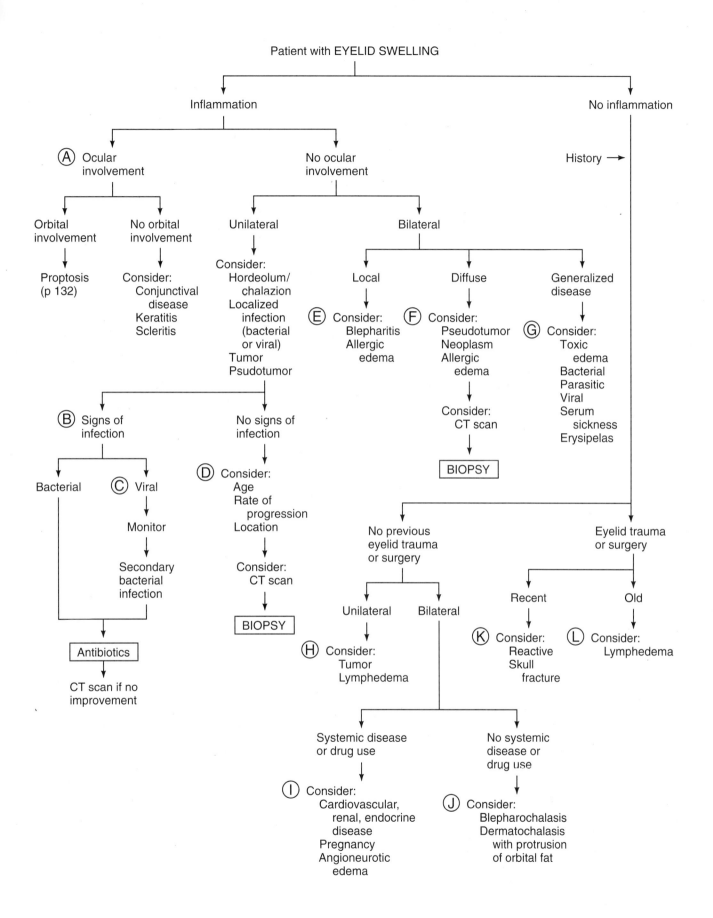

Patient with EYELID SWELLING

Inflammation

Ⓐ Ocular involvement

Orbital involvement → Proptosis (p 132)

No orbital involvement → Consider: Conjunctival disease, Keratitis, Scleritis

No ocular involvement

Unilateral → Consider: Hordeolum/chalazion, Localized infection (bacterial or viral), Tumor, Psudotumor

Ⓑ Signs of infection
- Bacterial
- Ⓒ Viral → Monitor → Secondary bacterial infection

Bacterial / Viral → Antibiotics → CT scan if no improvement

No signs of infection → Ⓓ Consider: Age, Rate of progression, Location → Consider: CT scan → BIOPSY

Bilateral

Local → Ⓔ Consider: Blepharitis, Allergic edema

Diffuse → Ⓕ Consider: Pseudotumor, Neoplasm, Allergic edema → Consider: CT scan → BIOPSY

Generalized disease → Ⓖ Consider: Toxic edema, Bacterial, Parasitic, Viral, Serum sickness, Erysipelas

No inflammation

History →

No previous eyelid trauma or surgery
- Unilateral → Ⓗ Consider: Tumor, Lymphedema
- Bilateral
  - Systemic disease or drug use → Ⓘ Consider: Cardiovascular, renal, endocrine disease, Pregnancy, Angioneurotic edema
  - No systemic disease or drug use → Ⓙ Consider: Blepharochalasis, Dermatochalasis with protrusion of orbital fat

Eyelid trauma or surgery
- Recent → Ⓚ Consider: Reactive, Skull fracture
- Old → Ⓛ Consider: Lymphedema

113

RETRACTION OF THE UPPER EYELID

Kenneth L. Piest, M.D.

The upper eyelid normally covers the superior limbus by 1–2 mm. The upper lid is considered retracted if the sclera is visible between the superior limbus and the upper lid.

A. Increased neuromuscular stimulation to the ptotic eye may produce a contralateral lid retraction. Perform an alternative cover test to assess the lid position of each eye.

B. Scarring or excessive skin removal in eyelid surgery can produce lid retraction. The shortage of skin requires grafting. Good donor sites include contralateral lid and postauricular and preclavicular skin. If anterior and posterior lamellar tissue are lacking, both will need to be supplemented.

C. Lid retraction is most commonly caused by thyroid disease. The patient typically has widened palpebral fissures, producing a stare appearance and evidence of lid lag.

D. The term *lid lag* refers to the delay of the upper lid in following the eye as it moves in downward gaze. It is a common finding in patients with thyroid disease.

E. Lid retraction secondary to lesions in the upper dorsal midbrain demonstrates Collier's sign. Midbrain retraction is usually bilateral and symmetric. The distinguishing feature is the absence of lid retraction in downgaze, as in thyroid disease. The common association with upgaze palsies and light-near dissociation of the pupils represents Parinaud's syndrome.

References

Burde RM, Savino PJ, Trobe JD. Clinical decisions in neuroophthalmology. 2nd ed. St Louis: Mosby, 1992.

Gay AJ, Salmon ML, Windsor CE. Hering's law, the levators, and their relationship to disease states. Arch Ophthalmol 1967; 77:157–160.

Smith BC, Della Rocca RC, Nesi FC, Lisman RD, eds. Ophthalmic, plastic, and reconstructive surgery. St Louis: Mosby, 1998: 1135–1138.

Rootman J. Diseases of the orbit. Philadelphia: JB Lippincott, 1988: 241–280.

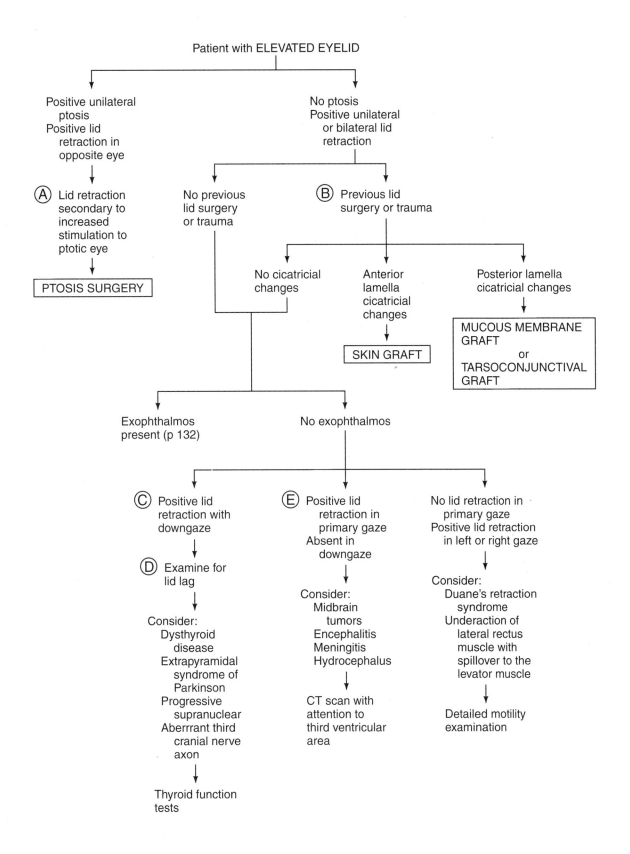

Patient with ELEVATED EYELID

Positive unilateral ptosis
Positive lid retraction in opposite eye

Ⓐ Lid retraction secondary to increased stimulation to ptotic eye

PTOSIS SURGERY

No ptosis
Positive unilateral or bilateral lid retraction

No previous lid surgery or trauma

Ⓑ Previous lid surgery or trauma

No cicatricial changes

Anterior lamella cicatricial changes

SKIN GRAFT

Posterior lamella cicatricial changes

MUCOUS MEMBRANE GRAFT
or
TARSOCONJUNCTIVAL GRAFT

Exophthalmos present (p 132)

No exophthalmos

Ⓒ Positive lid retraction with downgaze

Ⓓ Examine for lid lag

Consider:
Dysthyroid disease
Extrapyramidal syndrome of Parkinson
Progressive supranuclear
Aberrrant third cranial nerve axon

Thyroid function tests

Ⓔ Positive lid retraction in primary gaze
Absent in downgaze

Consider:
Midbrain tumors
Encephalitis
Meningitis
Hydrocephalus

CT scan with attention to third ventricular area

No lid retraction in primary gaze
Positive lid retraction in left or right gaze

Consider:
Duane's retraction syndrome
Underaction of lateral rectus muscle with spillover to the levator muscle

Detailed motility examination

DROOPING OF THE UPPER EYELID (PTOSIS)

Kenneth L. Piest, M.D.

Ptosis refers to a drooping of the upper eyelid. This can occur congenitally or be acquired from several causes. Various conditions that may either simulate a ptosis (pseudoptosis) or produce a secondary true ptosis (e.g., neurogenic, myogenic, mechanical) must be differentiated to ensure that proper correction and treatment are undertaken.

A. Ptosis is often described by several means: how much the upper eyelid covers the upper corneal limbus, the vertical lid fissure height, and the distance from the center of the pupil to the edge of the upper lid (marginal reflex distance) are the most common measurements. The marginal reflex distance is probably the best way to describe the degree of ptosis present.

B. Dermatochalasis may either simulate a ptotic condition or be present with true ptosis. The redundant skin may hang over the lid margin giving the appearance of a lowered eyelid. Motility disorders (e.g., Duane's retraction syndrome) may give the appearance that a ptosis is present. In all cases of ptosis, perform a detailed motility examination. Disorders that affect the globe position can also affect the lid position.

C. Congenital ptosis is thought to result from a defect in the development of the levator muscle or in its innervation. Of all cases of ptosis approximately 60% are believed to be congenital; bilaterality occurs 25% of the time. Simple congenital ptosis constitutes 75%–80% of all congenital ptosis. The Marcus Gunn jaw-winking syndrome occurs in 2%–6% of patients with congenital ptosis.

D. Myasthenia gravis is uncommon in childhood but should be thought of in ptosis cases. Three myasthenia syndromes are recognized in childhood. Transient neonatal myasthenia gravis is seen only in infants whose mothers have the disease. The infant is weak and hypotonic, has a feeble respiratory effort, and has ptosis. Persistent neonatal myasthenia gravis is identical to the transient form, but the disease is not present in the mother. The disease persists throughout life. The eyelids and extraocular muscles are usually severely affected. Juvenile myasthenia gravis is the third type. It usually presents after the age of 10 years, and females are affected six times more often than males. Ptosis and diplopia can be the presenting symptoms. The ptosis is variable and worsens with repetitive or sustained muscular contraction.

E. The Marcus Gunn jaw-winking syndrome is the most common congenital synkinetic ptosis condition. It is usually unilateral and more often involves the left side. It is rarely associated with other anomalies except a superior rectus weakness.

F. Ptosis may occur in a wide variety of syndromes. A few examples include blepharospasm and Homer's, Crouzon's, Saethre-Chotzen, and Goldenhar's syndromes.

G. Many disease states fall under the classification of acquired neurogenic ptosis. This ptosis results from the interruption of previously normally developed innervation. Homer's syndrome is relatively common and may be caused by tumors, aneurysms, inflammatory processes, injuries, or chest surgery. Ptosis may be produced by diseases of the third cranial nerve, multiple sclerosis, and various neurotoxins.

H. If a lid is thickened or misshaped, various lid tumors should be suspected. Neurofibromatosis commonly affects the lid. Fibromas, lipomas, dermoids, and tumors of the lacrimal gland may also involve the lid. Redundant skin in dermatochalasis may produce a ptosis or pseudoptosis.

I. Acquired myogenic ptosis results from either local or diffuse muscular disease such as muscular dystrophy, chronic progressive external ophthalmoplegia (CPEO), or oculopharyngeal dystrophy. Myasthenia gravis is actually a neuromuscular disorder but is considered myopathic in origin. Onset of myasthenia gravis may occur at any age and is most common in young women. It may be a generalized disease or localized to the eyes. Ptosis may be unilateral or bilateral. Variability and fatigability are the hallmarks. Perform Tensilon testing if myasthenia gravis is suspected. A negative Tensilon test does not exclude myasthenia gravis.

J. Acquired aponeurotic ptosis is caused by a disinsertion, dehiscence, or attenuation of the levator aponeurosis. The eyelid typically has a high lid crease with near normal levator function.

References

Callahan MA. Congenital ptosis. In: Smith BC, Nesi FA, Lisman RD, Levine MR, eds. Ophthalmic, plastic, and reconstructive surgery. St Louis: Mosby, 1998: 355–378.

Leone CR, Shore JW. The management of the ptosis patient: Part I. Ophthalmic Surg 1985; 16:666–670.

Leone CR, Shore JW. The management of the ptosis patient: Part II. Ophthalmic Surg 1985; 16:720–727.

Savino PJ, Schanzer B, Moster ML. Ptosis in neurological disease. In: Smith BC, Nesi FA, Lisman RD, Levine MR, eds. Ophthalmic, plastic, and reconstructive surgery. St Louis, Mosby, 1998: 345–354.

Siddens JD, Nesi FA. Acquired ptosis: Classification and evaluation. In: Smith BC, Nesi FA, Lisman RD, Levine MR, eds. Ophthalmic, plastic, and reconstructive surgery. St Louis, Mosby 1998: 379–394.

Siddens JD, Nesi FA. Management of acquired ptosis: Classification and evaluation. In: Smith BC, Nesi FA, Lisman RD, Levine MR, eds. Ophthalmic, plastic, and reconstructive surgery. St Louis, Mosby 1998: 395–407.

Small RG, Sabates NR, Burrows D. The measurement and definition of ptosis. Ophthalmic Plast Reconstr Surg 1989; 5:171–175.

Patient with DROOPY EYELID

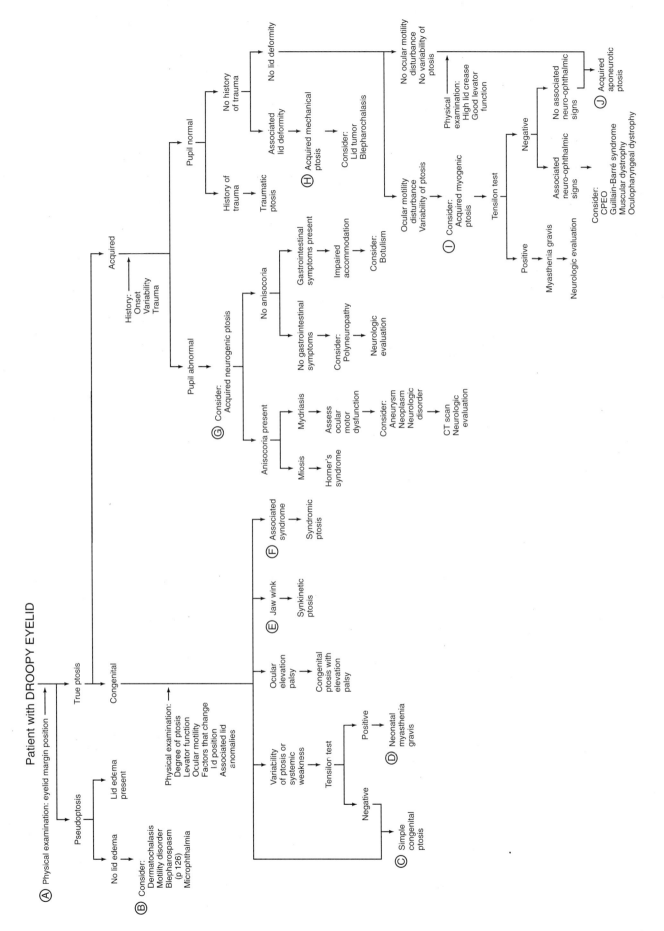

A. Physical examination: eyelid margin position

Pseudoptosis

B. Consider:
Dermatochalasis
Motility disorder
Blepharospasm (p 126)
Microphthalmia

No lid edema

Lid edema present

True ptosis

Congenital

Physical examination:
Degree of ptosis
Levator function
Ocular motility
Factors that change lid position
Associated lid anomalies

Variability of ptosis or systemic weakness → Tension test
- Positive → D. Neonatal myasthenia gravis
- Negative → C. Simple congenital ptosis

Ocular elevation palsy → Congenital ptosis with elevation palsy

E. Jaw wink → Synkinetic ptosis

F. Associated syndrome → Syndromic ptosis

Acquired

History:
Onset
Variability
Trauma

Pupil abnormal

G. Consider: Acquired neurogenic ptosis

Anisocoria present
- Miosis → Horner's syndrome
- Mydriasis → Assess ocular motor dysfunction → Consider: Aneurysm, Neoplasm, Neurologic disorder → CT scan, Neurologic evaluation

No anisocoria
- No gastrointestinal symptoms → Consider: Polyneuropathy → Neurologic evaluation
- Gastrointestinal symptoms present → Impaired accommodation → Consider: Botulism

Pupil normal

History of trauma → Traumatic ptosis

No history of trauma
- Associated lid deformity → H. Acquired mechanical ptosis → Consider: Lid tumor, Blepharochalasis
- No lid deformity

No ocular motility disturbance
No variability of ptosis

Ocular motility disturbance
Variability of ptosis → I. Consider: Acquired myogenic ptosis → Tension test
- Positive → Myasthenia gravis → Neurologic evaluation
- Negative
  - No associated neuro-ophthalmic signs → J. Acquired aponeurotic ptosis
  - Associated neuro-ophthalmic signs → Consider: CPEO, Guillain-Barré syndrome, Muscular dystrophy, Oculopharyngeal dystrophy

Physical examination:
High lid crease
Good levator function

117

ACQUIRED ECTROPION

Kenneth L. Piest, M.D.

A. Approximately 75% of patients who acquire a seventh nerve palsy have a complete or satisfactory return of function. If the palsy is of recent onset, lubrication and temporizing measures to protect the globe may be sufficient. If the lower lid function does not improve and the ectropion persists, it can be treated as a severe lower lid laxity.

B. A deficiency of lid skin produces a cicatricial ectropion. This shortage of anterior lamellar tissue must be replaced. It can have numerous causes, including skin removal after blepharoplasty, burns, irradiation, or inflammatory conditions.

C. Involutional ectropion is caused by laxity of the canthal tendons. Laxity of the lower eyelid is evaluated by pulling the lid downward and observing how quickly it snaps back into position. Lack of elevation upon release indicates horizontal laxity. Pinching full-thickness lid tissues together estimates the amount of redundant lid. Lateral laxity of the canthal tendon is measured by pulling the lateral canthus nasally. The lateral canthus should have only minimal movement. Displacement past the limbus indicates attenuation of the tendon. The medial canthal tendon is evaluated in a similar fashion by pulling laterally. A combination of medial and lateral laxity is common, and often both need to be corrected during eyelid repair.

D. Horizontal tightening of the lid can be performed in several ways. The exact method depends on the degree of laxity present. Mild cases may simply require plication of the tendon. Most often, removing a full-thickness segment of lateral lid is required.

E. Medial canthal laxity must be corrected before tightening the lateral canthal tendon. Otherwise, the punctum can be displaced temporally. If eversion of the punctum persists after correction of the medial or lateral laxity, additional techniques of punctal repositioning may be required.

References

Bosniak SL, Zilkha MC. Ectropion. In: Smith BC, Nesi FA, Lisman RD, Levine MR, eds. Ophthalmic, plastic, and reconstructive surgery. St Louis: Mosby, 1998: 290–307.

Jordan DR, Anderson RL. The lateral tarsal strip revisited. Arch Ophthalmol 1989; 107:604–606.

Neuhaus RW. Anatomical basis of "senile" ectropion. Ophthalmic Plast Reconstr Surg 1985; 1:87–89.

Patient with OUTWARD ROTATION OF (EVERTED) EYELID MARGIN

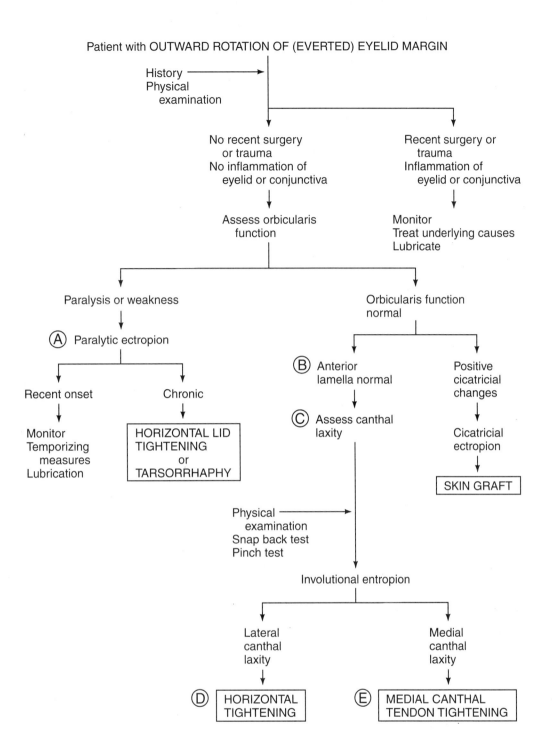

History ──────→
Physical
    examination

No recent surgery
or trauma
No inflammation of
eyelid or conjunctiva

Recent surgery or
trauma
Inflammation of
eyelid or conjunctiva

Assess orbicularis
function

Monitor
Treat underlying causes
Lubricate

Paralysis or weakness

Orbicularis function
normal

Ⓐ Paralytic ectropion

Ⓑ Anterior
lamella normal

Positive
cicatricial
changes

Recent onset

Chronic

Ⓒ Assess canthal
laxity

Cicatricial
ectropion

Monitor
Temporizing
    measures
Lubrication

HORIZONTAL LID
TIGHTENING
or
TARSORRHAPHY

SKIN GRAFT

Physical ──────→
examination
Snap back test
Pinch test

Involutional entropion

Lateral
canthal
laxity

Medial
canthal
laxity

Ⓓ HORIZONTAL
TIGHTENING

Ⓔ MEDIAL CANTHAL
TENDON TIGHTENING

ACQUIRED ENTROPION

Kenneth L. Piest, M.D.

A. Acute spastic entropion follows swelling of the eyelid from ocular irritation or inflammatory causes. The condition usually resolves when the cycle is broken by treating both the underlying cause and the entropion. Temporary measures such as taping the lid to evert the margin or everting suture techniques may be required until the edema resolves. Often, underlying involutional changes must be evaluated and treated appropriately.

B. The digital eversion test is a simple maneuver to help distinguish the cicatricial from the involutional entropion. Digital pressure near the inferior border of the tarsus easily everts the lid margin with involutional changes but not with cicatricial changes.

C. Involutional entropion is the most common type of entropion encountered. Many procedures have been described for correction of entropion. Several main factors are involved. The lower lid retractors have become attenuated and fail to pull the lower lid down and outward; the atrophy of orbital fat associated with aging produces a relative enophthalmos that reduces support of the lower lid against the globe; preseptal orbicularis becomes less fixed and overrides onto the tarsus inverting it; and the medial and lateral canthal tendons become lax, reducing horizontal support. One must examine all of these contributing factors and correct each to effect a cure.

D. Cicatricial entropion is caused by the shortening of the posterior lamella of the eyelid. The effectiveness of treatment depends primarily on the cause and severity. In inflammatory and autoimmune disorders, the prognosis is poor. In surgical or traumatic causes, the prognosis is much better. Management involves marginal rotation techniques and supplementation of the deficient posterior lamella.

References

Benger RS, Frueh BR. Involutional entropion: A review of the management. Ophthalmic Surg 1987; 18:140–142.

Kohn R. Textbook of ophthalmic plastic and reconstructive surgery. Philadelphia: Lea & Febiger, 1988.

Levine MR, El-Towchy E, Schaefer AJ. Entropion. In: Smith BC, Nesi FA, Lisman RD, Levine MR, eds. Ophthalmic, plastic, and reconstructive surgery. St Louis: Mosby, 1998: 271–289.

McCord CD, Tanenbaum M, Dryden RM, Doxanas MT. Eyelid malpositions: Entropion, eyelid margin deformity and trichiasis, ectropion, and facial nerve palsy. In: McCord CD, Tanenbaum M, eds. Oculoplastic surgery. 2nd ed. New York: Raven, 1987: 279–324.

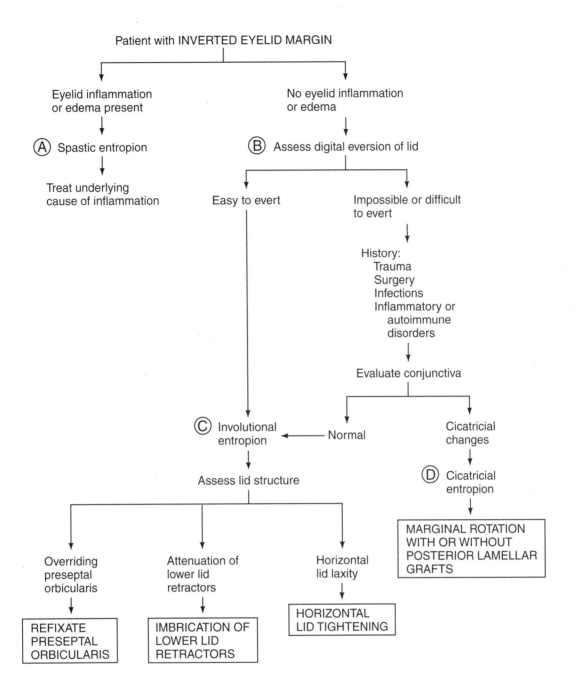

Patient with INVERTED EYELID MARGIN

Eyelid inflammation or edema present

Ⓐ Spastic entropion

Treat underlying cause of inflammation

No eyelid inflammation or edema

Ⓑ Assess digital eversion of lid

Easy to evert

Impossible or difficult to evert

History:
Trauma
Surgery
Infections
Inflammatory or autoimmune disorders

Evaluate conjunctiva

Normal

Cicatricial changes

Ⓒ Involutional entropion

Ⓓ Cicatricial entropion

Assess lid structure

MARGINAL ROTATION WITH OR WITHOUT POSTERIOR LAMELLAR GRAFTS

Overriding preseptal orbicularis

Attenuation of lower lid retractors

Horizontal lid laxity

REFIXATE PRESEPTAL ORBICULARIS

IMBRICATION OF LOWER LID RETRACTORS

HORIZONTAL LID TIGHTENING

UPPER EYELID RECONSTRUCTION

Kenneth L. Piest, M.D.

Closure of upper eyelid defects must not only provide the structural base of the lid but also maintain functional properties to ensure the integrity of the eye. Techniques can be grouped into those using adjacent tissue, opposing eyelid tissue, and remote tissue.

A. It is important to reconstruct the lateral canthal area if disrupted. If the inferior limb of the lateral canthal tendon remains, tissue can be sutured to the remaining tendon. Otherwise, posterior fixation must be accomplished by placing attachments to the orbital rim as close to the orbital tubercle as possible and securing them to periosteum. If placement is too anterior, the lid will be displaced away from the globe.

B. The lacrimal drainage system may be destroyed by medially located lesions. Reconstruction depends on the remaining segments. If the remaining portion of the canaliculus can be repaired, perform silicone intubation and anastomose the segments. If canalicular length is insufficient to allow full reconstruction, it is still useful to intubate the remaining system. Epithelialization around the tube is possible, and if additional reconstruction is performed later, the tube will serve as a guide in locating the remainder of the lacrimal system. Avoid violation of the periosteum and bone in the immediate postoperative period if the defect is caused by tumor excision. Reconstruction of the medial canthal attachments also requires posterior placement to maintain the correct globe-lid relationship.

C. Given the same defect size and lid laxity, direct closure cannot be accomplished on as large a defect in the upper lid as the lower lid even when a canthotomy and cantholysis are performed.

D. When the defect involves the central portion of the lid with remaining tarsus on either side, the Tenzel semicircular rotational flap works well. The curve of the flap is inferiorly directed in upper lid defects.

E. Isolated medial or lateral defects can be reconstructed without using lower lid tissue. A section of remaining tarsus and conjunctiva can be slid horizontally into the defect and the anterior lamella covered with a free skin graft or an adjacent skin-muscle flap. A lateral defect may also be closed with a lid-sharing Hewes-Beard tarsoconjunctival flap. A tarsoconjunctival strip is taken from the lower lid and swung into the upper lid defect. Blood supply comes from the lateral hinge, which is cut later. Anterior lamella is again reconstructed from skin-muscle flaps or grafts. A full-thickness rotational flap can be created by the Mustarde pedicle flap. A full-thickness lid pedicle flap is taken from the lower lid and rotated into the upper lid defect. This provides both good function and eyelashes. The lower lid is reconstructed with a rotational flap.

F. The Cutler-Beard or bridge flap can reconstruct large full-thickness eyelid defects. Because this graft does not contain tarsus, some have modified the technique by inserting cartilage. The Leone tarsoconjunctival flap also can be used for large defects using both residual upper tissue and a donor lower lid flap. Composite grafting is an alternative technique. Grafts can be harvested from the opposite lid. The musculocutaneous layer is removed, but the lid margin and lashes are preserved. The anterior lamella is closed by a skin-muscle flap, which also provides blood supply to the graft.

G. The Mustarde rotational cheek flap can be used to reform either the upper or lower lid. However, scarring may be significant. Often, a combination of techniques is required to reconstruct extensive defects.

References

Frueh BR. Upper eyelid reconstruction. In: Stewart WB, ed. Ophthalmic, plastic and reconstructive surgery. San Francisco: American Academy of Ophthalmology, 1984: 258–264.

Kohn R. Textbook of ophthalmic, plastic and reconstructive surgery. Philadelphia: Lea & Febiger, 1988.

Kwitko EM, Nesi FA. Eyelid and ocular adnexal reconstruction. In: Smith BC, Nesi FA, Lisman RD, Levine MD, eds. Ophthalmic, plastic, and reconstructive surgery. St Louis: Mosby, 1998: 576–608.

McCord CD, Wesley R. Reconstruction of the upper eyelid and medial canthus. In: McCord CD, Tanenbaum M, eds. Oculoplastic surgery. New York: Raven, 1987: 73–93.

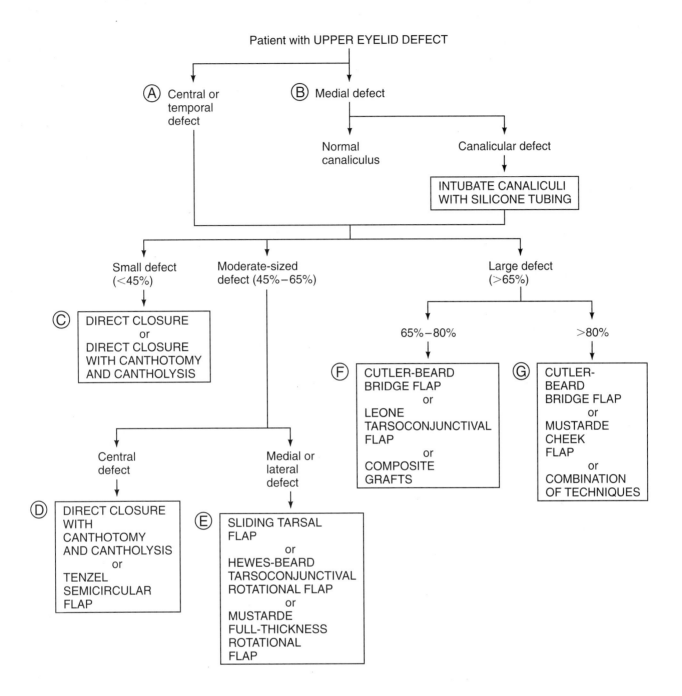

Patient with UPPER EYELID DEFECT

(A) Central or temporal defect

(B) Medial defect

Normal canaliculus

Canalicular defect

INTUBATE CANALICULI WITH SILICONE TUBING

Small defect (<45%)

Moderate-sized defect (45%–65%)

Large defect (>65%)

(C) DIRECT CLOSURE or DIRECT CLOSURE WITH CANTHOTOMY AND CANTHOLYSIS

65%–80%

>80%

(F) CUTLER-BEARD BRIDGE FLAP or LEONE TARSOCONJUNCTIVAL FLAP or COMPOSITE GRAFTS

(G) CUTLER-BEARD BRIDGE FLAP or MUSTARDE CHEEK FLAP or COMBINATION OF TECHNIQUES

Central defect

Medial or lateral defect

(D) DIRECT CLOSURE WITH CANTHOTOMY AND CANTHOLYSIS or TENZEL SEMICIRCULAR FLAP

(E) SLIDING TARSAL FLAP or HEWES-BEARD TARSOCONJUNCTIVAL ROTATIONAL FLAP or MUSTARDE FULL-THICKNESS ROTATIONAL FLAP

LOWER EYELID RECONSTRUCTION

Kenneth L. Piest, M.D.

Anatomically, the eyelid may be divided into two planes: the anterior lamella, consisting of skin and orbicularis muscle, and the posterior lamella, consisting of tarsus and conjunctiva. In reconstruction of the eyelid, this bilamellar construction must be respected. If an anterior lamellar defect has been created, it must be replaced with similar tissue from either a free graft or a flap. The same is true if posterior lamellar tissue is absent. If both lamellae have been sacrificed, both must be reconstructed. The lower lid is a less dynamic structure than the upper lid. Loss of a large area of the lower lid can be well tolerated, but loss of a small portion of the upper lid can lead to severe exposure problems and possible loss of the globe. Although lid-sharing techniques are available for both upper and lower lid reconstruction, some surgeons do not advocate using the upper lid for reconstruction of the lower lid. However, if done properly, lid-sharing procedures are time tested, giving excellent results. Many procedures and variations exist in lid repair. Only a few reliable examples are mentioned here.

A. Defects of any size in the nasal aspect of the lid may involve the canaliculus. If the canaliculus is involved and can be salvaged, intubate with silicone tubes. If the entire upper lacrimal system is lost and cannot be repaired, perform reconstruction without canalicular repair. While defects from tumor excision are being repaired, do not perform any further lacrimal surgery, other than canalicular intubation. Allow significant time to elapse to rule out tumor recurrence before violating the natural barriers of periosteum and bone.

B. Defects of <45% can often be repaired by direct closure. The exact size of the defect that can be reapproximated varies according to the degree of tissue elasticity. If the defect is too large for direct closure, the lower limb of the lateral canthal tendon can be released to mobilize additional tissue.

C. In defects that cannot be closed primarily, a semicircular rotational flap of Tenzel may be prepared. A semicircular sliding flap provides more tissue length than a horizontal incision. An inferior cantholysis is performed, and the flap advanced. The wound is then closed primarily. Canthal reconstruction is important in any repair to maintain normal appearance and function of the eyelid.

D. In large defects involving ≥65% of the lower lid, a number of procedures may be used. Lid-sharing techniques provide good tissue, but care must be taken not to threaten upper lid function. The modified Hughes tarsoconjunctival flap provides good cosmesis and lid function. This lid-sharing technique is a two-stage procedure. The first stage brings the tarsoconjunctival flap from the upper lid into the lower lid defect. Anterior lamella is reconstructed with a skin flap or graft. After 6–8 weeks the bridging flap is opened. This type of repair is not used in children in the amblyopic age range. A Hewes-Beard tarsoconjunctival flap, also a two-stage procedure, is useful in shallow defects in the temporal area. This bridging flap does not occlude the visual axis. Composite grafting may be used alone or in conjunction with other techniques. The free graft is taken from the contralateral lid. The anterior lamella is removed, leaving the lid margin and posterior lamella intact. After the graft is secured, a sliding skin-muscle flap is placed anteriorly. The Mustarde flap is a full-thickness rotational cheek flap that can be used to reconstruct large defects. It allows complete lid reconstruction in a one-stage procedure. After the flap is brought into the defect, the posterior lamella must be formed with grafts or flaps.

References

Kohn R. Textbook of ophthalmic plastic and reconstructive surgery. Philadelphia: Lea & Febiger, 1988.

Kwitko EM, Nesi FA. Eyelid and ocular adnexal reconstruction. In Smith BC, Nesi FA, Lisman RD, Levine MD, eds. Ophthalmic, plastic, and reconstructive surgery. St Louis: Mosby, 1998: 576–608.

McCord CD, Nunery WR. Reconstruction of the lower eyelid and outer canthus. In: McCord CD, Tanenbaum M, eds. Oculoplastic surgery. New York: Raven, 1987: 93–115.

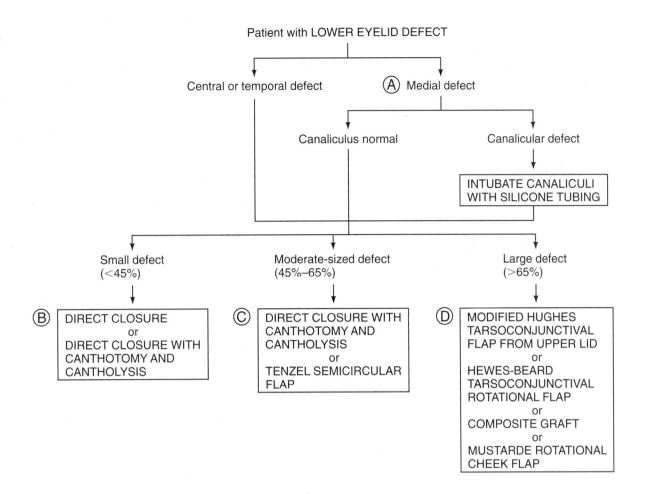

BLEPHAROSPASM

Kenneth L. Piest, M.D.

A. A careful drug history of all prescription and over-the-counter medications must be obtained. Dopamine stimulators, nasal decongestants containing antihistamines and sympathomimetics, and other drugs have been reported to cause blepharospasm.

B. Irritation of the fifth cranial nerve can cause blepharospasm. The ophthalmic division of the trigeminal nerve may be stimulated by meningeal inflammation or ocular irritation.

C. Ophthalmic factors are rarely the cause of blepharospasm but should be excluded. Keratitis, uveitis, scleritis, or an acute rise in intraocular pressure, as well as other causes of photophobia, may produce blepharospasm.

D. A benign tic consists of intermittent twitches of the eyelids. Often related to stress or fatigue, such tics are of no neurologic significance. Blepharospasm may present as unilateral, intermittent spasms with increased blinking. Progression is variable, ranging from months to years.

E. Ocular facial myokymia is characterized by unilateral, continuous, undulating movements of orbicularis and facial muscles. The movements are produced by intermittent contractions of adjacent muscle bundles. Myokymia is often caused by a brainstem lesion or multiple sclerosis.

F. Hemifacial spasms are unilateral, involuntary muscle contractions that last seconds to minutes and involve the periocular and facial muscles innervated by the seventh cranial nerve. Often, there is an underlying facial weakness with hemifacial spasm, whereas in blepharospasm, normal or increased facial strength is the rule. Many cases of hemifacial spasm are caused by intracranial lesions that compress the facial nerve anywhere along its pathway.

G. Essential blepharospasm is the involuntary contraction of the entire orbicularis muscle. It is bilateral but may show asymmetric involvement. As the contractions increase in frequency, significant visual disability results. Pharmacotherapy has been disappointing. Current treatments involve botulinum toxin injections, myectomy, and selective seventh cranial nerve sectioning.

H. Blepharospasm may also occur as part of a spectrum of craniocervical dystonias. When lower facial muscle involvement occurs with blepharospasm, it is termed *Meige's syndrome* (orofacial dystonia). Extensive mandibular involvement suggests Brueghel's syndrome (oromandibular dystonia). The tongue, pharynx, neck, and respiratory muscles may be involved. When several cranial nerves become affected, the term *craniocervical dystonia* is used. *Nuchal dystonia* refers to persistent tonic head deviations that may accompany Meige's or Brueghel's syndrome. Some investigators believe that blepharospasm and the dystonias represent variable expressions of a similar underlying process.

I. Apraxia of eyelid opening occurs in diseases involving the basal ganglion. It may mimic blepharospasm, but the orbicularis is not in spasm. Reflex blepharospasm may also be elicited in basal ganglion disease by touching the lids or brows. In myotonic dystrophy the facial muscles become weak and a severe ptosis may develop. In addition, eyelid opening is delayed after forced closure.

References

Burde RM, Savino PL, Trobe ID. Clinical decisions in neuroophthalmology. 2nd ed. St Louis: Mosby, 1992: 365–378.

Jordan DR, Patrinely JR, Anderson RL, Thiese SM. Essential blepharospasm and related dystonias. Surv Ophthalmol 1989; 34:123–132.

Miller NR, Gittinger JW, Keltner JL, Burde RM. "Squeezing eyes": A clinical pathological conference. Surv Ophthalmol 1981; 26:97–100.

Patel B, Weinstein GS, Anderson RL. Diagnosis and treatment of blepharospasm. In: Smith BV, Nesi FA, Lisman RD, Levine MR, eds. Ophthalmic, plastic, and reconstructive surgery. St Louis: Mosby, 1998: 319–335.

Roy FH. Ocular differential diagnosis. 3rd ed. Philadelphia: Lea & Febiger, 1984.

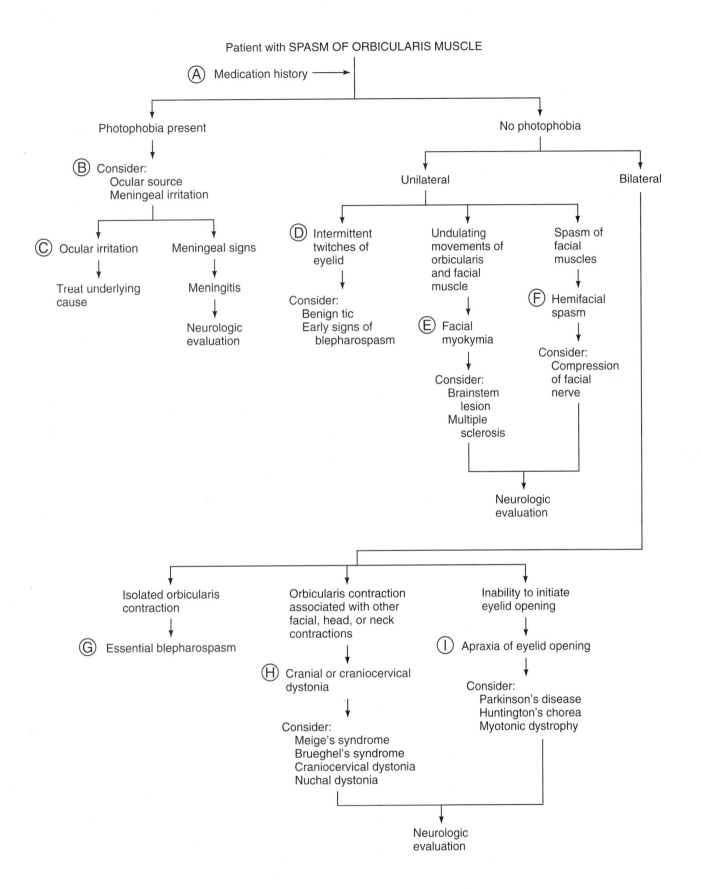

Patient with SPASM OF ORBICULARIS MUSCLE

Ⓐ Medication history

Photophobia present

Ⓑ Consider:
Ocular source
Meningeal irritation

Ⓒ Ocular irritation

Treat underlying
cause

Meningeal signs

Meningitis

Neurologic
evaluation

No photophobia

Unilateral

Ⓓ Intermittent
twitches of
eyelid

Consider:
Benign tic
Early signs of
blepharospasm

Undulating
movements of
orbicularis
and facial
muscle

Ⓔ Facial
myokymia

Consider:
Brainstem
lesion
Multiple
sclerosis

Spasm of
facial
muscles

Ⓕ Hemifacial
spasm

Consider:
Compression
of facial
nerve

Neurologic
evaluation

Bilateral

Isolated orbicularis
contraction

Ⓖ Essential blepharospasm

Orbicularis contraction
associated with other
facial, head, or neck
contractions

Ⓗ Cranial or craniocervical
dystonia

Consider:
Meige's syndrome
Brueghel's syndrome
Craniocervical dystonia
Nuchal dystonia

Inability to initiate
eyelid opening

Ⓘ Apraxia of eyelid opening

Consider:
Parkinson's disease
Huntington's chorea
Myotonic dystrophy

Neurologic
evaluation

ORBITAL FLOOR FRACTURE (BLOW-OUT FRACTURE)

Kenneth L. Piest, M.D.

It is not unusual for orbital trauma to involve the eyelid, lacrimal system, globe, bones, sinuses, and brain. Orbital fractures can be direct fractures that involve the orbital rim or indirect fractures, in which the rim is intact and the fractures involve the bones within the orbital cavity.

A. Many ocular injuries are associated with midface fractures. Repair of a serious ocular injury (e.g., corneoscleral laceration, retinal detachment) takes precedence over the fracture repair. The presence of a hyphema or vitreous hemorrhage necessitates waiting for the condition to stabilize before bony manipulation.

B. The inferior rectus muscle is often involved in floor fractures. The muscle or its connective tissue may be entrapped in the fracture, inhibiting the motion of the globe.

C. Diplopia and decreased range of motion are indications for forced duction testing. A positive forced duction test demonstrating restricted motion suggests entrapment of the inferior rectus muscle (less often the inferior oblique). In acute conditions, restriction may also be caused by orbital edema and hemorrhage. If the eye moves freely with forced duction testing but decreased motility is present, a primary injury to the muscle or nerve is likely.

D. A true blow-out fracture of the orbital floor consists of a floor fracture with an intact orbital rim. Secondary orbital floor fractures occur almost invariably if a rim fracture is present. The blow-out fracture is the most common type of fracture that confronts the ophthalmic surgeon. The most common site of the fracture is in the thin portion of the maxillary bone in the posterior medial portion of the orbital floor. Involvement of the ethmoid bones producing an associated medial wall fracture is common.

E. Signs suggesting an insult significant enough to produce bony injury include periorbital ecchymosis, subcutaneous emphysema, enophthalmos, inferior displacement of the globe, flattening of the malar region, displacement of a portion of the orbital rim, and infraorbital nerve dysfunction.

F. If forced duction testing is negative and associated signs do not suggest a fracture, monitor the patient for 1–2 weeks. This allows edema, hemorrhage, or contusion injury to resolve partially. If the motility or diplopia continues to improve and the patient is not troubled, continued observation is warranted. However, if the conditions do not improve or the patient remains symptomatic, CT imaging is recommended.

G. CT scanning is the most valuable imaging technique because it visualizes both the bones and soft tissues, including the extraocular muscles. In requesting a CT scan in the evaluation of orbital trauma, specify coronal and axial thin orbital sections. Sagittal reconstructions may also be helpful. MRI does not image bone well and is not as useful. If only standard radiologic means are available, the Waters's view is best in visualizing the orbital floor.

H. If a fracture site is not discovered on CT scanning, the restricted eye movements may be caused by orbital edema, hemorrhage, or a small fracture with entrapped orbital tissue. Monitoring is appropriate for 1–2 weeks because the motility may improve. Improvement may occur as the edema and hemorrhage resolve and as entrapped fat stretches, reducing tension on the ocular muscles.

I. The persistence of a motility problem in the presence of normal forced ductions suggests a primary neuromuscular injury. Consider ocular muscle surgery if the diplopia is visually handicapping.

J. Absolute indications for surgery are somewhat controversial. General guidelines for surgical intervention include persistent diplopia within 30 degrees of primary position or in downgaze, positive forced ductions, a large defect, and enophthalmos >2 mm. As mentioned, diplopia and positive forced ductions in the presence of a floor fracture are strong indications for surgery. Repair large fractures that involve half of the floor or more. The large defects have a high incidence of developing significant enophthalmos and motility problems. Enophthalmos commonly is masked initially by the orbital edema. Therefore, if enophthalmos is present immediately after the injury, it will likely worsen. Enophthalmos >2 mm is an indication for surgery. In general, the best time for surgical intervention is within the first 2 weeks after injury. Early surgery can be performed (and is advocated by some) if clear indications for repair are present. After 2–3 weeks, fibrosis sets in. Subsequent repairs require sharp dissection to free entrapped tissue.

References

Dortzbach RK, Segrest DR. Blowout fractures of the orbital floor. In: Stewart WB, ed. Ophthalmic, plastic and reconstructive surgery. 4th ed. San Francisco: American Academy of Ophthalmology, 1984: 387–399.

Grove AS, McCord CD. Acute orbital trauma: diagnosis and management. In: McCord CD, Tanenbaum M, eds. Oculoplastic surgery. New York: Raven, 1987: 129–154.

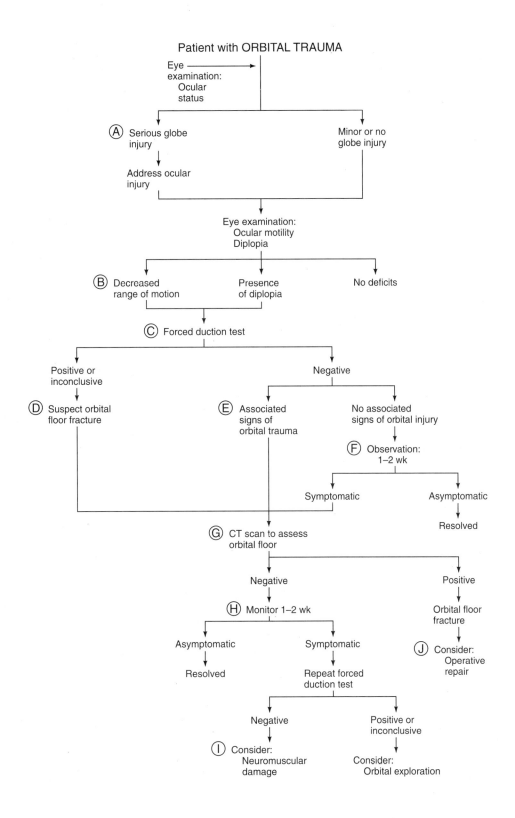

Patient with ORBITAL TRAUMA

Eye examination:
Ocular status

Ⓐ Serious globe injury

Minor or no globe injury

Address ocular injury

Eye examination:
Ocular motility
Diplopia

Ⓑ Decreased range of motion

Presence of diplopia

No deficits

Ⓒ Forced duction test

Positive or inconclusive

Negative

Ⓓ Suspect orbital floor fracture

Ⓔ Associated signs of orbital trauma

No associated signs of orbital injury

Ⓕ Observation: 1–2 wk

Symptomatic

Asymptomatic

Resolved

Ⓖ CT scan to assess orbital floor

Negative

Positive

Ⓗ Monitor 1–2 wk

Orbital floor fracture

Asymptomatic

Symptomatic

Ⓙ Consider: Operative repair

Resolved

Repeat forced duction test

Negative

Positive or inconclusive

Ⓘ Consider: Neuromuscular damage

Consider: Orbital exploration

Hornblass A, Gross ND. Fractures of the floor of the orbit. In: Hornblass A, ed. Oculoplastic, orbital, and reconstructive surgery. Baltimore: Williams & Wilkins, 1990: 1155–1167.

Putterman AM, Smith BC, Lisman RD. Blowout fractures. In: Smith BC, Nesi FA, Lisman RD, Levine MR, eds. Ophthalmic, plastic, and reconstructive surgery. St Louis: Mosby, 1998: 209–223.

ENOPHTHALMOS

Kenneth L. Piest, M.D.

Enophthalmos is a posterior displacement of the globe. It is an important and often overlooked or ignored sign. Three main mechanisms, separately or in combination, can produce an enophthalmic condition: structural abnormalities, cicatricial changes, and atrophy of orbital fat. The structural abnormalities concern the bony orbit. Cicatrization of the orbital contents can cause traction on the globe and produce a posterior displacement. Atrophy of orbital fat can be caused by a number of entities.

A. If an orbital structural abnormality is present or suspected, obtain a CT scan to evaluate the bony architecture. Trauma with fractures of the orbital walls produces an increased volume of the orbit. This increased orbital volume, along with prolapsing of the orbital contents through the fracture sites, produces an enophthalmic condition. Similarly, destruction of the orbital walls by a chronic sinusitis, sinus mucocele, or invasive malignancy can cause enophthalmos. Absence of the sphenoid wing in neurofibromatosis can also produce enophthalmos by the same mechanism. Many syndromes manifest an enophthalmic condition. In addition, a microphthalmic eye may be thought to be solely an enophthalmic problem at first.

B. Enophthalmos may be produced by traction on the globe by a cicatrization process. Certain metastatic adenocarcinomas can produce this. Breast carcinoma is the most widely recognized neoplastic disease exhibiting this property, but it can also be produced by lung, prostate, and stomach tumors. Orbital inflammatory disease (sclerosing pseudotumor) and post-traumatic conditions can also cause orbital cicatrization. Motility disturbances are common. Orbital imaging (CT scan or MRI) is required to delineate the problem.

C. Fat atrophy can be produced by several causes. It may simply be the result of aging, often producing a deep superior sulcus. Wasting diseases deplete total body tissue, orbital fat included. Irradiation in the head area for any reason (neoplasm or pseudotumor) may result in a secondary atrophy of orbital fat. A distensible orbital varix may cause pressure necrosis of surrounding tissue. If a varix is suspected, MRI differentiates tissues well. Ultrasonography or CT may also be helpful. Venograms can be obtained but are usually not required.

References

Jackson IT. Enophthalmos. In: Hornblass A, ed. Oculoplastic, orbital and reconstructive surgery. Baltimore: Williams & Wilkins, 1990: 1299–1312.

Rootman J. Diseases of the orbit. Philadelphia: JB Lippincott, 1988.

Spencer WH, ed. Ophthalmic pathology: An atlas and textbook. 3rd ed. Vol. 3. Philadelphia: WB Saunders, 1986.

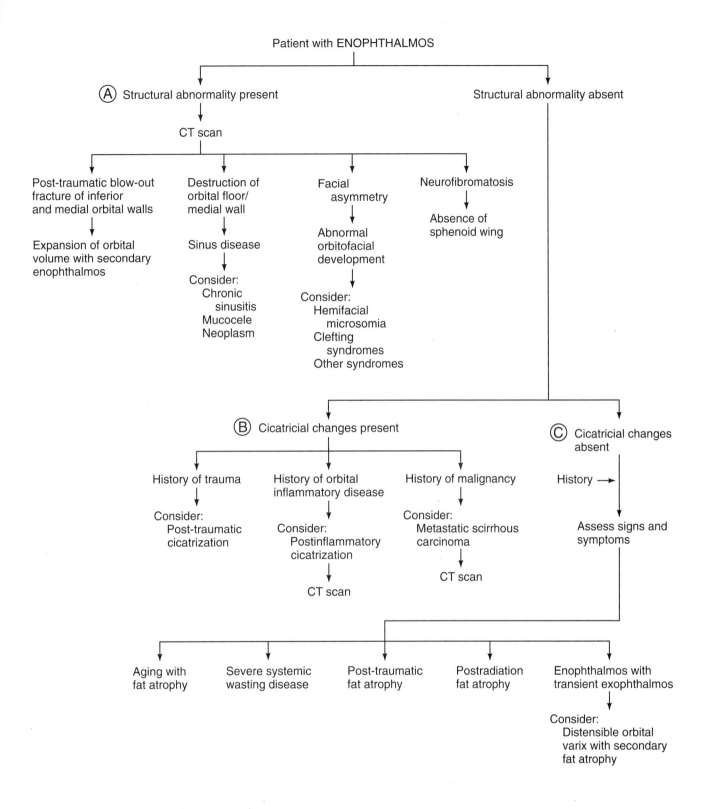

Patient with ENOPHTHALMOS

A Structural abnormality present

CT scan

Post-traumatic blow-out fracture of inferior and medial orbital walls

Expansion of orbital volume with secondary enophthalmos

Destruction of orbital floor/ medial wall

Sinus disease

Consider:
Chronic sinusitis
Mucocele
Neoplasm

Facial asymmetry

Abnormal orbitofacial development

Consider:
Hemifacial microsomia
Clefting syndromes
Other syndromes

Neurofibromatosis

Absence of sphenoid wing

Structural abnormality absent

B Cicatricial changes present

History of trauma

Consider:
Post-traumatic cicatrization

History of orbital inflammatory disease

Consider:
Postinflammatory cicatrization

CT scan

History of malignancy

Consider:
Metastatic scirrhous carcinoma

CT scan

C Cicatricial changes absent

History →

Assess signs and symptoms

Aging with fat atrophy

Severe systemic wasting disease

Post-traumatic fat atrophy

Postradiation fat atrophy

Enophthalmos with transient exophthalmos

Consider:
Distensible orbital varix with secondary fat atrophy

EXOPHTHALMOS

Kenneth L. Piest, M.D.

An abnormally prominent eye should call attention to the possibility of an orbital problem. Of most concern are infections and neoplastic processes, which may endanger the patient's life. In children the most common cause of unilateral proptosis is orbital cellulitis, and bilateral proptosis is most often from leukemia or metastatic neuroblastoma. Dermoids and capillary hemangiomas are the most common benign tumors in children, and rhabdomyosarcoma is the most common primary malignancy. In adults Graves' disease is the most common cause of unilateral and bilateral proptosis. Cavernous hemangiomas are the most common benign lesions, and the most common malignant process is caused by metastasis or extension from the paranasal sinuses of a malignant neoplasm.

A. The history and examination are extremely important in guiding the work-up of a patient with a suspected orbital problem. Proptosis is a common presenting sign of an orbital abnormality. The direction of the displacement of the globe can provide a clue to the location of the lesion. Decreased visual acuity, motility disturbances, pupillary abnormalities, pulsation, and pain are also signs of orbital involvement.

B. Pseudoproptosis results from a simulation of ocular prominence or asymmetry and not from an increase in orbital contents.

C. The most common ocular abnormality in Graves' disease is lid retraction. In addition, Graves' disease is the most common cause of proptosis in adults. If lid retraction is present, initiate a work-up for thyroid disease.

D. Proptosis, or exophthalmos, is the forward displacement of one or both globes. The usual amount of ocular protrusion as measured from the lateral orbital rim to the corneal apex is 14–21 mm in adults. Protrusion >21 mm or a 2-mm asymmetry is generally abnormal. However, individual and racial variations must be taken into account. In the presence of proptosis or other orbital signs, CT scanning (or MRI) is essential in understanding the process.

E. Structural abnormalities can decrease orbital volume, producing secondary exophthalmos. This is common in craniofacial syndromes (e.g., Crouzon's disease). Post-traumatic conditions may produce a similar situation. Orbital or midface advancements are usually required to increase the orbital volume.

F. Orbital inflammation produces nearly 60% of the orbital problems. Presentation is usually acute or subacute, producing lid erythema, edema, conjunctival injection, and chemosis, in addition to orbital signs.

G. Thyroid ophthalmopathy is the most common cause of unilateral or bilateral proptosis in adults, with women affected more often than men. Exophthalmos, lid retraction, chemosis, inflammation, and motility disturbances all can be present. All of the extraocular muscles can be affected, but there is a predilection for the inferior and medial recti. Visual loss may occur from a compressive optic neuropathy.

H. Both children and adults may present with an orbital inflammatory syndrome or pseudotumor. Any orbital structure may be affected, or it may present as a diffuse process. In children approximately half have bilateral involvement. Bilateral involvement in adults, however, suggests a systemic lymphoproliferative disorder or systemic vasculitis.

I. In children, proptosis is most commonly produced by an orbital cellulitis secondary to sinusitis or respiratory infection. The CT scan may show an opacified ethmoid sinus, which is helpful in distinguishing cellulitis from an orbital inflammatory syndrome in which the sinuses are clear. If an abscess is detected, surgical drainage is required.

J. Neoplastic lesions account for approximately 20% of orbital disease. Virtually any tumor can occur in the orbit. However, most are rare. To determine what pathologic process is occurring, look at the pattern of involvement. The listed differential diagnosis gives guidelines for uncovering a cause but is not all-inclusive.

K. Diseases originating in the sinuses, face, or intracranial areas may invade the orbit and proptosis may be the presenting sign.

L. Rhabdomyosarcoma can occur anywhere in the orbit, but its rapid growth often masks the initiating site. It appears to arise from undifferentiated mesenchyma rather than actual formed muscle tissue. Rapid diagnosis is essential. Vascular lesions (hemangioma, varix, lymphangioma) usually have a more diffuse pattern of orbital involvement. An intralesional hemorrhage in a lymphangioma may produce a sudden increase in proptosis.

References

Burde RM, Savino PJ, Trobe JD. Proptosis and adnexal masses. In: Clinical decisions in neuro-ophthalmology. 2nd ed. St Louis: Mosby, 1992: 379–416.

Leone CR, Lloyd WC. Treatment protocol for orbital inflammatory disease. Ophthalmology 1985; 92:1325–1331.

Rootman I. Diseases of the orbit. Philadelphia: JB Lippincott, 1988.

Roy FH. Ocular differential diagnosis. 5th ed. Philadelphia: Lea & Febiger, 1993.

Spencer WH, ed. Ophthalmic pathology: An atlas and textbook. 3rd ed. Vol. 3. Philadelphia: WB Saunders, 1986.

Patient with PROMINENT-APPEARING GLOBE

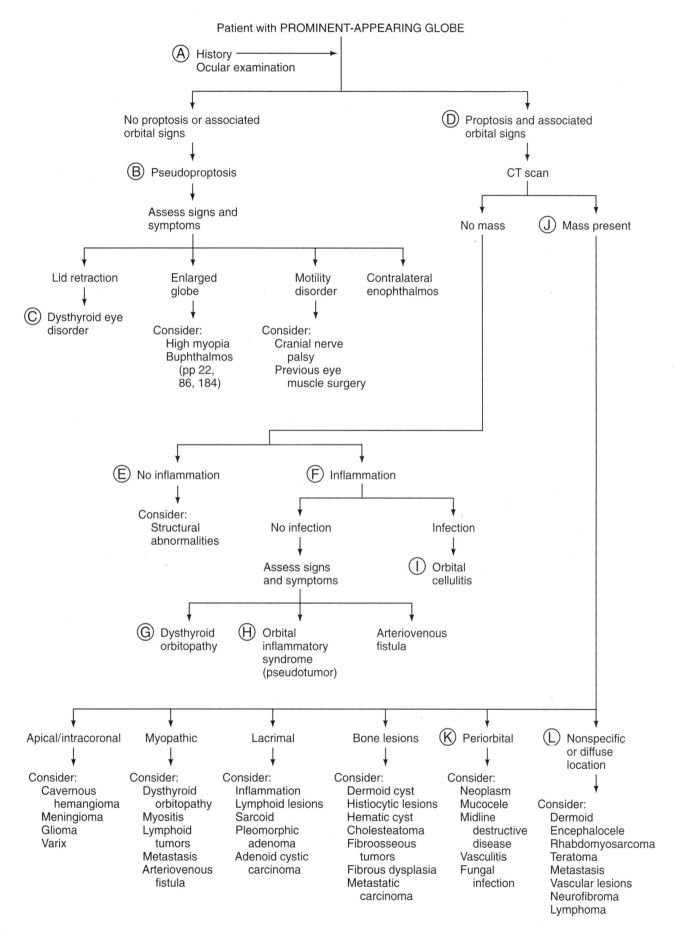

Ⓐ History ——→ Ocular examination

No proptosis or associated orbital signs

Ⓑ Pseudoproptosis

Assess signs and symptoms

Lid retraction

Ⓒ Dysthyroid eye disorder

Enlarged globe

Consider:
High myopia
Buphthalmos
(pp 22, 86, 184)

Motility disorder

Consider:
Cranial nerve palsy
Previous eye muscle surgery

Contralateral enophthalmos

Ⓓ Proptosis and associated orbital signs

CT scan

No mass

Ⓙ Mass present

Ⓔ No inflammation

Consider:
Structural abnormalities

Ⓕ Inflammation

No infection

Assess signs and symptoms

Ⓖ Dysthyroid orbitopathy

Ⓗ Orbital inflammatory syndrome (pseudotumor)

Arteriovenous fistula

Infection

Ⓘ Orbital cellulitis

Apical/intracoronal

Consider:
Cavernous hemangioma
Meningioma
Glioma
Varix

Myopathic

Consider:
Dysthyroid orbitopathy
Myositis
Lymphoid tumors
Metastasis
Arteriovenous fistula

Lacrimal

Consider:
Inflammation
Lymphoid lesions
Sarcoid
Pleomorphic adenoma
Adenoid cystic carcinoma

Bone lesions

Consider:
Dermoid cyst
Histiocytic lesions
Hematic cyst
Cholesteatoma
Fibroosseous tumors
Fibrous dysplasia
Metastatic carcinoma

Ⓚ Periorbital

Consider:
Neoplasm
Mucocele
Midline destructive disease
Vasculitis
Fungal infection

Ⓛ Nonspecific or diffuse location

Consider:
Dermoid
Encephalocele
Rhabdomyosarcoma
Teratoma
Metastasis
Vascular lesions
Neurofibroma
Lymphoma

SYMBLEPHARON

Charles R. Leone, M.D.

A *symblepharon* is an adhesion between conjunctival surfaces or between the conjunctiva and the cornea that can be congenital, traumatic, postsurgical, or inflammatory in etiology. When mucosal surfaces are abraded and come in contact with each other, they can become adherent.

A. A congenital symblepharon is rare and may be associated with Goldenhar's syndrome or a forme fruste of that disease. Dermolipomas and limbal dermoids, which occur commonly in this syndrome, can rarely be associated with abnormal adhesions. Symblepharon may occur after trauma, when a malpositioning of tissues or a loss of conjunctiva associated with denuded epithelial surfaces adjacent to each other can promote adhesions. It is thus important to avoid being too aggressive in debridement and save as much traumatized tissue as possible. Postsurgical symblepharon occurs most often after pterygium excision. In this situation raw surfaces are created on the cornea, limbus, and sclera, which, together with conjunctival shortening and shrinkage, produce adhesions, which may also involve the inner aspects of both the upper and lower eyelids. This may also occur after any conjunctival excision, particularly aggressive removal of dermolipomas. After removal of large eyelid tumors, there can be a paucity of conjunctiva to cover the reconstructed area, and bare epithelial surfaces may adhere. Symblepharon was also common after scleral buckling procedures, when the 360-degree conjunctival incision was several millimeters from the limbus. However, most retina surgeons now use limbal incisions.

B. Treat congenital symblepharon early, particularly if extraocular muscle movement is restricted or a strabismus results. Otherwise, amblyopia could ensue. Symblepharon after trauma or surgery can be prevented or reduced if realignment of malpositioned tissue is recognized and rectified in the immediate postoperative period. In these cases definitive surgical treatment can be delayed until the traumatic or inflammatory process has ceased and the tissues are stable for at least 6 months. If the symblepharon is small, a Z-plasty can be done to increase the fornix depth. Another technique is to separate the symblepharon from the globe, then mobilize the bulbar conjunctiva on either side of the symblepharon excision site. Next, slide the two sides toward each other and suture them together, and then transpose the remaining symblepharon, which is still attached to the palpebral conjunctiva, into the fornix and secure it with a through-and-through lid suture, which is tied on the outside of the lid (transposition).

C. For the more severe symblepharon associated with shrinkage, a split-thickness buccal mucosal graft (0.5-mm thickness) or a free conjunctival graft should be used to cover the raw surfaces after the symblepharon has been completely released and the globe and eyelids are fully mobile. A scleral shell is then used to keep the fornices intact and should be left in for 1–2 weeks. If the area is not too extensive, a thin silicone sleeve (0.005-inch thickness) can be draped over the lid margin, one surface on the fornix side and the other on the cutaneous side, with a through-and-through suture to stabilize it.

D. Inflammatory symblepharon is the most frustrating and difficult to treat because its activity may persist and any surgical intervention, although successful at first, may fail later. This is particularly true in ocular pemphigoid, a bilateral autoimmune inflammatory conjunctival disease with progressive, relentless shrinkage of the mucosal surfaces. It affects women twice as often as men and usually occurs after the age of 60. Cicatrizing conjunctivitis can cause a decrease in tear and goblet cell secretion, and there may even be restricted ocular motility. The most aggravating sequelae are cicatricial entropion and trichiasis. Stevens-Johnson syndrome (erythema multiforme) is an acute inflammatory vesicular reaction of the skin and mucous membranes. Although potentially fatal, this disease is self-limited, as opposed to ocular pemphigoid. However, during the acute stage there can be conjunctival shrinkage, surface membrane destruction, and permanent keratitis sicca. This condition is thought to occur most often as a result of drug sensitivity to sulfonamides, salicylates, or penicillin.

E. Progressive inflammatory symblepharon is treated medically to reduce the amount of inflammation and cicatrization. Systemic and topical corticosteroids are used; in ocular pemphigoid, antimetabolites (e.g., cyclophosphamide) together with corticosteroids have had limited success. Separating a newly formed symblepharon with a glass rod is sometimes helpful. Placement of scleral shells in the fornices also separates the palpebral from the bulbar conjunctiva, but it is sometimes traumatic and irritating to an eye that is already inflamed and may not really retard the process in the long run. Perform cryotherapy to relieve trichiasis. Definitive corrective surgery, such as grafts, usually produces limited and only temporary benefit, so it should be postponed until the disease process has ceased and the symblepharon has stabilized.

References

Belin MW, Hannush SB. Mucous membrane abnormalities. In: Abhott RL, ed. Surgical intervention in corneal and external diseases. Orlando: Grune & Stratton, 1987: 159–176.

Leone CR. Treatment of conjunctival diseases and chalazia. In: Stewart W, ed. Ophthalmic plastic surgery and reconstructive surgery. San Francisco, American Academy of Ophthalmology, 1984.

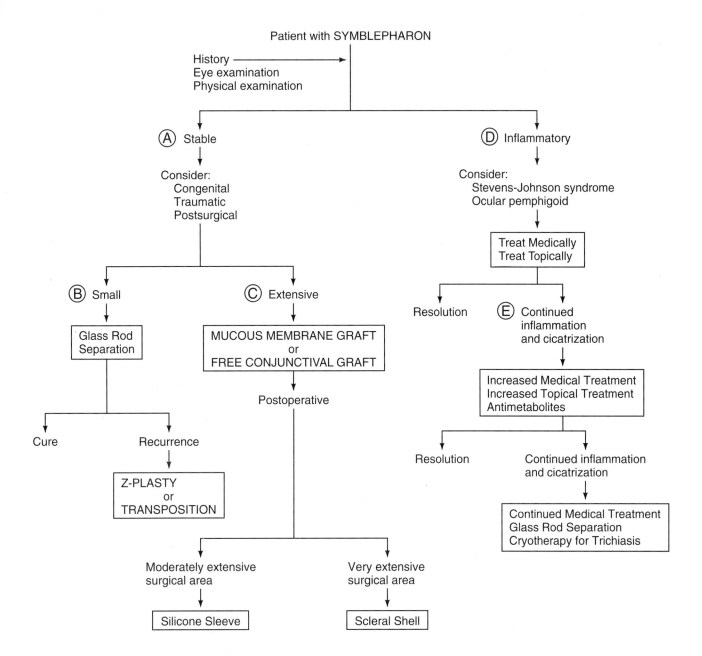

Patient with SYMBLEPHARON

History ⟶
Eye examination
Physical examination

(A) Stable

Consider:
Congenital
Traumatic
Postsurgical

(B) Small

Glass Rod
Separation

Cure   Recurrence

Z-PLASTY
or
TRANSPOSITION

(C) Extensive

MUCOUS MEMBRANE GRAFT
or
FREE CONJUNCTIVAL GRAFT

Postoperative

Moderately extensive
surgical area

Silicone Sleeve

Very extensive
surgical area

Scleral Shell

(D) Inflammatory

Consider:
Stevens-Johnson syndrome
Ocular pemphigoid

Treat Medically
Treat Topically

Resolution   (E) Continued
inflammation
and cicatrization

Increased Medical Treatment
Increased Topical Treatment
Antimetabolites

Resolution   Continued inflammation
and cicatrization

Continued Medical Treatment
Glass Rod Separation
Cryotherapy for Trichiasis

PEDIATRIC OPHTHALMOLOGY AND STRABISMUS

TREATMENT OF AMBLYOPIA SECONDARY TO A REFRACTIVE ERROR

James L. Mims III, M.D.

A. The degree of anisometropia that is likely to cause amblyopia is only moderately well known. The following is based on a poll of several experienced pediatric ophthalmologists. You should provide optical correction for these degrees of anisometropia: (1) >+1.25 diopter (D) sphere difference in hyperopia, (2) >−2.50 D sphere difference in myopia, (3) >1.25 D difference in astigmatism with parallel or symmetric axes of astigmatism,* and (4) >0.50 D astigmatism with one axis oblique and the other vertical or horizontal.*

B. Children with bilateral hyperopia of >+4.75 D sphere will have bilateral refractive amblyopia if they do not start wearing glasses by age 7 years, even if there is no anisometropia. If they are given the full correction, divergence fusional amplitudes will be reduced and iatrogenic accommodative esotropia can result. ("My child wasn't cross-eyed without glasses until he started wearing the glasses you prescribed, Doctor.") Giving 2 D less than the full spherical equivalence is safe in anticipation of patching, unless the child has a tiny esotropia ("flick ET," or a monofixation syndrome), in which case the full hyperopic correction should be given. An obsolete rule was to give 50% of a highly hyperopic correction. I have seen more than one child with +8.00 D hyperopia whose accommodative esotropia began when 50% of the full plus was prescribed by another practitioner. This left the child with +4.00 D residual, enough to produce accommodative esotropia. Children with bilateral myopia of −5.75 D sphere also need glasses to prevent bilateral refractive amblyopia, but if they are given the full myopic correction, they may reject it because of the new demands being made on their accommodative abilities. Also, a few may become esotropic as a result of new stimulation of accommodative convergence provided by the full myopic correction. Finally, there is evidence that in highly myopic children a widely dilated pupil after cycloplegia may give an excessively high myopic reading on retinoscopy because of aberrations in the peripheral lens. (Children usually have larger pupils after cycloplegia than adults.) These are three good reasons to underminus a highly myopic child's first pair of glasses, generally by about 2 D. In moderate myopia overcorrection by 0.50 D is preferred by some practitioners, anticipating that the myopia will worsen.

C. Because adults may develop headaches or other symptoms of asthenopia when they are first given an optical correction for their astigmatism, many practitioners do not realize the importance of giving the full astigmatic correction to a child. Not only can the child readily adapt to the full correction, but it is required if amblyopia is to be treated effectively.

D. Once the determination has been made whether glasses should be prescribed, the next question is how to occlude the better eye. Babies 6–14 months old are extremely sensitive to patching, and severe iatrogenic amblyopia can result from overpatching in infancy. Interestingly, severe strabismic amblyopia in infancy can be associated with eccentric fixation, but severe amblyopia from too much patching is not associated with eccentric fixation. If the infant is being seen in a charity clinic context or the parents have to travel an unusually long distance for the office visits, it is wise to prescribe a course of alternate patching, the right eye one day followed by the left eye the next day, to follow the string of days when only the dominant eye is patched. For each month of age of the infant, the dominant eye should be patched no more than 1 day for 6–8 hours daily without checking.

E. When a child reaches 14 months of age, he or she enters the developmental period known as the "terrible two's." (A poll of 18 pediatricians and 2 pediatric specialists led to the unanimous response that the terrible two's starts at age 14 months and ends at age 27–36 months.) During this period, seriously consider atropine penalization.

F. After the third birthday, patching all but 2 hours daily, 1 week per year of age, is standard. Many eye care practitioners do not routinely prescribe enough hours of patching each day. When the amblyopia is severe in a child aged 6–9 years, the dominant eye should be patched all waking moments for a full 10 weeks. If no improvement occurs after the 10 weeks, it is reasonable to stop patching. When patching is discontinued, it should be withdrawn gradually, reducing the hours of patching each week by 1 hour daily. Calendar sheets given to the parents are helpful. It has been demonstrated that if the original visual acuity at the start of patching was very poor (20/100 or worse) or if the best visual acuity obtained after prolonged patching was 20/50 or worse, maintenance patching 2 hours daily after school until the tenth birthday is important

---

*Parallel axes can be judged simply by looking at the refractor, phoropter, or trial frame and judging whether the axis of astigmatism of one eye is within 20 degrees of parallel with the axis of astigmatism of the other eye. *Symmetric axes of astigmatism* refers to mirror image astigmatism (e.g., 45 degrees in one eye and 135 degrees in the other eye). If the axes are 30 degrees or more away from parallel or mirror image symmetry, a very minor amount of astigmatism will cause amblyopia, even if the amount of astigmatism is the same in each eye.

TREATMENT OF AMBLYOPIA SECONDARY TO A REFRACTIVE ERROR

(A) >+1.25D sphere difference in hyperopia?
    >−2.50D sphere difference in myopia?
    >1.25D difference in astigmatism with
       parallel or symmetric axes of astigmatism?
    >0.50D astigmatism with one axis oblique
       and the other vertical or horizontal?

No significant optical asymmetry   Significant optical asymmetry

Hyperopia >+4.75D?
Myopia >−5.75D?

(C) Prescribe Glasses with the Full Astigmatic Correction

Yes   No

(B) Prescribe Glasses with 2 Diopter Underminus or Underplus

No Glasses Needed

(D) Age 6 mo–14 mo

Patch 6–8 hr Daily, 1 Day per Month of Age

(E) Age 14 mo–36 mo

Consider: Atropine Penalization

(F) Age 37 mo–6 yr

Patch All But 2 hr Daily, 1 Week per Year of Age

to prevent a return of severe amblyopia. When the amblyopia is severe, it may be unreasonable to ask one adult to initiate patching. Having one parent set up a schedule of several concerned adults (e.g., grandparents) so that each one can spend an hour with the child on a Saturday (simply keeping him or her from touching the patch) is more effective than elaborate restraints, punishments, and so on, when the patching is started. Filling up a large desk pad calendar with the patches as they are removed and giving a reward for each week of good patching behavior is another effective technique.

References

Attebo K, Mitchell P, Cumming R, et al. Prevalence and causes of amblyopia in an adult population. Ophthalmology 1998; 105:154–159.

Lam GC, Repka MX, Guyton D. Timing of amblyopia therapy relative to strabismus surgery. Ophthalmology 1993; 100:1751–1756.

Pratt-Johnson JA, Tillson G. Management of strabismus and amblyopia. New York: Thieme, 1994: 74–90.

von Noorden GK. Binocular vision and ocular motility. St Louis: Mosby, 1996: 206–274.

THE DIAGNOSIS OF STRABISMUS

Johan Zwaan, M.D., Ph.D.

When a parent brings a child with a suspected misalignment of the eyes to the ophthalmologist, a complete eye examination, including a dilated fundus examination and cycloplegic retinoscopy or refraction, is imperative. Attention needs to be paid to significant refractive errors, to abnormalities in the media (p 182), and to possible lesions of the fundus. As noted elsewhere (p 192), one in five children with retinoblastoma presents with strabismus. Once the causes of secondary strabismus have been eliminated, the examiner can concentrate on the ocular motility problem.

The diagnostic scheme proposed here is somewhat dogmatic. It does not take into account that conditions may coexist. For instance, a positive angle kappa, giving an appearance of exotropia, may be combined with a true esotropia, which then is more difficult to detect. Alternatively, esotropia is commonly associated with overaction of the inferior oblique muscles, which turns a primarily comitant strabismus transiently into an incomitant one, mostly in adduction.

A. Misalignment of the visual axes with full motility and basically the same deviation in all directions of gaze occurs by far in the largest group of children with strabismus. The epidemiology of strabismus is rather deficient, but up to 5% of the entire population may have strabismus. In addition, children with pseudostrabismus also have comitant and full motility.

B. Sometimes, a phoria is difficult to bring out with the cover and uncover test. Repeated alternate cover testing may be needed to break up fusion.

C. A head tilt indicates a cyclovertical muscle palsy or a disorder of the sternocleidomastoid muscle or cervical spine. Their differentiation is important (pp 156 and 158) for the institution of proper treatment. If a child with a fourth cranial nerve palsy is unnecessarily treated by surgery or physical therapy, as if the torticollis were caused by a sternocleidomastoid abnormality, amblyopia can be induced.

D. Microstrabismus covers a range of abnormalities in which the deviation is so small that it is difficult to demonstrate a shift of the eye with the usual cover test. One type is characterized by a minimal misalignment with a complete sensory adaptation. Unilateral amblyopia is often caused by anisometropia and parafoveal fixation. Peripheral fusion and modest stereoacuity are demonstrable.

E. The angle kappa is the angle between the visual axis (from point of fixation to fovea) and the pupillary axis (through the center of the pupil perpendicular to the cornea). Its interest lies mainly in the confusion it may cause in the recognition of strabismus. It can simulate an exodeviation or esodeviation or obscure a true strabismus in the opposite direction.

F. Ectopia of the macula by dragging is mostly caused by severe retinal scarring seen with retinopathy of prematurity. It may be bilateral. It can also be associated with the retinitis caused by *Toxocara canis* infection and with familial exudative vitreoretinopathy.

G. The limited data available indicate that perhaps only 1 in 1000 strabismus patients has an incomitant type (excluding the rather common overaction of the inferior obliques and dissociated vertical deviation).

H. The transient vertical deviations seen in association with congenital (infantile) esotropia and sometimes exotropia (i.e., overaction of the inferior obliques and dissociated vertical deviations) are perhaps the most common reason for a vertical deviation. They are discussed in detail elsewhere (p 146).

I. Double elevator palsy is demonstrated by an inability to elevate the eye in any direction of gaze. Although this disability may result from a paralysis of both superior rectus and inferior oblique muscle, more likely the paralysis of the superior rectus causes contraction of the inferior rectus, which then mechanically limits upgaze in all directions.

J. Brown's syndrome is congenital or acquired. Its hallmark is an inability to elevate the eye in adduction, which becomes progressively less the more the eye is abducted. The congenital variety may be caused by an anomaly of the superior oblique tendon (too short) or by an abnormality of the trochlea or tendon sheath. All types mechanically restrict elevation. The acquired variety can be caused by inflammation, trauma, or rarely other causes such as a metastasis.

K. The differential diagnosis of cranial nerve VI palsies can be confusing. The most common type is Duane's syndrome type I, in which the palsy is combined with retraction of the eye and narrowing of the lid fissure on adduction. Congenital isolated palsy of the sixth cranial nerve is usually benign and transient, resolving before age 2 months. In the absence of other neurologic abnormalities, the prognosis is excellent. An acquired sixth cranial nerve palsy can also be benign and transient. It may occur 1–3 weeks after a febrile illness, after immunization, or without a recognized precipitating factor, and it may recur. The paralysis generally resolves within 2–3 months, but recovery may take several months. Persistence of the palsy for several months without any improvement is a reason for concern and neurologic and otolaryngologic evaluations, CT scanning, and/or MRI should be done. Hydrocephalus and pseudotumor may be associated with sixth cranial nerve palsy, but a tumor, usually a pontine glioma, must be excluded.

L. In Möbius' syndrome congenital palsies of the sixth cranial nerve are combined with facial diplegia, resulting in a flat expressionless face. Other neurologic and other anomalies may be present.

M. Frozen globes with little or no motility can be the result of congenital fibrosis of the extraocular muscles (CFEOM), of which several varieties exist. Recent research has shown that the most common type, with the eyes fixed in downgaze and associated with ptosis, is caused by an autosomal-dominant locus on chromosome 12. A second type with the eyes frozen in exotropia and with ptosis is caused by an autosomal-recessive gene on chromosome 11q13. In both types the third cranial nerve and its nucleus is (partially) absent. Other causes for frozen globes include orbital fibrosis, following severe orbital pseudotumor, and very high myopia.

References

Afifi AK, Bell WE, Bale JF, et al. Recurrent lateral rectus palsy in childhood. Pediatr Neurol 1990; 6:315–318.

Brodsky MC, Pollock SC, Buckley EG. Neural misdirection in congenital ocular fibrosis syndrome: Implications and pathogenesis. J Pediatr Ophthalmol Strabismus 1989; 26:159–161.

Clarke WN, Noel LP. Stereo acuity testing in the monofixation syndrome. J Pediatr Ophthalmol Strabismus 1990; 27:161–163.

Helveston EM. Classification of superior oblique muscle palsy. Ophthalmology 1992; 99:1609–1615.

Hotchkiss MD, Miller NR, Clark AW, et al. Bilateral Duane's retraction syndrome: A clinicopathological case report. Arch Ophthalmol 1980; 98:870–874.

Metz HS. Double elevator palsy. J Pediatr Ophthalmol Strabismus 1981; 18:31–35.

Raab EL. Clinical features of Duane's syndrome. J Pediatr Ophthalmol Strabismus 1986; 23:64–68.

Wang SM, Zwaan J, Mullaney PB, et al. Congenital fibrosis of the extraocular muscles Type 2, an inherited exotropic strabismus fixus, maps to distal 11q13. Am J Hum Genet 1998; 63:517–525.

Wilson ME, Parks MM. Primary inferior oblique overaction in congenital esotropia, accommodative esotropia and intermittent exotropia. Ophthalmology 1989; 96:950–955.

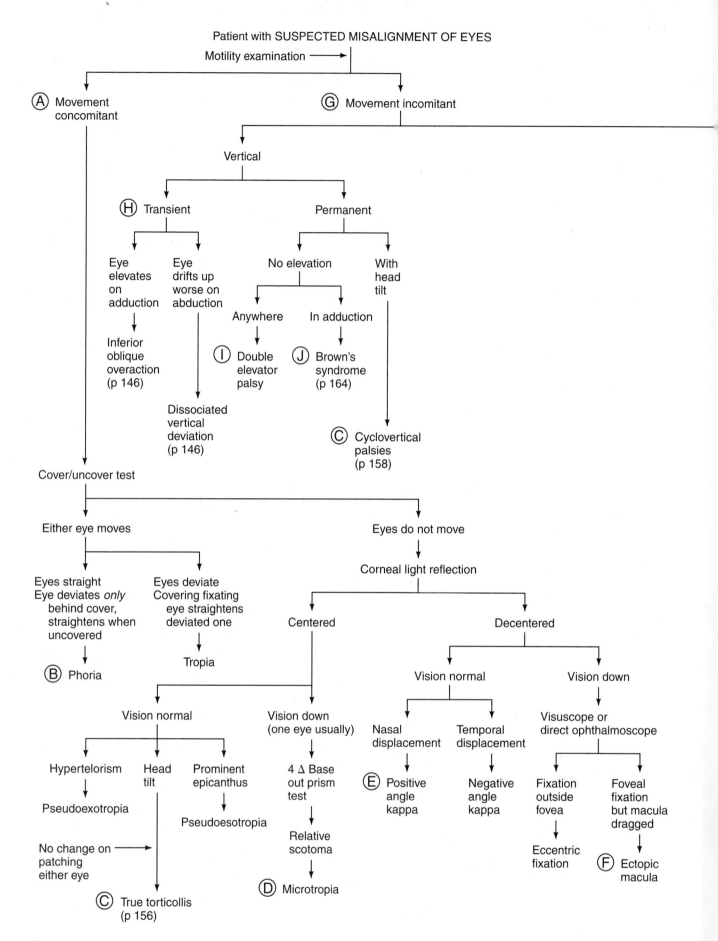

Patient with SUSPECTED MISALIGNMENT OF EYES

Motility examination →

Ⓐ Movement concomitant

Ⓖ Movement incomitant

Vertical

Ⓗ Transient

Permanent

Eye elevates on adduction
↓
Inferior oblique overaction (p 146)

Eye drifts up worse on abduction
↓
Dissociated vertical deviation (p 146)

No elevation

With head tilt

Anywhere
↓
Ⓘ Double elevator palsy

In adduction
↓
Ⓙ Brown's syndrome (p 164)

Ⓒ Cyclovertical palsies (p 158)

Cover/uncover test

Either eye moves

Eyes straight
Eye deviates *only* behind cover, straightens when uncovered
↓
Ⓑ Phoria

Eyes deviate
Covering fixating eye straightens deviated one
↓
Tropia

Vision normal

Hypertelorism
↓
Pseudoexotropia

Head tilt

Prominent epicanthus
↓
Pseudoesotropia

No change on → patching either eye

Ⓒ True torticollis (p 156)

Vision down (one eye usually)
↓
4 Δ Base out prism test
↓
Relative scotoma
↓
Ⓓ Microtropia

Eyes do not move
↓
Corneal light reflection

Centered

Decentered

Vision normal

Nasal displacement
↓
Ⓔ Positive angle kappa

Temporal displacement
↓
Negative angle kappa

Vision down
↓
Visuscope or direct ophthalmoscope

Fixation outside fovea
↓
Eccentric fixation

Foveal fixation but macula dragged
↓
Ⓕ Ectopic macula

142

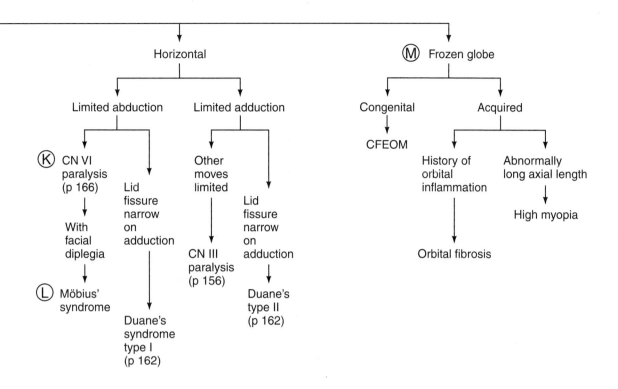

Horizontal

Ⓜ Frozen globe

Limited abduction

Limited adduction

Congenital

Acquired

Ⓚ CN VI paralysis (p 166)

Lid fissure narrow on adduction

Other moves limited

Lid fissure narrow on adduction

CFEOM

History of orbital inflammation

Abnormally long axial length

With facial diplegia

CN III paralysis (p 156)

Duane's type II (p 162)

Orbital fibrosis

High myopia

Ⓛ Möbius' syndrome

Duane's syndrome type I (p 162)

INFANTILE ESOTROPIA

James L. Mims III, M.D.

A. Infants believed by referring physicians, nurses, or family to have esotropia should be examined by age 5 months to rule out defects of the fundi or ocular media, including retinoblastoma. Primary care physicians should be taught to use the red reflex test with the direct ophthalmoscope, as well as the corneal reflection test (Hirschberg) when esotropia is suspected. Many infants with esotropia have only a small or intermittent deviation by age 6 months, which grows into a large, constant deviation by age 10 months.

B. A deviation in infants that is intermittent or spasmodic and <25 prism diopters (PD) in size may simply resolve with no treatment and deserves several months of simple observation.

C. Incomitant esotropia with limited abduction of one eye may be a sign of Duane's syndrome if the palpebral fissure narrows on adduction and the degree of esotropia is relatively small compared with the severity of the limitation of abduction. True lateral rectus palsies, with a 25–35 PD esotropia combined with severe limitation of abduction and little or no narrowing of the palpebral fissure on adduction, are less common than Duane's syndrome, require neurologic examination, and may clear spontaneously in 6 weeks.

D. Atropine refraction is mandatory unless office drops in a blue-eyed child indicate significant myopia. Glasses are prescribed if the spherical equivalent is ≥+3.25 diopter (D) hyperopic or if there is a significant optical difference between the two eyes (p 138). Preoperative glasses generally do not straighten the eyes in infantile esotropia, but if glasses prove to be needed postoperatively, the parents will never say, "Doctor, my child didn't need glasses until you did your surgery."

E. Patching to equal vision means free alternation of fixation, or at least maintenance of fixation of the cross-fixating eye until at least the midline as it follows a horizontally moving target.

F. Avoid cul-de-sac technique and recess conjunctiva if preoperatively the fixing eye is in adduction to null nystagmus with a face turn or if the esotropia persists under anesthesia.

G. Recess the medial recti according to a dose-response curve, with minor modifications for the deviation observed under anesthesia if the deviation is substantially more or less than expected. Amounts of medial rectus recession in classic textbooks have previously been too small. If the measurement is made with calipers from the apex of the insertional ridge present after disinsertion of the muscle, the following amounts of surgery (bimedial recessions, both eyes) are now popular: 15 PD = 3.4 mm, 20 PD = 4.1 mm, 25 PD = 4.6 mm, 30 PD = 5.1 mm, 35 PD = 5.5 mm, 40 PD = 5.7 mm, 45 PD = 5.8 mm, 50 PD = 6.0 mm, 55 PD = 6.2 mm, 60 PD = 6.4 mm, 65 PD = 6.5 mm, 70 PD = 6.7 mm, 75 PD = 6.9 mm, 80 PD = 7.0 mm, 85 PD = 7.2 mm. The ideal age for surgery is 9–11 months.

References

Ing MR. Early surgical alignment for congenital esotropia. Pediatr Ophthalmol Strabismus 1983; 20:11–18.

Kushner BJ, Lucchese NJ. Should recessions of the medial recti be graded from the limbus or the insertion? Arch Ophthalmol 1989; 107:1755–1758.

Mims JL III, Treff G, Kincaid M, et al. Quantitative surgical guidelines for bimedial recession for infantile esotropia. Binocular Vision 1985; 1:7–22.

Mims JL III, Wood RC. Verification and refinement of surgical guidelines for infantile esotropia: A prospective study of 40 cases. Binocular Vision 1989; 4:7–14.

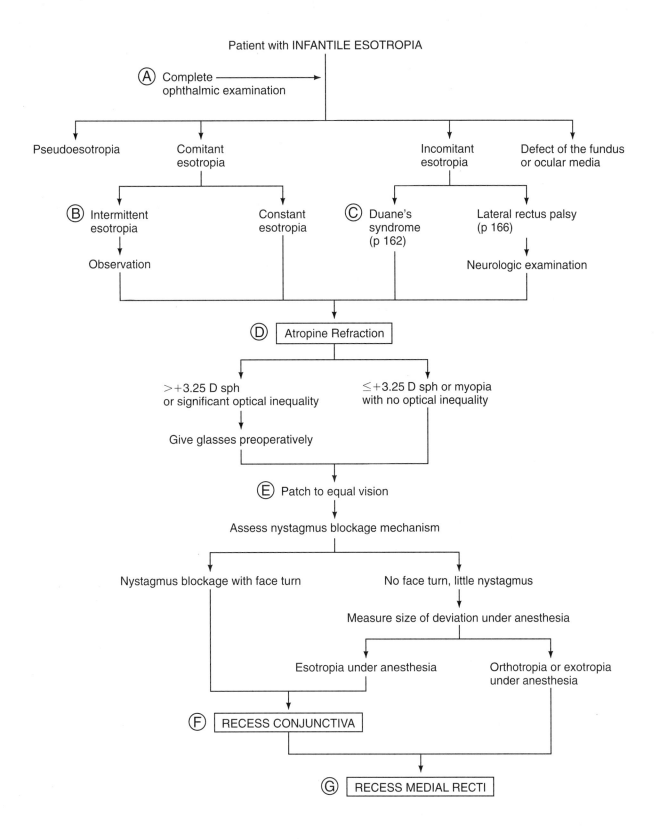

Patient with INFANTILE ESOTROPIA

(A) Complete ophthalmic examination

Pseudoesotropia

Comitant esotropia
- (B) Intermittent esotropia → Observation
- Constant esotropia

Incomitant esotropia
- (C) Duane's syndrome (p 162)
- Lateral rectus palsy (p 166) → Neurologic examination

Defect of the fundus or ocular media

(D) Atropine Refraction
- >+3.25 D sph or significant optical inequality → Give glasses preoperatively
- ≤+3.25 D sph or myopia with no optical inequality

(E) Patch to equal vision

Assess nystagmus blockage mechanism
- Nystagmus blockage with face turn
- No face turn, little nystagmus → Measure size of deviation under anesthesia
  - Esotropia under anesthesia
  - Orthotropia or exotropia under anesthesia

(F) RECESS CONJUNCTIVA

(G) RECESS MEDIAL RECTI

OVERACTION OF THE INFERIOR OBLIQUE MUSCLES AND DISSOCIATED VERTICAL DEVIATION

James L. Mims III, M.D.

A. The most common disorders producing transient or incomitant vertical deviation in a young child are dissociated vertical deviation (DVD) and primary overaction of the inferior obliques (OAIO). Both are common in children who have had infantile esotropia. Numerous remote-controlled toys at the end of a 20-foot eye lane and several toys for near fixation are essential to obtain good alternate cover test measurements in all cardinal positions with good fixation and attention. In DVD, the other eye does not move when the elevated eye regains fixation (no hypotropia of the fellow eye when the hypertropic eye fixes). In primary OAIO, however, the other eye moves downward when the elevated eye regains fixation (hypotropia of the fellow eye when the hypertropic eye fixes). DVD occurs as a slow, upward drift of the affected eye, often with some extorsion as the eye drifts upward. It may be spontaneous or may occur only behind cover. In OAIO a hypertropia of the fixing eye always occurs in adduction. In DVD the elevation in abduction is generally (not always) greatest; in OAIO the elevation in adduction is always greatest. DVD is intermittently manifest in the primary (straight-ahead) position early, whereas in OAIO the deviation is not present in the primary position until late in the course of the disorder. The vertical deviation of DVD is present (and may be greatest) in downgaze; the vertical deviation of OAIO is usually absent in downgaze. If there is no elevation of the adducting eye on direct sidegaze in the patient who has significant upshoot of the adducting eye when the fixing abducted eye looks up and into abduction, suspect a variant of the co-contraction syndromes (e.g., Duane's syndrome; p 162). In this case bilateral lateral rectus recessions with supraplacement are the appropriate surgical therapy.

B. Once the diagnosis of DVD has been made, give careful attention to the spectacle correction. In many cases optical correction of astigmatism controls the DVD. If the deviation is uncontrolled with glasses and the DVD is much worse in one eye than in the other, the eyes of some children <5 years of age may be patched so thoroughly that the eye with the greater tendency to DVD can be made to become the fixing (dominant) eye. If this can be accomplished, the DVD remains latent. If the DVD is symmetric or objectionably large in both eyes even after glasses and patching, carefully look for an association of OAIO. If even a little OAIO is present, recession of the inferior obliques with anteriorization to a point 2 mm anterior to the lateral end of the inferior rectus eliminates both the DVD and the OAIO. If simply no OAIO is present, the most popular procedure is bilateral 10-mm recession of the superior recti. This may be done by the "hang loose" technique, which is technically easy and leaves the superior rectus on the nasal side of the vertical axis of Fick, a detail important in the prevention of the secondary exotropia that could otherwise be produced by a large superior rectus recession. One complication of the hang loose technique has been lack of adherence of the superior rectus to the globe, especially if it falls over the superior oblique tendon. A more reliable procedure is to attach the end of the superior rectus directly to the globe with a 10-mm recession and 3–4 mm of nasal transposition. Whatever technique of superior rectus recession is used, it is essential to dissect the dorsal surface of the superior rectus 16–18 mm posterior to its insertion to sever the frenulum that connects the superior rectus to the levator. If this connection is not severed, severe lid retraction can result postoperatively.

C. If the incomitant vertical deviation has been determined primarily to be OAIO, some DVD is often present also. If the child has had infantile esotropia, DVD may develop in the future. In either of these situations, the best surgical procedure is recession of the inferior obliques with anteriorization to a point 2 mm anterior to the lateral end of the inferior rectus. In some children >5 years of age (too old to develop DVD if it has not already occurred) who have overaction of the inferior obliques with no associated DVD, other weakening procedures of the inferior obliques may be used, such as myectomy, extirpation, or recession without anteriorization.

D. Recession of the inferior obliques with anteriorization to a point 2 mm anterior to the lateral end of the inferior rectus eliminates not only the OAIO but also the DVD. It should never be done unilaterally; unilateral anteriorization produces a significant restrictive hypotropia.

References

Kushner BJ. Pseudo inferior oblique overaction associated with Y- and V-patterns. Ophthalmology 1991; 98:1500–1505.

Magoon E, Cruciger M, Jampolsky A. Dissociated vertical deviation: An asymmetric condition treated with large bilateral superior rectus recession. J Pediatr Ophthalmol Strabismus 1982; 19:152–156.

Mims JL III, Wood RC. Bilateral anterior transposition of the inferior obliques. Arch Ophthalmol 1989; 107:41–44.

Parks MM, Parker JE. Atlas of strabismus surgery. New York: Harper & Row, 1983: 167–181.

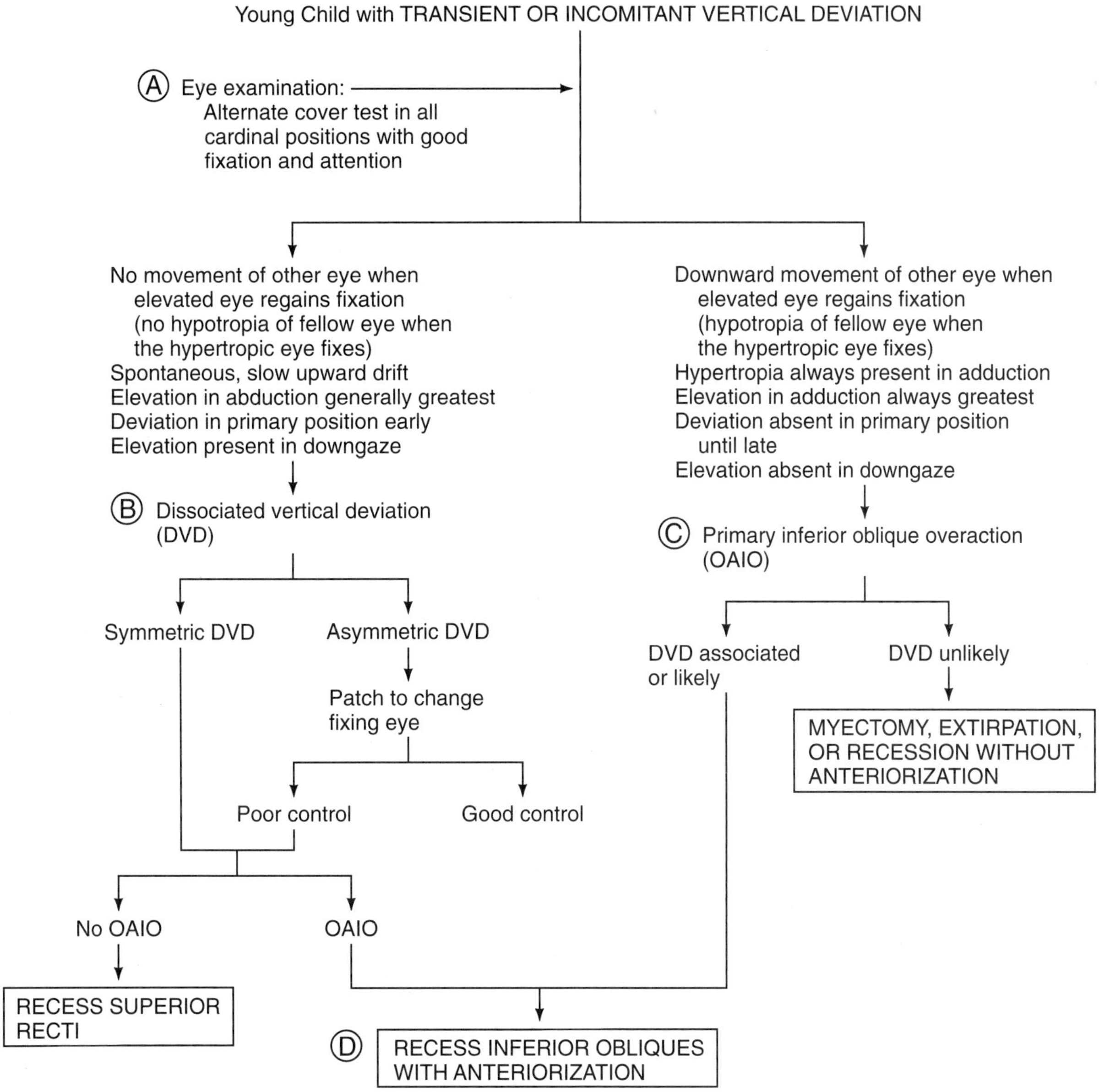

Young Child with TRANSIENT OR INCOMITANT VERTICAL DEVIATION

Ⓐ Eye examination:
    Alternate cover test in all
    cardinal positions with good
    fixation and attention

No movement of other eye when
    elevated eye regains fixation
    (no hypotropia of fellow eye when
    the hypertropic eye fixes)
Spontaneous, slow upward drift
Elevation in abduction generally greatest
Deviation in primary position early
Elevation present in downgaze

Downward movement of other eye when
    elevated eye regains fixation
    (hypotropia of fellow eye when
    the hypertropic eye fixes)
Hypertropia always present in adduction
Elevation in adduction always greatest
Deviation absent in primary position
    until late
Elevation absent in downgaze

Ⓑ Dissociated vertical deviation
    (DVD)

Ⓒ Primary inferior oblique overaction
    (OAIO)

Symmetric DVD   Asymmetric DVD

DVD associated   DVD unlikely
or likely

Patch to change
fixing eye

MYECTOMY, EXTIRPATION,
OR RECESSION WITHOUT
ANTERIORIZATION

Poor control   Good control

No OAIO   OAIO

RECESS SUPERIOR
RECTI

Ⓓ   RECESS INFERIOR OBLIQUES
    WITH ANTERIORIZATION

RECURRENT ESOTROPIA AFTER BIMEDIAL RECESSION FOR INFANTILE ESOTROPIA

James L. Mims III, M.D.

A. In the first 2 months after strabismus surgery, the preoperative atropine refraction (retinoscopy) generally is closer to the refraction the child is likely to have after healing is complete than a repeat cycloplegic retinoscopy performed early after surgery would be because there may be temporary changes in astigmatism the first few weeks after strabismus surgery. Significant optical asymmetry is >+1.25 diopter (D) sph difference on the hyperopic side, >−2.50 D sph difference on the myopic side, >1.25 D difference in symmetric or parallel axes of astigmatism, or >0.50 D difference if one axis of astigmatism is oblique and the other is vertical or horizontal.

B. Floropryl, recommended in the previous edition for recurrent high accommodative convergence/accommodation (AC/A) ratio esotropia in infants, is no longer available, and other miotics are not safe for infants. Fortunately, it recently has been realized that the currently popular large bilateral medial rectus recessions require 3 months to reach their full effect. Also, a child with <10 prism diopters (PD) of esotropia at near will preserve stereopsis.

C. Lack of availability of preoperative glasses or poor control of the distance or near deviation after placement of the preoperative glasses onto the child should lead to a repeat atropine refraction.

D. If the atropine refraction is to be repeated, once-daily administration of a tiny dab of 1% atropine ophthalmic ointment for 3 days before the office visit is adequate. Atropine overdose leading to late-night phone calls from anxious parents can be eliminated by teaching the parents to put a tiny dab of the ointment onto the fingertip and to place the dab directly into the cul-de-sac. Because of the previous bimedial recession, glasses with a spherical equivalent of only +2.00 D may eliminate residual esodeviation, even if the AC/A ratio is clinically high (10 PD greater esodeviation at near than at distance). If the spherical equivalent found on atropine refraction is <+2.00 D and the AC/A ratio is clinically high, prescribe a bifocal with ST-35 segments, with the segment line placed at the lower border of the upper lid margin, with a segment power of +2.00 D. If the AC/A ratio is not high and the spherical equivalent found on atropine refraction is <+1.50 D, prescribe glasses only for optical asymmetry. If the AC/A ratio is low and the spherical equivalent is +1.50 D or +1.75 D, prescribe single vision glasses. In all cases of recurrent esotropia in which the spherical equivalent is >+1.75 D, prescribe single vision glasses.

E. If single vision glasses do not control the distance deviation, consider a second operation. If single vision glasses control the distance deviation but there is an unexpected residual near deviation, a bifocal may be added.

F. The most common second operation for recurrent esotropia after bimedial recession is a bilateral lateral rectus resection. Bilateral resections of 4 mm for 15 ET, 5 mm for 20 ET, and 6 mm for 25 ET work well only if performed within 4 months after the original surgery. If the original bimedial recession was ≥6.2 mm, these numbers for bilateral resection should be reduced by 1 mm, or a unilateral lateral rectus resection of 5 mm for 10 ET, 6 mm for 12 ET, or 7 mm for 14 ET may be performed. If the original bimedial recession was performed >6 months before the bilateral resection, the amounts for bilateral resection should be increased by 1 mm, or rerecessions of the medial recti should be performed with respect for the increasing slope of the medial rectus recession dose-response curve.

References

Freeley DA, Nelson LB, Calhoun JH. Recurrent esotropia following early successful surgical correction of congenital esotropia. J Pediatr Ophthalmol Strabismus 1983; 20:68–71.

Mims JL III, Wood RC. A method for graduated re-recession of the medial recti for late recurrent esotropia: Results in 25 cases. Binocular Vision 1988; 3:77–84.

Parks MM, Jampolsky A, Crawford JS. Monocular and binocular vision: Expectations in treatment of strabismus. In: Pediatric ophthalmology and strabismus: Transactions of the New Orleans Academy of Ophthalmology. New York: Raven, 1986: 441–442.

Stager DR, Weakly DR, Everett M, Birch EE. Delayed consecutive exotropia following 7-millimeter bilateral medial rectus recession for congenital esotropia. J Pediatr Ophthalmol Strabismus 1994; 31:147–150.

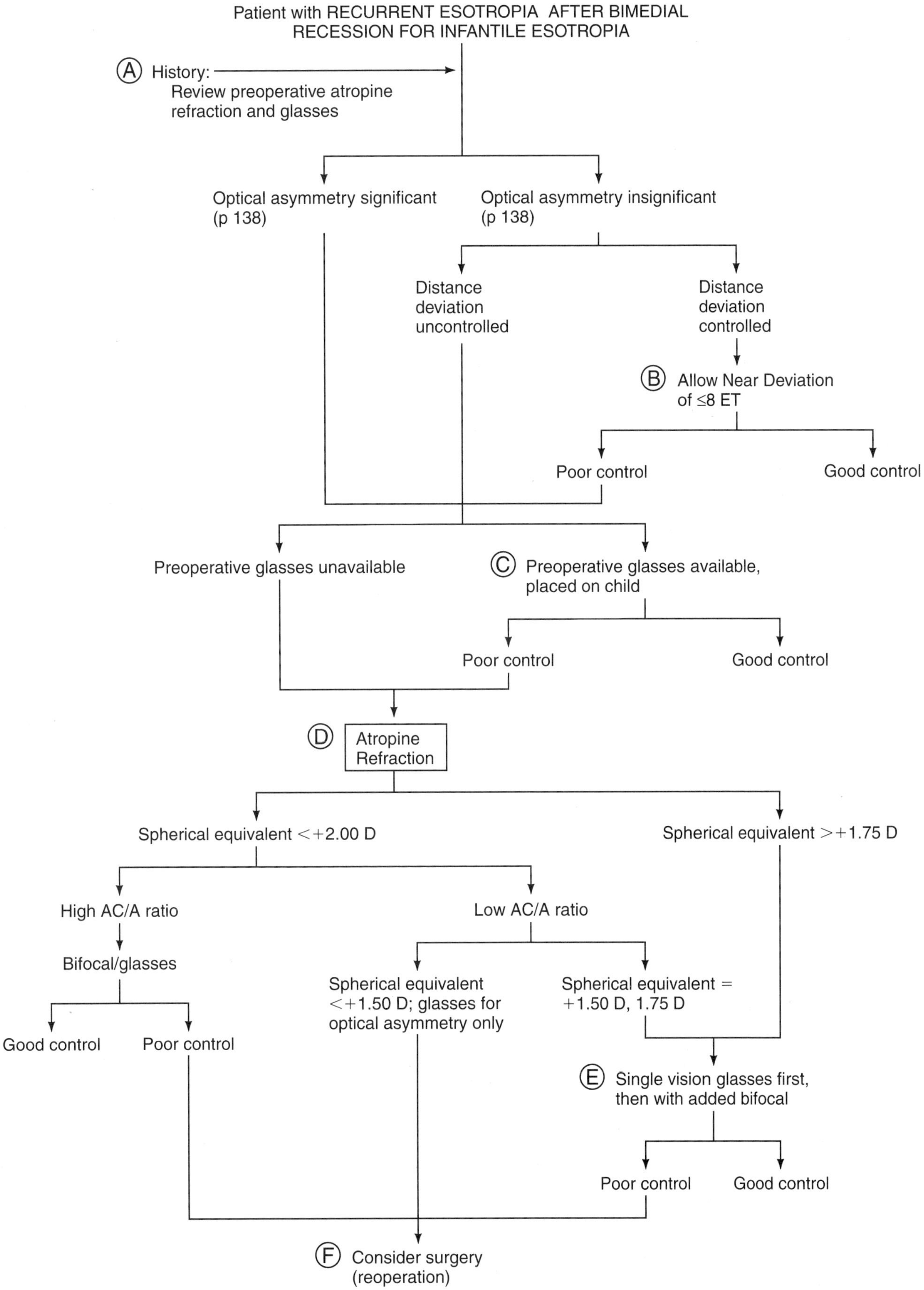

Patient with RECURRENT ESOTROPIA AFTER BIMEDIAL
RECESSION FOR INFANTILE ESOTROPIA

(A) History:
Review preoperative atropine
refraction and glasses

Optical asymmetry significant
(p 138)

Optical asymmetry insignificant
(p 138)

Distance
deviation
uncontrolled

Distance
deviation
controlled

(B) Allow Near Deviation
of ≤8 ET

Poor control

Good control

Preoperative glasses unavailable

(C) Preoperative glasses available,
placed on child

Poor control

Good control

(D) Atropine
Refraction

Spherical equivalent <+2.00 D

Spherical equivalent >+1.75 D

High AC/A ratio

Low AC/A ratio

Bifocal/glasses

Spherical equivalent
<+1.50 D; glasses for
optical asymmetry only

Spherical equivalent =
+1.50 D, 1.75 D

Good control   Poor control

(E) Single vision glasses first,
then with added bifocal

Poor control   Good control

(F) Consider surgery
(reoperation)

SURGICAL TREATMENT OF CONSECUTIVE EXOTROPIA

James L. Mims III, M.D.

Consecutive exotropia after bilateral medial rectus recession is common, occurring in up to 1 in 5 infantile esotropes and 1 in 10 acquired esotropes. Half of the cases occur in the first 2 years after the first surgery; the remainder can occur up to 20 years later. This chapter is based on a personal series of 136 patients treated surgically for consecutive exotropia, as well as on the listed references. Success rate is >90% at 6 months follow-up with this protocol.

A. About one third of children with consecutive exotropia will have a significant V- or Y-pattern with overaction of the inferior obliques (OAIO) or a significant A-pattern with overaction of the superior obliques (OASO). Alternating hypertropias as the child looks back and forth across the primary plane are the hallmark of both OAIO and OASO.

B. Weakening of the inferior obliques (IO) is indicated if hypertropia is seen as the child looks to the side >20 degrees. Most surgeons prefer recessions. In the context of consecutive exotropia with a V- or Y-pattern, it is important to remember that anteriorization of the posterior fibers of the IO will not collapse the V- or Y-pattern in one third of cases. Thus the posterior fibers must be reattached to the globe along the lateral edge of the inferior rectus, generally directly posterior to the point where the anterior fibers of the IO are reattached to the globe, to ensure collapse of the pattern. If the surgeon prefers myectomy, the collapse of the pattern is ensured, but oversewing Tenon's capsule may produce a powerful weakening effect on the IO, causing the superior obliques (SO) to overact years later.

C. If no hypertropias are seen in extreme sidegazes, the "OASO" appearance seen on the testing of versions may be simply the result of the vertical dimension of the orbital outlet being wider in the middle than at the sides, as pointed out by Guyton, and no SO tenotomies may be needed. This phenomenon has been called *pseudo-OASO*. If they are truly needed (as indicated by left hypotropia on extreme right gaze and right hypotropia on extreme left gaze), the tenotomies should be effective and on the temporal side. Silicone spacers will collapse the pattern but will not normalize the versions and may be associated with restrictive hypertropias on downgaze. (Wright silicone spacers are recommended for Brown's syndrome.) In a child with a history of infantile esotropia or in any child with enough instability of ocular alignment that consecutive exotropia (XT) with OASO has developed, dissociated vertical deviation (DVD) will be made significantly worse after SO tenotomy. Thus simultaneous with the SO tenotomies, the surgeon should almost always perform a bilateral superior rectus (SR) recession of 10 mm with 3 mm of nasal transposition. The nasal transposition prevents worsening of the consecutive exotropia because the secondary action of the SR is adduction. The SR should be directly sewn to the surface of the globe using a Parks' crossed swords or similar technique. Using a hang-back can result in lack of adherence of the SR to the globe (lost muscle) because of the SO tendon in this area. This complex surgery has had an 80% success with 1 year follow-up in 14 cases.

D. About one fourth of the cases, those with a distance deviation of ≥24 XT, are well treated with advancement of one medial rectus to the insertion in addition to whatever surgery is needed on the cyclovertical muscles for A- or V-pattern. This remarkably successful surgical plan was discovered only in the last 10 years. Many years ago it was discovered that advancement of both medial recti to the insertion led to a return of the original esotropia, even for consecutive exotropia angles as large as 45 XT. This distressing result led Cooper (1961) to recess lateral recti (LR) for consecutive exotropia and to "Cooper's Dictum," in which he advocated treating the consecutive exotropia as a new case, emphasizing recessions of one or two LR. This dictum is now obsolete in regard to bilateral LR recessions for consecutive exotropia; bilateral LR recessions have a low success rate with long-term follow-up. In an occasional case with a significant A-pattern without good evidence of OASO, advancement of one medial rectus will be successful if the near deviation is at least 15 XT'.

E. About half of the cases will return (or present) when the distance deviation is ≤23 XT because an exotropia of ≥8 XT is noticeable by most lay observers. These are well treated with recession of one lateral rectus in addition to whatever surgery is needed on the cyclovertical muscles for the A- or V-pattern. Recess one LR 7 mm for 10–12 XT, recess one LR 7.5 mm for 13–16 XT, and recess one LR 8 mm for 17–20 XT.

References

Biedner B, Yassur Y, David R. Advancement and reinsertion of one medial rectus as treatment for surgically overcorrected esotropia. Binocular Vision 1991; 6:197–200.

Bradbury JA, Doran RML. Secondary exotropia: A retrospective analysis of matched cases. J Pediatr Ophthalmol Strabismus 1993; 30:163–166.

Cooper EL. The surgical management of secondary exotropia. Trans Am Acad Ophthalmol Otol 1961; 65:595–608.

Ohtsuke H, Hasebe S, Tadokoro Y, et al. Advancement of one medial rectus to the original insertion for consecutive exotropia. J Pediatr Ophthalmol Strabismus 1993; 30:301–305.

SURGICAL TREATMENT OF CONSECUTIVE EXOTROPIA

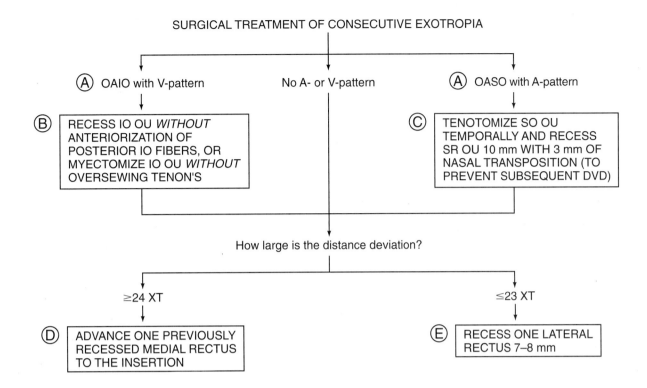

INTERMITTENT EXOTROPIA

James L. Mims III, M.D.

A. Intermittent exotropia of childhood generally begins at 1 or 2 years of age as a deviation seen only occasionally by the caregiver when the child is fixing on a distant object. The disorder progresses to the point that the distance deviation is often manifest by 3 or 4 years of age, the most common age of presentation in the ophthalmologist's office. Visual acuities (HOTV matching test; Allen cards) and careful refraction (retinoscopy) are essential. Amblyopia must be treated effectively before surgery to maximize success rates. If significant optical asymmetry or myopia of >-1.00 diopters (D) is present, prescribe glasses. Significant optical asymmetry is $>+1.25$ D sph difference on the hyperopic side, >-2.50 D sph difference on the myopic side, >1.25 D difference in symmetric or parallel axes of astigmatism, or >0.50 D difference if one axis of astigmatism is oblique and the other is vertical or horizontal.

B. A few children with intermittent exotropia may respond to stimulation of their accommodative convergence with small amounts of overminus in the glasses prescription. At age 2–6 years, a child with -1.00 D myopia may be given -2.00 D, a child with -2.00 D myopia may be given -2.75 D, and a child with -3.00 D myopia may be given -3.50 D. Children in this age group with myopia of ≥-4.00 D or ≤-0.75 D and those with hyperopia generally do not tolerate overminus in glasses more than briefly.

C. Six weeks of alternate-day patching (ADP)—patching of one eye for all except 2 waking hours for 1 day, followed by patching of the other eye the next day—is associated with an 87% success rate as preoperative therapy before lateral rectus recessions for intermittent exotropia. Occasionally, the ADP alone cures the disorder.

D. Persistent poor vision in one eye (20/80 or worse) is an indication for limiting strabismus surgery to the poorer eye.

E. If the child is <36 months of age and has a deviation of ≤25 XT, recession of one lateral rectus 8.0–9.5 mm works well.

F. For the child >36 months of age, bilateral lateral rectus recessions of 5 mm for 16–19 XT, 5.5 mm for 20 XT, 6.0 mm for 25 XT, 7.0 mm for 30 XT, and 8.0 mm for 40 XT work well (87% success in children 2–6 years old after 6 weeks of ADP). Add 1 mm to these guidelines if the near deviation is >10 XT or >50% of the distance deviation; avoid bilateral lateral rectus recessions of >8.0 mm in children. Success with symmetric lateral rectus recessions for patients with equal distance and near exodeviations was reported as long ago as 1840 (MacKensie) and as recently as 1988 (Kushner). Prognosis for cure with one operation is substantially better if the child is 10–20 ET at the first postoperative visit 4–6 days after bilateral lateral rectus recession. If >10 ET persists at 21 days after surgery, part-time ADP 8 hours daily for 2 or 3 weeks will usually eliminate the overcorrection. The anticipated need for full hyperopic correction with glasses or for bimedial rectus recession for consecutive esotropia is no more than 5% of those having received surgery.

G. If anatomic abnormality, disease, or amblyopia unresponsive to standard treatment is present and the poorer eye has 20/80 or worse acuity, treat the condition as an exotropia of disuse, with recess-resect surgery.

References

Jampolsky A. Management of exodeviations. In: Strabismus symposium: New Orleans Academy of Ophthalmology. St Louis: Mosby, 1962: 140–156.

Kushner BJ. Exotropic deviations: A functional classification and approach to treatment. Am Orthoptic J 1988; 38:81–93.

MacKensie W. The cure of strabismus by surgical operation. Appendix to a practical treatise on the diseases of the eye. 3rd ed. (with 1st ed. appendix). London: Longman, Orme, Brown, Green, and Longmans, 1840: 20 (appendix).

Mims JL III, Wood RC. The effect of preoperative alternate day patching on surgical results in intermittent exotropia: a retrospective study of 66 cases. Binocular Vision 1990; 4:189–195.

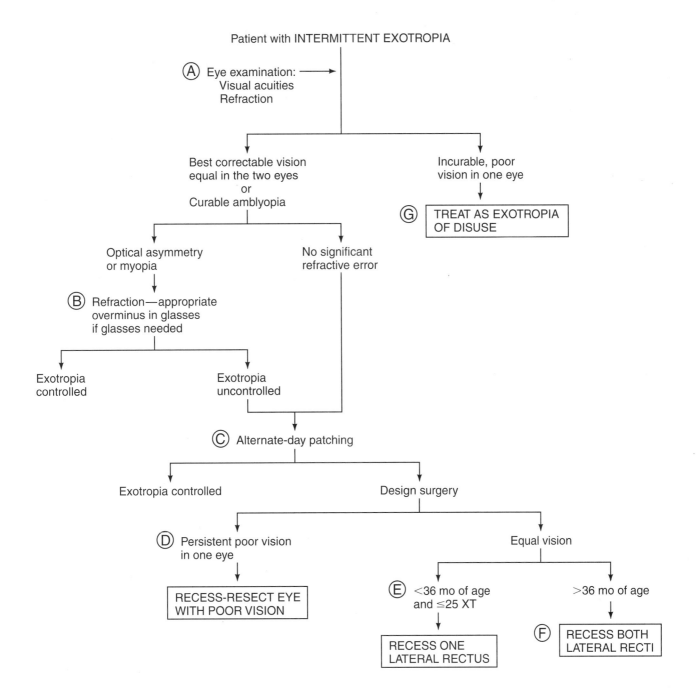

Patient with INTERMITTENT EXOTROPIA

Ⓐ Eye examination:
Visual acuities
Refraction

Best correctable vision
equal in the two eyes
or
Curable amblyopia

Incurable, poor
vision in one eye

Ⓖ TREAT AS EXOTROPIA
OF DISUSE

Optical asymmetry
or myopia

No significant
refractive error

Ⓑ Refraction—appropriate
overminus in glasses
if glasses needed

Exotropia
controlled

Exotropia
uncontrolled

Ⓒ Alternate-day patching

Exotropia controlled

Design surgery

Ⓓ Persistent poor vision
in one eye

RECESS-RESECT EYE
WITH POOR VISION

Equal vision

Ⓔ <36 mo of age
and ≤25 XT

>36 mo of age

RECESS ONE
LATERAL RECTUS

Ⓕ RECESS BOTH
LATERAL RECTI

153

ACQUIRED ESOTROPIA OF CHILDHOOD

James L. Mims III, M.D.

Success in management of acquired esotropia of childhood depends as much on care and vigilance in nonsurgical therapy as on performing the "right amount" of surgery.

A. Office cycloplegic retinoscopy follows instillation of a mixture that includes 0.5% cyclopentolate and 2.5% phenylephrine. Control with distance fixation on interesting toys is classified as good (esophoria only), fair (esotropia only occasionally), or poor (esotropia). Significant optical asymmetry is >+1.25 diopter (D) sph difference on the hyperopic side, >−2.50 D sph difference on the myopic side, >1.25 D difference in symmetric or parallel axes of astigmatism, and >0.50 D difference if one axis of astigmatism is oblique and the other is vertical or horizontal. Keep in mind that acquired esotropia can be the presenting sign of hydrocephalus and intracranial neoplasms. More esodeviation with distance than with near fixation, lateral incomitance, onset after 6 years of age, head circumference above the upper 2nd percentile, or other associated neurologic signs mandate referral to a neurologist and neuroimaging studies.

B. Full cylinder as well as full sphere are given; children adapt to the cylinder. As long as the full office cycloplegic retinoscopy controls the deviation, do not give a higher power because higher power makes the esotropia more frequent or constant when the glasses are removed. ("My child wasn't crossing her eyes all the time until she started wearing those glasses you prescribed, Doctor.")

C. Floropryl, recommended in the previous edition for high accommodative convergence/accommodation (AC/A) ratio acquired esotropia with good distance control, is no longer available. Phospholine Iodide 0.06%, one drop to each eye once nightly, has a number of unpleasant side effects, including enuresis, restlessness during sleep, asthma, and a rare skin rash, all of which I have seen. The side effects are produced by a decrease in the systemic cholinesterase. It is recommended only when the distance deviation is a small phoria and the near deviation is intermittently controlled with a phoria no larger than 16 ET'. Parents must be warned about possible interaction with succinylcholine. The latter will produce prolonged postanesthesia apnea (48 hours in one reported case), if it is used to aid intubation for general anesthesia in a patient who has been using Phospholine Iodide eye drops. In some patients Phospholine Iodide 0.06% will work well for 6–12 months. The development of cysts of the iris margin in brown-eyed children can be prevented or reduced by concurrent administration of 2.5% phenylephrine (Neo-Synephrine) eye drops. Such cysts are rare in blue-eyed children.

D. Once-daily administration of a tiny dab of 1% atropine ophthalmic ointment for 3 days before the office visit is adequate. Atropine overdose leading to late-night phone calls from anxious parents can be eliminated by teaching the parents to place a tiny dab of the ointment onto the fingertip and to place the dab directly into the cul-de-sac.

E. If the spherical equivalent is <+3.00 D and the AC/A ratio is clinically high (10 prism diopters [PD] greater esodeviation at near than at distance), prescribe bifocals before surgery, even if the spherical equivalent is myopic, in case bifocals are needed postoperatively for a residual deviation with near fixation. (This avoids the parental comment, "My child didn't need to wear bifocals until you did your surgery, Doctor.") ST-35 flat-top bifocal segments produce a lighter pair of glasses and work as well as executive segments if the segment line is placed high.

F. Surgery should not be considered until multiple examinations have been performed with multiple cycloplegic refractions. Often, a child can accept more hyperopic correction after a hyperopic correction has been worn for several months. Allow at least 6 weeks of wearing a lens prescription before concluding that a specific prescription will not straighten the eyes. If the clinical AC/A ratio is normal (approximately equal distance and near deviations) and the amount of bilateral medial rectus recession is measured from the apex of the insertion ridge after disinsertion of the muscle, the following amounts of surgery work well: 15 ET = 3.7 mm, 20 ET = 4.3 mm, 25 ET = 4.7 mm, 30 ET = 5.0 mm, 35 ET = 5.3 mm, 40 ET = 5.5 mm, 45 ET = 5.8 mm, 50 ET = 6.1 mm, 55 ET = 6.3 mm, 60 ET = 6.4 mm, 65 ET = 6.5 mm, and 70 ET = 6.6 mm. If the AC/A ratio is high, the formulas of Kushner for augmented bimedial recession work well. Kushner's basic surgical formula is 15 ET = 3.5 mm, 20 ET = 4.0 mm, 25 ET = 4.5 mm, and 30 ET = 5.0 mm, adding 1 mm to each medial rectus recession if the convergence excess is 10 PD, 1.5 mm for 15 PD, and 2 mm for ≥20 PD, up to 6.5 mm for each medial rectus recession.

References

Kushner BJ, Preslan MW, Morton GV. Treatment of partly accommodative esotropia with a high accommodative convergence-accommodation ratio. Arch Ophthalmol 1987; 105:815–818.

Leopold IH, Krishna N, Lehman RA. Effects of anticholinesterase agents on the blood cholinesterase levels of normal and glaucoma subjects. Trans Am Ophthalmol Soc 1959; 57:63–66.

Mims JL III, Treff C, Wood RC. Variability of strabismus surgery for acquired esotropia. Arch Ophthalmol 1986; 104: 1780–1782.

Preslan MW, Beauchamp GR. Accommodative esotropia: Review of current practices and controversies. Ophthalmic Surg 1987; 18:68–72.

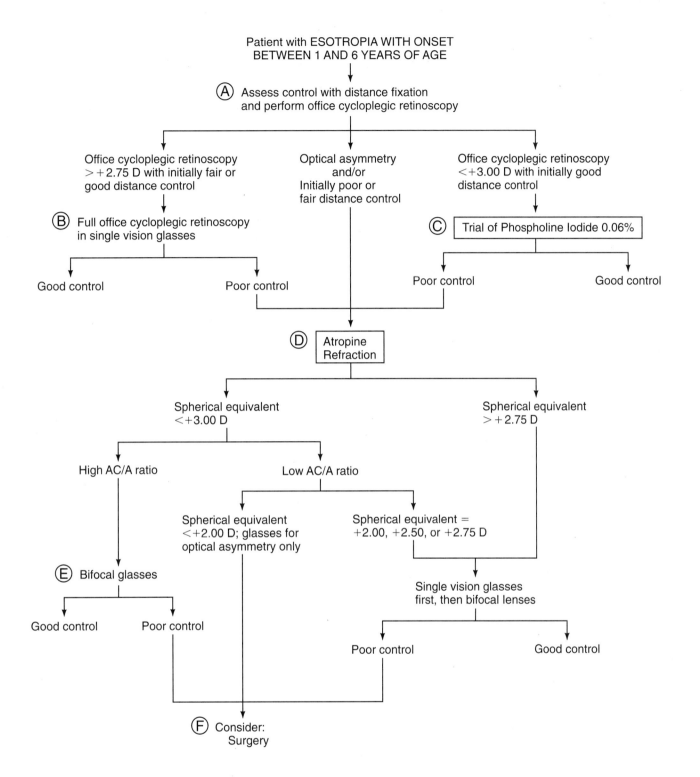

DIAGNOSIS OF HEAD TILTS AND FACE TURNS IN CHILDREN

James L. Mims III, M.D.

A. The ophthalmic examination of any child >6 months of age should begin with a study of the ductions and versions. This can be done with a series of interesting toys held in various cardinal positions. The versions (both eyes together and binocular) are checked first; if there is an abnormality in the versions, the examiner can then study the ductions (one eye and monocular) by holding his or her hand just in front of one eye without touching the child. At times the mother's hand may be needed to cover one eye. If the (monocular) ductions are limited in supraduction and in adduction, the child probably has Brown's superior oblique syndrome from either poor slippage of the superior oblique tendon through the trochlea or an abnormality of length or insertion of the superior oblique tendon. Children with progressive Brown's syndrome may also have a progressive face turn and an increasing exodeviation with time. Only if the face turn or chin elevation is progressive should children with Brown's syndrome receive superior oblique tenotomy. Limited adduction may be caused by a third cranial nerve palsy or by type II Duane's retraction syndrome. Exotropia is associated with both third cranial nerve palsies and with type II Duane's syndrome, but only the third cranial nerve palsy may occur with hypotropia. The palpebral fissure narrows on attempted adduction in Duane's syndrome; the palpebral fissure stays the same or widens on attempted adduction in third cranial nerve palsies. Third cranial nerve palsies in children mandate examination by a neurologist. If abduction is limited, the child may have a sixth cranial nerve palsy or type I Duane's retraction syndrome. The esotropia of a sixth cranial nerve palsy is typically much larger than that associated with most cases of type I Duane's syndrome. Narrowing of the palpebral fissure (caused by co-contraction of the horizontal recti in the eye with Duane's syndrome) occurs on attempted adduction in Duane's syndrome but not in sixth cranial nerve palsies. Sixth cranial nerve palsies in children may resolve without treatment in 6 weeks if caused by postinfectious neuritis, but the innocuous nature of CT scanning has led to widespread use of CT soon after the acute onset of sixth cranial nerve palsies. This allows early detection of the uncommon case with significant abnormality of the CNS.

B. If the versions (both eyes) are normal, the ductions (one eye) are also normal. The three most common causes of an abnormal face turn in a child with unlimited ductions are nystagmus with a null point in extreme sidegaze, hyperdeviation on gaze to one side absent or less on gaze to the other side, and refractive errors (astigmatism or myopia). The nystagmus may be grossly worse when the child's attention is forced toward the nonpreferred direction of gaze, or only micronystagmus may be present, necessitating direct ophthalmoscopy (and a cooperative patient) to confirm nystagmus as the cause of the face turn. More than 90% of children with congenital nystagmus have a disorder of the visual sensory system; children with acquired nystagmus may have CNS tumors. Hyperdeviation on gaze to one side absent or less on gaze to the other side commonly is caused by superior oblique palsy, less commonly by dissociated vertical deviation, and rarely by asymmetric primary inferior oblique overaction. Refractive errors such as astigmatism or myopia should not be overlooked as causes of face turns in children. The child may be using the edge of his or her nose to produce a pinhole camera effect to improve vision. If a child with some nystagmus is given glasses to correct the astigmatism and/or the myopia and the face turn persists to the extent that the child has difficulty using the glasses, a Kestenbaum or augmented Anderson procedure (10-mm recession of the medial rectus of the eye that is adducted during the preferred face turn, combined with 12-mm recession of the lateral rectus of the eye that is abducted during the preferred face turn) is indicated for the nystagmus.

C. A head tilt in a child may be the result of ocular or nonocular causes, such as spastic torticollis. If the child cooperates for alternate cover testing with the head tilted to either side, cyclovertical muscle palsy is diagnosed. A less cooperative child may allow patching of one eye for a time. If there is no change in the head tilt with either eye covered, the cause of the tilt is nonocular. If the tilt is little changed with one eye covered and improves significantly with the other eye covered, a cyclovertical muscle palsy is probably present.

References

Harley RD. Paralytic strabismus in children, etiologic incidence and management of the third, fourth, and sixth nerve palsies. Ophthalmology 1980; 87:24–43.

Kushner BJ. Ocular causes of abnormal head postures. Trans Am Acad Ophthalmol Otolaryngol 1979; 86:2115–2125.

Mitchell PR, Wheeler MB, Parks MM. Kestenbaum surgical procedure for torticollis secondary to congenital nystagmus. J Pediatr Ophthalmol Strabismus 1987; 24:94–96.

Weiss AH, Biersdorf WR. Visual sensory disorders in congenital nystagmus. Ophthalmology 1989; 96:517–523.

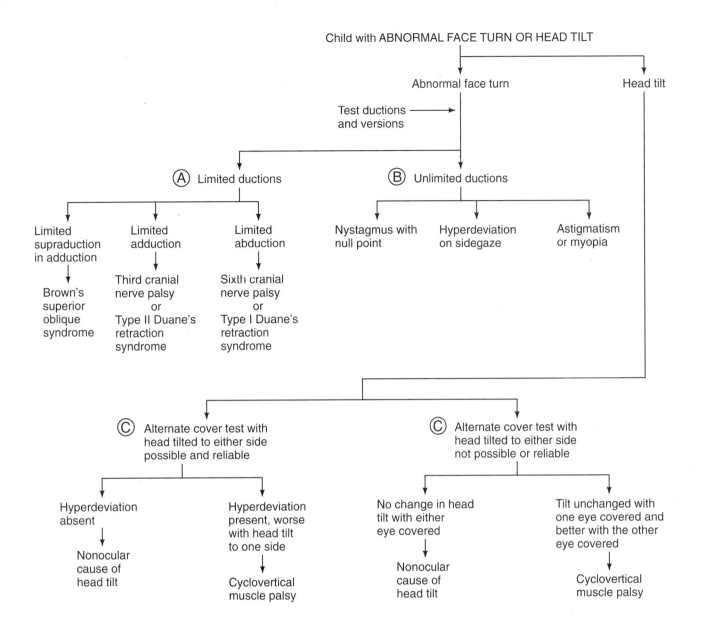

DIAGNOSIS OF CYCLOVERTICAL MUSCLE PALSIES

James L. Mims III, M.D.

Bielschowsky and Parks have popularized a three-step test for the diagnosis of cyclovertical muscle palsies. This test works only when the cause of the hyperdeviation is a paresis of a single cyclovertical muscle in a patient who has had no surgery. The first step is to determine whether the hypertropia is a right hypertropia (RHT) or a left hypertropia (LHT). The second step is to identify whether the hypertropia increases in right gaze (dextroversion) or in left gaze (levoversion). Finally, the third step is to determine whether the vertical deviation increases on tilting the head to the right or to the left.

A. If there is an RHT in the primary position, either the depressors of the right eye (the right inferior rectus [RIR] and the right superior oblique [RSO]) or the elevators of the left eye (the left superior rectus [LSR] and the left inferior oblique [LIO]) are paretic.

B. Among these four muscles, right gaze is the field in which the LIO and the RIR are acting more powerfully in the vertical direction and in which the other two muscles are acting more as tortors.

C. When the head is tilted to the right, there is a tendency toward extorsion of the left eye. The extortors of the left eye are the LIO and the left inferior rectus (LIR). A paretic LIO would be opposed by a normal LIR as these extortors were acting, thus increasing the RHT. When the head is tilted to the left, there is a tendency toward extortion of the right eye. The extortors of the right eye are the RIR and the right inferior oblique (RIO). A paretic RIR would be opposed by a normal RIO, thus increasing the RHT.

D. Again, when there is an RHT in the primary position, either the depressors of the right eye (the RIR and the RSO) or the elevators of the left eye (the LSR and the LIO) are paretic. Among these four muscles, left gaze is the field in which the RSO and the LSR are acting more powerfully in the vertical direction and in which the other two muscles are acting more as tortors. When the head is tilted to the right, there is a tendency toward intorsion of the right eye. The intortors of the right eye are the RSO and the right superior rectus (RSR). A paretic RSO would be opposed by a normal RSR as these intortors were acting, thus increasing the RHT. When the head is tilted to the left, there is a tendency toward intorsion of the left eye. The intortors of the left eye are the LSR and the left superior oblique (LSO). A paretic LSR would be opposed by a normal LSO, thus increasing the RHT.

E. An LHT could be caused by the left eye depressors LIR or LSO or by the right eye elevators RSR or RIO.

F. Among these four muscles, the LIR and the RIO act more powerfully in the vertical direction in left gaze.

G. On right head tilt, the left eye extortors LIR and LIO are stimulated, thus increasing the LHT if the LIR is paretic. On left head tilt, the right eye extortors RIO and RIR are stimulated, thus increasing the LHT if the RIO is paretic.

H. With an LHT greater in right gaze, the two suspect muscles are the RSR and the LSO. On right head tilt, the right eye intortors RSR and RSO are stimulated, thus increasing the LHT if the RSR is paretic. On left head tilt, the left eye intortors LSO and LSR are stimulated, thus increasing the LHT if the LSO is paretic.

References

Kushner BJ, Kraft S. Ocular torsional movements in normal humans. Am J Ophthalmol 1983; 95:752–762.

Parks MM. Isolated cyclovertical muscle palsy. Arch Ophthalmol 1958; 60:1027–1035.

Scott AB. Extraocular muscles and head tilting. Arch Ophthalmol 1967; 78:397–399.

von Noorden GK. Atlas of strabismus. St Louis: Mosby, 1983: 148–155.

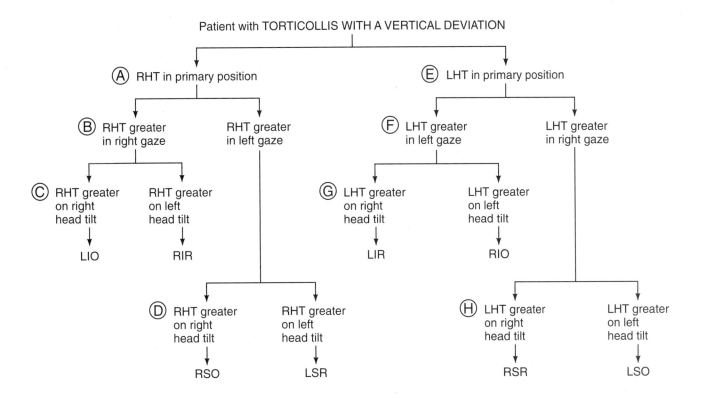

Patient with TORTICOLLIS WITH A VERTICAL DEVIATION

(A) RHT in primary position

(B) RHT greater in right gaze

RHT greater in left gaze

(C) RHT greater on right head tilt → LIO

RHT greater on left head tilt → RIR

(D) RHT greater on right head tilt → RSO

RHT greater on left head tilt → LSR

(E) LHT in primary position

(F) LHT greater in left gaze

LHT greater in right gaze

(G) LHT greater on right head tilt → LIR

LHT greater on left head tilt → RIO

(H) LHT greater on right head tilt → RSR

LHT greater on left head tilt → LSO

CHOICE OF SURGERY FOR UNILATERAL SUPERIOR OBLIQUE PALSY

James L. Mims III, M.D.

For simplicity and clarity, the decision tree is written for a unilateral right superior oblique (RSO) palsy.

Among the isolated extraocular muscle palsies, paresis of the superior oblique (SO) is the most common in most strabismus practices. Also, SO paresis is the most common cause of a vertical strabismus among patients who have not had infantile esotropia.

A. A head tilt of ≥6 degrees is objectionable to the patient; a head tilt smaller than this will be noticed more by the doctor than by the patient. For head tilts <6 degrees, weakening of the antagonist inferior oblique (IO) will make the patient very happy without any unpleasant side effects—such as a Brown's syndrome. As a physician, accept the patient's happiness gratefully in this situation and do not fret about a residual head tilt of <6 degrees. Alan Scott has stated that most of the patients with enough postoperative problems to be presented at a strabismus Grand Rounds had both a tuck and an IO weakening procedure simultaneously. On the other hand, if the head is tilted >6 degrees, the SO tendon must be strengthened directly with a tuck or a kink, or the head tilt will not be significantly improved postoperatively. For almost all other patients, an IO recession is the best first step. One technique for measuring the head tilt is to line up the occluder paddle with the center of the patient's nose and chin and then, without changing the angle, place the occluder paddle directly in front of a Green's I refractor or a similar refraction device, such as the phoropter. Then the degree of head tilt can be read easily from the dial for the angle of astigmatism on the machine.

B. Although a few surgeons have published series of SO tucks (notably Knapp, Saunders, and Flynn), for most surgeons, an SO tuck produces objectionable iatrogenic Brown's syndrome. For this reason in this decision tree, an alternative to the SO tuck is enthusiastically recommended. The Dyer anteriorization of the midportion of the entire SO tendon to the Harada-Ito point is a procedure that produces less severe Brown's syndrome than tucks because the Dyer "kink" of the tendon straightens out as the eye looks into adduction. Dyer originally recommended a disinsertion of the IO to be performed simultaneously with the "kink." In the hands of most surgeons, it is more predictable to do a controlled recession of the IO simultaneously with the Dyer kink, especially with techniques recently described by Stager, than to perform the disinsertion of the IO as originally described by Dyer. Significant overcorrection has resulted from combining an IO myectomy with a Dyer kink or an SO tendon tuck, although Saunders does recommend combining IO myectomy with a tuck when the primary position deviation is especially large. When an IO myectomy works well in patients with SO palsies, it does so by reattachment to the globe. If a tuck or a Dyer kink of the SO tendon has been performed and the myectomized IO does not reattach to the globe, severe overcorrection and iatrogenic Brown's syndrome will occur. (In patients with primary overaction of the IO, a myectomy will work well even if the IO does not reattach to the globe.) When a Dyer kink is indicated, simultaneously perform a recession of the IO without anteriorization.

C. Surgeons who perform SO tendon tucks usually recommend a simultaneous IO weakening procedure only if the primary position hypertropia is ≥25–30 prism diopters (PD).

D. If the head tilt is not objectionable but the right gaze hypertropia (the hypertropia out of the field of action of the paretic SO) is 5–15 PD and the only other surgery has been an IO recession, recess the right superior rectus a very small amount, generally 3 mm.

Special Note: Avoid recession of the inferior rectus (IR) of the other eye. There are three reasons for this. First, in most cases with a good early result of IR recession as a part of the surgery, overcorrections will develop in a few months or years. Second, recession of the IR of the other eye will theoretically make the head tilt worse by producing intorsion of the other eye. Third, contracture of the IR of the other eye will gradually lessen during the months after appropriate surgery on the eye with the paretic SO. Another obsolete recommendation that must be avoided is tenotomy of the other superior oblique in long-standing cases for whom the hypertropia is greatest in all three downgaze positions. In an occasional elderly patient, such as characterized by Helveston, there is mainly a slight underaction of the SO from a presumed microvascular accident. Such patients are best treated with prisms.

References

Bartley GB, Dyer JA. Strengthening the weak superior oblique muscle. Ophthalmic Surg 1987; 18:893–897.

Helveston EM. Surgical management of strabismus. St Louis: Mosby, 1993: 473–481.

Saunders RA. Treatment of superior oblique palsy with superior oblique tendon tuck and inferior oblique myectomy. Ophthalmology 1986; 93:1023–1027.

Scott WE, Kraft AP. Classification and surgical treatment of superior oblique palsies. In: Pediatric ophthalmology and strabismus: Transactions of the New Orleans Academy of Ophthalmology. New York: Raven, 1986: 15–38.

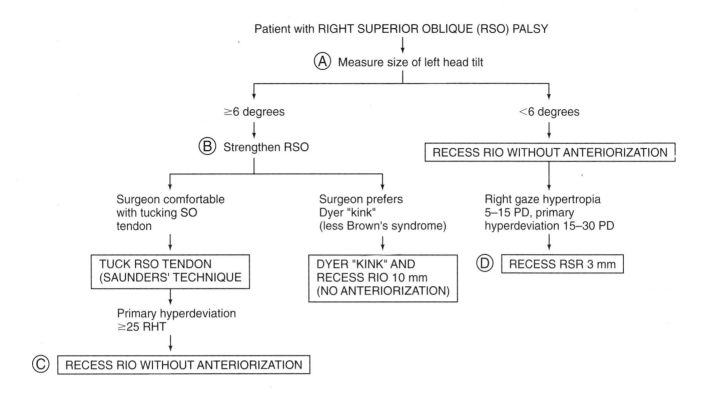

Patient with RIGHT SUPERIOR OBLIQUE (RSO) PALSY

Ⓐ Measure size of left head tilt

≥6 degrees

<6 degrees

Ⓑ Strengthen RSO

RECESS RIO WITHOUT ANTERIORIZATION

Surgeon comfortable
with tucking SO
tendon

Surgeon prefers
Dyer "kink"
(less Brown's syndrome)

Right gaze hypertropia
5–15 PD, primary
hyperdeviation 15–30 PD

TUCK RSO TENDON
(SAUNDERS' TECHNIQUE

DYER "KINK" AND
RECESS RIO 10 mm
(NO ANTERIORIZATION)

Ⓓ RECESS RSR 3 mm

Primary hyperdeviation
≥25 RHT

Ⓒ RECESS RIO WITHOUT ANTERIORIZATION

CHOICE OF SURGERY FOR DUANE'S RETRACTION SYNDROME

James L. Mims III, M.D.

A. Patients with all types of Duane's retraction syndrome have co-contraction of the medial and lateral recti on adduction with narrowing of the palpebral fissure on adduction. The narrowing of the palpebral fissure is caused by innervation of the Duane's lateral rectus (LR) with fibers from the medial rectus (MR) subnucleus of the third cranial nerve. Patients with type I Duane's syndrome have significantly limited abduction because of a congenital absence of the sixth cranial nerve on the affected side. Patients with the relatively rare type II Duane's syndrome have more limited adduction than those with type I because of co-contraction of the MR and an LR that has a dual innervation—both an abnormal innervation from the MR subnucleus of the third cranial nerve and the usual, normal, innervation from an intact sixth cranial nerve. Abduction is normal in type II Duane's syndrome. Most patients with Duane's syndrome fuse with a face turn and/or a chin elevation or depression. This decision tree is for patients with a face turn >10 degrees in the primary position, significant chin depression or elevation, or a face turn >8 degrees in reading downgaze. Patients with type I Duane's syndrome with exotropia in the primary position are uncommon, but they may be helped with recession of the non-Duane's LR 12 mm and posterior fixation suture on the MR of the non-Duane's eye as suggested by Saunders (1994). If the only problem is an exotropia in downgaze, both lateral recti should be infraplaced 4 mm. Patients with type II Duane's syndrome benefit from a 5-mm recession of the Duane's LR. Because the Duane's LR has a stiff length-tension curve, only a small amount of recession is required.

B. In most patients with type I Duane's syndrome with a face turn, the single binocular field (SBF) does not extend more than a few degrees into the side of the eye with Duane's syndrome. Twelve degrees is a functional minimum. When the field extends this far, recession of the Duane's MR 5 mm may be sufficient to change the face turn. This case is rare.

C. The Duane's LR in some patients is innervated not only with fibers from the MR subnucleus of the third cranial nerve but also with fibers from the superior rectus (SR) or from the inferior rectus (IR) subnucleus. Patients with innervation from the IR subnucleus may have a compensatory chin elevation head posture to take advantage of the normal width of the SBF in reading downgaze. Recession of both inferior recti 7 mm provides permanent relief from the necessity of this chin elevation. These recessed inferior recti must be nasally transposed 4 mm, and the recessions should not exceed 7 mm to prevent exotropia in downgaze. The in-

termuscular septum must be returned to its original position to prevent lid lag. Similarly, patients with significantly better abduction of the Duane's eye in upgaze and a chin tuck respond well to 10-mm recessions (attaching the SR directly to the sclera) with 3–4 mm nasal transpositions.

D. If abduction of the Duane's eye is not significantly better in upgaze or downgaze, either recess-resect of the Duane's eye or lateral transposition of the vertical recti of the Duane's eye as suggested by Rosenbaum will be required to change the face turn. Both of these types of surgery make the signs of co-contraction more severe, and these surgical options are limited by the severity of the co-contraction. Signs of co-contraction include (1) exodeviation in far gaze to the side opposite the eye with Duane's syndrome, (2) narrowing of the palpebral fissure of ≥1.5 mm on adduction, (3) defective adduction with corneal reflection >2 mm inside the lateral limbus by the Urist test, (4) noticeable enophthalmos on adduction, (5) 25% reduction in adduction saccadic velocities, (6) near point of convergence remote beyond 6 cm, and (7) upshoot or downshoot on adduction.

E. Minimal signs of co-contraction allow a small recess-resect (as originally suggested by Brown). Recess the MR 5 mm, and resect the LR 3 mm. The resection of the Duane's LR must not exceed 3 mm because of the very stiff length-tension curve of the Duane's LR.

F. When co-contraction is no more than moderate, lateral transposition of the vertical recti as described by Rosenbaum reduces the face turn and centralizes the SBF. If the forced ductions on abduction are positive at surgery or if the primary position esodeviation is >25 ET, it is more likely that a medial rectus recession (not to exceed 5 mm) must be added to the vertical rectus transposition at a second surgery. Care should be taken during the transposition surgery to place the superior rectus tendon at a point 2–3 mm superior to the lateral rectus insertion to avoid producing hyperdeviations. Warn parents that co-contraction signs may be slightly worse and that full abduction of the eye with Duane's syndrome will not be accomplished by any surgery to reduce the face turn.

G. Some patients have no face turn, and their primary reason for consulting an ophthalmologist is unsightly upshoot in adduction of the eye with the Duane's syndrome. Recess-recess of the MR and the LR of the Duane's eye has replaced posterior fixation sutures as the treatment of choice for upshoot in adduction.

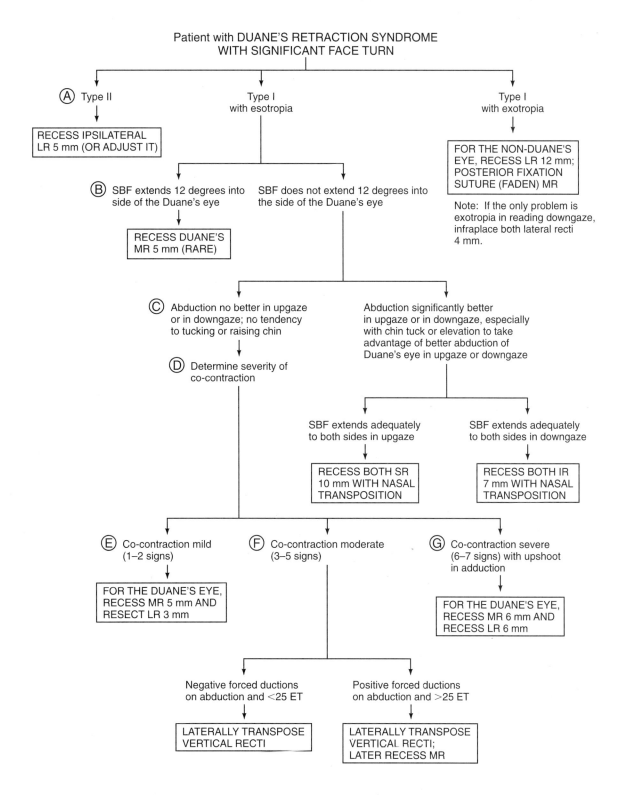

Patient with DUANE'S RETRACTION SYNDROME
WITH SIGNIFICANT FACE TURN

Ⓐ Type II

RECESS IPSILATERAL
LR 5 mm (OR ADJUST IT)

Type I
with esotropia

Type I
with exotropia

FOR THE NON-DUANE'S
EYE, RECESS LR 12 mm;
POSTERIOR FIXATION
SUTURE (FADEN) MR

Note: If the only problem is
exotropia in reading downgaze,
infraplace both lateral recti
4 mm.

Ⓑ SBF extends 12 degrees into
side of the Duane's eye

SBF does not extend 12 degrees into
the side of the Duane's eye

RECESS DUANE'S
MR 5 mm (RARE)

Ⓒ Abduction no better in upgaze
or in downgaze; no tendency
to tucking or raising chin

Abduction significantly better
in upgaze or in downgaze, especially
with chin tuck or elevation to take
advantage of better abduction of
Duane's eye in upgaze or downgaze

Ⓓ Determine severity of
co-contraction

SBF extends adequately
to both sides in upgaze

SBF extends adequately
to both sides in downgaze

RECESS BOTH SR
10 mm WITH NASAL
TRANSPOSITION

RECESS BOTH IR
7 mm WITH NASAL
TRANSPOSITION

Ⓔ Co-contraction mild
(1–2 signs)

Ⓕ Co-contraction moderate
(3–5 signs)

Ⓖ Co-contraction severe
(6–7 signs) with upshoot
in adduction

FOR THE DUANE'S EYE,
RECESS MR 5 mm AND
RESECT LR 3 mm

FOR THE DUANE'S EYE,
RECESS MR 6 mm AND
RECESS LR 6 mm

Negative forced ductions
on abduction and <25 ET

Positive forced ductions
on abduction and >25 ET

LATERALLY TRANSPOSE
VERTICAL RECTI

LATERALLY TRANSPOSE
VERTICAL RECTI;
LATER RECESS MR

References

Duane A. Congenital deficiency of abduction associated with impairment of adduction, retraction movements, contraction of the palpebral fissure and oblique movements of the eye. Arch Ophthalmol 1905; 34:133–159.

Miller NR, Kiel SM, Green WR, Clark AW. Unilateral Duane's retraction syndrome (type I). Arch Ophthalmol 1982; 100:1468–1472.

Molarte AB, Rosenbaum AL. Vertical rectus transposition surgery for Duane's syndrome. J Pediatr Ophthalmol Strabismus 1990; 27:171–177.

Saunders RA, Wilson ME, Bluestein EC, Sinatra RB. Surgery on the normal eye in Duane retraction syndrome. J Pediatr Ophthalmol Strabismus 1994; 31:162–169.

CHOICE OF SURGERY FOR LIMITED SUPRADUCTION IN A CHILD

James L. Mims III, M.D.

A. The cause of double elevator palsy (DEP) is poorly understood but is thought to be supranuclear. A patient with a paralyzed superior rectus (SR) with a normal inferior oblique (IO) cannot elevate the eye convincingly even in adduction; it is useful to think of a DEP as an SR palsy. Indeed, vertical saccades are often subnormal in this disorder. Children with DEP have limitation of elevation in up, up-and-left, and up-and-right ductions and a consequent hypotropia in the involved eye that increases in upgaze. They may have a chin-up position with fusion in downgaze (more common) or amblyopia in the hypotropic affected eye. Ptosis or pseudoptosis may be present in the primary position. As with other vertical deviations, it is important to level the eyes before considering ptosis surgery. In some patients with DEP the primary defect is restriction of the inferior rectus (IR); in others the primary defect is the SR palsy. If the vertical forced ductions are tight (positive going into supraduction) at surgery, the best procedure is an 8-mm recession of the IR with adequate separation of the IR from the underlying tissues and suspension of the palpebral head of the IR to prevent lid retraction. If the vertical forced ductions are normal, the accepted procedure is a vertical transposition of the horizontal recti as popularized by Knapp. This generally corrects 25 prism diopters (PD) of vertical deviation.

B. Brown's superior oblique (SO) syndrome includes inability of the patient to look up and in with positive forced ductions in this direction. Usually, the patient exhibits depression on adduction of the involved eye and normal or near-normal elevation when the eye is in abduction. Also, overaction of the SO is usually absent. Brown's SO syndrome can be progressive or stable. In the more severe, progressive form, the chin elevation and face turn are progressive, and there may also be a progressively larger exodeviation in the primary position. In this type the insertion of the SO may be abnormally nasal and posterior, and a tenotomy of the SO may be significantly more difficult than usual as a result of the abnormal insertion. The best procedure for the progressive and severe form is tenotomy of the SO. Although some have advocated simultaneous weakening of the IO, this may compromise the success of the tenotomy and is not generally recommended. In up to 40% of children who have had SO tenotomy for Brown's syndrome, the head tilt and vertical deviation of an iatrogenic SO palsy appear months to years after the tenotomy. This may require one or two subsequent operations for correction, including an IO weakening procedure or even a rotational procedure involving supraplacement of the medial rectus (MR) and infraplacement of the lateral rectus (LR). Clearly, SO tenotomy should be reserved for the more severe and progressive form of Brown's syndrome. When there is no face turn or chin elevation and there is fusion in reading downgaze, serious consideration should be given to avoiding surgery. The only procedure reported to be safe for the less severe form of Brown's syndrome is the silicone tendon extender (retinal band) devised by Wright.

C. The treatment of traumatic blow-out fracture of the orbital floor remains controversial, but most surgeon/authors agree that some delay is appropriate to see whether the patient improves spontaneously. Although the mechanism probably does not involve deformation of the globe, up to 30% of patients with blow-out fractures also have serious intraocular abnormality. The IR muscle may have become paretic, and a hypertropia may result after freeing the muscle from the fracture. This can be predicted by preoperative saccadic velocities. In many cases this paresis of the IR proves temporary.

D. The key to success for surgery for third cranial nerve palsies is tenotomy of the SO on the involved side. In an acquired third nerve palsy, injection of botulinum A toxin (Oculinum) into the LR and patching early may speed recovery. Beware of the MR in congenital third nerve palsies; it may have a very stiff length-tension curve, even stiffer than the Duane's LR. Avoid resections when possible. If the MR is not fibrotic and stiff with positive forced ductions in abduction, a large recess-resect can work well. If the MR is stiff and fibrotic, 12-mm bilateral LR recessions are appropriate.

References

Harley RD. Paralytic strabismus in children, etiologic incidence and management of the third, fourth, and sixth nerve palsies. Ophthalmology 1980; 87:24–43.

Metz HS. Double elevator palsy. Arch Ophthalmol 1979; 97:901–903.

Wilkins RB, Havens WE. Current treatment of blowout fractures. Ophthalmology 1982; 89:464–467.

Wright DW. Superior oblique silicone expander for Brown syndrome and superior oblique overaction. J Pediatr Ophthalmol Strabismus 1991; 28:101–107.

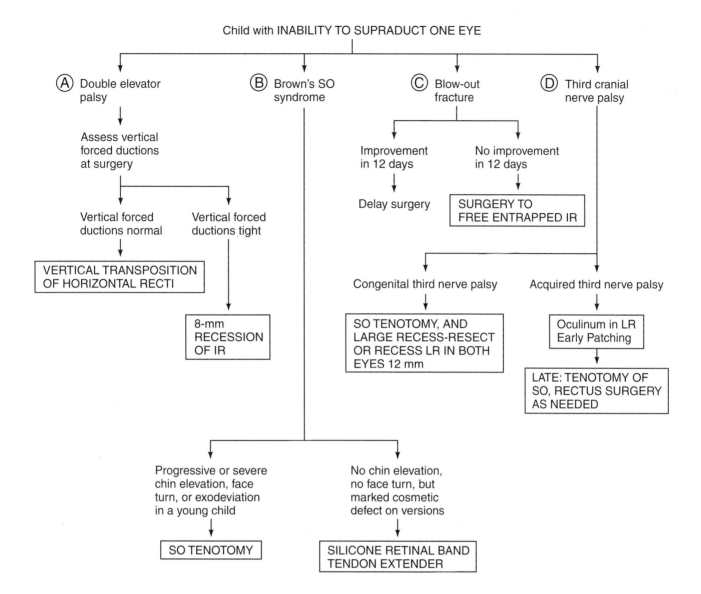

Child with INABILITY TO SUPRADUCT ONE EYE

(A) Double elevator palsy

Assess vertical forced ductions at surgery

Vertical forced ductions normal

VERTICAL TRANSPOSITION OF HORIZONTAL RECTI

Vertical forced ductions tight

8-mm RECESSION OF IR

(B) Brown's SO syndrome

Progressive or severe chin elevation, face turn, or exodeviation in a young child

SO TENOTOMY

No chin elevation, no face turn, but marked cosmetic defect on versions

SILICONE RETINAL BAND TENDON EXTENDER

(C) Blow-out fracture

Improvement in 12 days

Delay surgery

No improvement in 12 days

SURGERY TO FREE ENTRAPPED IR

Congenital third nerve palsy

SO TENOTOMY, AND LARGE RECESS-RESECT OR RECESS LR IN BOTH EYES 12 mm

(D) Third cranial nerve palsy

Acquired third nerve palsy

Oculinum in LR Early Patching

LATE: TENOTOMY OF SO, RECTUS SURGERY AS NEEDED

CHOICE OF SURGERY FOR SIXTH CRANIAL NERVE PALSY

James L. Mims III, M.D.

A. Limited abduction of one eye is most commonly Duane's retraction syndrome; surgical options for this condition are covered in another chapter (p 162). The experienced ophthalmologist usually makes a diagnosis of type I Duane's syndrome in the first 10 seconds of the examination. Usually, the examiner is impressed by the severe lack of abduction of one eye in the presence of a relatively small angle of esotropia. The diagnosis is confirmed by the narrowing of the palpebral fissure on adduction of the affected eye. Upshoots or downshoots in adduction, V-patterns, limitation of adduction of the affected eye, and reduced saccadic velocity on adduction as well as on abduction of the affected eye are commonly seen in Duane's syndrome.

B. Congenital sixth nerve palsies in the neonate are almost always self-limited and resolve without treatment. Infantile esotropia usually develops at age 4–7 months, not earlier. Large-angle infantile esotropia may have limited abduction of both eyes, and conjunctival recessions may be indicated to improve results of bimedial recessions in such infants. After successful recession of both medial recti, abduction is full and a diagnosis of bilateral lateral rectus palsy is no longer entertained.

C. Children with acute-onset lateral rectus palsies who fuse with a face turn generally have a benign postinfectious neuritis of the nerve that spontaneously resolves by 6 weeks after onset. If such a child begins to lose his or her face turns and fusion, part-time patching of the nonaffected eye may be indicated (2–5 hours daily). If the palsy is persistent for 6 weeks, diagnostic imaging studies of the CNS (CT or MRI) and consultation with a neurologist are mandatory. Some neurologists advocate obtaining imaging studies earlier.

D. Sixth nerve palsies in adults require consultation with a neurologist. Diabetic sixth nerve palsies are self-limited, but diabetes is so common that diabetic sixth nerve palsy is a diagnosis of exclusion. In adults, be careful to rule out thyroid eye disease, medial orbital wall fracture, and an over-resected medial rectus (or a lost lateral rectus) from previous strabismus surgery. Hypertrophy of the medial rectus may be seen on CT in thyroid eye disease. A lost lateral rectus is associated with widening of the palpebral fissure on attempted abduction.

E. CNS diagnostic imaging studies are mandatory in all adults with sixth nerve palsies (even diabetic adults) and among all children whose acute-onset sixth nerve palsy has persisted beyond 6 weeks. Obviously, a positive finding leads to consideration of neurosurgical intervention.

F. If the diagnostic imaging studies are negative and the lateral rectus palsy is <3 months old, the antagonist medial rectus may be injected with botulinum A toxin (Oculinum), which causes a temporary weakening of muscles. Oculinum in this context can be a great convenience to the adult, who may return to work with some binocularity, and it may help maintain binocular function in selected pediatric patients. In some patients the Oculinum causes an overeffect for several months; the best results are generally seen 4–8 months after injection.

G. A patient with mild sixth nerve palsy retains some abduction, but the amount of sclera still showing at the lateral limbus on attempted abduction is distinctly more on the affected side. Saccadic velocities show ≤20% reduction in adduction-abduction comparisons. A large recess-resect of the affected eye is indicated.

H. A moderate sixth nerve palsy shows little abduction beyond the midline with a moderately large esotropia. Lateral transposition of the vertical recti, the full tendon, gives the best results, but care should be taken to place the superior rectus tendon 2 mm posterior and 2 mm superior to the superior end of the lateral rectus insertion, or a hyperdeviation results. The medial rectus may be weakened simultaneously (or later) with an adjustable suture or with Oculinum (method of Rosenbaum). Do not use Oculinum and a recession simultaneously; this produces an overeffect.

I. A severe sixth nerve palsy with inability to abduct even to the midline and a large-angle esotropia respond to the treatment outlined for a moderate sixth nerve palsy, with the addition of a large recess-resect of the other (nonaffected) eye (method of Kushner).

References

Metz HS, Scott AB, Scott WE. Horizontal saccadic velocities in Duane's syndrome. Am J Ophthalmol 1975; 80:901–906.

Rosenbaum AL, Foster RS, Ballard E, et al. Complete superior and inferior rectus transposition with adjustable medial rectus recession for abducens palsy. In: Reinecke RD, ed. Strabismus II, Proceedings of the Fourth Meeting of the International Strabismological Association. Asilomar, Calif: Grune & Stratton, 1982: 599–605.

Scott AB. Botulinum toxin injection into extraocular muscles as an alternative to strabismus surgery. Ophthalmology 1980; 87:1044–1049.

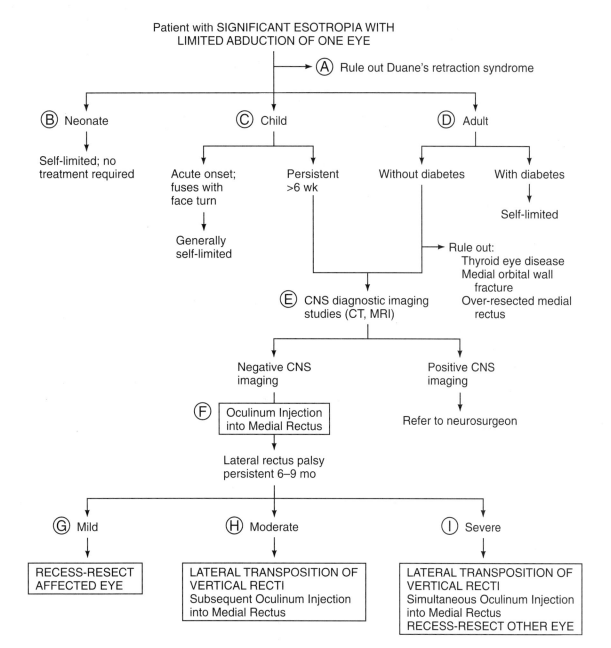

Patient with SIGNIFICANT ESOTROPIA WITH
LIMITED ABDUCTION OF ONE EYE

(A) Rule out Duane's retraction syndrome

(B) Neonate

Self-limited; no
treatment required

(C) Child

Acute onset;
fuses with
face turn

Generally
self-limited

Persistent
>6 wk

(D) Adult

Without diabetes

With diabetes

Self-limited

Rule out:
  Thyroid eye disease
  Medial orbital wall
    fracture
  Over-resected medial
    rectus

(E) CNS diagnostic imaging
    studies (CT, MRI)

Negative CNS
imaging

(F) Oculinum Injection
    into Medial Rectus

Lateral rectus palsy
persistent 6–9 mo

Positive CNS
imaging

Refer to neurosurgeon

(G) Mild

RECESS-RESECT
AFFECTED EYE

(H) Moderate

LATERAL TRANSPOSITION OF
VERTICAL RECTI
Subsequent Oculinum Injection
into Medial Rectus

(I) Severe

LATERAL TRANSPOSITION OF
VERTICAL RECTI
Simultaneous Oculinum Injection
into Medial Rectus
RECESS-RESECT OTHER EYE

CHOICE OF SURGERY FOR A- AND V-PATTERN STRABISMUS

James L. Mims III, M.D.

Up to 25% of patients with a horizontal strabismus have an A- or a V-pattern, a horizontal deviation that changes in size with upgaze and downgaze. Fairly extreme positions of upgaze and downgaze (25 degrees) are best for measuring the patterns; usually, the patient's chin is elevated for downgaze and depressed for upgaze. A clinically significant A-pattern has a difference between upgaze and downgaze of ≥10 prism diopters (PD). A clinically significant V-pattern has a difference between upgaze and downgaze of ≥15 PD.

A. Patients with A-patterns have increasing convergence (decreasing divergence) in upgaze. For all patients with A-pattern horizontal strabismus, it is important to look for overaction of the superior oblique (OASO) muscles. In downgaze, the superior oblique (SO) muscles have a powerful abducting capacity because the SO tendon unwraps from the globe as the eye looks down, and the effective point of contact of the SO tendon is more and more posterior to the vertical axis of Fick as the tendon unwraps from the globe.

B. A-patterns with OASO require surgery on the SO for correction. A-pattern exotropias usually have OASO; A-pattern esotropias often do not. One type of patient who has been frustrating in the past is the patient with demonstrable fusion with better than gross stereopsis who also has an intermittent exotropia with OASO and an A-pattern. If no surgery is performed on the SO, horizontal surgery for the intermittent exotropia generally produces only a temporary or incomplete correction. If SO tenotomies are performed, asymmetric effect of the tenotomies may produce a serious postoperative complication, a cyclovertical deviation that may be compensated for by a new and objectionable head tilt that the patient must adopt to avoid diplopia. Wright has devised a solution to this problem. A 6- or 7-mm length of no. 240 silicon retinal band is attached to the cut ends of the SO tendon as a "tendon expander" bilaterally. If the patient has no better than gross stereopsis or has no fusion, an SO tenotomy is safe. One may anticipate that a bilateral SO tenotomy corrects 35–45 PD of A-pattern. Also, bilateral SO tenotomies may increase the variability of the correction of simultaneous horizontal surgery, but on average they do not have a predictable esotropic or exotropic effect.

C. A-patterns without OASO may be treated with supraplacement of the medial recti (MR) or infraplacement of the lateral recti (LR) with the expectation of correcting approximately 15 PD of the upgaze-downgaze difference. Patients undergoing bilateral MR recessions for esotropia with A-pattern should not have >2 mm of supraplacement of the MR. Supraplacement more than this usually, in time, produces a secondary exotropia. LR may be infraplaced 4 mm with good result. Why does supraplacement or infraplacement work? Recession of a rectus muscle decreases the pull of a muscle by shortening it and placing it lower on its length-tension curve. After recession and infraplacement of an LR muscle, the LR becomes even shorter as the eye moves into downgaze, thus increasing the effect of the recession in downgaze. In nondominant eyes the MR may be supraplaced and the LR may be infraplaced as part of a recess-resect procedure.

D. Patients with V-patterns have increasing divergence (decreasing convergence) in upgaze. For all patients with V-pattern horizontal strabismus, look for overaction of the inferior oblique (OAIO) muscles. In upgaze the inferior oblique (IO) muscle and tendon unwrap from the globe as the eye looks up, and the effective point of contact of the IO is more and more posterior to the vertical axis of Fick as it unwraps from the globe.

E. V-pattern strabismus with OAIO should have a weakening procedure of the IO. If dissociated vertical deviation (DVD) is present or likely to develop in the future (as in infantile esotropia), anteriorize the IO. Otherwise, denervation and extirpation of the IO may be performed for severe OAIO, and IO recession or myectomy may be performed for mild OAIO.

F. For V-patterns without OAIO, supraplacement of the LR 4 mm or infraplacement of the MR 4 mm will correct 15 20 PD of upgaze-downgaze difference.

References

Knapp P. A and V patterns. In: Symposium on strabismus. Transactions of the New Orleans Academy of Ophthalmology. St Louis: Mosby, 1971: 242–254.

Mims JL III, Wood RC. Bilateral anterior transposition of the inferior obliques. Arch Ophthalmol 1989; 107:41–44.

Robin SE, Nelson LB, Harley RD. A complication of weakening the superior oblique muscle in A-pattern exotropia. Ophthalmic Surg 1984; 15:134–135.

von Noorden GK. A- and V-patterns. In: Binocular vision and ocular motility. 4th ed. St Louis: Mosby, 1990: 351–365.

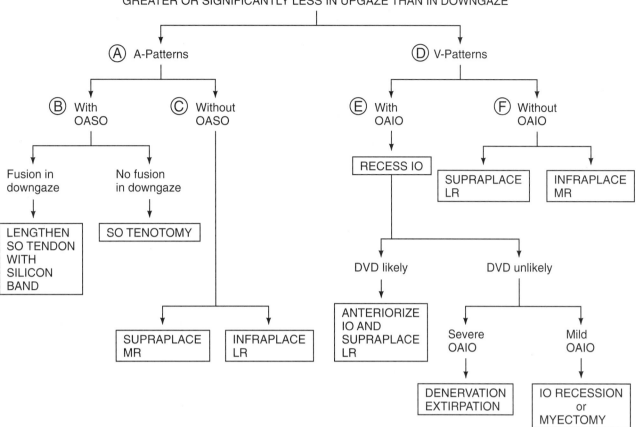

Patient with HORIZONTAL STRABISMUS SIGNIFICANTLY
GREATER OR SIGNIFICANTLY LESS IN UPGAZE THAN IN DOWNGAZE

Ⓐ A-Patterns

Ⓑ With OASO

Ⓒ Without OASO

Ⓓ V-Patterns

Ⓔ With OAIO

Ⓕ Without OAIO

Fusion in downgaze

No fusion in downgaze

RECESS IO

SUPRAPLACE LR

INFRAPLACE MR

LENGTHEN SO TENDON WITH SILICON BAND

SO TENOTOMY

SUPRAPLACE MR

INFRAPLACE LR

DVD likely

DVD unlikely

ANTERIORIZE IO AND SUPRAPLACE LR

Severe OAIO

Mild OAIO

DENERVATION EXTIRPATION

IO RECESSION or MYECTOMY

SURGICAL TREATMENT OF NYSTAGMUS

James L. Mims III, M.D.

The surgical treatment of nystagmus began in controversy because the objective parameters of improvement after surgery that can be measured in adults using routine eye lane equipment are unimpressive. Videotapes and electro-oculography (EOG) recordings show only slight improvement even after maximal recessions, and the improvement in visual acuity in an adult may be only one or two Snellen lines. Among young children from 4–6 years of age, however, Reinecke and I have seen several cases of visual acuity improvements of up to four or five lines, an impressive change that unquestionably goes beyond the placebo effect of surgery. Some adults report that they can do specific tasks much more easily, such as a front office worker in a medical office who says the time it takes her to find a chart has been cut in half after large recessions of all four horizontal recti. This corresponds to dramatically improved performance on the Speedioscope, a device used to teach speed reading by flashing a series of words onto a small screen. The types of surgeries described in this decision tree improve visual function in patients because they decrease the amplitude (not the frequency) of the nystagmus and thereby increase the momentary foveation time that occurs with each sweep of the moving eye as the nystagmoid macula moves back and forth across the image of the fixation target.

A. The first question that must be answered in planning surgery for nystagmus is whether the patient always turns his or her face the same way. This evaluation takes at least 20 minutes of examination time, during which multiple measurements are made of the face turn. The best method is to use a pocket laser or other lecture pointer held above the child's head in line with the nose anteriorly and the vertex of the back of the head posteriorly. It is best to stand behind the child and to use a good distance fixation target, such as a small cartoon movie or a videotape appealing to children. The position of the projected spot indicates the direction and size of the face turn. Classical trigonometry reveals that with the small movie screen or television 20 feet away, 5 degrees is 21 inches away from the center of the screen or television (to the right or left side, depending on the direction of the face turn), 10 degrees is 42 inches from the center, and 15 degrees is 64 inches from the center of the fixation movie. Reinecke has said that the total time required for an extreme right face turn to become an extreme left face turn in periodic alternating nystagmus (PAN) is rarely >4 minutes. I have seen one case for whom this change required 7 minutes. In most cases of PAN the time that the patient spends in transition from one extreme face turn to the opposite face turn is minimal. PAN is much more common than was initially realized.

B. If the face turn is <8 degrees to one side or if the patient has PAN, recessions of the two horizontal recti of both eyes (OU) are indicated. In his early cases, Helveston recessed all four horizontal recti to just posterior to the equator; many of these patients eventually became significantly exotropic. Also, I have seen two cases of drying of the inferior cornea, requiring artificial tears and periodic corneal ulcer treatment after maximal recessions of all four horizontal recti in children. Both cases were cured after advancement of one muscle. The amounts of surgery recommended here have been successful in improving visual acuity in patients without PAN and in reducing the sizes of the face turn in patients with PAN. They have not been associated with induced, iatrogenic exotropias or corneal ulcers resulting from keratitis sicca.

- Recess lateral recti (LR) 11 mm, and recess medial recti (MR) 6.7 mm.
- Recess LR 11.5 mm, and recess MR 7.0 mm.
- Recess LR 12.5 mm, and recess MR 7.3 mm.
- Recess LR 13 mm, and recess MR 7.6 mm.

For each case of nystagmus appropriately receiving recessions of all four horizontal recti (no objectionable face turn in one direction only or PAN), first recess a LR as much as possible without sewing the LR to the inferior oblique. Once the maximum possible LR recession is known, choose the corresponding MR recession from the above list. For PAN, Reinecke is currently trying even larger MR recessions coupled with sewing the LR to the inferior oblique.

C. In the Augmented Anderson procedure, a 10-mm recession of the MR of the eye adducted during the routine face turn is balanced with a 12-mm recession of the yoke LR of the other eye. Augmented Anderson procedures are currently preferred over Kestenbaum procedures for two major reasons: (1) Reinecke has shown that large recessions of horizontal muscles reduce the amplitude of nystagmus, whereas large resections do not, and (2) Helveston has interviewed several patients after bilateral large recess-resect (Kestenbaum) procedures, and these patients "confessed" that they routinely were uncomfortable with their faces in the straight ahead position and usually simply turned their face the other way for comfort, simply tolerating rather than "nulling" the nystagmus. Any improvement they were enjoying in this situation is clearly from the recessions. Amazingly, I have seen seven patients with infantile esotropia who had previously received bilateral MR recessions of 5–6.5 mm who remained orthotropic after their previously recessed MR was placed 10 mm from its original insertion and the yoke LR was recessed 12 mm. One of these patients had previously had a resection of one LR. Another had previously had a small recession of one LR, and that LR was placed 12 mm from its original insertion when the yoke MR was recessed 10 mm. The measured face change in the face turn with the patient maximally challenged (reading letters or iden-

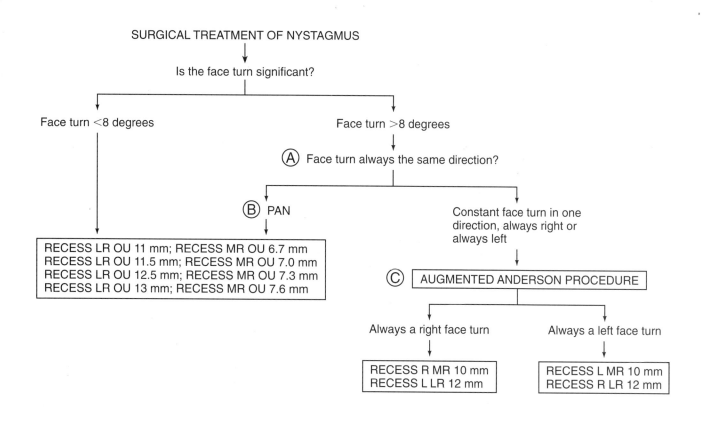

SURGICAL TREATMENT OF NYSTAGMUS

Is the face turn significant?

Face turn <8 degrees

Face turn >8 degrees

Ⓐ Face turn always the same direction?

Ⓑ PAN

Constant face turn in one direction, always right or always left

RECESS LR OU 11 mm; RECESS MR OU 6.7 mm
RECESS LR OU 11.5 mm; RECESS MR OU 7.0 mm
RECESS LR OU 12.5 mm; RECESS MR OU 7.3 mm
RECESS LR OU 13 mm; RECESS MR OU 7.6 mm

Ⓒ AUGMENTED ANDERSON PROCEDURE

Always a right face turn

Always a left face turn

RECESS R MR 10 mm
RECESS L LR 12 mm

RECESS L MR 10 mm
RECESS R LR 12 mm

tifying Allen figures in the eye lane) averages only 11 degrees. The parents are happy after the Augmented Anderson because even when the preoperative face turn is a full 30 degrees, the frequency of the maximal face turn (as observed on a typical day by the parents) is dramatically decreased. Future research should include the artifical divergence approach, not yet popular in the United States.

References

Helveston EM. Surgical management of strabismus. 4th ed. St Louis: Mosby, 1993: 542–547.

Helveston EM, Ellis FD, Plager DA. Large recessions of the horizontal recti for treatment of nystagmus. Ophthalmology 1991; 98:1302–1305.

Zubcov AA, Stark N, Weber A, et al. Improvement of visual acuity after surgery for nystagmus. Ophthalmology 1993; 100:1488–1497.

DEVELOPMENTAL GLAUCOMA

Johan Zwaan, M.D., Ph.D.

When an infant presents with significant photophobia, persistent tearing, blepharospasm, and hazy or enlarged cornea, developmental glaucoma should always be considered, even though none of these symptoms by themselves are pathognomonic for glaucoma. The developmental glaucoma are a heterogeneous group of disorders in which the aqueous outflow system is anatomically abnormal, leading to an increase in intraocular pressure (IOP) and subsequent damage to the optic nerve. The most common type is primary congenital glaucoma, in which the anomaly is limited to the trabecular meshwork and which may be caused by mutation of a cytochrome (CYP1B1). Regardless of the cause, the symptoms and signs of developmental glaucoma are very similar, as is the treatment.

A. The normal horizontal diameter of a newborn is 10.0–10.5 mm, increasing to 11.0–12.0 mm by 1 year of age. Because the fibrotic coat (cornea, sclera) of the infant eye is thinner and less rigid than in the adult, increased IOP will lead to expansion of the size of the eye and thus to enlarged corneal diameter and axial length. The earlier the IOP is high and the longer this persists, the more the eye will stretch. If the IOP remains uncontrolled, the diameter of the cornea may reach 15–16 mm. This increase and increasing myopia are useful indicators that the glaucoma is not controlled, regardless of normal or close to normal IOP readings. Enlarged corneal diameter by itself does not prove that glaucoma is present. The cornea is also larger, although clear, in megalocornea (p 86), and if the cornea was smaller to begin with, enlargement will lead to normalization of its size.

B. Although the conjunctiva may be diffusely injected in developmental glaucoma, more commonly the deep perilimbal vessels are involved, leading to a violaceous color of the area immediately around the cornea, the ciliary flush.

C. A history of increasing haziness and of the eye "getting bigger" is helpful. Many types of developmental glaucoma are heritable, making the family history important. Examination of the child in the clinic is usually adequate to make the diagnosis, even if no accurate IOP measurement can be obtained. Pacifying the infant by giving him or her a bottle or chloral hydrate sedation may facilitate IOP determination.

D. Detailed examination of the eye often requires anesthesia. If the diagnosis of glaucoma is confirmed, immediately proceed with surgery. The examination should include measurement of horizontal and vertical corneal diameter, a recording of the clarity of the cornea, the status of the anterior chamber, gonioscopy, ophthalmoscopy to determine the cup/disk ratio (C/D), and refraction.

E. It is important to realize that anesthetic agents influence the IOP. Succinyl choline can increase IOP because it first depolarizes muscle fibers before their paralysis. The resulting contraction of the extraocular muscles raises the IOP. Halothane reduces the IOP. Pressure readings should be taken early and under light anesthesia, before intubation. The normal IOP of infants is up to 15 mm Hg, and an IOP in the low twenties is high. Because the infant eye is distensible, the IOP never rises as high as it does in acute glaucoma in adults. Thus a normal IOP by itself is not enough to exclude a diagnosis of glaucoma if other signs are present.

F. The anterior chamber angle is always abnormal in developmental glaucoma. The iris has a flat appearance and inserts more anterior than usual, in front of the scleral spur, or it may sweep up to cover the trabecular meshwork. The ciliary body is obscured by this anterior insertion. Other anomalies often visible are thinning of the peripheral iris from stretching, exaggerated Schwalbe's line or posterior embryotoxon, iris processes inserting into Schwalbe's line, and abnormalities of the iris stroma.

G. The C/D ratio of the optic nerve is rarely >0.3 in infants. A difference in value between the two eyes of ≥0.2 is also highly suspicious for glaucoma. Cupping develops much more quickly in infants than in adults. Control of IOP will lead to stabilization of cup size, or the cup may even become smaller. Increase in cup size between examinations indicates poor control.

H. Start medical therapy as soon as a diagnosis of congenital glaucoma is made. However, developmental glaucoma is a surgical disease, and in almost all patients, topical or systemic medications cannot substitute for surgical intervention. They are useful for reducing or preventing further damage while surgical arrangements are made. They may also be necessary for the long-term management of complex cases, which have not responded adequately to surgery.

Primary drug therapy for infantile glaucoma includes carbonic anhydrase inhibitors and β blockers. The first is given orally in a dose of 10–15 mg/kg divided in three equal doses. Topical carbonic anhydrase inhibitors have recently become available and, in adults, are equally effective as the oral medication. Timolol is an effective drug for developmental glaucoma but can cause respiratory, cardiovascular, and other side effects. Complications may be less common with other β blockers. Sympathomimetic (epinephrine, dipivefrin) and parasympathomimetic agents (pilocarpine, choline esterase inhibitors) are not a first choice for the treatment of congenital glaucoma, but they have a role as adjunct therapy when used with other medications.

I. Goniotomy and trabeculotomy have been found to be equally effective as initial surgery for developmental glaucoma. Some surgeons prefer to always use trabeculotomy, even if the cornea is clear. A combination with trabeculectomy also has been advocated.

J. Generally, an IOP of ≤21 mm Hg is considered adequate control. If optic nerve damage has already occurred, a lower pressure may be preferable.

K. In primary congenital glaucoma, repeating trabeculotomy or goniotomy is the common approach. In more complex glaucomas it may be preferable to skip this step and go directly to trabeculectomy or valve implantation.

L. When the risk for failure is higher than usual, as in repeat surgeries for prior failures, in inflamed eyes, in eyes with thick Tenon's capsule, or in African-Americans, the use of mitomycin C (MMC) during the trabeculectomy should be considered. Another antimetabolite, 5-fluorouracil, is not practical for use in children because subconjunctival injections are required for up to 2 weeks.

M. Glaucoma valve implants or setons are generally reserved for difficult cases, in which other approaches have failed. Experience with these implants in children with glaucoma is limited, but increasing, and in the future, a more liberal application may become acceptable.

N. Cyclodestructive procedures are indicated when other methods to control the IOP have failed or when the potential for useful vision is very low. There is a risk for complete visual loss or phthisis bulbi.

O. Developmental glaucoma is a chronic disease, and many patients need multiple procedures before the IOP is normalized. Any of the surgeries listed here may need to be repeated one or more times.

P. There are many reasons why children with glaucoma need to be followed closely. Despite initial success of surgery, failure of IOP control may occur at any time. Because glaucomatous infant eyes often are highly myopic, refractions and, if indicated, amblyopia treatment are an essential, yet often overlooked, aspect of the care of these patients. Corneal decompensation can be caused by edema, scarring, or amyloid deposition, necessitating corneal surgery. Genetic advice to the family regarding recurrence risks should not be forgotten.

References

Al-Hazmi A, Zwaan J, Awad A, et al. Effectiveness and complications of Mitomycin-C use during pediatric glaucoma surgery. Ophthalmology 1998; 105:1915–1920.

Anderson DR. Trabeculotomy compared to goniotomy for glaucoma in children. Ophthalmology 1983; 90:805–806.

Hoskins HD, Hetherington J, Magee SD, et al. Clinical experience with timolol in childhood glaucoma. Arch Ophthalmol 1985; 103:1163–1165.

Mullaney PB, Selleck C, Al-Awad A, et al. Combined trabeculotomy and trabeculectomy as an initial procedure in uncomplicated congenital glaucoma. Arch Ophthalmol 1999; 117:457–460.

Reynolds JD. Pediatric glaucoma. In: Wright KW, ed. Pediatric ophthalmology and strabismus. St Louis: Mosby, 1995: 393–408.

Walton DS. Aniridic glaucoma: The results of goniosurgery to prevent and treat this problem. Trans Am Ophthalmol Soc 1986; 84:59–70.

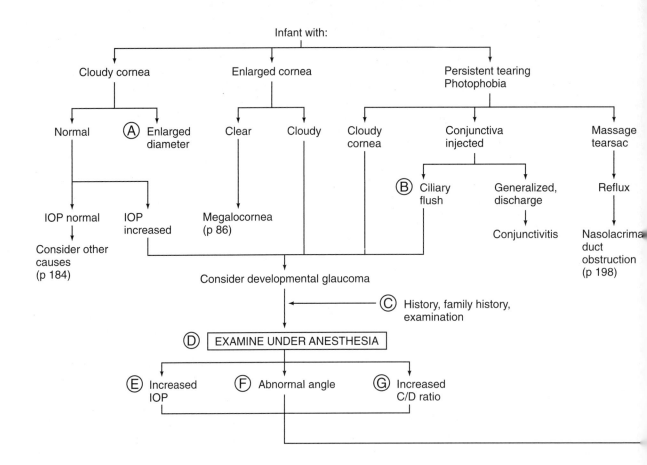

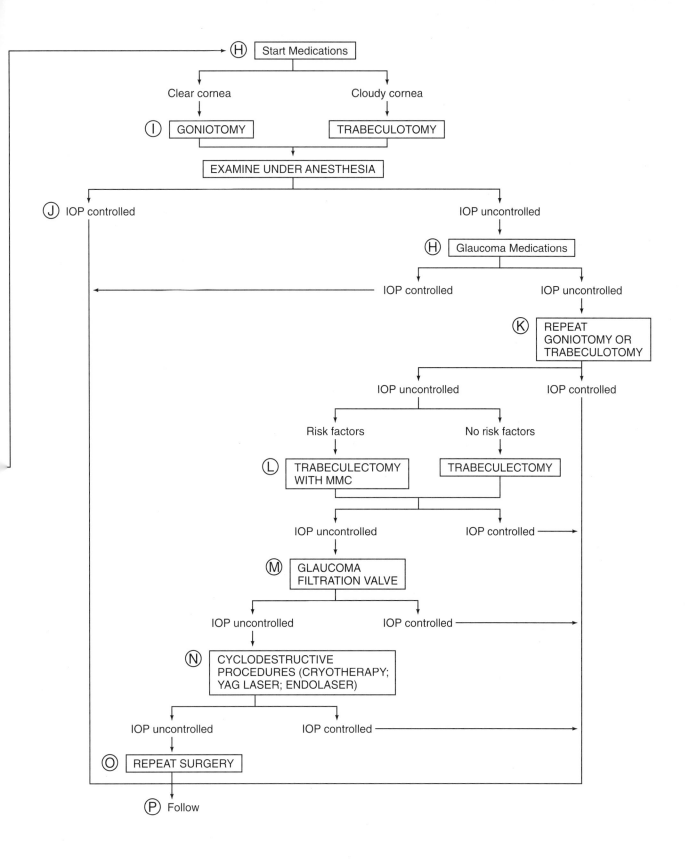

OPHTHALMIA NEONATORUM

Johan Zwaan, M.D., Ph.D.

Conjunctivitis in the first few weeks of life, with purulent discharge, lid edema, conjunctival hyperemia, and occasionally preauricular adenopathy, is common. In the United States 1%–2% of newborns may be affected. In less developed countries, the incidence is much higher and the pathogens are different. The time of onset after birth and the clinical characteristics of the conjunctivitis are helpful adjuncts in reaching a tentative diagnosis. However, there is a large overlap in time periods and clinical manifestations, and laboratory studies are essential in establishing the exact diagnosis.

A. The administration of 1% silver nitrate in the eye to prevent gonococcal conjunctivitis is mildly irritating and often causes some hyperemia and chemosis of the conjunctiva. Rarely, the cornea is affected, leading to a chemical keratitis. The conjunctivitis always occurs within 24 hours of birth and is mild and self-limiting (3–5 days). No treatment is required. Irrigation of the eyes may cause more irritation and should be avoided. The incidence of this problem is decreasing with the increasing use of erythromycin ointment or povidone-iodine for prophylaxis.

B. Bacterial conjunctivitis occurs mostly in the first week of life. It is fairly severe and characterized by purulent discharge. Obtain Gram and Giemsa stains of conjunctival scrapings, and initiate cultures and sensitivities.

C. If gram-negative diplococci are found in a conjunctival scraping, the most likely diagnosis is gonococcal conjunctivitis, although *Neisseria meningitidis* infection presents the same way. In either case urgent treatment is indicated; do not await the results of cultures. The clinical findings are dramatic, and corneal ulceration and even perforation develop rapidly if appropriate treatment is not instituted. The meningococcus can also penetrate intact tissues and rapidly cause disseminated disease, including meningitis.

D. Penicillin-resistant *Neisseria gonorrhoeae* is now endemic, and the use of systemic penicillin for gonococcal ophthalmia neonatorum is no longer the first choice. If it is used, an IV dose of 50,000 units penicillin G per kilogram body weight per day in divided doses twice daily for 7 days is recommended. Ceftriaxone in a single IM or IV dose of 25–50 mg/kg for 7 days is the best drug available. For children sensitive to β-lactam antibiotics, substitute spectinomycin hydrochloride. Adjunctive topical treatment with erythromycin or bacitracin ointment is helpful.

E. Mild bacterial conjunctivitis is usually self-limited, and postponement of treatment is acceptable until a specific diagnosis is available. Indeed, in many patients, lid hygiene and saline washes are adequate therapy.

However, antibiotics may shorten the course of the infection and prevent recurrence and spread.

F. Treat more severe conjunctivitis with a topical broad-spectrum antibiotic until a targeted choice of therapy can be made. Chloramphenicol gives broad coverage and is still popular in other countries, but in the United States it is no longer used as a primary medication because of the very small risk of aplastic anemia. Neosporin (polymyxin-bacitracin-neomycin) is a good choice, but it tends to cause allergic reactions. Bacitracin and erythromycin are usually effective; gentamicin can be used for gram-negative infections, although resistant strains of *Haemophilus influenzae* and *Pseudomonas aeruginosa* are common. Newer topical medications with broad coverage and few adverse reactions are Polytrim (trimethoprim-polymyxin) and fluoroquinolones such as Ciloxan (ciprofloxacin).

G. Mild to moderate conjunctivitis in the first few weeks of life points to *Chlamydia trachomatis* as a cause. In babies treated with prophylactic erythromycin ointment, the onset may be delayed more. *Chlamydia* is now the most important cause of ophthalmia neonatorum in the United States. In contrast to the situation in adults, in whom a work-up is often negative, the positive yield of laboratory tests in infants is high. Intracytoplasmic basophilic inclusion bodies on Giemsa preparations are typical. Immunofluorescent techniques are available and allow a rapid and accurate diagnosis.

H. Oral erythromycin is the drug of choice for chlamydial ophthalmia because it also treats the nasopharyngeal colonization, which can lead to reinfection. It may prevent the chlamydial pneumonia syndrome. Do not use tetracycline because of its deleterious effects on growing bones and teeth. Adjuvant treatment with topical erythromycin is beneficial.

I. Recognition of conjunctivitis caused by herpes simplex virus is important because of the possibility of disseminated infection with CNS involvement. Systemic treatment with acyclovir may reduce the risk for a generalized infection. In addition, topical idoxuridine or vidarabine is helpful. Up to 50% of babies with herpes simplex conjunctivitis develop keratitis with typical dendrites or punctate staining. If the keratitis is severe, cycloplegics are indicated.

J. Many, if not most, of the cases of ophthalmia neonatorum are caused by infection during passage through the birth canal. Thus the clinician must think of these diseases as a family problem rather than just an infection of an individual baby. Asymptomatic parental colonization with *Chlamydia* can be a source for reinfection of the infant. Treat parents with oral erythromy-

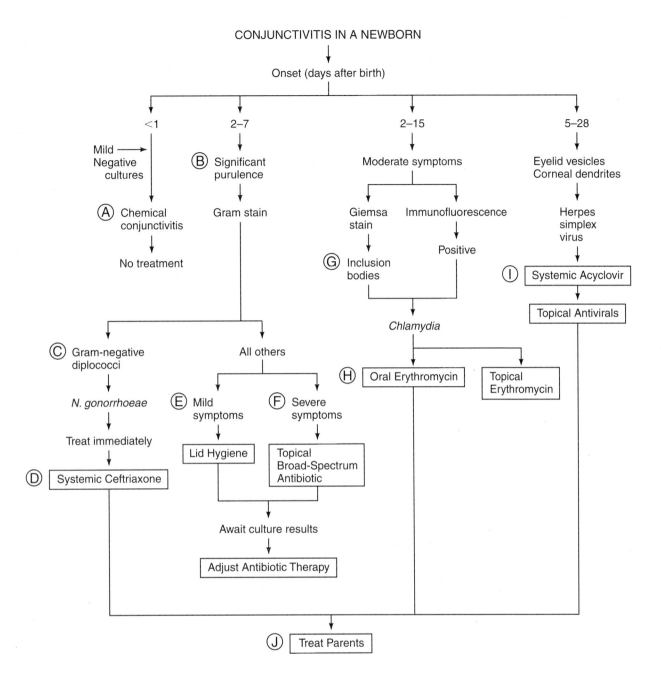

CONJUNCTIVITIS IN A NEWBORN

Onset (days after birth)

<1
Mild → Negative cultures
(A) Chemical conjunctivitis
No treatment

2–7
(B) Significant purulence
Gram stain

(C) Gram-negative diplococci
N. gonorrhoeae
Treat immediately
(D) Systemic Ceftriaxone

All others
(E) Mild symptoms
Lid Hygiene
(F) Severe symptoms
Topical Broad-Spectrum Antibiotic
Await culture results
Adjust Antibiotic Therapy

2–15
Moderate symptoms
Giemsa stain
(G) Inclusion bodies
Immunofluorescence
Positive
Chlamydia
(H) Oral Erythromycin
Topical Erythromycin

5–28
Eyelid vesicles
Corneal dendrites
Herpes simplex virus
(I) Systemic Acyclovir
Topical Antivirals

(J) Treat Parents

cin or tetracycline. However, do not give the latter to nursing mothers. Treat maternal (and usually paternal as well) gonococcal infections with a single IM dose of 1 g ceftriaxone. Maternal venereal herpes simplex is of particular concern because of the risk of neonatal disseminated infection. CNS involvement can lead to severe psychomotor retardation of the baby. Although prophylaxis is too late for the newborn with herpes simplex ophthalmia, subsequent deliveries should be done by cesarean section to prevent infection of additional children.

References

Grosskreutz C, Smith LBH. Neonatal conjunctivitis. Int Ophthalmol Clin 1992; 32:71–85.

Haase DA, Nash RA, Nsanze H, et al. Single-dose ceftriaxone therapy of gonococcal ophthalmia neonatorum. Sex Transm Dis 1986; 13:53–55.

Haimovici R, Roussel TJ. Treatment of gonococcal conjunctivitis with single-dose intramuscular ceftriaxone. Am J Ophthalmol 1989; 107:511–514.

Isenberg SJ, Apt L, Wood M. A controlled trial of povidone-iodine as prophylaxis against ophthalmia neonatorum. N Engl J Med 1995; 332:562–565.

Sandstrom KI. Treatment of neonatal conjunctivitis. Arch Ophthalmol 1987; 105:925–928.

Sandstrom KI, Bell TA, Chandler JW, et al. Microbial causes of neonatal conjunctivitis. J Pediatr 1984; 105:706–711.

Winceslaus J, Goh BT, Dunlop EM, et al. Diagnosis of ophthalmia neonatorum. Br Med J 1987; 295:1377–1379.

Zwaan J. Ophthalmia neonatorum. In: Dershewitz RA, ed. Ambulatory pediatric care. 3rd ed. Philadelphia: Lippincott-Raven, 1999: 535–538.

DOES THIS BABY SEE?

Johan Zwaan, M.D., Ph.D.

A. Although the acuity in Snellen equivalents in a newborn baby is low—around 20/1000—normal development progresses rapidly, and at 1 month, it has increased to 20/600. By 4 months, acuity is 20/200, and at 1 year, at least 20/50. At 6–8 weeks and often even earlier, clear fixation and following reflexes should be present. Before this age it may be unclear whether the baby sees or not. However, parents are quite aware if the visual development deviates from the norm, and this is obviously a reason for major concern. Relatively few ocular conditions cause apparent blindness in babies with normal appearing eyes: achromatopsia, all types of albinism, retinal degeneration, and bilateral optic nerve hypoplasia. The poor vision may have a central mechanism. Babies may also be "pseudoblind."

B. The scheme proposed here, based on eye movements, is useful as a starting point, but in all patients with suspected blindness, perform a complete examination, often including electrophysiology (EEG, electroretinogram [ERG], visually evoked response [VER]). CT scan and/or MRI can be helpful. Close cooperation with the pediatric neurologist, pediatrician, and geneticist may be indicated. Because it may be difficult to reach a diagnosis immediately, it is better to postpone a definitive answer to the parents until the clinical picture is unequivocal. Nothing is worse than to inform parents that their baby is blind (or normal) and to be forced later to reach the opposite conclusion.

C. In Leber's congenital amaurosis (LCA), the fundus first appears entirely normal, although a pigmentary retinopathy may eventually develop. High hyperopia is typical in uncomplicated LCA, in which the abnormalities are restricted to the eye. Pupillary reactions are sluggish or even paradoxical. The ERG is extinguished in both light- and dark-adapted conditions. Other retinal degenerations may have similar effects, but they are usually not evident in the neonate.

D. Although diagnosing hypoplasia of the optic nerves seems simple, the changes can be subtle and are sometimes overlooked. The small disc is often surrounded by a yellow halo, the "double-ring" sign. The nerve fiber layer is thinner than usual, and the foveal reflex may be decreased. Sometimes, the hypoplasia is segmental. The latter is particularly true for the children of diabetic mothers.

E. Severe optic nerve hypoplasia (ONH) causes random eye movements, if bilateral. It may be isolated or combined with CNS abnormalities. The classical combination is with sagittal midline defects, such as agenesis of the anterior commissure and septum pellucidum. Septooptic dysplasia is often associated with hypopituitarism; therefore endocrine evaluation is essential. Early recognition and appropriate hormonal replacement therapy allow reversal of the growth retardation commonly seen in these patients. Other often-associated anomalies are hydranencephaly, anencephaly, and encephaloceles. There is evidence that some cases of ONH may be caused by environmental factors. Drugs, such as anticonvulsants and quinidine, and maternal diabetes mellitus have been implicated.

F. At least 10 syndromes are characterized by oculocutaneous or ocular albinism. All have reduced pigmentation of the ocular pigment epithelia, hypoplasia of the fovea, reduced vision, and nystagmus. Their differentiation is beyond the scope of this chapter. However, a precise diagnosis is important because some types are associated with systemic disorders of significant morbidity. It is also required for genetic counseling. Foveal hypoplasia is also seen in aniridia.

G. Juvenile retinoschisis is almost always X-linked and thus manifested only in males. It has rarely been found in females, compatible with autosomal-recessive inheritance. There is a splitting of the nerve fiber layer at the posterior pole and in the peripheral retina. The macular changes can be subtle and difficult to detect. The expression is variable, and vision may be as good as 20/50. Vitreous abnormalities may be present. The ERG is helpful: A waves are normal, but the amplitudes of both scotopic and photopic B wave are usually reduced.

H. Vision is severely reduced in achromatopsia. Color vision is lost. Almost pathognomonic is severe photophobia. The disease is rare and is autosomal recessive. The ERG flicker response is absent; photopic flash response is reduced, but the scotopic response is normal. The nystagmus has a very low amplitude and at times is difficult to detect.

I. Congenital stationary night blindness (CSNB) is hereditary, although all three major inheritance patterns have been described, indicating genetic heterogeneity. In the X-linked variety, vision is reduced and nystagmus as well as (moderately) high myopia is present. Color vision is normal. The ERG shows a reduced scotopic B wave. Autosomal-dominant CSNB does not show reduced vision and nystagmus; the autosomal-recessive type is variable.

J. If no nystagmus is present, babies fall into two major groups once large refractive errors have been excluded and corrected. The first group has evidence of CNS abnormalities; the second has a negative history and essentially normal examination.

K. Very high degrees of myopia or hyperopia can lead to behavior that makes one suspect blindness. Therefore always perform retinoscopy. In addition, some other causes of reduced vision are typically associated with refractive errors, such as myopia in CSNB or hyperopia in LCA.

L.   Premature birth and/or low birth weight, a history of perinatal asphyxia, developmental anomalies, or a seizure disorder may all indicate possible damage to the occipital cerebral cortex. CT scan, MRI, and referral to the pediatric neurologist are necessary.

M.   If all test results are normal in a seemingly blind baby, the natural history may help. Waiting until the baby is 6 months old or so may yield a diagnosis.

N.   Ocular motor apraxia is usually congenital but can be acquired. Because of the lack of oculomotor response, the apraxia is often mistaken for visual unresponsiveness, particularly in the first several months, when the typical horizontal head jerks (to change fixation) have not yet appeared. The syndrome is characterized by a failure to elicit saccades on command, although saccades may be initiated by some visual reflexes (i.e., optokinetic stimulation). In the congenital variety, only the horizontal saccades are involved. The congenital condition improves with time.

O.   Delayed visual maturation (DVM) may occur in babies whose ocular and systemic examinations are otherwise normal. EEG and ERG are normal, but pattern onset/offset visual evoked responses may be mildly delayed. Most of these children will have "caught up" by age 6 months, and their subsequent development—

visual, neurologic, and otherwise—should be entirely normal. Premature babies or babies with psychomotor retardation may also show DVM. Finally, children with an ocular abnormality, explaining a reduction in sight, may have much poorer vision than expected on the basis of the eye findings. Although the prognosis for the last two groups is not as favorable as for the patients with isolated DVM, vision often improves with time.

References

Catalano RA. Nystagmus. In: Nelson LB, Calhoun JH, Harley RD, eds. Pediatric ophthalmology, 3rd ed. Philadelphia: WB Saunders, 1991.

Hoyt C, Nickel B, Billson F. Ophthalmological examination of the infant. Surv Ophthalmol 1982; 26:177–189.

Lambert SR, Kriss A, Taylor D. Delayed visual maturation, a longitudinal clinical and electrophysiological assessment. Ophthalmology 1989; 96:524–529.

Lambert SR, Taylor D, Kriss A. The infant with nystagmus, normal appearing fundi, but an abnormal ERG. Surv Ophthalmol 1989; 34:173–186.

O'Donnell FE, Green WR. The eye in albinism. In: Duane TD, Jaeger EA, eds. Clinical ophthalmology. Philadelphia: Harper & Row, 1988.

Rosenberg ML, Wilson E. Congenital ocular motor apraxia without head thrusts. J Clin Neurol Ophthalmol 1987; 7:26–28.

Teller D, McDonald M, Preston K, et al. Assessment of visual acuity in infants and children: The acuity card procedure. Dev Med Child Neurol 1986; 28:779–790.

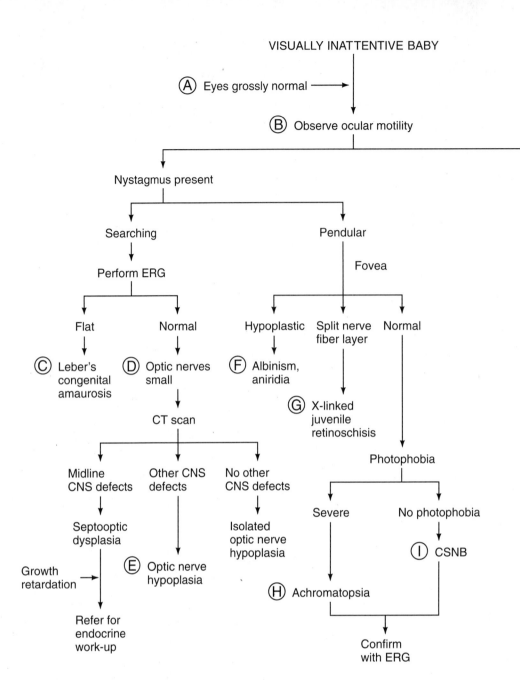

VISUALLY INATTENTIVE BABY

Ⓐ Eyes grossly normal ⟶

Ⓑ Observe ocular motility

Nystagmus present

Searching

Perform ERG

Flat

Ⓒ Leber's congenital amaurosis

Normal

Ⓓ Optic nerves small

CT scan

Midline CNS defects

Septooptic dysplasia

Growth retardation ⟶

Refer for endocrine work-up

Other CNS defects

Ⓔ Optic nerve hypoplasia

No other CNS defects

Isolated optic nerve hypoplasia

Pendular

Fovea

Hypoplastic

Ⓕ Albinism, aniridia

Split nerve fiber layer

Ⓖ X-linked juvenile retinoschisis

Normal

Photophobia

Severe

Ⓗ Achromatopsia

No photophobia

Ⓘ CSNB

Confirm with ERG

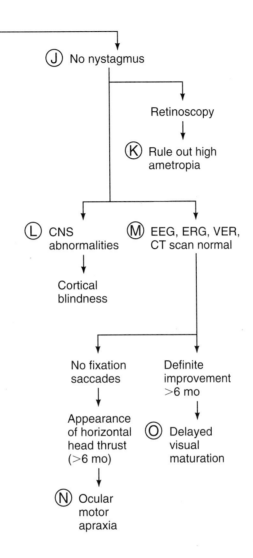

J No nystagmus

Retinoscopy

K Rule out high
ametropia

L CNS
abnormalities

M EEG, ERG, VER,
CT scan normal

Cortical
blindness

No fixation
saccades

Definite
improvement
>6 mo

Appearance
of horizontal
head thrust
(>6 mo)

O Delayed
visual
maturation

N Ocular
motor
apraxia

LEUKOCORIA

Johan Zwaan, M.D., Ph.D.

Leukocoria in a child requires urgent attention, primarily because in most patients with retinoblastoma it is the first sign noticed. Secondarily, a white pupil indicates a severely amblyopiogenic condition, which may be treatable. The history, including that of the family, can be extremely helpful in the differential diagnosis. In addition to eye examinations, special tests, such as ultrasonography, CT scanning, and MRI, may be required.

The scheme presented here is oversimplified because there is significant overlap in the pathologic expression of the multiple causes of leukocoria. Moreover, the findings depend on the stage of the clinical problem. Each patient should be evaluated individually, taking into account all information provided by history, eye and systemic examinations, and special tests.

A. Anatomic location is important in the differential diagnosis of leukocoria. The "vitreous" category includes structures displaced into the normal location of the vitreous gel (i.e., detached retinas).

B. Normally, only the lens is found immediately behind the pupil, so an opacity here indicates a cataract. Advanced cases of persistent hyperplastic primary vitreous (PHPV) can also present with a posterior or total cataract. A cataract does not exclude other causes of leukocoria. Therefore thoroughly examine the remainder of the eye.

C. Cells or clumps in the vitreous indicate hemorrhage, infection, or tumor, in particular retinoblastoma. Although seedlings from an endophytic retinoblastoma are not easily missed, the diffuse infiltrating type is insidious and often misdiagnosed as uveitis or endophthalmitis.

D. The most common expression of the congenital toxoplasmosis syndrome is chorioretinitis. Other causes for posterior uveitis in children are CMV, *Toxocara canis* or *catis,* and rarely *Candida albicans* (in immunosuppressed children) and congenital syphilis, sympathetic ophthalmia, and sarcoidosis.

E. Retinal detachments commonly present as leukocoria in children. There often is an overlap between the types of detachment. For instance, dominant exudative vitreoretinopathy has exudates, yet the associated detachment is usually caused by traction.

F. Coats' disease is almost always unilateral and occurs primarily in older boys, although it sometimes occurs at an early age and in females. At late stages subretinal lipid and cholesterol crystals may be seen.

G. Calcium in a retinal mass is highly typical for retinoblastoma, although not entirely pathognomonic.

H. *T. canis,* or rarely *T. catis,* can cause a chorioretinal granuloma in the peripheral retina or the macula, or it can masquerade as endophthalmitis. Systemic manifestations are rare. The ELISA test for *Toxocara* has its limitations: 10% of patients with the disease have a negative test, and the test can be positive when *Toxocara* is not present.

I. The serious forms (more than stage 2) of retinopathy of prematurity (ROP) affect mostly premature babies, whose birth weight is <1500 g. In stage 3 extraretinal neovascularization is seen, and in stage 4 a subtotal retinal detachment, tractional or exudative.

J. The appearance of dominant exudative vitreoretinopathy is similar to that of ROP, but there is an autosomal-dominant inheritance pattern and the children are not premature.

K. The hallmarks of PHPV are persistent hyaloid vessels and a retrolental fibrovascular membrane with traction, which pulls the ciliary processes behind the lens, making them visible. The lens may be cataractous, the posterior capsule may be ruptured, and blood vessels may invade the lens. The eye is usually microphthalmic. In posterior PHPV the retina is folded from the disc to the periphery, at times all the way to the ora serrata. Abnormal vessels are seen in the fold, and the adjacent vitreous is condensed.

L. The ocular manifestations of the different vitreoretinal dysplasias are similar, and a definitive diagnosis cannot be made on the basis of the eye examination alone. Systemic examination and history provide the major clues. Warburg's syndrome is autosomal recessive and combines brain and eye malformations. Brain abnormalities include agyria, hydrocephalus, and variably encephalocele; there is severe mental retardation. Ocular findings include retinal dysplasia. Because Norrie's disease is X-linked recessive, it is found in males only. The vitreoretinal dysplasia usually is progressive and leads to total retinal detachment and blindness. Many affected patients are retarded; others have hearing loss. Incontinentia pigmenti is X-linked dominant and presumed lethal in the male. Affected females develop skin bullae postnatally, which leave a pattern of pigmented lines upon resolution.

M. Both *Toxoplasma gondii* and CMV cause indistinguishable atrophic chorioretinal scars, surrounded by pigmentation.

N. Chorioretinal colobomas vary from very small to encompassing most of the fundus and optic nerve. They are always located inferonasally, reflecting the embryonic position of the choroidal fissure. If the coloboma is large, the eye is usually microphthalmic.

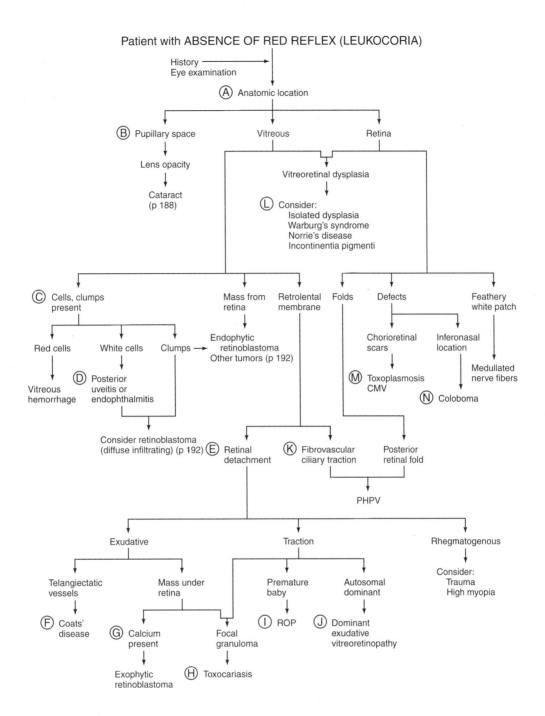

Patient with ABSENCE OF RED REFLEX (LEUKOCORIA)

History → Eye examination

Ⓐ Anatomic location

Ⓑ Pupillary space → Lens opacity → Cataract (p 188)

Vitreous

Retina

Vitreoretinal dysplasia

Ⓛ Consider:
Isolated dysplasia
Warburg's syndrome
Norrie's disease
Incontinentia pigmenti

Ⓒ Cells, clumps present

Mass from retina

Retrolental membrane

Folds

Defects

Feathery white patch

Red cells

White cells

Clumps →

Endophytic retinoblastoma Other tumors (p 192)

Chorioretinal scars

Inferonasal location

Medullated nerve fibers

Vitreous hemorrhage

Ⓓ Posterior uveitis or endophthalmitis

Ⓜ Toxoplasmosis CMV

Ⓝ Coloboma

Consider retinoblastoma (diffuse infiltrating) (p 192) Ⓔ Retinal detachment

Ⓚ Fibrovascular ciliary traction

Posterior retinal fold

PHPV

Exudative

Traction

Rhegmatogenous

Telangiectatic vessels

Mass under retina

Premature baby

Autosomal dominant

Consider:
Trauma
High myopia

Ⓕ Coats' disease

Ⓖ Calcium present

Focal granuloma

Ⓘ ROP

Ⓙ Dominant exudative vitreoretinopathy

Exophytic retinoblastoma

Ⓗ Toxocariasis

References

Char DH, Hedges TR, Norman D. Retinoblastoma CT diagnosis. Ophthalmology 1984; 91:686–695.

Ellis GS, Pakalnis VA, Worley G, et al. Toxocara canis infection: Clinical and epidemiological associations with seropositivity in kindergarten children. Ophthalmology 1986; 93:1032–1037.

Flynn JT, Bancalari E, Bachynski BN, et al. Retinopathy of prematurity: Diagnosis, severity, and natural history. Ophthalmology 1987; 94:620–629.

Karr DJ, Scott WE. Visual acuity results following treatment of persistent hyperplastic primary vitreous. Arch Ophthalmol 1986; 104:662–664.

Katz NK, Margo CE, Dorwart RH. Computerized tomography with histopathological correlation in children with leukocoria. J Pediatr Ophthalmol Strabismus 1984; 21:50–57.

Lieberfarb RM, Eavey RD, DeLong GR, et al. Norrie's disease: A study of two families. Ophthalmology 1985; 92:1445–1451.

Noble K, Carr R. Disorders of the fundus: toxoplasma retinochoroiditis. Ophthalmology 1982; 89:1289–1291.

Zwaan J. Leukocoria. In: Dershewitz RA, ed. Ambulatory pediatric care. 3rd ed. Philadelphia: Lippincott-Raven, 1999: 562–565.

CLOUDY CORNEA IN A NEONATE

Johan Zwaan, M.D., Ph.D.

A cornea cloudy at birth, if not very transient, always indicates a significant ocular problem. Although some of the underlying causes do not require immediate intervention, a detailed history and eye examination should be given immediately to identify babies who need treatment, such as congenital glaucoma patients. The prognosis for visual development depends greatly on the pathogenesis of the corneal opacity. The corneal abnormality can be a tip-off for the existence of systemic or genetic disease.

A. The appearance of the corneal opacity is one of the most important indications of the underlying pathogenesis.

B. A ground-glass appearance almost always indicates edema. It is important to differentiate the three major causes—congenital glaucoma, congenital hereditary endothelial dystrophy (CHED), and forceps injury—because the first requires immediate treatment.

C. The corneal diameter is enlarged in congenital glaucoma, unless the disease is in an early stage. Additional tests are required for a definitive diagnosis: measurement of the intraocular pressure (IOP), inspection of the anterior segment (gonioscopy), and examination of the optic nerves (optic cup size). The enlarged cornea in glaucoma should not be confused with megalocornea (p 86).

D. Tremendously increased corneal thickness is the hallmark of CHED. This is an autosomal-recessive condition characterized by absence or insufficiency of the corneal endothelium, resulting in massive corneal edema. It is rare in the United States but much more common in the Middle East. The abnormally thick cornea often results in what appears to be a moderately elevated IOP. This makes the differentiation from congenital glaucoma even more difficult. It is helpful that the corneal diameter does not increase, even in the presence of greatly increased thickness. If goniotomy or trabeculotomy is erroneously performed, the corneal edema will not improve in patients with CHED, whereas it usually will when congenital glaucoma is surgically controlled.

E. Congenital hereditary stromal dystrophy (CHSD) is autosomal dominant and not progressive. The stroma has a ground-glass appearance at birth or may be flaky white. Congenital syphilis can cause an interstitial keratitis, but this is almost never present at birth; the child usually is several years old before the problem manifests. Rubella can cause a congenital corneal haze, which may be more or less severe (see section K). Exposure, usually from eyelid abnormalities, is not apparent immediately at birth but shows up quickly, particularly if a portion of the lid is missing (see section Q). Immediate protection of the cornea with lubricants and patching is mandatory. Follow this as soon as practical by surgical eyelid reconstruction.

F. Horizontal breaks in the endothelium and Descemet's membrane (Haab's striae) are typical for congenital glaucoma. Even if the disease is arrested, the enlarged corneae of these patients, with or without Haab's striae, are always at risk for endothelial decompensation and often become edematous later in life.

G. Endothelial cracks from forceps deliveries are generally vertically or obliquely oriented because they are caused by compression of the eye against the superior orbital rim. The diagnosis is facilitated by the birth history and the presence of other signs of facial injury.

H. The use of contact lenses or hypertonic saline ointment may reduce the edema that follows the injury to the corneal endothelium. Because this edema resolves spontaneously in a few weeks to months when the endothelium heals, the actual benefit of these treatments is difficult to prove. In these babies significant astigmatism and myopia develop in the affected eye, and careful refraction and amblyopia therapy are most important.

I. With the exception of tyrosinemia, metabolic genetic diseases such as mucopolysaccharidoses, mucolipidoses, and cystinosis, uncommonly cause a congenitally cloudy cornea. If such a diagnosis is suspected, other findings such as dysmorphic features or psychomotor retardation are usually more important.

J. Conjunctival biopsy, combined with electron microscopy of the specimen, can often accurately pinpoint the diagnosis of these metabolic diseases. It is a simple procedure with low morbidity and is not used enough.

K. The congenital rubella syndrome can be associated with a keratopathy, which presents as a more or less dense haze. The cloudiness generally clears spontaneously in a few months. It should be differentiated from congenital glaucoma, which can occur in up to 10% of babies with rubella.

L. If the entire cornea is replaced with an ectatic and opaque structure or with a dermoidlike choristoma, the prognosis for restoration of useful vision is guarded.

M. Consider grafting, particularly when both eyes are affected, even though the outcome of penetrating keratoplasty (PKP) in children is not as favorable as in adults. Perform the surgery very early to minimize amblyopia. I also have the impression that the rejection rate is less if the keratoplasty is performed when the child is no more than a few months old. In some cases a lamellar keratoplasty gives a good cosmetic result.

N. A cosmetic shell or a painted contact lens may be used if the corneal lesion is not too elevated.

O. Enucleation should rarely be necessary. If the eye does not see and is unsightly, replacement with a hydroxyapatite implant or a dermis-fat graft can be considered. Effects of enucleation on orbital growth should be taken into account.

P. Limbal dermoids can be treated by simple excision (lamellar keratectomy). Occasionally, they take up the entire thickness of the cornea or sclera, and the surgeon must be prepared to do a corneal patch graft. Careful examination, including gonioscopy, warns the clinician of this possibility in most if not all cases.

Q. If the dermoid is associated with an eyelid coloboma, the latter needs to be repaired to prevent exposure keratitis.

R. Peters' anomaly is characterized by a central corneal leukoma with a relatively clear periphery. It often occurs bilaterally, in which case surgical treatment is indicated in at least one eye. Before the attempted repair, do a full evaluation, including ultrasound and perhaps CT scanning, to find the extent of iris and lens involvement and the possible presence of persistent hyperplastic primary vitreous, which may cloud the prognosis.

S. Surgical treatment of these patients is controversial because the results have been limited. With or without treatment, vision is usually severely reduced. If both eyes are involved an attempt at surgical improvement of the vision is warranted, as long as the parents understand that the prognosis is guarded. If congenital glaucoma is also present, it should be controlled first. In many patients an optical sector iridectomy will allow them to look around the corneal opacity. This much less invasive procedure does not require the intensive follow-up necessary after PKP.

T. PKP in patients with Peters' anomaly is often complicated by adhesions between the cornea and the iris or lens. This may necessitate lensectomy and anterior vitrectomy, which further diminishes an already poor prognosis.

U. In sclerocornea the peripheral cornea is opaque; the center is clear or at least less opaque.

V. In anterior chamber cleavage syndromes other than Peters' anomaly, corneal opacities are usually mild and do not require therapeutic intervention. Glaucoma is often present and must be treated.

References

Ahmad M, Barber J, Reinecke RD. Ocular choristomas. Surv Ophthalmol 1989; 33:339–358.

Angell LK, Robb RM, Berson FG. Visual prognosis in patients with ruptures in Descemet's membrane due to forceps injuries. Arch Ophthalmol 1981; 99:2137–2144.

Cotran PR, Bajart AM. Congenital corneal opacities. Int Ophthalmol Clin 1992; 32:93–105.

Kenyon KR. Lysosomal disorders affecting the ocular anterior segment. In: Nicholson DH, ed. Ocular pathology update. New York: Masson, 1980.

Kirkness CM, McCartney A, Rice NS, et al. Congenital hereditary corneal oedema of Maumenee: Its clinical features, management and pathology. Br J Ophthalmol 1987; 71:130–145.

Mulet M, Caldwell DR. Corneal abnormalities. In: Wright KW, ed. Pediatric ophthalmology and strabismus. St Louis: Mosby, 1995: 321–348.

Parmley VC, Stonecipher KG, Rowsey JJ. Peters' anomaly: A review of 26 penetrating keratoplasties in infants. Ophthalmic Surg 1993; 24:31–35.

Stein RM, Cohen EJ, Calhoun JH, et al. Corneal birth trauma managed with a contact lens. Am J Ophthalmol 1987; 103:596–597.

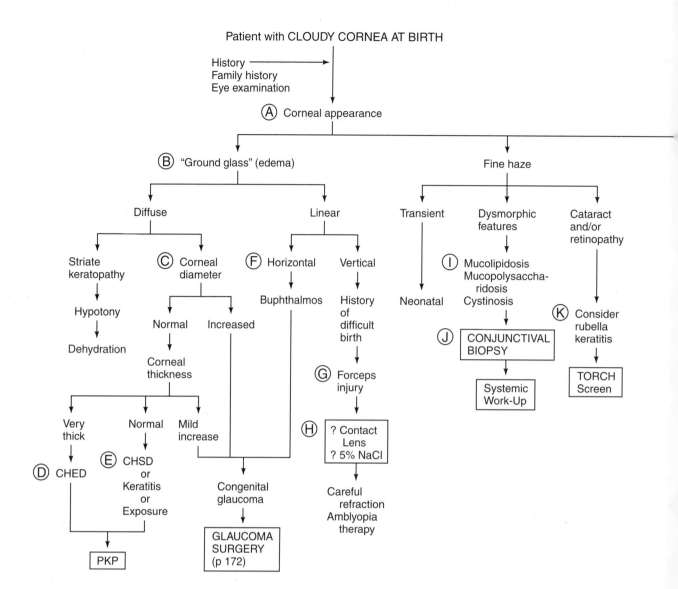

Patient with CLOUDY CORNEA AT BIRTH

History
Family history
Eye examination

Ⓐ Corneal appearance

Ⓑ "Ground glass" (edema)

Diffuse

Striate keratopathy

Hypotony

Dehydration

Ⓒ Corneal diameter

Normal

Corneal thickness

Very thick

Ⓓ CHED

Normal

Ⓔ CHSD or Keratitis or Exposure

PKP

Mild increase

Increased

Congenital glaucoma

GLAUCOMA SURGERY (p 172)

Linear

Ⓕ Horizontal

Buphthalmos

Vertical

History of difficult birth

Ⓖ Forceps injury

Ⓗ ? Contact Lens ? 5% NaCl

Careful refraction Amblyopia therapy

Fine haze

Transient

Neonatal

Dysmorphic features

Ⓘ Mucolipidosis Mucopolysaccharidosis Cystinosis

Ⓙ CONJUNCTIVAL BIOPSY

Systemic Work-Up

Cataract and/or retinopathy

Ⓚ Consider rubella keratitis

TORCH Screen

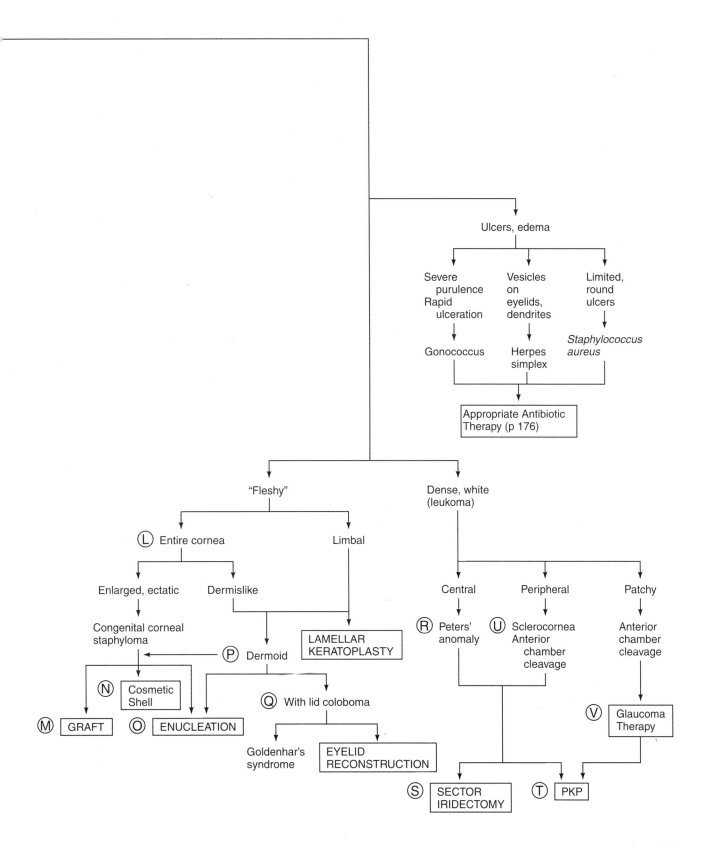

Ulcers, edema

Severe purulence Rapid ulceration → Gonococcus

Vesicles on eyelids, dendrites → Herpes simplex

Limited, round ulcers → *Staphylococcus aureus*

Appropriate Antibiotic Therapy (p 176)

"Fleshy"

Ⓛ Entire cornea

Limbal

Enlarged, ectatic → Congenital corneal staphyloma

Dermislike

LAMELLAR KERATOPLASTY

Ⓟ Dermoid

Ⓝ Cosmetic Shell

Ⓜ GRAFT

Ⓞ ENUCLEATION

Ⓠ With lid coloboma

Goldenhar's syndrome

EYELID RECONSTRUCTION

Dense, white (leukoma)

Central

Peripheral

Patchy

Ⓡ Peters' anomaly

Ⓤ Sclerocornea Anterior chamber cleavage

Anterior chamber cleavage

Ⓥ Glaucoma Therapy

Ⓢ SECTOR IRIDECTOMY

Ⓣ PKP

CATARACT IN A CHILD: DIAGNOSIS

Johan Zwaan, M.D., Ph.D.

A congenital cataract is found in about 1 in 250 live births. Roughly one third is associated with a syndrome or metabolic disease, one third is clearly hereditary, and the cause of the remainder is unknown. Congenital cataract is still one of the leading causes of blindness in children (20%).

A. A family history and particularly a careful eye examination of parents and other family members can be very helpful in establishing a diagnosis.

B. A work-up normally need not be extensive. If a baby has a cataract secondary to a metabolic deficiency, the child also fails to thrive, is sickly, and has come to the attention of the pediatrician well before the diagnosis of cataract is made. There is one exception to this: galactose kinase deficiency can result in lens opacification in an otherwise perfectly healthy child. It is usually more than adequate to obtain a fasting blood sugar (hypoglycemia), urine for reducing sugars (galactosemia), serum calcium and phosphate (hypoparathyroidism, severe vitamin D deficiency), and urinary amino acids (Lowe's syndrome). If an infectious process is suspected, order a TORCH screen and a VDRL.

C. Zonular cataracts are restricted to certain zones within the lens, although they may be accompanied by "riders." Most are either nuclear or lamellar, although sutural, stellate, floriform, and other morphologic types also fall under this category. The position of the cataract gives to an extent an indication of the timing of cataractogenesis, reflecting the way in which the lens fibers are laid down during development. A nuclear cataract dates back to early embryogenesis, and lamellar cataracts (typically with a clear nucleus inside and a clear cortical shell outside) originate later in prenatal or postnatal life.

D. A nuclear cataract is often familial. In a sick infant it should lead to the suspicion of rubella, although other viruses, notably varicella, can cause a similar lens opacity.

E. Lamellar lens opacities are often autosomal dominant. The cataracts associated with metabolic diseases are usually lamellar.

F. Galactosemia comes in two distinct types. In galactokinase deficiency, children have no systemic illness, whereas children with a deficiency of galactose-1-phosphate uridyltransferase are quite ill. The cataract appears the same in both; an oil drop configuration in the center of the lens is caused by a refractive change in the nucleus. It is secondary to osmotic changes and is reversible in an early stage. More permanent lamellar opacities appear if galactose is not removed from the diet.

G. Axial cataracts, as the name indicates, are located around the anteroposterior axis of the lens.

H. Anterior lenticonus is often found in Alport's syndrome (chronic renal failure and sensorineural deafness). Other eye findings include a flecked retina and corneal arcus.

I. Anterior polar cataracts are often small and until recently were thought to be nonprogressive. However, some progress to a point at which they interfere greatly with vision, making removal necessary.

J. Lowe's syndrome shows severe lens anomalies. In addition to having posterior lenticonus, the lens is often shaped like a flat disc and is always cataractous. The syndrome is X-linked recessive; carriers have fine punctate lens opacities. The children are severely retarded and have a dysmorphic face with chubby cheeks.

K. Patients with neurofibromatosis type 2 (bilateral central acoustic neuromas) have a high incidence (at least 80% in our series) of posterior subcapsular cataracts, often somewhat off-center, or sectorial cataracts. This finding may be a useful marker for genetic counseling.

L. Steroid therapy can cause posterior subcapsular cataracts. In an early stage these cataracts have little effect on vision. Given the choice of developing a cataract or omitting an often lifesaving therapy, the answer is clear. If the cataract interferes significantly with visual performance, it can always be removed. Juvenile rheumatoid arthritis, which can occur at an early age, may result in posterior subcapsular cataracts.

References

Brocklebank JT, Harcourt RB, Meadows SR. Corticosteroids-induced cataracts in idiopathic nephrotic syndrome. Arch Dis Child 1982; 57:30–35.

Cibis GW, Waeltermann JM, Whitcraft CT, et al. Lenticular opacities in carriers of Lowe's syndrome. Ophthalmology 1986; 93:1041–1046.

Crouch ER, Parks MM. Management of posterior lenticonus complicated by unilateral cataracts. Am J Ophthalmol 1978; 85:503–507.

Govan JAA. Ocular manifestations of Alport's syndrome. Br J Ophthalmol 1983; 67:493–503.

Jaafar MS, Robb RM. Congenital anterior polar cataract. A review of 63 cases. Ophthalmology 1984; 91:249–251.

Lambert SR, Drack AV. Infantile cataracts. Surv Ophthalmol 1996; 40:427–458.

Lambert SR, Taylor D, Kriss A, et al. Ocular manifestations of the congenital varicella syndrome. Arch Ophthalmol 1989; 107:52–56.

Child with CATARACT

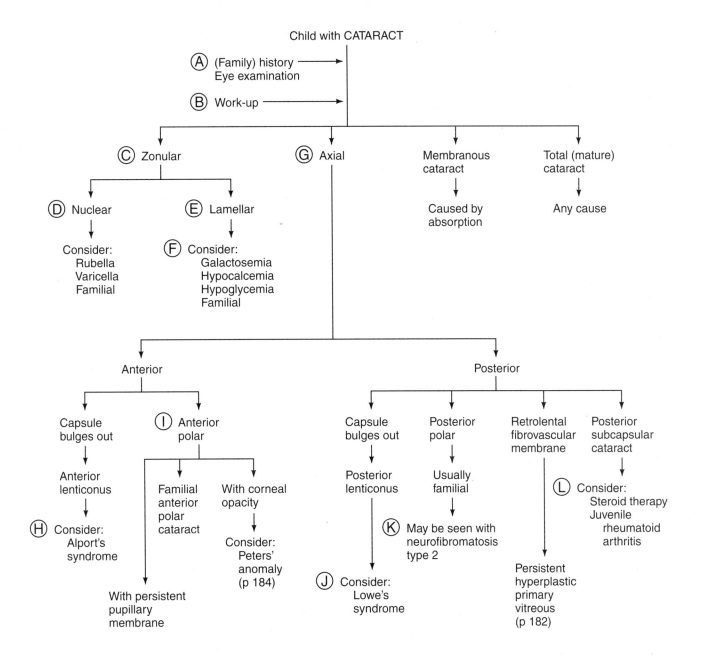

CATARACT IN A CHILD: TREATMENT

Johan Zwaan, M.D., Ph.D.

The treatment of pediatric cataracts has made great strides in the last 15 years. The availability of operating microscopes and cutting vitrectomy instruments; better correction of iatrogenic aphakia after cataract surgery, particularly with increasingly accepted intraocular lens implants in children; and rigorous amblyopia therapy has led to much improved results. The visual outcome now depends on the density of the cataract at and before the time of surgery, the age at which the cataract became significant, and very important, the commitment of the patient's parents. Pediatric cataract surgery should not be undertaken unless the parents or guardians of the child fully understand what is required of them and what the visual prognosis is. This includes frequent follow-up visits and compliance with amblyopia therapy and with optical correction as necessary.

A. The timing of cataract surgery is a major factor in visual rehabilitation.

B. Before the age of 2 months, nystagmus is generally not present and the visual prognosis is good, provided that aggressive correction of aphakia and amblyopia therapy take place. Bilateral cataracts have a better outcome than monocular ones. The best time for surgery within these first 2 months is still being debated, with some surgeons advocating surgery as early as possible (i.e., in the first week of life).

C. If the optic disc is visible with the direct ophthalmoscope or if a good retinoscopy can be performed, visual acuity is potentially at least 20/60 and surgery should probably not be undertaken because the visual rehabilitation to be anticipated may not be better than at this level.

D. If the decision has been made not to operate immediately, frequent and careful follow-up is imperative. If no formal visual acuity can be obtained, note visual behavior and ocular preference. If asymmetry between the eyes exists, such as a small monocular cataract, it may be helpful to prophylactically patch the better eye a few hours per day. A child can sometimes "look around" an axial cataract if the pupil is dilated with mydriatics. Bifocal glasses are then required to maintain near vision.

E. If the cataract worsens, as evidenced by the development of strabismus or reduction in vision, schedule lensectomy immediately.

F. Babies with dense cataracts who are not operated before the age of 2 months almost invariably get nystagmus, and the prognosis for visual rehabilitation drops: acuity may never be better than 20/200. The nystagmus and poor vision may be reversed if the nystagmus has existed for only a short while. Therefore perform surgery as soon as possible.

G. If the dense cataract develops later, the prognosis improves because the risk for deprivation amblyopia decreases with age. For instance, infants with posterior lenticonus usually do not get the associated cataract until they are a little older. They generally do well.

H. Lensectomy results, of course, in aphakia, which is as amblyopiogenic as the cataract was. Therefore aggressive treatment of the aphakia is essential. There has been a major change in the approach to aphakia correction in the last few years. The placement of intraocular lenses (IOLs) is now accepted by a significant number of ophthalmologists as a reasonably safe and effective alternative for aphakia correction.

I. After the age of 2 years most of the growth of the eye has taken place, although it levels off more after the age of 3 years. Therefore IOLs, although widely accepted for use in children after age 2 years, are still controversial for children younger than this age. A reasonable compromise is to perform the surgery in young infants in such a way that placement of a secondary IOL at a later age is facilitated. This can be done by doing a relatively small posterior capsulotomy and leaving a peripheral rim of the capsular bag in the eye. This rim can later serve as support for an IOL.

J. If an IOL has not been placed, initially correct the aphakia with a contact lens. Usually, I overcorrect the young infant by 2–3 diopters because near vision has more impact than vision at distance. When the contact lens wear fails, other options can be considered. Epikeratophakia is used occasionally, but some suppliers of the lenticules no longer make them available. The procedure is not recommended for children younger than 1 year of age because it has been shown that significant undercorrections occur with this age group.

K. Glasses have a role to play even in the correction of unilateral aphakia, although fusion will be impossible. For bilateral aphakes the fitting and wearing of glasses is much easier because the problem of aniseikonia does not occur. Fusion and stereopsis may be demonstrable in this group.

L. Secondary IOLs have been used with success in children. Placement of the implant in the sulcus, rather than the capsular bag, appears equally safe and effective, at least in the short run. Long-term follow-up is still lacking. At this time, I do not recommend sutured-in posterior chamber IOLs or anterior chamber IOLs for the pediatric age group.

M. If technically possible, placement of a primary IOL in the capsular bag is now the method of choice. It needs to be pointed out that the pediatric use of IOLs has not been sanctioned by the FDA. Parents should be made

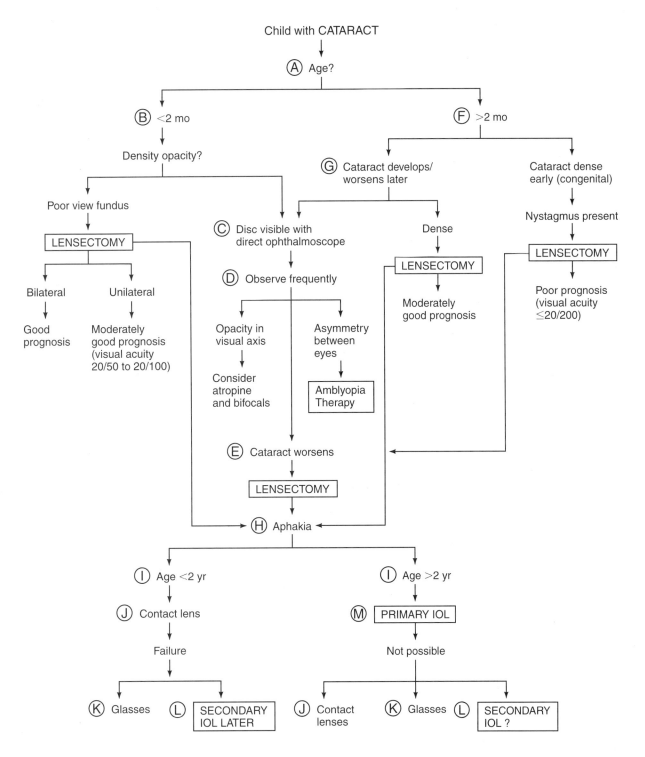

aware of this, and their informed consent is mandatory. Even bilateral IOL implants are not contraindicated.

References

Beller R, Hoyt CS, Marg E, et al. Good visual function after neonatal surgery for congenital monocular cataracts. Am J Ophthalmol 1981; 91:559–565.

Dutton JJ, Baker JD, Hiles DA, Morgan KS. Visual rehabilitation of aphakic children. Surv Ophthalmol 1990; 34:365–384.

Knight-Nanan D, O'Keefe M, Bowell R. Outcome and complications of intraocular lenses in children with cataracts. J Cataract Refract Surg 1996; 22:730–736.

Moore BD. Pediatric aphakic contact lens wear. Rates of successful wear. J Pediatr Ophthalmol Strabismus 1993; 30:253–258.

Zwaan J, Mullaney PB, Awad A, et al. Pediatric intraocular lens implantation: Surgical results and complications in more than 300 patients. Ophthalmology 1998; 105:112–119.

RETINOBLASTOMA

Johan Zwaan, M.D., Ph.D.

Retinoblastoma (RB) is relatively rare (the worldwide incidence is about 11 per 1 million children <5 years), but it is the most common malignant intraocular tumor in children. The alert pediatrician or family physician plays the most important role in early detection of the tumor. Although the diagnosis is occasionally made later than desirable, the combination of aware primary care providers, improved diagnostic methods, and aggressive treatment has yielded a cure rate of >90%. The care of these patients is best concentrated in centers where pediatric oncologists, radiologists, genetic counselors, and pediatric ophthalmologists are readily available.

A. About 60% of children with RB present with leukocoria and another 20% with strabismus, equally divided between esotropia and exotropia. In infants with these signs, always consider RB, especially if the child has a positive family history. Atypical clinical presentations include hypopyon, hyphema, glaucoma, and preseptal cellulitis. They may lead to a missed diagnosis.

B. A detailed history and a thorough eye and general physical examination should precede any more specialized tests. An examination under anesthesia is always indicated to thoroughly evaluate the peripheral retina, which requires scleral depression. The diagnosis of RB is primarily based on the ophthalmoscopic appearance of the tumor(s).

C. Although detailed counseling need not and probably should not be done immediately after the diagnosis is made, parents ought to be told that RB may be a genetic disease. RB behaves as an autosomal-dominant disease with a very high penetration rate. About 25% of patients have a positive family history; they are assumed to have the genetic disease. For the remaining 75% of patients, it is important to determine whether they had a germinal mutation and risk passing the RB gene to their children. Patients with multiple tumors and with bilateral disease had a germinal mutation. Most patients with one unilateral tumor probably had a somatic mutation, but 10%–15% have the genetic disease. Although laboratory screening (DNA polymorphism, gene locus analysis) can be helpful in making the distinction, unfortunately, these tests are least informative for the last group of patients, for which they are most needed. Table 1, based on available statistics but simplified in that it assumes 100% penetrance, is useful for determining approximate recurrence risk in family members of RB patients.

D. Once extraocular tumor is present, the prognosis becomes poor. If tumor cells are found at the surgical transection of the optic nerve after enucleation, survival used to be <20%. Advances in chemotherapy have improved the survival rate significantly in recent years.

E. Usually, combinations of irradiation and multiple agent chemotherapy are used. Recently used combinations of VP-16, carboplatin, vincristine, and others are meeting with much higher success.

F. A general physical examination helps in the differential diagnosis and, in advanced cases, may aid in the diagnosis of metastatic disease. Children suspected of having RB with a deletion of chromosomal region 13q14 show developmental delay and facial dysmorphism.

G. A CT scan is helpful in diagnosing RB and establishing possible extension in the orbit or the cranium.

H. Spinal taps, bone marrow biopsy or aspiration, and bone scans are no longer routinely obtained by most practitioners, unless metastases are suspected. MRI does not contribute to the understanding, unless the RB shows extrascleral extension.

I. Treatment choice depends on the tumor's size and location, the presence or absence of extraocular RB, and the local availability of treatment modalities. Treatment should always be individualized, and the listed choices should not be interpreted rigorously. The first goal is to save the child's life, the second to save the eyes and vision.

J. Tumors >3.0–4.0 mm in diameter and 2.0–2.5 mm in thickness are usually not fully destroyed by cryotherapy.

K. Photocoagulation is more appropriate for posterior tumors, which are not easily accessible for cryotherapy, but it is restricted by the same size limitations as cryotherapy.

TABLE 1   Risk for Recurrence of Retinoblastoma in Family Members of Affected Patients

	Bilateral tumors or positive family history (%)	Unilateral tumors and no family history (%)
Patient's child	50	8
Patient's brother or sister	5	0.8
Child of unaffected sibling	0.5	0.08
First cousin	0.05	0.008
Identical twin	100	15
Nonidentical twin	5	0.8

Modified from Musarella MA, Gallie BL. A simplified scheme for genetic counseling in retinoblastoma. J Pediatr Ophthalmol Strabismus 1987; 24:124–125.

L. The major advantage of local radioactive plaque therapy is the reduction of irradiation of normal tissue, although local scleral breakdown is possible. The therapy is not effective when the tumor is >10 mm or when significant vitreous seeding is present. When used anterior to the equator, radiation exposure of the lens may lead to cataract.

M. Effects of treatment should be checked in 3–5 weeks. This requires examination under anesthesia. Additional treatment may be applied at this time if viable tumor is still present. The frequency of examinations should depend on the success of the treatment.

N. Up to ages 3–4 years, perform examinations under anesthesia every 4 months, and from ages 5–6, every 6 months. Yearly examinations after age 6 may still require general anesthesia. After age 8 clinical examinations with scleral depression are usually tolerated and should be done yearly. Patients with genetic RB are at significant risk for other malignancies. Although some authors have recommended periodic CT scans or bone scans to rule out these tumors, this practice may not be necessary because clinical symptoms are usually present well before these tests yield results. Moreover, the radiation received may be tumorigenic by itself. Annual MRI scanning might be considered, but its value for periodic screening has not been established.

O. If a tumor is close to the optic nerve or fovea, avoid brachytherapy.

P. When multiple tumors or vitreous seeds are found, cryotherapy or photocoagulation are not effective. Although radioactive plaques are helpful, their radiation may not penetrate far enough into the vitreous. External beam irradiation is the method of choice, perhaps in combination with chemoreduction (see section Q).

Q. Chemoreduction or neoadjuvant chemotherapy is a promising new approach to the treatment of extensive intraocular RB. It aims at shrinking the tumors, rather than eliminating them, by the use of several (up to six) cycles of treatment with a combination of newer chemotherapeutic drugs, which enter the eye more efficiently than previously used drugs. Once the size of the tumors has been reduced, they can be treated by standard methods.

R. It is essential that a large segment of optic nerve be obtained during the enucleation to avoid having viable RB cells at the transection plane.

S. If the optic nerve is involved, particularly if tumor cells are found up to the end of the nerve stump, assume that the child is at risk for metastatic disease, even in the absence of other signs. Most clinicians agree that external beam irradiation is indicated.

T. Additional use of chemotherapy is still being debated. Although clear-cut evidence for benefit is not available, probably because of the small number of patients scattered over different centers, use of chemotherapy seems prudent.

References

Gallie BL, Budning A, DeBoer G, et al. Chemotherapy with focal therapy can cure intraocular retinoblastoma without radiotherapy. Arch Ophthalmol 1996; 114:1321–1328.

Kopelman JE, McLean IW, Rosenberg SH. Multivariate analysis of risk factors for metastasis in retinoblastoma treated by enucleation. Ophthalmology 1987; 94:371–377.

McCormick B, Ellsworth R, Abramson D, et al. Results of external beam radiation for children with retinoblastoma: A comparison of two techniques. J Pediatr Ophthalmol Strabismus 1989; 26:239–243.

Murphree AL, Christensen LE. Retinoblastoma and malignant intraocular tumors. In: Wright KW, ed. Pediatric ophthalmology and strabismus. St Louis: Mosby, 1995: 495–509.

Musarella MA, Gallie BL. A simplified scheme for genetic counseling in retinoblastoma. J Pediatr Ophthalmol Strabismus 1987; 24:124–125.

Roarty JD, McLean IW, Zimmerman LE. Incidence of second neoplasms in patients with retinoblastoma. Ophthalmology 1988; 95:1583–1587.

Shields CL, DePotter P, Himelstein BP, et al. Chemoreduction in the initial management of intraocular retinoblastoma. Arch Ophthalmol 1996; 114:1330–1338.

Shields CL, Shields JA, DePotter P, et al. Plaque radiotherapy in the management of retinoblastoma. Ophthalmology 1993; 100:217–224.

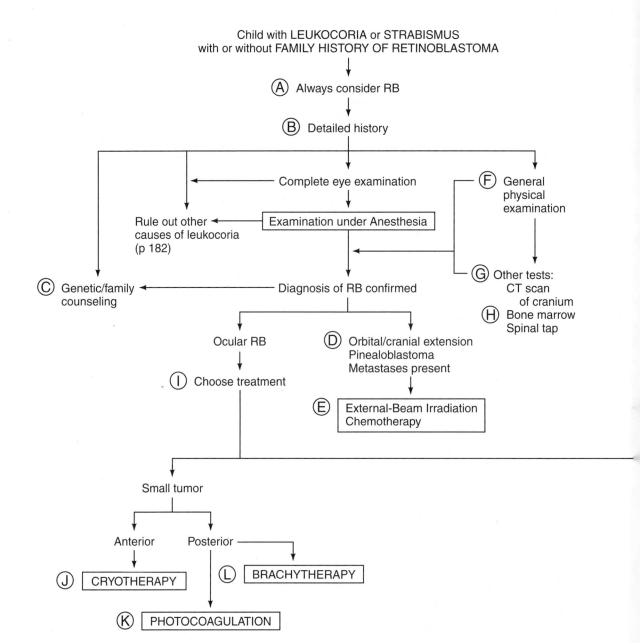

Child with LEUKOCORIA or STRABISMUS
with or without FAMILY HISTORY OF RETINOBLASTOMA

(A) Always consider RB

(B) Detailed history

Complete eye examination

(F) General physical examination

Rule out other causes of leukocoria (p 182)

Examination under Anesthesia

(C) Genetic/family counseling

Diagnosis of RB confirmed

(G) Other tests:
CT scan of cranium
(H) Bone marrow
Spinal tap

Ocular RB

(D) Orbital/cranial extension
Pinealoblastoma
Metastases present

(I) Choose treatment

(E) External-Beam Irradiation
Chemotherapy

Small tumor

Anterior

Posterior

(J) CRYOTHERAPY

(L) BRACHYTHERAPY

(K) PHOTOCOAGULATION

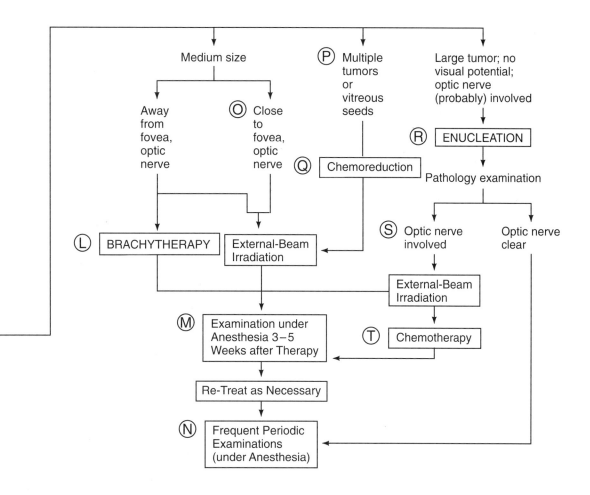

Medium size

Ⓟ Multiple tumors or vitreous seeds

Large tumor; no visual potential; optic nerve (probably) involved

Away from fovea, optic nerve

Ⓞ Close to fovea, optic nerve

Ⓡ ENUCLEATION

Ⓠ Chemoreduction

Pathology examination

Ⓛ BRACHYTHERAPY

External-Beam Irradiation

Ⓢ Optic nerve involved

Optic nerve clear

External-Beam Irradiation

Ⓜ Examination under Anesthesia 3−5 Weeks after Therapy

Ⓣ Chemotherapy

Re-Treat as Necessary

Ⓝ Frequent Periodic Examinations (under Anesthesia)

UNCORRECTABLE POOR VISION IN A CHILD

Johan Zwaan, M.D., Ph.D.

When one is confronted with a child with apparently uncorrectable poor vision, it is important to determine the duration of the condition. Congenital anomalies of the visual system often go unrecognized until later in life, particularly when only one eye is involved. A young child does not complain of decreased vision unless the loss is acute and bilateral. The earlier the loss, the more effective the compensatory mechanisms are. About half of pediatric vision loss is caused by genetic disease.

A.   The time of onset of vision loss is important in the differential diagnosis. Take a careful history to try to determine whether the presumed acquired problem actually may have been present since birth. In addition to structural abnormalities such as a large chorioretinal coloboma, there are other, not so obvious causes of decreased vision from birth (p 178).

B.   Nystagmus is associated with reduced visual acuity, moderately so in congenital motor nystagmus and more severely in secondary nystagmus associated with such disorders as albinism (p 178) or unoperated or late operated congenital cataract (p 188). The existence of nystagmus indicates the age at which the visual problem arose. Before age 2 years nystagmus will result, after age 6 definitely not; in between it can go either way. Nystagmus does not appear until about 2 months after birth.

C.   Retinoscopy is extremely useful, not only for refraction but also for detection of abnormalities in the media. For instance, very early keratoconus is often first detected by a distortion of the retinoscopic reflection. Opacities in the media are easily seen as well.

D.   A refractive error may be found in combination with strabismus. Microtropia is often associated with anisometropia. Similarly, a difference in refractive error between the two eyes may trigger a preference for one eye and amblyopia in the other.

E.   For simplicity, refractive errors and amblyopia and other causes of reduced vision are separated here, yet they often are combined. For instance, patients with retinal dystrophies commonly also have significant refractive errors, and the reduction in vision caused by optic nerve hypoplasia or cataract may be compounded by amblyopia or refractive errors.

F.   Retinal detachments may occur in high myopia, retinopathy of prematurity, and some vitreoretinal dystrophies and dysplasias, among others. Also consider trauma, including child abuse.

G.   Retinal dystrophies rarely present with reduced vision as a primary complaint. More commonly, night vision, peripheral vision, and color perception may be disturbed. Relatively few neurometabolic disorders affecting both brain and eyes first present with vision complaints (see section K).

H.   Macular dystrophies (e.g., Best's vitelliform dystrophy, Stargardt's disease) often present with vision loss. Particularly in Stargardt's disease, the early retinal changes may be so subtle that they are overlooked and the patient may be considered "functionally" blind.

I.   Leukemia may cause retinal hemorrhages, white patches, and even infarctions. It can also infiltrate the optic nerve, resulting in a picture difficult to separate from papilledema from other causes.

J.   Reduced vision resulting from a conversion disorder (this term is considered preferable to hysterical blindness) is a diagnosis of exclusion. If all testing is negative, this possibility can be entertained. Children with this problem may have some social difficulties (at home or at school) but are generally normal without evidence for psychiatric disease. The prognosis is excellent. Münchausen's syndrome and clear malingering are rare in children. Several tests are available for the diagnosis of conversion disorder. Most are based on making the child believe that he or she is using the "good" eye, whereas in reality the "bad" one is being used.

K.   Neurometabolic disorders often show eye abnormalities, but the systemic findings overshadow the visual ones. Exceptions are juvenile Batten's disease, juvenile metachromatic leukodystrophy, adrenoleukodystrophy, and sialidosis type 1, in which at least initially reduced vision is the major symptom.

L.   Optic neuritis presents with profound and acute vision loss. The picture can be dramatic. There is an afferent pupillary defect, and the optic disc is swollen. If it is not, retrobulbar optic neuritis may be present. CT scan and CSF studies should clarify the diagnosis. The visually evoked response (VER) is most helpful. Both the visual and systemic prognoses are good; most children with this disorder have good visual recovery and no neurologic sequelae.

M.   Dominant optic atrophy has its onset usually around 10 years of age, Leber's more commonly in young adulthood. The latter is preponderantly seen in young men and is the result of mitochondrial inheritance, possibly combined with an external factor. Several autosomal-recessive syndromes are characterized by optic atrophy. An example is DIDMOAD syndrome, combining optic atrophy with diabetes mellitus and diabetes insipidus. Deafness may also occur.

N.   Keratoconus often has its onset in the early teens, with increasing amounts of astigmatism and myopia.

POOR VISION IN A CHILD

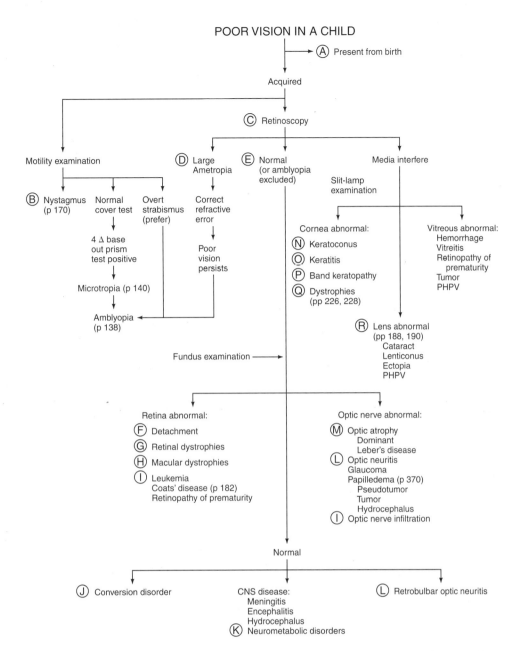

O. Acute forms of keratitis are easily detected; syphilitic interstitial keratitis with characteristic stromal blood vessels and "ghost" vessels must be separated from Cogan's syndrome, in which keratitis is combined with vestibular hearing loss.

P. Band keratopathy indicates ocular inflammation or systemic disease such as sarcoidosis. Juvenile rheumatoid arthritis (JRA) is insidious in its course, and band keratopathy may be the first sign of the disease. By then the low grade uveitis of JRA may have done severe damage to the eyes.

Q. A child with epithelial or stromal corneal dystrophies rarely has decreased vision. This contrasts with endothelial dystrophies (congenital hereditary endothelial dystrophy [CHED] and posterior polymorphous endothelial dystrophy [PPMD]), which can significantly interfere with normal vision (p 184). Corneal problems

are discussed in more detail in the section "Corneal Disorders."

R. For lens abnormalities, see pp 188 and 190.

References

Droste PJ, Archer SM, Helveston EM. Measurement of low vision in children and infants. Ophthalmology 1991; 98:1513–1518.

Kerrison JB, Howell N, Miller NR, et al. Leber hereditary optic neuropathy. Electron microscopy and molecular genetic analysis of a case. Ophthalmology 1995; 102:1509–1516.

McDonald MA. Assessment of visual acuity in toddlers. Surv Ophthalmol 1986; 31:189–210.

Repka MX, Miller NR. Optic atrophy in children. Am J Ophthalmol 1988; 106:191–194.

Taylor D. Non-organic ocular disorders. In: Taylor D, ed. Pediatric ophthalmology. 2nd ed. Oxford: Blackwell Scientific, 1996.

NASOLACRIMAL DUCT OBSTRUCTION IN CHILDREN

Johan Zwaan, M.D., Ph.D.

Nasolacrimal duct obstruction (NLDO) is present in about 5% of newborn infants. Tear production is not fully developed at birth, and epiphora may not be obvious until the child is a few weeks old. NLDO results from a blockage anywhere in the nasolacrimal drainage system, which may be caused by an incomplete opening of the duct between the inner canthus and the inferior turbinate of the nasal cavity or, rarely, by the absence of parts of the system. In most patients, it results from an obstruction at the lower end of the nasolacrimal duct, where the duct joins the nasal mucosa at the valve of Hasner. The infant presents with an overflow of tears, and the eye looks wet. A variable amount of mucopurulent discharge may be present. Although the diagnosis should be self-evident, it is commonly mistaken for conjunctivitis, particularly by nonophthalmologists, even though the conjunctiva is usually quiet. Rare causes of epiphora, such as congenital glaucoma, must be excluded.

A. Clinical signs are usually enough to make the diagnosis of NLDO, but it may be helpful to test the lacrimal drainage by instilling fluorescein in the conjunctival sac. If the yellow solution does not clear from the eye in a few minutes or if the clearance lags considerably behind that of the fellow eye, a complete or partial NLDO is present. A formal Jones test (p 48) is not practical in children. There is usually no need to perform sophisticated diagnostic work-up such as dacryoscintigraphy.

B. Occasionally, a newborn has a bluish swelling in the area of the nasolacrimal sac. Kinking of the canaliculi prevents backflow from the sac, and a clear mucoid fluid accumulates. This mucocele, also called *congenital dacryocystocele* or *amniotocele,* should not be mistaken for a hemangioma or a midline encephalocele. Sometimes, the mucocele drains spontaneously or after massage, but if drainage does not occur within a few days, do a probing to prevent secondary infection. If such an infection occurs, hospitalization for treatment with systemic antibiotics is usually necessary to control the dacryocystitis and the commonly associated preseptal cellulitis.

C. If evidence for infection is present, initiate proper antibiotic treatment. Erythromycin ointment or 10% sodium sulfacetamide are a rational first choice and should be applied topically three to four times daily until the infection clears. Some ophthalmologists prefer to use an antibiotic chronically.

D. If the tear sac becomes infected, the resulting abscess may drain through the skin or the infection may spread, causing a cellulitis of the periorbita. Systemic and topical antibiotics are required. Probing can be performed after the infectious process has quieted down. To prevent fistula formation, avoid surgical drainage by a stab incision through the skin or through the inferonasal conjunctival cul-de-sac deep to the canaliculi.

E. Chronic wetness of the lower eyelid and toxic effects of mucopurulent drainage can cause dermatitis of the eyelids, which is very irritating (a "diaper rash of the eyelid"). Early probing is indicated.

F. Although some physicians probe all infants with NLDO early, I prefer to wait because ≥90% of the obstructions resolve spontaneously by the age of 1 year. Massage of the nasolacrimal sac helps decompress it and reduce the amount of discharge. Massage can be curative when the distal obstruction "pops" as the contents of the sac are driven through the duct.

G. If NLDO is still present at age 10–12 months, it will probably not clear on its own. The disadvantage of waiting is that probing requires general anesthesia in the older child. An infant <6 months can be mummified, and probing can be done safely in the office under topical anesthesia. Nevertheless, the high spontaneous resolution rate justifies being patient and thereby saving most infants from an unnecessary procedure. Of course, this reasoning applies only if the NLDO is uncomplicated.

H. Rarely, other anatomic abnormalities cause epiphora. Occluded puncta can be opened by rupturing the occluded membrane or by snipping the tissues between the distal end of the canaliculus and the cul-de-sac. It may be possible to intubate the canaliculi retrograde from a dacryocystotomy incision. Usually, a (conjunctival) dacryocystorhinostomy (DCR) becomes necessary if parts of the nasolacrimal drainage system are missing.

I. Well-done probings are almost always successful in infants with NLDO. Patients requiring a DCR should be the exception rather than the rule.

J. If the first probing does not work, one or two repetitions are called for. The repeat procedure may be combined with fracturing of the inferior turbinate, which may block the lower opening of the nasolacrimal duct. I have not found this to be useful. A technically more complex method of probing by means of balloon catheter dilation has recently been reported but should rarely be necessary.

References

Becker BB, Berry FD, Koller H. Balloon catheter dilatation for treatment of congenital nasolacrimal duct obstruction. Am J Ophthalmol 1996; 124:304–309.

Mansour AM, Cheng KP, Mumma JV, et al. Congenital dacryocele. A collaborative review. Ophthalmology 1991; 98:1744–1751.

EPIPHORA IN AN INFANT

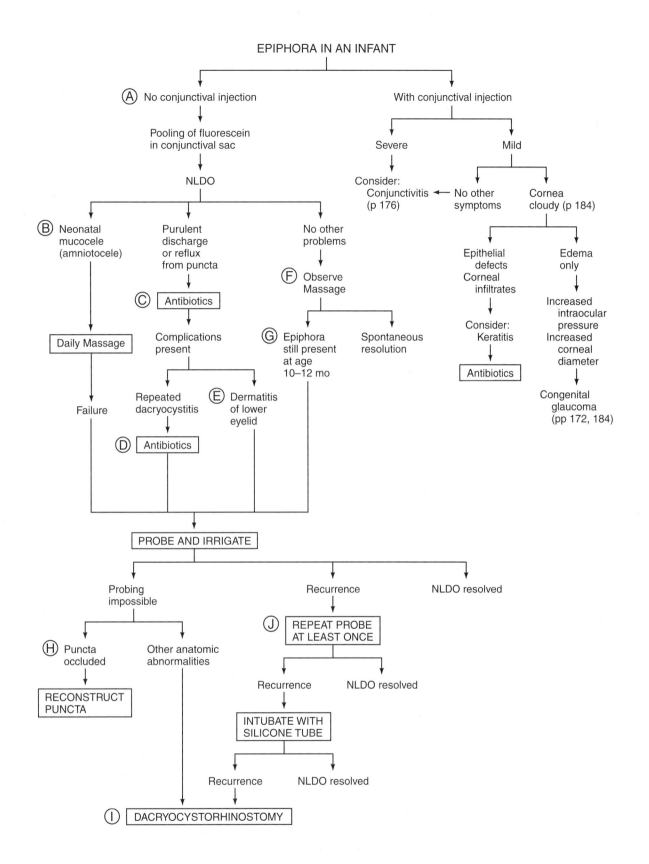

Robb RM. Probing and irrigation for congenital nasolacrimal duct obstruction. Arch Ophthalmol 1986; 104:378–379.
Zwaan J. The anatomy of probing and irrigation for congenital nasolacrimal duct obstruction. Ophthalmic Surg Lasers 1997; 28:71–73.

Zwaan J. Treatment of congenital nasolacrimal duct obstruction before and after the age of one year. Ophthalmic Surg Lasers 1997; 28:932–936.

CORNEAL DISORDERS

PUNCTATE CORNEAL STAINING

Mark L. McDermott, M.D.
Elmer Y. Tu, M.D.

A. Punctate corneal staining is a common endpoint for myriad ocular surface diseases. A detailed medical and drug history is important in distinguishing its cause. Question patients specifically about a history of collagen vascular diseases, mucous membrane disorders, neurologic disease, previous eye infections, and atopy, and elicit details of onset and exacerbating and alleviating factors. In addition, take a complete, exacting medication history of all medications with specific attention to all topical ophthalmic preparations. Patients often do not consider eyedrops to be medication. Many ocular medications and over-the-counter tear substitutes contain preservatives toxic to the cornea epithelium, and drugs with anticholinergic side effects may reduce tear secretion, causing a dry eye.

B. A careful adnexal examination is of great help in finding the cause of punctate corneal staining. Eyelid abnormalities are one of the most common sources of ocular surface disease. Examination of the face and eyelid margins may uncover the stigmata of rosacea. Careful examination of the eyelids may reveal molluscum lesions, misdirected lashes, or lid position abnormalities predisposing to corneal staining. Examination of the bulbar conjunctiva may show raised lesions such as pterygia or pingueculae, which result in drying of the adjacent cornea, causing staining. Examine the conjunctival fornix for the presence of follicles, which suggests an infectious or toxic cause; papillae, which suggest a bacterial or atopic cause; or subepithelial scarring from cicatricial pemphigoid. A thorough slit-lamp examination should differentiate between the three distinct entities that exhibit punctate staining: punctate epithelial erosions, superficial punctate keratitis, and subepithelial infiltrates. Location of the lesions is often suggestive of the underlying disease process and will help in diagnosis. Traditionally, punctate staining refers to fluorescein; other vital dyes such as rose bengal, lissamine green B, and sulforhodamine B may help elucidate the underlying disease.

C. Superficial punctate epithelial erosions (PEE) are tiny focal areas of epithelial discontinuity. They are subtle on unaided slit-lamp examination, but instillation of fluorescein will clearly reveal them. They appear as tiny brilliant green areas restricted to the epithelial surface. Without dye these areas are nearly transparent. The distinct lack of inflammatory elements should suggest a mechanical or toxic cause rather than an infectious or inflammatory disorder. The patient may be asymptomatic or have photophobia, foreign body sensation, lacrimation, and reactive blepharospasm. A variety of insults can result in these erosions, and a thorough history is particularly useful. History of topical drug use, ocular discharge, ultraviolet light exposure, or allergies must be specifically elicited. The pattern of corneal involvement can be useful in the differential diagnosis.

D. Generalized punctate erosions are often caused by medicamentosa consisting of extended use, overdosage, or an already compromised ocular surface. Offending agents include cycloplegics, aminoglycoside antibiotics, and preserved ophthalmic solutions. Atopic disease in vernal keratoconjunctivitis, as well as early bacterial conjunctivitis, may also produce a generalized pattern. The popularization of antimetabolites, such as 5-FU and mitomycin C, for ocular pathology induces a diffuse pattern of PEE. Systemic oncolytic medications like cytarabine may precipitate erosions. As with all of these drugs a delay between administration and observed effects will be seen. Conjunctivalization of the cornea may lead to PEE in various limbal deficiency syndromes, as well as in vitamin A deficiency.

E. Central erosions are typical of ultraviolet (UV) light burns and contact lens overwear, and symptoms are often delayed. Before the formation of subepithelial infiltrates, adenoviral conjunctivitis may produce a central pattern of noninflammatory erosions. UV photokeratopathy may be central or inferior in boaters from water-surface reflection.

F. Distribution in the inferior half or "exposure zone" should suggest disorders in which exposure might decompensate an already compromised surface or in which mechanical factors prevent proper tear distribution. Exposure keratitis should be suspected not only in anatomic lid abnormalities but also in incomplete blink states and decreased blink rate states such as Parkinson's disease. Neurotrophic keratitis and keratoconjunctivitis sicca (KCS) would be expected to have the most prominent findings in this area of least protection.

G. Distribution in the superior third of the cornea is unusual but should implicate disorders of the upper eyelid or upper conjunctiva such as superior limbic keratitis (SLK), molluscum lesions of the upper eyelid margin, and infection with *Chlamydia trachomatis*. Atopic and vernal keratoconjunctivitis have their greatest effects on the upper eyelid palpebral conjunctiva with expected consequences to the superior cornea.

H. Focal erosions, especially if present in a linear configuration, suggest trauma from a foreign body. A vertical configuration suggests that a careful search be performed to rule out a retained foreign body lodged in the upper tarsus. Thoroughly investigate focal lesions near the limbus because early corneal intraepithelial neoplasia (CIN) is often related to adjacent limbal CIN.

I. Unlike erosions, which represent focal epithelial defects without surrounding inflammation, superficial punctate epithelial keratitis (SPK) is the result of accumulated epithelial cells surrounded by inflammatory cells, which results in discrete gray-white lesions, visible without the aid of vital dyes. These lesions will also stain with fluorescein. However, instillation of rose bengal stains these areas strongly. An inflammatory component should suggest an infectious or immune-mediated cause. The size of the lesions varies and may be useful.

J. Fine punctate keratitis is present in earlier stages of adenoviral infections and chlamydial infections and is also commonly seen in KCS. The presence or absence of preauricular adenopathy, conjunctival follicles, or micropannus may differentiate these entities. Adenoviral infections commonly have preauricular adenopathy, conjunctival follicles, and no micropannus. Chlamydial infections characteristically have micropannus and variable adenopathy and conjunctival follicles. Dry eyes are not associated with follicular conjunctival response or preauricular adenopathy.

K. Coarse punctate keratitis is characteristic of Thygeson's keratitis, early adenoviral keratitis, herpes simplex infection, and herpes zoster infection. Differentiation among these entities depends on unilateral or bilateral involvement, presence or absence of corneal sensation, adnexal examination, and patient history. Herpes simplex and zoster are almost always unilateral and associated with diminished corneal sensation. Herpes zoster has an antecedent history of severe pain associated with cutaneous vesicles or scarring in a unilateral, dermatomal, trigeminal nerve pattern. Herpes simplex, by contrast, has minimal pain and few vesicles, if any, which do not respect a specific dermatome. Thygeson's superficial punctate keratitis is an entity of unknown cause that results in recurrent bilateral episodes of superficial punctate keratitis exquisitely responsive to topical corticosteroids. In this disease, cornea sensation is normal and there are no conjunctival follicles or preauricular adenopathy. The disease may persist in a waxing and waning cycle for many years. Both the appearance and clinical course will distinguish it from other entities. A viral cause is suspected.

L. Filamentary keratitis results from epithelial cell proliferation forming a cord of epithelium and mucus that remains adherent to the epithelial surface. These filaments stain with fluorescein and with rose bengal. Presence of filaments is common after patching and surgery. Filaments are also commonly seen in the dry eye and in SLK. SLK is a bilateral condition characterized by punctate keratitis of the upper third of the cornea with or without filaments, as well as keratinization, punctate staining, and vertical, straight-vessel hyperemia of the adjacent limbal conjunctiva and upper palpebral conjunctiva. A micropannus is often present. SLK is much more common in women in the fifth decade, and there is an associated absence of deep tendon reflexes. There is a high association with thyroid disease, making a thorough evaluation for thyroid dysfunction mandatory if SLK is suspected. The staining of adjacent cornea and bulbar and palpebral conjunctiva differentiates this diagnosis from other causes of filaments. Various medical treatments, including mast cell stabilizers and retinoids, have been proposed as therapy, as has surgical intervention with silver nitrate, punctal occlusion, and conjunctival resection.

M. Combined epithelial and subepithelial punctate keratitis has features of superficial punctate keratitis with the added finding of inflammatory deposits in the subepithelial or anterior stromal space. This combination is most characteristic of later-stage adenoviral keratitis. This combination may also be seen in other viral infections, such as those in the herpes family. However, herpes simplex is more commonly unilateral and focal or diffuse, whereas adenoviral disease may more often be bilateral and central. Staphylococcal hypersensitivity reactions may produce epithelial and subepithelial punctate keratitis as a precursor to a marginal ulcer in the classic 10, 2, 4, or 8 o'clock positions near the limbus. Adult inclusion conjunctivitis may also have similar cornea findings, although the lesions are associated with a micropannus and are more peripherally located.

References

Arffa R, ed. Grayson's diseases of the cornea. 3rd ed. St Louis: Mosby, 1991: 48–52.

Chodosh J, Dix RD, Howell RC, et al. Staining characteristics and antiviral activity of sulforhodamine B and lissamine green B. Invest Ophthalmol Vis Sci 1994; 35:1046–1058.

Friedland S, Loya N, Shapiro A. Handling punctate keratitis resulting from systemic cytarabine. Ann Ophthalmol 1993; 25:290–291.

Kadramas EF, Bartley GB. Superior limbic keratoconjunctivitis. A prognostic sign for severe Graves ophthalmopathy. Ophthalmology 1995; 102:1472–1475.

Krachmer JH, Mannis MJ, Holland EJ, eds. Cornea. St Louis: Mosby, 1997: 275–277, 668–670.

Pettit TH, Meyer KT. The differential diagnosis of superficial punctate keratitis. Int Ophthalmol Clin 1984; 24:79–92.

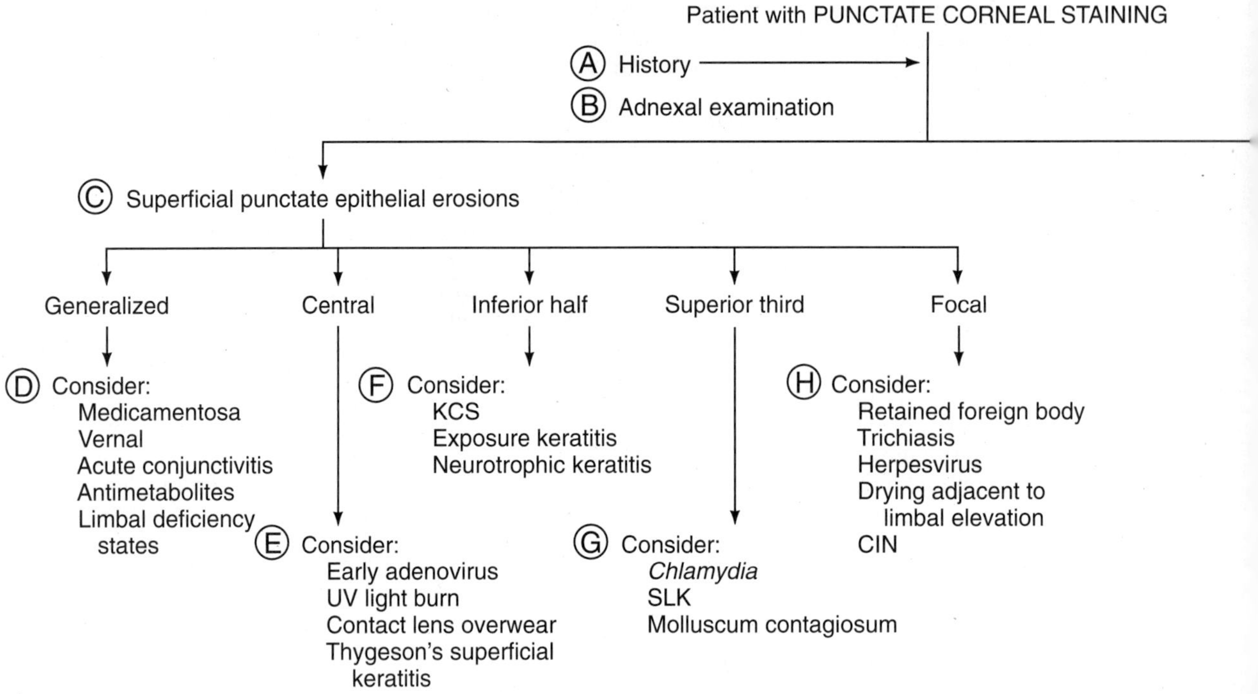

Patient with PUNCTATE CORNEAL STAINING

(A) History ⟶

(B) Adnexal examination

(C) Superficial punctate epithelial erosions

Generalized   Central   Inferior half   Superior third   Focal

(D) Consider:
    Medicamentosa
    Vernal
    Acute conjunctivitis
    Antimetabolites
    Limbal deficiency
      states

(F) Consider:
    KCS
    Exposure keratitis
    Neurotrophic keratitis

(E) Consider:
    Early adenovirus
    UV light burn
    Contact lens overwear
    Thygeson's superficial
      keratitis

(G) Consider:
    Chlamydia
    SLK
    Molluscum contagiosum

(H) Consider:
    Retained foreign body
    Trichiasis
    Herpesvirus
    Drying adjacent to
      limbal elevation
    CIN

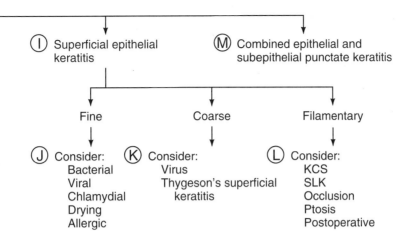

CORNEAL DENDRITIC LESIONS

Cameron K. Shields, M.D.
Richard W. Yee, M.D.

A. Determining the cause of a corneal dendrite or branch-shaped corneal lesion requires careful history taking and physical examination. Emphasis should be placed on obtaining a history of skin lesions, prior trauma or surgery, and the use of topical medications or contact lenses.

B. Skin lesions can be very helpful in the differential diagnosis. The primary episode of herpes simplex virus may be present; single or grouped painful vesicles with clear to yellow fluid may appear on the lids, lips, face, nose, and trunk. These lesions usually crust and resolve in 2 weeks. Herpes zoster ophthalmicus skin lesions begin as grouped vesicles on a painful erythematous base. These lesions are usually unilateral, respect the midline, and are limited to one to two dermatomes. They become pustular in 3–4 days and crust by days 7–10. Permanent deep-pitted scars may result.

Varicella primary infection produces lesions characterized by crops of pruritic small vesicles with pink halos on the scalp, face, mouth, and trunk. The lesions begin as macules and progress into papules, vesicles, and pustules that then crust. They usually heal without scarring.

Keratosis follicularis (Darier's disease) is an autosomal-dominant disorder of keratinization. Typical skin lesions are yellow-brown crusted papules that appear on the face, scalp, retroauricular areas, neck, axilla, and trunk. Keratotic papules of the palms and soles may be seen. Mucous membrane involvement occurs less commonly. Tyrosinemia type 2 (Richner-Hanhart syndrome) is an autosomal-recessive disorder characterized by partial or complete absence of hepatic tyrosine aminotransferase. Patients have increased levels of tyrosine in the plasma and urine. Hyperkeratotic skin lesions are seen on the palms, soles, and elbows.

C. The morphology of the corneal dendrite may help in differentiating between herpes simplex virus and herpes zoster virus. The dendrite of herpes simplex is characterized by single or multiple branching linear lesions that may exhibit a beadlike projection (terminal bulb) at the end of the branches. Fluorescein dye stains the central ulceration, and rose bengal dye stains the epithelial edges containing actively replicating virus. A superficial stromal infiltrate may appear localized under the dendrite. The cornea is focally anesthetic. In contrast, herpes zoster virus produces gray-white dendrites that are often more stellate, broader, and more plaquelike than those of herpes simplex virus. They do not have terminal bulbs and stain with rose bengal, but they exhibit only poor to moderate staining with fluorescein dye. There is no ulceration of the epithelium.

D. Keratosis follicularis corneal lesions are characterized by peripheral opacities and central epithelial irregularities appearing in radiating or cobweb patterns that pool fluorescein. In tyrosinemia type 2, the pseudodendrites are bilateral, thick, and plaquelike and lack terminal bulbs.

E. Varicella dendrites are raised, coarse, and gray-white and do not stain well with fluorescein. They are made up of swollen epithelial cells that contain intracellular viral particles. The dendrites have been reported to occur months after the skin lesions of varicella during use of topical corticosteroid, idoxuridine, and atropine for disciform keratitis. Vaccinia has been reported to cause linear or maplike lesions with branching extensions that resemble herpetic keratitis.

F. Topical β blockers, including betaxolol and levobunolol, have been reported to cause dendriform corneal epithelial lesions that are gray-white and stain faintly with rose bengal. These lesions rapidly improve after cessation of the topical drops. Idoxuridine has been reported to cause dendriform lesions.

G. Acanthamoeba keratitis may present with a dendriform pattern of edematous corneal epithelium that stains with fluorescein. A small amount of anterior stromal inflammation may be present under the epithelial keratopathy. Soft contact lens wear has been reported to cause dendritic corneal lesions. These lesions have been described as annular sinuous epithelial dendritic figures in the midperipheral cornea or as large branching subepithelial dendrites. The lesions lack the typical herpes simplex virus end bulbs and may stain lightly with fluorescein. The keratitis disappears after discontinuation of soft contact lens wear.

H. Thygeson's superficial punctate keratitis is a bilateral epithelial keratitis that is characterized by spontaneous remissions and exacerbations. The corneal lesions are round to oval gray-white intraepithelial dots that may exhibit a stellate pattern. During exacerbations the lesions may have an elevated epithelium that stains centrally with rose bengal and fluorescein. During remissions the lesions may remain flat with no stain. Epstein-Barr virus has been implicated in dendritic keratitis. It has been cultured from the conjunctiva and tears, and virus DNA has been detected from dendritic epithelial cells. The lesions have been described as multiple small stellate microdendrites of opaque epithelial cells that stain with rose bengal involving the central and peripheral cornea.

I. Microsporidial keratitis is associated with immunosuppression. Microsporidia are obligated intracellular protozoan parasites that are becoming increasingly recog-

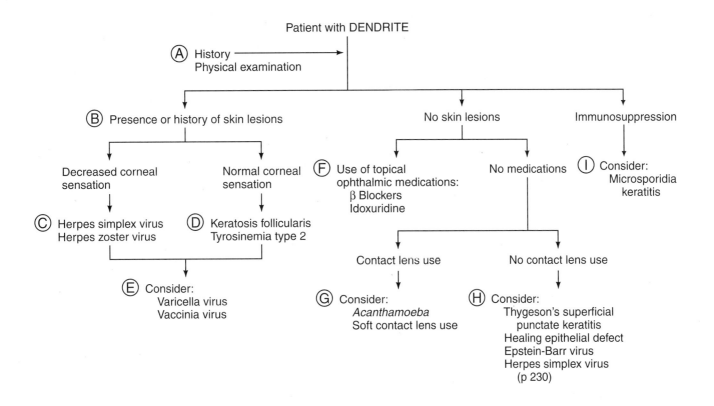

Patient with DENDRITE

(A) History ———————→
Physical examination

(B) Presence or history of skin lesions

(F) Use of topical ophthalmic medications:
β Blockers
Idoxuridine

No skin lesions

Immunosuppression

No medications

(I) Consider:
Microsporidia
keratitis

Decreased corneal sensation

Normal corneal sensation

(C) Herpes simplex virus
Herpes zoster virus

(D) Keratosis follicularis
Tyrosinemia type 2

(E) Consider:
Varicella virus
Vaccinia virus

Contact lens use

No contact lens use

(G) Consider:
Acanthamoeba
Soft contact lens use

(H) Consider:
Thygeson's superficial punctate keratitis
Healing epithelial defect
Epstein-Barr virus
Herpes simplex virus
(p 230)

nized as opportunistic pathogens in patients with AIDS. They have been associated with enteritis, hepatitis, peritonitis, and recently, superficial keratoconjunctivitis and stromal keratitis. The clinician's suspicion should be raised when a patient has a positive risk factor for acquiring HIV or is HIV positive. History of recent travel to the tropics or close contact with domestic animals such as cats and birds, which are known microsporidial hosts, are also risk factors. Systemic symptoms depend on the organ involved. Slit-lamp examination reveals punctuate epithelial opacities with irregular fluorescein uptake that can acquire a dendritic shape. Corneal ulceration may occur, with superficial stromal focal infiltrates being the most common. An associated anterior uveitis may be present.

Hematoxylin and eosin, Giemsa, Gram stain, and Warthin-Starry stain can demonstrate the presence of this organism on light microscopy sections. The specific diagnosis features that distinguish Microsporidia from other small nonspore forming organisms are best demonstrated by electron microscopy, which shows the pathognomonic coiled polar filament or tubule. Confocal microscopy demonstrates many small intraepithelial opacities of the corneal epithelium. Treatment includes topical dibromopropamidine isethionate (Brolene) and Fumagillin (Fumagillin bicyclohexylammonium salt).

References

Arffa R. Grayson's diseases of the cornea. 3rd ed. St Louis: Mosby, 1991.

Berger CA, White CR. Exudative papulosquamous diseases. In: Sams WM Jr, Lynch PJ, eds. Principles and practice of dermatology. New York: Churchill Livingstone, 1990: 357–358.

Elliot GW, Sams WM. Viral vesicular diseases. In: Sams WM, ed. Principles and practice of dermatology. New York: Churchill Livingstone, 1990: 99–107.

Kaufman HE, Rayfield MA. Viral conjunctivitis and keratitis. In: Kaufman HE, Barron BA, McDonald MB, Waltman SR. eds. The cornea. New York: Churchill Livingstone, 1988: 299–331.

Liesegang TJ. Corneal complications from herpes zoster ophthalmicus. Ophthalmology 1985; 92:316–324.

McCluskey PJ, Goonan PV, Marriott DJ, Field AS. Microsporidial keratoconjunctivitis in AIDS. Eye 1993; 7:80–83.

Rastrelli PD, Didier E, Yee RW. Microsporidial keratitis. Ophthalmologic clinics of North America. Cec 1994; 7:617–633.

Uchida Y, Kaneko M, Hayashi K. Varicella dendritic keratitis. Am J Ophthalmol 1980; 89:259–262.

MARGINAL CORNEAL ULCERS

Jeffrey T. Liegner, M.D.
Richard W. Yee, M.D.

There are several causes of marginal corneal thinning, with or without infiltrate. Patients may have pain or photophobia or be asymptomatic.

A. History (onset, eye care, trauma), a physical examination (tear quality, eyelids, or corneal sensitivity), dermatologic evaluation (facial rash, acne rosacea, or psoriasis), and systemic assessment (connective tissue disorder, arthritis, vasculitis, immune status, diabetes, or oral or genital lesions) often provide a diagnosis. Debridement of necrotic corneal tissue for special stains and culture is essential to rule out infection. After removing debris, dry the area thoroughly and place a cyanoacrylate glue patch if thinning is severe. A bandage soft contact lens may reduce discomfort and promote healing but should not be used over an infected ulcer. Keratoplasty may be needed for severe thinning or for a descemetocele.

B. Frequent instillation of fortified antibiotics for gram-positive (cefazolin, 50 mg/ml) and gram-negative coverage (gentamicin or tobramycin, 14 mg/ml) may be necessary. The initial goal is treatment of the infection and promotion of wound repair.

C. Mooren's ulcer is painful and bilateral and is characterized by an aggressive, grayish, overhanging advancing edge of an epithelial and stromal defect with vascularization of the ulcer base. It may respond to systemic steroids and immunosuppression; topical steroids are often useless. Perforation is rare, requiring a corneal graft, which may melt or become vascularized. Conjunctival excision with or without cryotherapy may arrest progression. Corneal graft rejection, characterized by keratic precipitates, an endothelial rejection line, stromal or epithelial edema with or without infiltrates, and anterior segment inflammatory signs, requires prompt aggressive management. Elevated intraocular pressure or a suture abscess may be inciting and should be corrected. Topical, subtenon, and systemic steroids are effective.

D. Correct eyelid and eyelash abnormalities (e.g., entropion, cicatricial exposure, lagophthalmos, neuroparalytic cornea) to prevent deterioration of ocular surface integrity. A temporary tarsorrhaphy may help. Chemical injuries may cause only peripheral corneal inflammation. Immediate copious irrigation, confirmed with tear pH measurements, is essential. Blepharitis from staphylococcal hypersensitivity can cause peripheral corneal inflammation and mild corneal thinning, separated from the limbus by clear cornea at the 10, 2, 8, and 4 o'clock positions. Acne rosacea can affect the cornea in patients with characteristic erythema and telangiectasis of the eyelid margin, nose (rhinophyma), cheeks, and forehead. Treatment includes topical steroids, improved lid hygiene, and systemic doxycycline (100 mg PO twice daily). Sutures or foreign bodies may cause corneal inflammation. Removal is curative.

E. Noninflamed degenerative corneal changes can be striking on observation but rarely require treatment. Terrien's marginal degeneration, a bilateral degeneration of the superior peripheral cornea, may show superficial vascularization with lipid deposits at the leading edge. Pellucid marginal degeneration is a non-vascularized, noninfiltrative inferior band of corneal thinning located 1–2 mm from the limbus. Irregular or high astigmatism warrants refractive surgery. Furrow degeneration is found in elderly patients, peripheral to an arcus senilis. No epithelial defect is present, and problems are rare. Dellen is corneal thinning at the limbus adjacent to a surface elevation, which creates poor spreading of the tear film with stromal desiccation under an intact epithelium. Lubrication or pressure patching should cure the defect. Exposure keratitis, often inferior and caused by malpositioned lid margins, improves with lubrication. Phlyctenulosis presents as a small, white, painful nodule at the limbus, with dilated conjunctival vessels. Often bilateral, it migrates centrally and may produce neovascularization. Topical steroids, hygiene, and antibiotic ointments suppress this delayed hypersensitivity reaction to *Staphylococcus* antigen. Localized tuberculosis infection may also cause phlyctenulosis.

F. Once an infectious process is excluded, antibiotics can be stopped. Laboratory studies can be tailored to find associated systemic disorders.

G. Primary keratoconjunctivitis sicca (KS) produces low-grade irritation with reflex tearing. Schirmer's tests have variable reliability. The height of the tear meniscus (<0.3 mm), the quality of the tears (thin aqueous zone with rapid dehydration), and rose bengal staining are more reliable. Exclude drug-induced tear hyposecretion (antihistamines, diuretics, phenothiazines, or anticholinergics). Sjögren's syndrome with KS and xerostomia may be associated with rheumatoid arthritis (15%). Graft-versus-host disease, associated with bone marrow transplants, can be extensive, with lacrimal failure, lymphocytic conjunctival infiltration, and goblet cell depletion. Symblepharon and corneal scarring require vigorous lubrication and mechanical treatment. Systemic immunosuppression is required.

H. Cicatricial pemphigoid produces chronic conjunctivitis, trichiasis, ankyloblepharon, and symblepharon. Bilateral red eyes with foreign body sensation, tearing, and photophobia associated with a superficial punctate keratitis in an elderly person with a history of remissions and exacerbations are characteristic of pemphigoid. All mucous membranes (mouth, nose, larynx, and vagina) may be involved. It may mimic a severe

Patient with MARGINAL CORNEAL ULCER

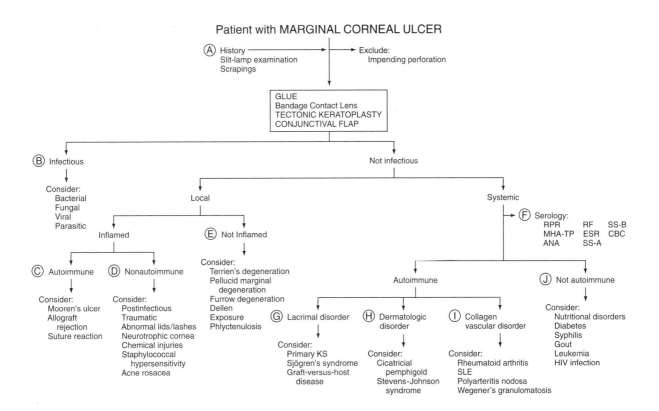

chemical burn, and conjunctival biopsy for immuno-fluorescence studies may be necessary. Local care with lubrication, antibiotic ointments, hygiene, and topical steroids is appropriate. Systemic immunosuppression may be required for progressive disease. Stevens-Johnson syndrome (erythema multiforme) is more acute, with purulent conjunctivitis, uveitis, and more widespread dermatologic disruption. Significant scarring may occur. Frequent lubrication and anti-inflammatory drugs are necessary to minimize symblepharon, keratinization, and lid distortion. Conjunctival or oral mucosal autografts may help restore surface quality. Systemic and topical steroids may reduce ocular inflammation and corneal melting.

I. Rheumatoid arthritis is a chronic inflammatory disorder characterized by symmetric joint pain, morning stiffness, and increased fatigability. Seventy-five percent of patients are women, and symptoms commonly appear in the third or fourth decade. The metacarpophalangeal and proximal interphalangeal joints are distorted. Systemic lupus erythematosus (SLE) is also a chronic systemic inflammatory autoimmune disorder of unknown cause, characterized by facial erythema (butterfly rash), photosensitivity, mucocutaneous ulcerations, proteinuria, arthritis, and/or blood dyscrasias. The ANA test is often positive. Polyarteritis nodosa, an inflammatory disorder of medium-sized arterioles, is associated with fever, weight loss, fatigue, systemic hypertension, and multiple organ dysfunction. All ages and sexes are affected. There is neutrophilic leukocytosis, anemia, elevated ESR, and thrombocytosis. Wegener's granulomatosis produces the triad of severe constitutional symptoms, respiratory tract disease, and glomerulonephritis. Destruction of

collagen-containing structures as a result of complement and T-cell activation can occur at the corneoscleral junction with rheumatoid arthritis, SLE, and other collagen vascular disease. Topical steroids cause collagenase release by granulocytes and may accelerate ulceration. Oral immunosuppressive agents are appropriate, as are topical nonsteroidal preparations (flurbiprofen, cyclosporine). Resection of local perilimbal conjunctiva debulks the area of antibody-antigen complexes. Vigorous lubrication with preservative-free methylcellulose may help epithelial repair. Autoimmune dysregulation, with deposition of antigen-antibody complexes, activation of complement, and vascular disruption, may cause rapid corneal ulceration and perforation. Patients may have several concurrent autoimmune disorders.

J. Deficient nutritional status (e.g., alcoholism, vitamin A deficiency) or impaired glucose management (diabetes) interferes with epithelial migration, fibroblastic proliferation, and wound repair. Immunodeficiencies also retard healing and should always be suspected.

References

Aronson SB, Elliott JH, Moore TE Jr, O'Day DM. Pathogenetic approach to therapy of peripheral corneal inflammatory disease. Am J Ophthalmol 1970; 70:65–90.

Robin JB, Schanzlin DJ, Verity SM, et al. Peripheral corneal disorders. Surv Ophthalmol 1986; 31:1–29.

Wagoner MD, Kenyon KR, Foster CS. Management strategies in peripheral ulcerative keratitis. Int Ophthalmol Clin 1986; 26:147–157.

CENTRAL CORNEAL ULCERS

Richard W. Yee, M.D.
Christine J. Cheng, B.S.

Most central corneal infiltrations and ulcerations cause symptoms of a red eye: ocular pain, photophobia, decreased vision, and discharge. The ulceration may be sterile or infectious in origin and caused by a variety of viruses, fungi, bacteria, and parasites. Because corneal infections do not have absolute pathognomonic appearances, clinical diagnosis requires experience and skill in differentiating infectious keratitis from other types of ulcerative and infiltrative keratitis.

A. A history of trauma or previous corneal abnormalities (keratomalacia, neurotrophic keratopathy, or bullous keratopathy); contact lens wear, especially when associated with homemade saline solutions; previous corneal ulcerations; nasal, oral, or genital ulcerations; or systemic diseases (e.g., rheumatoid arthritis with associative immunosuppressive therapy) may help one to make the diagnosis and know the predisposing factors that promote microbial keratitis. The initial slit-lamp examination should consist of a detailed drawing denoting the ulcer size and shape and stromal infiltration; a slit beam ruler or eyepiece reticle is used. Photographic documentation is also helpful. Often, laboratory verification is needed to confirm the diagnosis and guide therapy.

B. Obtain corneal scrapings from advancing borders of the ulcer where actively replicating organisms most likely exist. Stain two slides with Gram and Giemsa stains, respectively. Reserve two other slides for special stains when needed. Gram stain helps identify bacteria and fungi; Giemsa stain helps identify bacteria, fungi, and *Acanthamoeba*. Gomori's methenamine silver and PAS are special stains for fungi; acid-fast staining is for *Mycobacterium* and *Nocardia;* PAS stained smear and calcofluor-white help identify *Acanthamoeba* when a fluorescent light microscope is used.

C. During the initial evaluation, culture material from the conjunctiva and lid margins of both eyes using calcium alginate swabs. Moisten the swabs with liquid media before obtaining culture material. Anesthetize the cornea with 0.5% proparacaine hydrochloride. Using a flame-sterilized Kimura spatula, place the inoculum on the surface of the media, not penetrating the agar, in C-shaped rows. It is important to be aware of ulcer depth to avoid inducing perforation. Routine media include blood agar for most bacteria, Sabouraud's medium without cycloheximide for fungi, thioglycollate broth for aerobic and anaerobic bacteria, and chocolate agar for *Haemophilus* and *Gonococcus.* Optional media include Weinstein-Jensen medium for *Mycobacterium* and *Nocardia* and non-nutrient agar with *Escherichia coli* overlay for *Acanthamoeba.*

D. The initial antimicrobial therapy, based on the corneal smear, has been advocated by Jones. One bacterial agent is necessary for one type of bacterium. Two or more types of bacteria may necessitate multiple specific antibacterial agents. The presence of hypha fragments or pseudohyphae may require a 5% suspension of natamycin. When no microorganisms are noted on corneal smears, one may, depending on clinical impressions, select combined broad-spectrum antibacterial therapy (cefazolin, 50 mg/ml, and gentamicin, 14 mg/ml) when considering bacterial keratitis. Defer therapy when considering fungal keratitis until cultures are obtained, or defer therapy to consider noninfectious causes. Most antibacterial drops should be administered every half-hour during the first 24–48 hours of therapy. Bacterial corneal ulcer treatment may warrant subconjunctival injections (cefazolin, 100 mg, and/or gentamicin, 20 mg), especially in the initial therapy of severe keratitis. Systemic therapy may be reserved for scleral suppuration and pending or existing corneal perforation. Treatment of *Acanthamoeba* consists of one or more of the following drops: Neosporin (neomycin sulfate), Brolene (propamidine isethionate), 1% clotrimazole, or 1% miconazole and/or paromomycin every 2 hours. New effective drugs for *Acanthamoeba* keratitis effective in vitro and in vivo include chlorhexidine biguanide 0.02%, pentamidine isethionate, hexamidine diisethinate (Desomedine) 0.1%. First-line therapy includes 0.02% chlorhexidine and Brolene (propamidine) 0.1% every hour for 1 week, reduced to every 2 hours with progressive tapering to every 4–6 hours within 3 months. (These two drugs have been proven to have an additive in vitro effect against cysts and trophozoites.). The related compound polyhexamethylene biguanide (PHMB) is also acanthamoebicidal, and its use can result in early and effective treatment. PHMB is not licensed, however, for medical use, although it has gained approval for inclusion as a disinfectant in certain soft contact lens solutions. The role of steroid therapy remains controversial. Ketoconazole, 200 mg twice a day, can be given systemically. A cycloplegic is vital to prevent synechia formation and to relieve pain.

Confocal microscopy is a rapid, noninvasive method of identifying *Acanthamoeba* keratitis. It is capable of providing high-contrast in vivo images of the cornea at different depths from the epithelium to the endothelium. Magnifications of 240× or more can see an individual cell, including *Acanthamoeba* in the cornea. *Acanthamoeba* cysts are visualized as high-contrast, round structures measuring between 10 and 25 microns. In certain circumstances, because of extensive corneal scarring, the double-walled nature of the cysts is apparent. Trophozoites extending pseudopodia may also be detected, but they appear to be more variable in size and shape than cysts. Inflammation of a corneal nerve in the anterior to midcorneal stroma, known as radial keratoneuritis, consisting of irregularly swollen nerve fibers caused by disruption of

Patient with CENTRAL CORNEAL ULCER

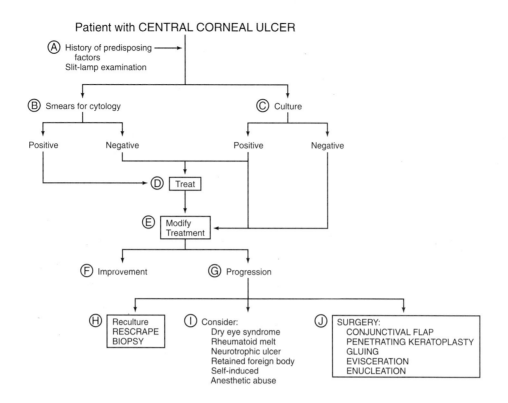

the neural membrane with amoebic infiltration can also be identified.

E. The decision to modify treatment is based on the clinical response to initial therapy, preliminary culture results, tolerance of the antimicrobial agent, and in vitro susceptibility to the antimicrobial agents. Regardless of the findings from smears and cultures, it is essential to continue the initial therapy for the first 48 hours if there is clinical improvement. If susceptibility testing from the corneal cultures shows a substantially more effective agent than the initial selection, that drug may be substituted. If the smears and cultures are negative, the possibility of noninfectious causes may be considered and antibiotics may be discontinued to initiate corticosteroid or other therapy.

F. Judge improvement by daily slit-lamp examinations and corneal drawings, noting the size of the epithelial defect, the stromal infiltrate, anterior chamber reaction, and stromal white cell reaction. The stromal infiltrate demonstrates improvement when the density decreases, the borders are more distinct, and the size and depth of the infiltrate become smaller or show no change. When improvement is noted, the frequency of antibiotics can be reduced after 48 or 72 hours. Early tapering or reduction of topical medications is probably the most common error in the management of corneal ulcers.

G. If the corneal ulcer progresses or worsens, consider the possibility of a fungal, amebic, or herpetic keratitis or an organism that did not grow in culture.

H. Obtain repeat scrapings and cultures, and consider stopping the antimicrobials for 24 hours until a new diagnosis can be made. Toxicity from concentrated antibiotics can be a causative factor in a worsening clinical picture. Hospitalization is needed if there is an indication of noncompliance or self-induced disease.

I. If repeated cultures, scrapings, and biopsies remain negative, consider noninfectious causes. Antibiotics can be discontinued and corticosteroid or other treatments can be started.

J. A conjunctival flap has been reported to be beneficial, especially in peripheral fungal ulcers. If corneal perforation is impending, corneal transplant or patch graft can be considered. Lamellar keratoplasty is contraindicated in fungal keratitis. Cyanoacrylate glue may also be a useful adjunct. In the event of severe progressive suppuration (e.g., pseudomonas), evisceration or enucleation may be the only cure.

References

D'Aversa G, Stern GA, Driebe WT Jr. Diagnosis of successful medical treatment of *Acanthamoeba* keratitis. Arch Ophthalmol 1995; 113:1120–1123.

Groden LR, Brinser JH. Outpatient treatment of microbial corneal ulcers. Arch Ophthalmol 1986; 104:84–86.

Jones DB. Decision-making in the management of microbial keratitis. Ophthalmology 1981; 88:814–820.

Pfister DR, Cameron JD, Krachmer JH, Holland EJ. Confocal microscopy findings of *Acanthamoeba* keratitis. Am J Ophthalmol 1996; 121:119–128.

Wilson LA. Acute bacterial infection of the eye: Bacterial keratitis and endophthalmitis. Trans Ophthalmol Soc UK 1986; 105:43.

CORNEAL EDEMA

Richard W. Yee, M.D.
Neil Lalani, B.S.

The cornea has three important layers: epithelium, stroma, and endothelium. Excess water in the epithelium or stroma results in corneal edema. Corneal water content depends on the equilibrium between forces driving water into the cornea and those pushing water out. The forces driving water into the cornea include the swelling pressure of the stroma and the intraocular pressure (IOP). The factors that keep the cornea from swelling are the barrier function and metabolic pump of the endothelium. Less important factors are the epithelial barrier and evaporation from the corneal surface. If any of these factors are not functional or damaged, corneal edema and increased corneal thickness can develop, with complaints of blurred vision most severe in the morning and improving as the day goes on. As the edema worsens, epithelial microcysts and bullae may form, leading to sharp, stabbing pain, photophobia, and redness. Prolonged edema can lead to scarring of Bowman's membrane and stroma, as well as pannus and stromal vascularization.

A. Increased IOP does not directly damage the endothelium but disrupts the balance of forces of transport across the cornea. Congenital glaucoma can be present and increase corneal thickness, corneal diameter, and produce horizontal linear tears of Descemet's membrane.

B. Acute glaucoma can be diagnosed if there is epithelial edema, pain, closed chamber angles, and fixed mid-dilated pupils. Usually the pressure is >60 mm Hg. The patient sees a halo around bright objects. Once the pressure is treated, the symptoms generally clear. However, untreated, increased pressure causes irreversible endothelial damage and chronic edema.

C. Endothelial dystrophies are hereditary diseases of the endothelium. Some are apparent at birth; others appear later in life. Peter's anomaly is recognized by a bilateral central corneal leukoma, with edema in the affected areas, which is caused by defects in the posterior stroma, Descemet's membrane, and endothelium. Congenital hereditary endothelial dystrophy (CHED) can have two forms: dominant and recessive. The recessive is recognized at birth as a diffuse, bilaterally symmetric corneal edema and generally does not advance. The dominant form is not evident at birth. Edema develops in the first year and may advance in later life to severe edema, band keratopathy, and epithelial erosion. *Fuchs' endothelial dystrophy* occurs later in life and can be diagnosed if corneal edema accompanied by many corneal guttae are seen posterior to Descemet's membrane. Corneal guttae are focal, refractive collagen deposits. In posterior polymorphous dystrophy (PPD), several small lesions surrounded by faint halos or fewer large, blisterlike lesions with dense halos are seen on Descemet's membrane. Corneal guttae are not present. Iridocorneal endothelial syndrome (ICE) is a spectrum of primary proliferative endothelial disorders, including iris nevus syndrome of Cogan-Reese, Chandler's syndrome, and essential iris atrophy. These disorders are characterized by an attenuated endothelium, an extensive posterior collagenous layer, and development of an ectopic basement membrane over the iris. Although these diseases form a spectrum, they can be recognized individually. In iris nevus syndrome, iris stromal tissue herniates through the ectopic basement membrane. In Chandler's syndrome the posterior collagenous layer is associated with a diffuse corneal edema. Essential iris atrophy is characterized by a gray posterior collagenous layer, peripheral anterior synechiae, distorted pupil, and holes in the iris.

D. The endothelium may be damaged during or after surgery. Intraoperative damage may be caused by corneal contact with surgical instruments or the intraocular lens or by toxic effects of intraocular drugs, preservatives, or irrigating solutions. Postoperative damage can be caused by intraocular hemorrhage, increased IOP, and contact lens–induced hypoxia, as well as by corneal endothelial contact with vitreous, the intraocular lens, or its sutures.

E. Perforation of the cornea by a foreign body can cause endothelial damage and reduce cell count, producing corneal edema. Forceful contact of a foreign body with the cornea can cause a 0.5- to 0.1-mm diameter ring-shaped opacity on the posterior corneal surface. These rings are caused by fibrin and leukocyte deposits in the corneal endothelium and disappear in a few days.

F. In patients with advanced keratoconus, Descemet's membrane can break centrally. The aqueous humor can enter and cause edema. However, endothelial cells grow, and the wound soon heals so that the edema subsides within several months. All that persists is a small scar.

G. Breaks on Descemet's membrane can occur at birth from forceps injury and typically appear vertically or in oblique orientation. Depending on the extent of injury, corneal edema may clear and recur later in life.

H. Sensorimotor trigeminal neuropathy, from surgical procedures, neoplasms, and other processes, can influence corneal hydration and result in corneal edema during exposure to low environmental temperatures.

I. Diabetic keratopathy can occur following the undue stress of intraocular surgery or photocoagulation. Corneal endothelium of a diabetic exhibits abnormalities in cell morphology, so corneal edema tends to persist postoperatively.

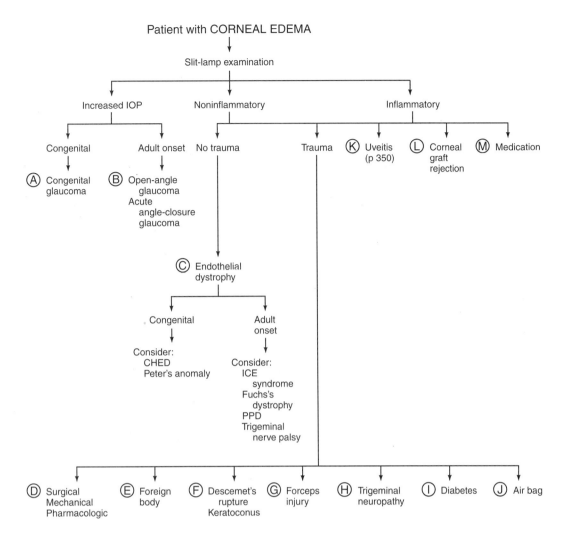

Patient with CORNEAL EDEMA

Slit-lamp examination

Increased IOP — Noninflammatory — Inflammatory

Increased IOP:
- Congenital → (A) Congenital glaucoma
- Adult onset → (B) Open-angle glaucoma / Acute angle-closure glaucoma

Noninflammatory:
- No trauma → (C) Endothelial dystrophy
- Trauma

Inflammatory:
- (K) Uveitis (p 350)
- (L) Corneal graft rejection
- (M) Medication

(C) Endothelial dystrophy:
- Congenital → Consider: CHED, Peter's anomaly
- Adult onset → Consider: ICE syndrome, Fuchs's dystrophy, PPD, Trigeminal nerve palsy

Trauma:
- (D) Surgical Mechanical Pharmacologic
- (E) Foreign body
- (F) Descemet's rupture Keratoconus
- (G) Forceps injury
- (H) Trigeminal neuropathy
- (I) Diabetes
- (J) Air bag

J. Multiple reports have described cases of corneal decompensation after air bag trauma. Scanning electron microscopy reveals localized areas of complete endothelial destruction associated with areas of endothelium cell count <1000 cells/mm². Some persistent corneal edema may fail to resolve, requiring corneal transplantation.

K. Uveitis is inflammation of any part of the uveal tract of the eye, including the iris, ciliary body, and choroid. Inflammation of the iris and ciliary body, also called *anterior uveitis,* is usually painful and can cause visual impairment, sometimes blindness. Although the relationship is unclear, corneal edema often accompanies uveitis. Uveitis can be diagnosed if specular photomicroscopy shows dark areas on the endothelium. These dark areas may be caused by keratitic precipitates or localized endothelial edema. This damage is caused by invading microbes and by cells of the immune system. Corneal edema is secondary to the immunologic response. The edema typically is stromal and monocular. The organisms capable of eliciting this response include herpes simplex and herpes zoster viruses, some bacteria, and some fungi.

L. After a corneal graft, lymphocytes may migrate to the endothelium and form a line that moves toward the center, destroying the endothelial cells in its path. By about 3 months after the graft, the line has disappeared and the damage is visible as many keratic precipitates and uniform graft edema.

M. Reversible corneal edema has been associated with keratitis during treatment with levodopa. Perfluorodecalin is a liquid used intraoperatively in retinal detachment surgery. Residual amounts may be retained in the anterior chamber in contact with the endothelium, causing corneal decompensation.

References

Geggel HS, Griggs PB, Freeman MI. Irreversible bullous keratopathy after air bag trauma. CLAO J 1996; 22:148–150.

Levenson JE. Corneal edema: Cause and treatment. Surv Ophthalmol 1976; 20:190–204.

Nakamagoe K, Ohkashi N, Fujita T, et al. Keratitis and corneal edema associated with levodopa use. A case report. Rinsho Shinkeigaku 1996; 36:886–888.

Waring GO, Bourne NM, Edelhauser HF, Kenyon KR. The corneal endothelium, normal and pathologic structure and function. Ophthalmology 1982; 89:531–590.

Wilbanks GA, Apel AJ, Jolly SS, et al. Perfluorodecalin corneal toxicity: Five case reports. Cornea 1996;15:129–334.

INTERSTITIAL KERATITIS

Constance L. Fry, M.D.
Richard W. Yee, M.D.

Active interstitial keratitis (IK) is any inflammation located in the corneal interstitial space or stroma. Symptoms include decreased vision, redness, pain, photophobia, and tearing. Superficial and deep stromal blood vessels and stromal edema can be seen diffusely or sectorially. Anterior chamber cells or flare may or may not be present. Inactive or old IK demonstrate deep corneal haze or scarring, lipid deposition, empty stromal blood vessels (ghost vessels), and corneal stromal thinning.

A. The approach to a patient with active IK should be to search for and treat associated systemic conditions, particularly syphilis, and to treat active inflammation of the anterior segment with topical steroids. In cases of active inflammation of uncertain cause not responding to steroids, consider cytologic examination on corneal biopsies. In patients with inactive IK, the goal is to ascertain whether a treatable systemic disease is involved.

B. Syphilis is by far the most common cause of IK (90% of cases). Therefore serologic studies must be obtained. Distinguishing congenital from acquired syphilis is possible by history and physical examination. In congenital syphilis, ocular symptoms usually begin between the ages of 5 and 15. Patients present with bilateral red eye, photophobia, and decreasing vision. Other manifestations are pigmentary mottling of the fundus, Hutchinson's teeth, mulberry molars, eighth nerve deafness, saber shins, frontal bossing, saddle nose, mental retardation, and tabes dorsalis. IK resulting from acquired syphilis usually occurs in an older age group, is unilateral, and does not have the associated physical findings. The evaluation of IK should, with few exceptions, always include laboratory testing for syphilis, taking care to exclude neurosyphilis by evaluation of the CSF when indicated.

C. Numerous toxins and medications can result in IK. Toxic exposures range from acid and alkali burns to metal exposure (i.e., gold and arsenic).

D. In patients who live in or travel to developing countries, do not overlook syphilis. Once this cause has been ruled out, the differential diagnosis of bilateral IK in this setting includes helminths, protozoans, and *Mycobacterium leprae*. Onchocerciasis is caused by a helminth commonly found along rapid streams in equatorial Africa and parts of Central and South America. The microfilaria may be seen in the peripheral cornea, anterior chamber, and less often, the vitreous. It causes a punctate keratitis, severe anterior uveitis, sclerosing keratitis, and chorioretinitis, as well as IK. Onchocerciasis is diagnosed by finding microfilaria in skin snips, nodules, body fluids, or the anterior chamber. The protozoa are uncommon culprits in IK. A diffuse bilateral IK has rarely been associated with

Trypanosoma gambiense, which causes African sleeping sickness. When corneal involvement occurs, a mild iritis is common but severe necrosis and scarring of the cornea are rare. Along with the clinical picture of African sleeping sickness, the diagnosis can be made by demonstration of the parasite in serum or spinal fluid. The most common type of leishmaniasis to involve the eye is the American form, *Leishmania braziliensis*. A sectorial or nodular diffuse superficial interstitial process of the cornea may become vascularized, ulcerated, and opaque without prompt systemic therapy. Conjunctival manifestations include large ulcerative granulomas and trachoma-like follicles.

E. Leprosy, caused by *M. leprae*, usually creates a bilateral IK, either diffuse or sectorial. Ophthalmologic characteristics include nasolacrimal duct obstruction, ptosis, supraciliary ridge thickening, loss of eyebrows, lid thickening, madarosis, keratoconjunctivitis sicca, facial nerve dysfunction, and uncommonly, trigeminal nerve involvement. Cranial nerves III, IV, and VI are usually spared. Lepromatous leprosy causes a superficial punctate keratopathy with an avascular keratitis in the supertemporal quadrant. This is the most characteristic lesion of leprosy. "Beads on a string," or thickened corneal nerves, as well as limbal granulomas, scleritis, episcleritis, scleromalacia, and severe uveitis, may also occur. There are two forms of IK in leprosy. The first is caused by an autoimmune reaction that begins superiorly with occasional ghost vessels seen in middle to deep stroma. The second type is secondary to direct bacterial invasion and is characterized by inflammation, necrosis, and vascular invasion starting superiorly and superficially.

F. In the Third World, the most common causes of unilateral IK are tuberculosis (TB) and malaria. Unilateral IK caused by TB may appear similar to that of acquired syphilis. In addition to skin testing and a systemic work-up, some clinical clues help make this distinction. The ocular inflammatory attacks in TB are more common than in syphilis and are more likely to occur peripherally and sectorially. They usually spare the central cornea, and unlike the deep involvement of lues, this infiltration is seen mainly in the superficial and middle layers of the cornea. Also, vascularization occurs more superficially and later than in syphilitic infiltration. Malaria ocular involvement is uncommon and usually manifests a unilateral dendritic keratitis; IK occurs less commonly as a superficial unilateral keratitis with little or no vascularization. The inflammatory process usually lasts several months and leaves residual scarring. The diagnosis is made by examination of serial thick blood smears.

G. Lyme disease, caused by *Borrelia burgdorferi,* may cause a bilateral diffuse IK. The lesions are multiple, fo-

Patient with INTERSTITIAL KERATITIS

(A) Serologic tests for syphilis

(B) Positive

Treat IK
Refer for
treatment
of syphilis

Negative

History
Physical examination

(C) Toxin exposure / Self-medication

Observe
Discontinue
offending
agent

Third World travel

(D) Bilateral

Sectorial

Glaucoma
Uveitis
Chorioretinal
scarring

(E) Refer for
evaluation
for helminths
and protozoans

Corneal
thickening
Eyelid
thickening
Madarosis

Refer for
evaluation
for leprosy

Diffuse

(F) Unilateral

Sectorial

Chest film
PPD skin test

Positive
for TB

Refer for
treatment
of TB

Negative
for TB

Go to (G)

Diffuse

Peripheral
blood smear

Positive for
protozoa

Refer for
treatment
of malaria

Negative

Go to (G)

(G) Other

Unilateral
Sectorial or
diffuse

Consider:
Foreign body
Previous
surgery
Herpes zoster/
simplex
LGV
Trauma
Lyme disease
EBV

Bilateral
Sectorial or
diffuse

Consider:
Herpes zoster/
simplex
EBV
Lyme disease
Collagen
vascular
disease
Cogan's
syndrome
Mumps
Measles

Refer
to
ENT

Treat IK and
underlying
condition

(H) Consider:
Corneal biopsy
Culture/scraping
for active disease
of unclear cause

---

cal, nebular opacities in the stroma. Corneal neovascularization, edema, and scarring also occur. Systemic treatment may include tetracycline, 250 mg PO four times daily for 3 weeks. Lymphogranuloma venereum (LGV), caused by *Chlamydia trachomatis,* begins as a segmental IK of the upper third of the cornea and may spread, resulting in dense vascularization throughout. Herpes simplex virus type 1 and herpes zoster can cause unilateral stromal involvement. Epstein-Barr virus (EBV) demonstrates both deep and superficial changes. The IK of mumps and measles usually resolves with time in the absence of intervention. However, severe cases of measles in underdeveloped countries may result in significant corneal scarring, secondary infection, and ocular perforation. Cogan's syndrome is an ill-defined entity causing nonsyphilitic IK and vestibuloauditory symptoms. Typically, young adults, after an upper respiratory tract infection, develop a bilateral subepithelial keratitis in the peripheral and posterior half of the cornea. Treatment with topical steroids usually prevents progression to IK. The systemic findings are varied, including cardiovascular, gastrointestinal, and central nervous systems. The hearing loss, unlike that of congenital syphilis, rapidly progresses toward deafness without steroid treatment. Infectious crystalline keratopathy is an invasion of the corneal stroma by microbial pathogens clinically characterized by crystal-like opacities. *Streptococcus viridans* is the most common pathogen recovered in culture, but other pathogens have been isolated, including *Haemophilus, Mycobacterium fortuitum, Pseudomo-*

nas species, staphylococcal species, *Propionibacterium acnes,* and fungi. The lesions are needlelike, crystalline opacities with little or no inflammation. Also consider *Acanthamoeba* keratitis and microsporidial keratitis. Interstitial keratitis is also associated with the initial phase of Wegener's granulomatosis.

H. In cases of active IK of unclear cause, consider biopsy and/or culture to ascertain the diagnosis.

References

Grant WM. Ocular complication of malaria. Arch Ophthalmol 1946; 35:48–54.

Kornmehl EW, Lesser RL, Jaros P, et al. Bilateral keratitis in Lyme disease. Ophthalmology 1989; 96:1194–1197.

Maisler DM. Infectious crystalline keratopathy. Ophthalmology clinics of North America. 1994; 7:577–582.

Roizenblatt J. Interstitial keratitis caused by American (mucocutaneous) leishmaniasis. Am J Ophthalmol 1979; 87: 175–179.

Spaide R, Nattis R, Lipka A, D'Amico R. Ocular findings in leprosy in the United States. Am J Ophthalmol 1985; 100:411–416.

Tabbara KF, Hyndiuk RA, eds. Interstitial keratitis. Infections of the eye: Diagnosis and management. Boston: Little, Brown, 1986: 601–612.

Tooker CW. Allergic phenomena in tuberculous keratitis. Arch Ophthalmol 1929; 2:540–544.

CORNEAL NEOVASCULARIZATION

Rebecca J. Brock, M.D.
Richard W. Yee, M.D.

Capillaries invade the cornea in many diseases that cause poor visual acuity and blindness. Corneal vascularization is the result of disease or injury. In some cases, however, vessels are not considered a complication but are desirable for healing the underlying disease. For example, in chemical burns, vascularization may be an obligate component of surface healing. Corneal vascularization has been induced by a variety of experimental situations, including injuries to the cornea from microorganisms, chemicals, physical methods, intracorneal inoculations, nutritional deficiencies, toxic states, and immunologic reactions. These experiments have led to several important observations about the cause of corneal neovascularization. Possible causative factors include corneal edema, leukocyte invasion, trauma, hypoxia, prostaglandin E, and tumor angiogenic factor.

Recently, corneal argon laser photocoagulation has been used successfully to treat superficial and deep stromal vascularization. The 577-nm yellow dye laser has also been reported to reduce the neovascularization in patients with corneal neovascularization and active graft rejection, with resolution of the graft rejection, and in patients with lipid keratopathy.

A. The perilimbal plexus called the *superficial marginal arcade* is formed from anterior (episcleral) branches of the anterior ciliary arteries. From this plexus, superficial neovascularization and invasion of the cornea occur. Superficial neovascularization is often called a *pannus,* which is measured in millimeters from the limbus. The normal arcade is often seen against the clear cornea to the extent of 1 mm; superficial vessels >2–3 mm are considered abnormal. Variations from normal are common, and the superior limbal segment often has a more pronounced marginal arcade resembling a pannus. Normal arcades are elongated in contrast to true pannus, which are often multiplied, irregular arcades.

B. Common infectious causes of micropannus include childhood trachoma, inclusion conjunctivitis, and molluscum contagiosum. All of these infections are most commonly located in the superior cornea. Staphylococcal keratoconjunctivitis and phlyctenulosis tend to be found as a peripheral wedge. Adult inclusion conjunctivitis appears with acute follicular conjunctivitis and mucopurulent discharge and usually occurs in sexually active adults. In molluscum contagiosum, inspect the eyelids for small, elevated, pearly, umbilicated nodules representing molluscum. There is often associated chronic follicular conjunctivitis.

C. Common noninfectious causes of micropannus are vernal conjunctivitis, rheumatoid keratoconjunctivitis, superior limbic keratoconjunctivitis (SLK), and contact lens wear. Micropannus from the last two causes tends

to be located superiorly in the cornea. A good history and physical examination are important in differentiating the aforementioned causes. Vernal conjunctivitis is generally found in children and young adults with a history of atopy. These patients often have a bilateral inflammation of the conjunctiva with associated symptoms of itching and mucopurulent discharge. SLK is associated with superior limbus and corneal filaments, and a thickened, keratinized upper bulbar and palpebral conjunctiva.

D. Common infectious causes of gross pannus include trachoma, staphylococcal keratoconjunctivitis or phlyctenulosis, and herpes simplex keratitis. In herpes simplex keratitis the pannus is usually fascicular and associated with dendritic scars and decreased corneal sensitivity. In trachoma there is often superior tarsal conjunctival scarring and limbal follicles, or Herbert's pits. Less common infectious causes are lymphogranuloma venereum, rubeola, tularemia, and leprosy. Leprosy is similar in appearance to phlyctenular pannus and is associated with limbal granulomas.

E. Common noninfectious causes of gross pannus are atopic keratoconjunctivitis of atopic dermatitis, contact lens wear, superficial inflammation from chemical and toxic keratitis, and acne rosacea. An inferior or sector pannus is usually seen in acne rosacea. An epithelial keratitis in combination with subepithelial keratitis may occur, causing a dense white leukomatous scar with heavy vascularization. In addition, there may be associated blepharitis and conjunctivitis. Acne rosacea characteristically appears in the central third of the face and is seen in both sexes. Comedones are lacking, and the acne pustules are associated with telangiectasia and persistent flush. Less common noninfectious causes of gross pannus are hyperlipidemia; Refsum's disease; skin diseases (e.g., psoriasis and ichthyosis); and immune and mucous membrane diseases, including pemphigus, benign mucous membrane pemphigoid, toxic epidermal necrosis, scalded skin syndrome, rheumatoid arthritis (adults), and vernal catarrh. Hodgkin's disease, Marfan's syndrome, mucolipidosis, myotonic dystrophy, Klinefelter's syndrome, ariboflavinosis keratopathy, hypoparathyroidism, vitamin B deficiency, and pellagra have all been reported to cause a pannus. A degenerative pannus can be caused by glaucoma, Fuchs's dystrophy, or blind degenerative eyes, often associated with bullous keratopathy.

F. Deep corneal vascularization arises from anastomoses of the anterior and posterior ciliary vessels and tends to run a fairly straight course in a single plane of the cornea.

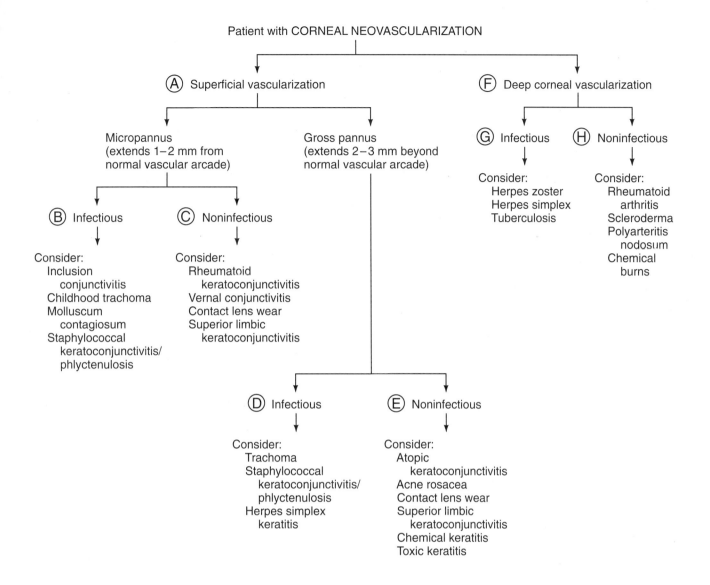

Patient with CORNEAL NEOVASCULARIZATION

Ⓐ Superficial vascularization

Micropannus
(extends 1–2 mm from
normal vascular arcade)

Gross pannus
(extends 2–3 mm beyond
normal vascular arcade)

Ⓑ Infectious

Consider:
  Inclusion
    conjunctivitis
  Childhood trachoma
  Molluscum
    contagiosum
  Staphylococcal
    keratoconjunctivitis/
    phlyctenulosis

Ⓒ Noninfectious

Consider:
  Rheumatoid
    keratoconjunctivitis
  Vernal conjunctivitis
  Contact lens wear
  Superior limbic
    keratoconjunctivitis

Ⓓ Infectious

Consider:
  Trachoma
  Staphylococcal
    keratoconjunctivitis/
    phlyctenulosis
  Herpes simplex
    keratitis

Ⓔ Noninfectious

Consider:
  Atopic
    keratoconjunctivitis
  Acne rosacea
  Contact lens wear
  Superior limbic
    keratoconjunctivitis
  Chemical keratitis
  Toxic keratitis

Ⓕ Deep corneal vascularization

Ⓖ Infectious

Consider:
  Herpes zoster
  Herpes simplex
  Tuberculosis

Ⓗ Noninfectious

Consider:
  Rheumatoid
    arthritis
  Scleroderma
  Polyarteritis
    nodosum
  Chemical
    burns

G. Infectious causes of deep stromal vascularization of the cornea include herpes zoster, herpes simplex, vaccinia, tuberculosis, syphilis, sleeping sickness, malaria, onchocerciasis, and leishmaniasis (American) (see p 214 on interstitial keratitis).

H. Noninfectious causes of deep stromal vascularization include the rheumatic diseases of adult rheumatoid arthritis, Behçet's syndrome (rare), scleroderma, polyarteritis nodosum, Wegener's granulomatosis, systemic lupus erythematosus, and discoid lupus erythematosus. Other causes are hyperlipidemia, Refsum's disease, Cogan's interstitial keratitis syndrome, diabetes (rare), and chemical burns (see p 214 on interstitial keratitis).

References

Arffa R, ed. Grayson's diseases of the cornea. 3rd ed. St Louis: Mosby, 1991.

Bare JC, Foster CS. Corneal laser photocoagulation for treatment of neovascularization. Ophthalmology 1992; 99: 173–179.

Duane T, Jaeger E. Clinical ophthalmology. Vols. 4 and 5. Philadelphia: JB Lippincott, 1991.

Klintworth GK. The cornea: Structure and macromolecules in health and disease. Am J Pathol 1977; 89:719–785.

Mayer W. Corneal neovascularization. In: Fraunfelder FT, Roy FH, eds. Current ocular therapy. 3rd ed. Philadelphia: WB Saunders, 1990: 443–444.

Ruben M. Corneal vascularization. Int Ophthalmol Clin 1980; 21:27–38.

Smolin G, Thoft RA. The cornea. Boston: Little, Brown, 1987: 601–602.

BAND KERATOPATHY

J. Alberto Martinez, M.D.
Richard W. Yee, M.D.

Band keratopathy (BK) is a common, nonspecific corneal condition that can occur at any age. It consists of a grayish haze that begins at the peripheral cornea at the 3 and 6 o'clock meridians. The haze is caused by the deposits of calcium in Bowman's membrane in the interpalpebral region. A clear interval is usually seen between the forming band and the limbus. Characteristically, the band is not uniform but has multiple holes that give it a Swiss cheese appearance. As the deposition advances centrally, vision can be diminished. Other symptoms include photophobia, irritation, and epithelial erosion in the more advanced stages. The formation of the band may take years or, in some cases, only a matter of weeks. BK is most commonly associated with uveitis, chronic glaucoma, and phthisis bulbi. Diffuse deposition of calcium involving the entire cornea is called *calcareous degeneration*. This condition is rare and may be associated with severe hypercalcemia or advanced phthisis with intraocular bone formation.

A. BK can be associated with genetically determined disorders. Among these are Norrie's disease (bilateral blindness, eventual phthisis, psychosis, and hearing loss), Hallerman-Doering syndrome (deafness, abnormal calcium metabolism, and BK), Parry-Romberg syndrome (progressive facial hemiatrophy), Rothmund-Thomson syndrome (BK, bilateral cataracts, skin pigmentation, and telangiectasia), hypophosphatasia, tuberous sclerosis, and anterior mosaic dystrophy (primary type). There are also reports of autosomal-recessive and sex-linked forms of BK.

B. Exposure to many toxic substances has been implicated in the cause of BK. One of the most common substances is mercury. Mercury derivatives such as calomel, thimerosal, and benzalkonium chloride are common preservatives in many eye preparations. Medications for glaucoma and dry eye are more likely to be associated with BK because of the frequency and chronicity of their use. Heavy use of lasers can cause severe uveitis followed by BK.

C. Conduct a careful review of systems aimed primarily at dermatologic, articular, and renal problems. Look for the butterfly rash of lupus, the dryness and epidermal scales of ichthyosis vulgaris, and the joint swelling and deformities of rheumatoid conditions.

D. Hypercalcemia is an important cause of BK. The most common causes of hypercalcemia are hyperparathyroidism, excessive intake of vitamin D, milk-alkali syndrome, idiopathy, malignancy, Paget's disease, hypophosphatasia, renal failure, sarcoidosis, adrenal insufficiency, immobilization, and thiazide drugs. An internist should conduct a work-up of hypercalcemia.

E. When BK causes visual loss, irritation, recurrent erosion, or photophobia, treatment is indicated. BK is most commonly treated by chelation of the calcium deposits with a 0.05-M solution of disodium ethylenediaminetetraacetic acid (EDTA).* The procedure is as follows: Topical application of 4% cocaine or 4% lidocaine hydrochloride (Xylocaine) provides anesthesia and facilitates removal of the corneal epithelium (EDTA does not penetrate an intact epithelium). A wire lid speculum keeps the eyelids open. The globe is fixated with toothed forceps, and the epithelium is removed. Next, a cellulose sponge is soaked with EDTA and applied to the area to be chelated. The sponge is kept moistened by replacing it with freshly soaked ones or by dropping the EDTA solution on it. Care is taken to confine EDTA contact to the abnormal areas because EDTA irritates the ocular surface. The length of the application depends on the severity of the disease. After several minutes, the remaining calcium deposits may be gently scraped with a blade or polished with a diamond bur. Cycloplegics are instilled, and patching with an antibiotic ointment is used until the cornea is re-epithelialized. Treatment may need to be repeated. Alternatively, some ophthalmologists advocate simple scraping of the epithelium with a no. 15 blade without chelation. Occasionally, a lamellar or penetrating keratoplasty may be needed. However, if the underlying condition still exists, BK may recur in the graft.

Excimer laser phototherapeutic keratectomy (PTK) has also been used to remove superficial stromal opacities. Complications include recurrent erosions, irregular astigmatism, and recurrence of keratopathy.

References

Arffa R, ed. Grayson's diseases of the cornea. 3rd ed. St Louis: Mosby, 1991: 346–349.

Kaufman HE, Barron BA, McDonald MB, eds. The cornea. New York: Churchill Livingstone, 1988.

O'Brart DPS, Gartry DS, Lohmann CP, et al. Treatment of band keratopathy by excimer laser phototherapeutic keratectomy: Surgical techniques and long term follow up. Br J Ophthalmol 1993; 77:702–708.

O'Connor RG. Calcific bank keratopathy. Trans Am Ophthalmol Soc 1972; 70:58–81.

---

*To obtain a 0.05-M, 1.7% solution of neutral disodium EDTA, a 20-ml, 150-mg/ml ampule of Endrate is diluted to 175 ml with water.

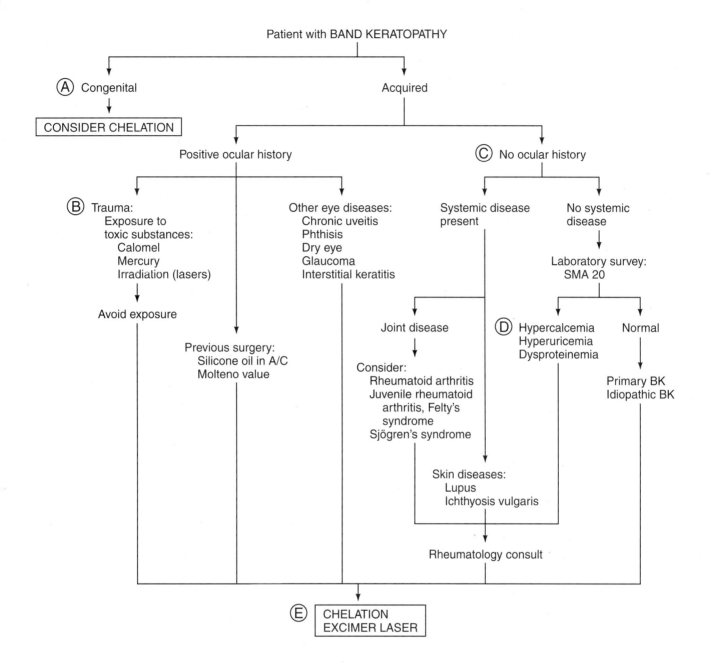

Patient with BAND KERATOPATHY

Ⓐ Congenital

CONSIDER CHELATION

Acquired

Positive ocular history

Ⓒ No ocular history

Ⓑ Trauma:
Exposure to
toxic substances:
Calomel
Mercury
Irradiation (lasers)

Avoid exposure

Other eye diseases:
Chronic uveitis
Phthisis
Dry eye
Glaucoma
Interstitial keratitis

Previous surgery:
Silicone oil in A/C
Molteno value

Systemic disease
present

No systemic
disease

Laboratory survey:
SMA 20

Joint disease

Ⓓ Hypercalcemia
Hyperuricemia
Dysproteinemia

Normal

Consider:
Rheumatoid arthritis
Juvenile rheumatoid
arthritis, Felty's
syndrome
Sjögren's syndrome

Primary BK
Idiopathic BK

Skin diseases:
Lupus
Ichthyosis vulgaris

Rheumatology consult

Ⓔ CHELATION
EXCIMER LASER

CORNEAL PIGMENTATION

Mark L. McDermott, M.D.
Elmer Y. Tu, M.D.

Corneal pigmentation may result from local or systemic processes. Pigmentation represents an abnormal deposition of a substance in the cornea, which manifests in an identifiable corneal opacity that may or may not be vision-threatening. The two major characteristics of pigmentation, color and location, can be reliably determined by slit-lamp biomicroscopy. The location of a lesion is usually categorized by the most involved layer of the corneal anatomy, and color may vary by form and extent of involvement.

A. Brown pigmentation restricted to the corneal epithelium is most likely caused by iron or melanin deposition. Iron may be deposited in a variety of patterns reflecting different areas of tear distribution; for example, a horizontal line at the junction of the upper two thirds and the lower one third of the cornea (Hudson-Stähli line), a complete or partial ring at the base of the cone in keratoconus (Fleischer's ring), an arclike deposition adjacent to a filtering bleb (Ferry's line), or an arclike area adjacent to a pterygium (Stocker's line). An iron line may form in any area of corneal surface irregularity that disrupts tear distribution. Stellate iron lines may be seen in radial keratotomy, whereas central iron deposition may be seen in phototherapeutic keratectomy beds as either a central dot or surrounding central islands. Iron may also be deposited in a dense, rust-colored area where a ferruginous foreign body has been removed. In darkly pigmented patients, limbal conjunctival melanosis may result in injection of melanin pigment into the juxtalimbal corneal epithelium; the pigment then spreads onto the corneal surface in a whorl-like pattern, creating striate melanokeratitis. In a white adult patient with an acquired brown conjunctival plaque or nodule adjacent to the limbus, the adjacent corneal epithelium and stroma may be pigmented. In acquired melanosis, there is injection of melanin into the adjacent corneal epithelium, causing a whorl-like or plaque distribution. With an adjacent conjunctival pigmented nodule, frank corneal stromal invasion by presumed malignant melanoma is possible. In more highly pigmented races, inflammation surrounding a squamous cell carcinoma may result in pigment deposition, rendering the lesion brown or black. This same pigment deposition may spread onto adjacent corneal areas. Drug-induced or metabolic verticillata may occasionally appear brown (see section C).

B. Gray-white epithelial opacities in a variety of distributions suggest superficial punctate keratitis (p 202).

C. Long-term use of amiodarone, chlorpromazine, chloroquine, tamoxifen, or indomethacin can cause epithelial deposits arranged in a whorl-like pattern usually centered on the inferior two thirds of the cornea.

The deposits are bilateral, seldom affect vision, and gradually disappear with cessation of therapy. Their appearance is indistinguishable from that seen in X-linked α-galactosidase deficiency (Fabry's disease). Fabry's disease is an X-linked recessive inborn error of metabolism characterized by elevated urinary ceramide trihexoside levels. The cornea shows dustlike epithelial deposits in a whorl-like distribution. Vision is unaffected. Associated ocular findings include tortuous vessels in the conjunctiva and retina, as well as lens opacities. Systemic manifestation includes cutaneous angiokeratomas in a bathing suit distribution. Female carriers may be detected by a leukocyte α-galactosidase assay that shows levels to be reduced to 15%–40% of normal.

D. Intraepithelial deposits may be found in Meesmann's dystrophy consisting of "peculiar" substance. Ophthalmic ointment used in the treatment of corneal abrasions and mucin may become temporarily trapped in intraepithelial cysts. Epithelial cysts may also be found in recurrent erosion syndromes, as well as in certain forms of acanthamoeba epithelitis and microsporidia infection.

E. Urate keratopathy may produce an orange-brown band keratopathy in addition to corneal crystals. Although more common in the conjunctiva, adrenochrome deposition from the use of topical epinephrine or, more uncommonly, dipivefrin may appear near the limbus as black subepithelial deposits. Spheroidal degeneration manifests as brown subepithelial nodules in the interpalpebral zone and may look similar to adrenochrome deposition. Alkaptonuria (ochronosis) is an autosomal-recessive disorder characterized by the absence of the enzyme homogentisic acid oxidase. The primary ocular manifestations are brown pigmentation of the sclera and episclera, especially at the insertions of the horizontal recti. In peripheral anterior corneal stroma, however, focal accumulations of light brown to black pinhead-size droplets may be seen. Vision is unaffected.

F. In degenerative diseases affecting the anterior segment (e.g., chronic iridocyclitis), calcium may accumulate, forming deposits in Bowman's membrane. Initially, these deposits cause a peripheral ground-glass haze at the temporal and nasal horizontal meridian. With progression the haze extends and becomes more opaque centrally. This may also result from the use of topical phosphate-containing medications. Other ocular medications (e.g., ciprofloxacin) may precipitate in chronic epithelial defects. Gelatinous deposits as found in Salzmann's nodular degeneration and amyloid deposition may create grayish blue subepithelial nodules. Excess basement membrane elements may accumulate in Reis-Bückler's dystrophy and other basement membrane dystrophies.

G. In the rare amino acid disorder tyrosinemia type 2, caused by tyrosine aminotransferase deficiency, infants present with recurrent episodes of superficial central corneal ulceration. Characteristically, these ulcers assume stellate, pseudodendritic, or geographic patterns. With time a central corneal opacity with thickening develops in the epithelium and subepithelial space. The corneal lesions may provide evidence for an early diagnosis. If the diagnosis is made early enough, dietary restriction of tyrosine results in resolution of the corneal opacities.

H. Long-term phenothiazine use may result in deposition of yellow-white granules in the central corneal stroma at the level of Descemet's membrane. A more common ocular finding is deposition of similar fine granules in a dendriform pattern beneath the anterior lens capsule. The most serious ocular finding is a bull's eye pigmentary maculopathy. Large hyphemas with elevated intraocular pressure refractory to treatment often result in deposition of hemoglobin and later hemosiderin in the corneal stroma. The pigmentation may appear rusty to greenish black to greenish yellow. Characteristically, the blood staining is most dense centrally and clears from the peripheral cornea, closest to the limbal vasculature. Bilirubinemia may cause deposits in the deep corneal stroma, beginning in the periphery from the limbal circulation. Conjunctival involvement normally precedes corneal involvement. Siderosis from a retained intraocular foreign body or, less commonly, from hemochromatosis causes brown iron deposition in the posterior stroma.

I. With aging or in rare disorders affecting lipoprotein levels, cholesterol and phospholipids may accumulate in the peripheral corneal stroma. The accumulation begins superiorly and inferiorly and later spreads circumferentially. Vision is unaffected. Refer younger patients with cornea arcus formation for lipoprotein electrophoresis and lipid determinations; unilateral arcus may indicate contralateral ocular ischemic disease. Schnyder's corneal dystrophy is the accumulation of cholesterol in the corneal stroma, resulting in a gray-white haze with scattered crystals. Bilateral, diffuse, corneal clouding appearing to affect all layers in a child prompts an evaluation for metabolic storage diseases. Mucopolysaccharidoses I H (Hurler), I S (Scheie), I HIS (Hurler-Scheie), IV-A (Morquio-classic), IV-B (Morquio-like), VI-A (Maroteaux-Lamy), VI-B (Maroteaux-Lamy, mild form), and VII (β-glucuronidase deficiency) all have variable degrees of corneal clouding. Mucolipidoses (ML), ML I, ML I variant, ML II, MLIII, ML IV, metachromatic leukodystrophy, mannosidosis, and fucosidosis have cornea clouding. The most severe clouding is seen in ML III and ML IV.

J. In an asymptomatic patient receiving gold salts for rheumatoid arthritis, dustlike glittering gold or purple granules may be seen throughout the stroma. The deposition of gold may disappear after cessation of therapy. Vision is unaffected. Various colored pigments can also be introduced intentionally into the stroma to hide corneal scars and decrease glare in patients with large iris defects. Stromal cystine crystals can be found in cystinosis (p 224).

K. Golden-brown, greenish-yellow, or blue-green pigmentation at the level of Descemet's membrane in the corneal periphery is usually caused by copper deposition. Typically, the deposition begins as a superior arcus, later accumulates inferiorly, and then forms a complete ring. If there is accompanying neurologic and hepatic disease (Wilson's disease), the ring is called a *Kayser-Fleischer ring*. However, patients with non-Wilsonian liver disease may have similar peripheral pigmented rings. Pigmentation resolves with chelation therapy. Intraocular copper foreign bodies with >85% copper content will cause chalcosis. Chalcosis is very similar in appearance to Wilson's disease but is unilateral. Greenish-gray posterior stromal deposition of mercury can be found after long-term exposure to mercurial vapors. Both superficial and deep deposition can be found with old topical phenylmercurial nitrate medications.

L. Long-term exposure to silver-containing compounds may result in a gray-blue-green discoloration of Descemet's membrane and deep stroma. Because silver-containing eye drops are seldom used, cases of argyrosis in developed countries are usually related to industrial exposure to organic silver salts. X-linked ichthyosis may cause deep stromal gray-white opacities shaped as punctuation marks.

M. A fine dusting of brown pigment in a vertical spindle pattern on the endothelial surface—a Krukenberg spindle—is a characteristic feature of pigmentary dispersion syndrome. Accompanying findings include myopia, slitlike transillumination defects of the iris, and pigment dispersion upon mydriasis (p 72). Some patients have a secondary glaucoma. Intraocular surgery and blunt and penetrating trauma may result in iridocorneal touch, transferring pigment to the endothelium. Similarly, anterior uveitis and Fuch's dystrophy may result in endothelial pigment phagocytosis.

N. Gray-white endothelial replacement may occur, extending from a site of surgical or traumatic ocular perforation, with epithelial or fibrous downgrowth. Prognosis is usually poor. Bilateral endothelial opacities consisting of vesicles and scalloping sometimes associated with iris abnormalities may be found in posterior polymorphous dystrophy. Unilateral findings may indicate iridocorneal endothelial (ICE) syndrome.

References

Arffa R, ed. Grayson's diseases of the cornea. 3rd ed. St Louis: Mosby, 1991: 364–409.

Barraquer-Somers F, Chan CC, Green WR. Corneal epithelial iron deposition. Ophthalmology 1983, 90:729–734.

Duane TD, ed. Clinical ophthalmology. Philadelphia: Harper & Row, 1985.

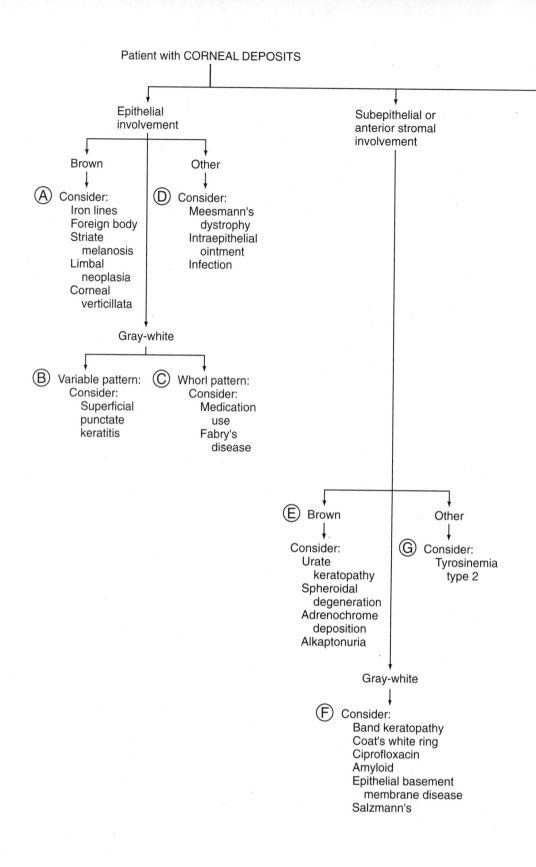

Patient with CORNEAL DEPOSITS

Epithelial involvement

Subepithelial or anterior stromal involvement

Brown

Other

Ⓐ Consider:
Iron lines
Foreign body
Striate
melanosis
Limbal
neoplasia
Corneal
verticillata

Ⓓ Consider:
Meesmann's
dystrophy
Intraepithelial
ointment
Infection

Gray-white

Ⓑ Variable pattern:
Consider:
Superficial
punctate
keratitis

Ⓒ Whorl pattern:
Consider:
Medication
use
Fabry's
disease

Ⓔ Brown

Other

Consider:
Urate
keratopathy
Spheroidal
degeneration
Adrenochrome
deposition
Alkaptonuria

Ⓖ Consider:
Tyrosinemia
type 2

Gray-white

Ⓕ Consider:
Band keratopathy
Coat's white ring
Ciprofloxacin
Amyloid
Epithelial basement
membrane disease
Salzmann's

Krachmer JH, Mannis MJ, Holland EJ, eds. Cornea. St Louis: Mosby, 1997: 417–428, 897–924.

Krueger RR, Tersi I, Seiler T. Corneal iron line associated with steep central islands after photorefractive keratectomy. J Refractive Surg 1997; 13:401–403.

Spencer WH, ed. Ophthalmic pathology: An atlas and text-book. Philadelphia: WB Saunders, 1986: 369–380.

Steinberg EB, Wilson LA, Waring GO III, et al. Stellate iron lines in the corneal epithelium after radial keratotomy. Am J Ophthalmol 1984; 98:416–421.

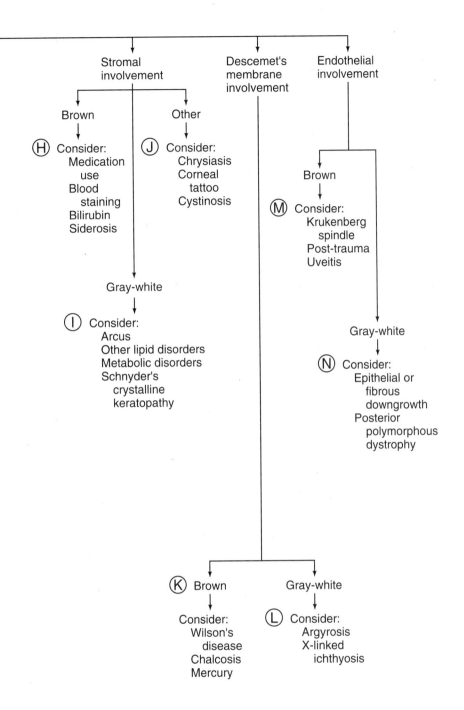

Stromal
involvement

Descemet's
membrane
involvement

Endothelial
involvement

Brown

Other

(H) Consider:
Medication
use
Blood
staining
Bilirubin
Siderosis

(J) Consider:
Chrysiasis
Corneal
tattoo
Cystinosis

Brown

(M) Consider:
Krukenberg
spindle
Post-trauma
Uveitis

Gray-white

(I) Consider:
Arcus
Other lipid disorders
Metabolic disorders
Schnyder's
crystalline
keratopathy

Gray-white

(N) Consider:
Epithelial or
fibrous
downgrowth
Posterior
polymorphous
dystrophy

(K) Brown

Gray-white

Consider:
Wilson's
disease
Chalcosis
Mercury

(L) Consider:
Argyrosis
X-linked
ichthyosis

CORNEAL CRYSTALS

Mark L. McDermott, M.D.
Elmer Y. Tu, M.D.

The discovery of crystals in the cornea may be expected, as in known cases of infantile cystinosis, or totally unexpected, as in cases of undiagnosed plasma cell dyscrasias. Careful attention to the location and distribution of the crystals is useful in considering diagnostic possibilities.

A. Unilateral, white, large crystals in a cornea with neovascularization are caused by accumulation of cholesterol and other lipids that leak out of incompetent blood vessels. This is usually found in stromal vascularization related to chronic corneal transplant rejection, interstitial keratitis, or infectious keratitis. If there is encroachment on the visual axis, argon laser photocoagulation to the feeder vessels may arrest the progression or reduce the size of the lipid keratopathy.

B. Unilateral, white, branching accumulations of crystals in an eye postoperatively, especially after keratoplasty or in an eye receiving topical corticosteroid eye drops, suggest infectious crystalline keratopathy. In this disorder, streptococci of the viridans group insinuate themselves between the anterior stromal lamellae of the cornea. Recently, other organisms, including coagulase-negative *Staphylococcus,* fungi, and a host of other bacterial pathogens, have been implicated. Remarkably little inflammation and corneal neovascularization is present. Treatment with fortified antibiotics is successful in 50% of cases, with the remaining cases requiring therapeutic keratoplasty. A common house plant of the species *Dieffenbachia* may eject high-speed, needlelike calcium oxalate crystals into the cornea and conjunctiva, creating a keratoconjunctivitis. Similar symptoms may be seen in the oral mucosa.

C. Brown monosodium urate crystals in the interpalpebral epithelium and extending to the limbus are typical of urate keratopathy. In some instances crystals are found in the anterior corneal stroma. There is associated conjunctival hyperemia, which may be severe. These crystals may be irritating, causing erosions or vascularization. Simple epithelial debridement can result in substantial improvement in vision. However, the keratopathy does recur. A pigmented bandlike keratopathy may also be a manifestation of gout keratopathy. The serum uric acid level is almost always elevated.

D. Schnyder's crystalline dystrophy, also called *central stromal crystalline dystrophy,* is an autosomal-dominant disorder characterized by central accumulations of fine, polychromatic, randomly oriented, needlelike crystals at the level of Bowman's membrane and the anterior stroma. The overlying epithelium is uninvolved, and the intervening areas of stroma are usually clear. The crystals consist of predominantly cholesterol esters and are strongly correlated with hy-percholesterolemia. There is no definite association between this disorder and hyperlipidemia, but investigation should include a systemic work-up. Penetrating keratoplasty or phototherapeutic keratectomy is indicated when sufficient clouding has occurred to incapacitate the patient visually. Tissue obtained at keratoplasty for suspected cases of this disorder should be submitted as frozen sections for neutral fat (oil red 0) staining.

E. In rare instances, patients with porphyria cutanea tarda have displayed white-tan nonrefractile crystals in Bowman's layer at the peripheral cornea. Other cornea changes include diffuse opacification of Bowman's membrane and the deep stromal lamellae. These findings are associated with high levels of urinary porphyrins.

F. In this rare autosomal-recessive condition, Bietti's crystalline dystrophy exhibits crystals in the superficial stroma in a paralimbal distribution. In the cases described, there was an association with fundus albipunctatus and choroidal sclerosis. The progressive disorder may lead to visual loss secondary to retinal disease.

G. In the autosomal-recessive disorder of lecithin cholesterol acetyltransferase deficiency (LCAT), free plasma cholesterol and lecithin are elevated. Ocular findings include diffuse, fine, gray dots at all stromal levels and a dense peripheral arcus. Occasionally, crystals are present at the level of Descemet's membrane peripheral to the area of arcus formation. Vision is rarely affected. Tangier's disease is also an autosomal-recessive disorder that results in significantly reduced HDL levels with findings similar to LCAT deficiency.

H. Hypergammaglobulinemia states, including multiple myeloma, benign monoclonal gammopathy, cryoglobulinemias, Waldenstrom's macroglobulinemia, dysproteinemia, and paraproteinemia, are all associated with bilateral cornea opacities. These opacities consist of amorphous and crystallized immunoglobulin. Immunoglobulin crystals may appear as polychromatic, fine, punctate, or needlelike. They may be present in the corneal epithelium and anterior or posterior stroma. Crystals have been described centrally, paracentrally, and paralimbally in location. Noncrystalline corneal opacities have also been described. Associated findings include tortuosity of the conjunctival vasculature, conjunctival crystals, pars plana cysts, and hyperviscosity retinopathy.

I. The presence of sparkling polychromatic crystals in the anterior corneal stroma of a photophobic child with growth retardation and renal failure is highly sug-

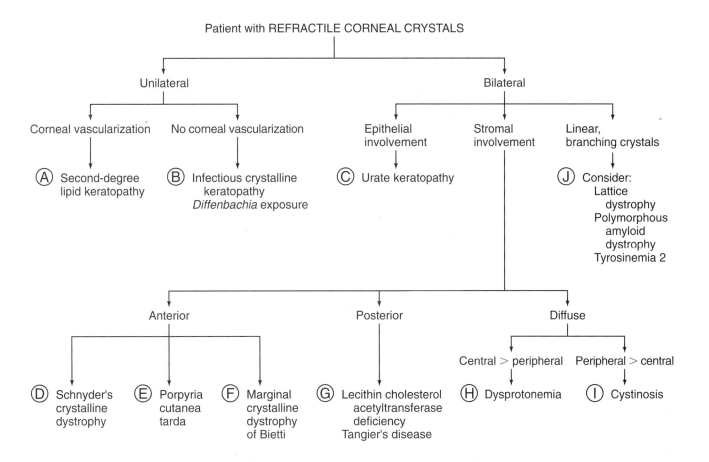

gestive of type 1 cystinosis. The crystals appear linear, have sharp edges, and are more concentrated in the peripheral corneal stroma, where they are present in both anterior and posterior stroma. They are less concentrated centrally and tend to lie more superficially in the stroma. Recurrent erosions may occur secondary to the anterior location of some deposits. Associated ocular findings include crystal formation in the conjunctiva, sclera, extraocular muscles, aqueous humor, and uvea. A pigmentary retinopathy may precede crystal formation. In type 2 (juvenile) and type 3 (adult) cystinosis, the systemic manifestations are less severe, and in the adult form corneal crystals may be the only finding. The inheritance of all three types is believed to be autosomal recessive. The crystals are water soluble, and biopsy specimens must be placed in absolute ethanol to prevent dissolution of the crystals. The use of topical cysteamine has some reported success in reversing corneal crystal deposition.

J. Long, linear branching refractile crystals are found in amyloid deposition in the form of lattice dystrophy and polymorphous amyloid dystrophy. The location of the branching filaments varies in lattice dystrophy types 1–3, with type 2 having significant systemic manifestations. Tyrosinemia type 2 may also exhibit long branching lines in the superficial stroma resembling

dendrites with superficial plaques. This autosomal-recessive disorder is caused by a deficiency in tyrosine aminotransferase and is treatable with a low-tyrosine, low-phenylalanine diet. Reduction in corneal opacities may occur with this treatment.

References

Arrfa R, ed. Grayson's diseases of the cornea. 3rd ed. St Louis: Mosby, 1991: 364–401.

Jones NP, Postlethwaite RJ, Noble JL. Clearance of corneal crystals in nephropathic cystinosis by topical cysteamine 0.5%. Br J Ophthalmol 1991; 75:311–312.

Kaufman HE, Barron BA, McDonald MB, et al, eds. The cornea. New York: Churchill Livingstone, 1988: 361–382.

Meisler DM, Langston RHS, Naab TJ, et al. Infectious crystalline keratopathy. Am J Ophthalmol 1984; 97:337–343.

Seet B, Chan WK, Ang CL. Crystalline keratopathy from *Diefenbachia* plant sap. Br J Ophthalmol 1995; 79:98–99.

Spencer WH. Ophthalmic pathology: A textbook and atlas. Philadelphia: WB Saunders, 1985: 363–367.

Weisenthal RW, Krachmer JH, Folberg R, et al. Postkeratoplasty crystalline deposits mimicking bacterial infectious crystalline keratopathy. Am J Ophthalmology 1988; 105: 70–74.

CORNEAL EPITHELIAL DYSTROPHY

Richard W. Yee, M.D.

The epithelial dystrophies consist of abnormalities in the epithelium basement membrane and, in some cases, Bowman's layer. They are easily diagnosed by history and thorough slit-lamp examination. Family history and slit-lamp examination of immediate family members help elucidate the genetic pattern and aid in the classification.

A. Intraepithelial microcysts can occur confluently or in isolated groups, either unilaterally or bilaterally, depending on the associated cause. They can be associated with localized areas of epithelial healing or recurrent erosions. Cystic spaces can occur in the epithelium with or without corneal edema. Typically, no staining occurs with fluorescein. Microcysts are nonspecific responses of the epithelium and occur with contact lens wear and long-term drug use. Typically, no symptoms occur unless there are actual epithelial erosions from the microcyst. Treatment consists of resolving the associated conditions. Meesmann's epithelial dystrophy (also called *Stocker-Holt dystrophy*) is dominantly inherited with incomplete penetrance and is evident in the first few months of life. Patients are asymptomatic, demonstrating anterior epithelial cysts, which, on focal lumination, appear as small, clear to gray-white punctate precipitates. They do not stain with fluorescein. The cysts have been shown to contain degenerate cellular material, "peculiar" substance, which is PAS positive. No treatment is necessary unless irritation or decreased vision occurs.

B. Vortex corneal dystrophy is probably a degenerative disorder, in which pigmented whorl-shaped lines are seen in the epithelial and subepithelial tissues. These have been seen in Fabry's disease, in toxic keratopathy, and in patients who are taking a variety of systemic medications such as chloroquine, amiodarone, phenothiazine, or indomethacin. Striate melanokeratosis can also mimic vortex dystrophy. Melanotic cells growing from the limbus, particularly in African-Americans, can also penetrate the central cornea as a response to a variety of noxious stimuli. Treatment is seldom necessary.

C. Anterior epithelial basement membrane dystrophy is also called *map-dot-fingerprint dystrophy, anterior basement membrane dystrophy,* and *Cogan's microcystic dystrophy.* It is bilateral and epithelial and is characterized by various patterns of dots, lines, and irregularities. It occurs more commonly in women after the fourth decade and is autosomal dominant with incomplete expression. Pathologic study shows a thickened basement membrane extending into the epithelium, abnormal epithelial cells with microcysts, and fibrillar material between the basement membrane and Bowman's layer. Most patients are asymptomatic. When symptoms are present, blurring of vision and foreign body sensation are common. Recurrent erosions can occur, typically in the early morning, when the patient awakes and has sharp stabbing pain. Treatment is necessary only when recurrent erosions occur.

D. Recurrent corneal erosions typically follow corneal trauma that involves the epithelium and epithelial basement membrane. They can also occur with anterior basement membrane dystrophy. The disorder results from defects in basement membrane healing or failed or faulty production by the basement membrane. Symptoms can occur days to years after the injury. Treatment is aimed at encouraging re-epithelialization and at preventing recurrences. Acute erosions are treated with topical antibiotics, cycloplegic drops, and a pressure patch. Sometimes, 5% sodium chloride may help promote adherence of the epithelial cells to the underlying tissue to minimize epithelial edema. Lubricating ointments with no preservatives are helpful, especially in patients with lagophthalmos. Treatment should continue to minimize recurrences and allow repair of the abnormal basement membrane. If recurrences persist, contact lenses may be helpful. Anterior stromal puncture has also been advocated in patients in whom other modes of therapy have failed. Debridement of abnormal epithelium may be effective occasionally when accompanied by use of a diamond bur on the irregular surface of the anterior basement membrane.

E. Reis-Bückler's dystrophy is an autosomal-dominant superficial corneal dystrophy that affects Bowman's membrane. The dystrophy is bilaterally symmetric and becomes evident in the first or second decade of life, with recurring erosions and decreased vision. The opacities spare the peripheral 2 mm of the cornea. Slit-lamp examination demonstrates irregular epithelium with subepithelial fibrous tissue in the region of Bowman's layer. Opacities appear to be reticular in pattern. Treatment is similar to that for recurrent erosions. The surgical procedure of choice is subepithelial fibrous dissection from the superficial cornea. Occasionally, a lamellar keratoplasty or penetrating keratoplasty can be performed after dissection of the subepithelial fibrous tissue layer if vision is not satisfactory. Recurrences are possible.

References

McLean EN, MacRae SSM, Rich LF. Recurrent erosion: Treatment by anterior stromal puncture. Ophthalmology 1986; 93:784–788.

Waring GO III, Rodrigues MM, Laibson PR. Corneal dystrophies. I. Dystrophies of the epithelium, Bowman's layer and stroma. Surv Ophthalmol 1978; 23:71–122.

Wood TO, Fleming IC, Dotson RS, Cotten MS. Treatment of Reis-Bückler's corneal dystrophy by removal of subepithelial fibrous tissue. Am J Ophthalmol 1978; 85:360–362.

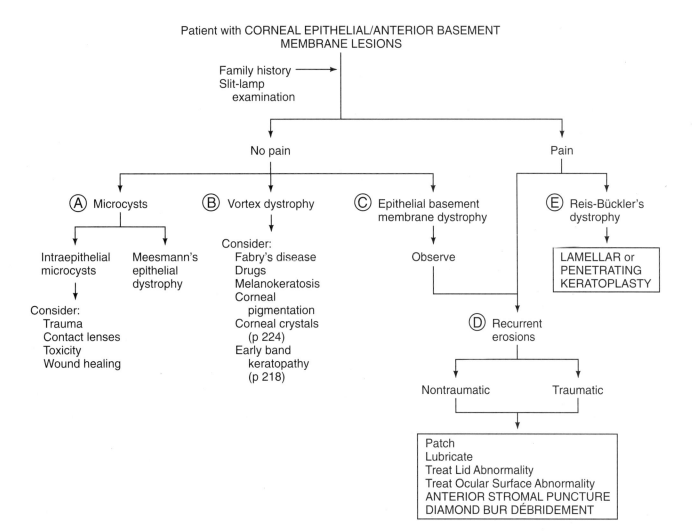

Patient with CORNEAL EPITHELIAL/ANTERIOR BASEMENT
MEMBRANE LESIONS

Family history ⟶
Slit-lamp
   examination

No pain

Pain

Ⓐ Microcysts

Intraepithelial
microcysts

Meesmann's
epithelial
dystrophy

Consider:
 Trauma
 Contact lenses
 Toxicity
 Wound healing

Ⓑ Vortex dystrophy

Consider:
 Fabry's disease
 Drugs
 Melanokeratosis
 Corneal
  pigmentation
 Corneal crystals
  (p 224)
 Early band
  keratopathy
  (p 218)

Ⓒ Epithelial basement
membrane dystrophy

Observe

Ⓔ Reis-Bückler's
dystrophy

LAMELLAR or
PENETRATING
KERATOPLASTY

Ⓓ Recurrent
erosions

Nontraumatic

Traumatic

Patch
Lubricate
Treat Lid Abnormality
Treat Ocular Surface Abnormality
ANTERIOR STROMAL PUNCTURE
DIAMOND BUR DÉBRIDEMENT

CORNEAL STROMAL DYSTROPHY

Richard W. Yee, M.D.
Matthew B. Mills III, M.D.

Corneal stromal dystrophies generally involve a genetically transmitted metabolic defect, which results in the deposition of an excessive amount of some metabolic product in the keratocytes. The accumulation of these deposits causes signs and symptoms ranging from essentially asymptomatic opacities to complete functional visual impairment. Accurately diagnosing a specific dystrophy early in its course better prepares both the physician and patient to manage the condition as it progresses.

A. Present at birth, congenital hereditary stromal dystrophy is an autosomal-dominant disorder manifested by bilateral, symmetric, nonprogressive, cloudy opacification of the cornea. The flaky or feathery opacities are most dense in the superficial central stroma, becoming progressively less dense in the deep peripheral regions. The early visual impairment may result in nystagmus, esotropia, and amblyopia. Very early penetrating keratoplasty should be considered.

B. In granular dystrophy, white breadcrumb-like opacities develop in the superficial central corneal stroma during the first decade. The opacities enlarge, coalesce, increase in number, and extend into the deeper stroma as the disease progresses through the fifth decade. At that time, a diffuse ground-glass haze appears in the intervening stroma, resulting in the onset of visual impairment. A 2- to 3-mm paralimbal zone remains clear, and epithelial erosions are rare. The opacities consist of a hyaline substance and are bilateral and symmetric. Penetrating keratoplasty may be necessary late in the disease, and opacities tend to recur in the donor graft.

C. In central crystalline dystrophy, minute polychromatic crystals, arranged in a discoid or ring configuration, appear in the central superficial stroma during the first year of life. Patients (80%) develop a limbal girdle and a dense corneal arcus by the fourth decade. Treatment is rarely indicated because visual acuity is seldom severely impaired. The crystals consist largely of cholesterol, and the disorder is often associated with hyperlipidemia and genu valgum. Therefore evaluate serum cholesterol and triglyceride levels in these patients.

D. Patients with gelatinous droplike dystrophy complain of photophobia, lacrimation, foreign body sensation, and impaired visual acuity in the first decade as a result of protuberant, opaque, subepithelial mounds that are located centrally and give the cornea a "mulberry-like," irregular surface. Amyloid deposits are present in the epithelial basal cells. Sporadic and autosomal-recessive patterns have been observed. Total deep lamellar keratoplasty is the treatment of choice; recurrences are common.

E. In lattice dystrophy a branched lattice network of refractile lines, white punctate opacities, and a diffuse central superficial stromal haze appears during the first and second decades. Recurrent, painful epithelial erosions also occur. Visual acuity deteriorates progressively through the fourth and fifth decades as central subepithelial opacities develop. Penetrating keratoplasty is often necessary, and recurrences of the disease with donor grafts are common. The inheritance pattern is autosomal dominant. The opacities contain amyloid deposits. The lattice lines fluoresce under cobalt blue (365 nm) ultraviolet light in advanced cases. Lattice dystrophy type 2 is associated with systemic amyloidosis and a more favorable visual outcome. Types 3 and 3A have recently been described.

F. Progressive corneal dystrophy of Waardenburg, a variant of granular dystrophy, is characterized by an earlier onset, a more rapid progression of opacification, more frequent epithelial erosions, and a poorer visual prognosis.

G. In macular dystrophy, diffuse, central, superficial, stromal cloudiness develops during the first decade. During the second decade, this diffuse ground-glass opacification extends to involve the posterior and peripheral stroma as well. Focal, irregular, white opacities develop by the third decade. Later in the disease, irregularities of Descemet's membrane and painless epithelial erosions are common. Visual acuity is often significantly impaired by the fourth decade. Penetrating keratoplasty is often necessary by 30 years of age. Recurrences with donor grafts are less common than in granular and lattice dystrophies. The inheritance pattern is autosomal recessive, and the primary defect is accumulation of excess acid mucopolysaccharides in the keratocytes.

H. In central cloudy dystrophy, small, indistinct, ovoid opacities—most dense posteriorly and restricted to the central third of the cornea—are the classic findings. Visual acuity is rarely impaired, and the opacities are usually incidental findings.

I. Fleck dystrophy is a benign disorder in which discrete, flat, white, dandrufflike flecks are present throughout all stromal layers, involving both central and peripheral regions. These opacities may be congenital, and the inheritance pattern is autosomal dominant. This disorder has been associated with cortical lens opacities in certain families. Visual acuity remains normal.

J. Polymorphic stromal dystrophy is probably a degenerative disorder featuring gray-white punctate and filamentous opacities involving the entire cornea. Onset is after 50 years of age, and visual acuity is spared.

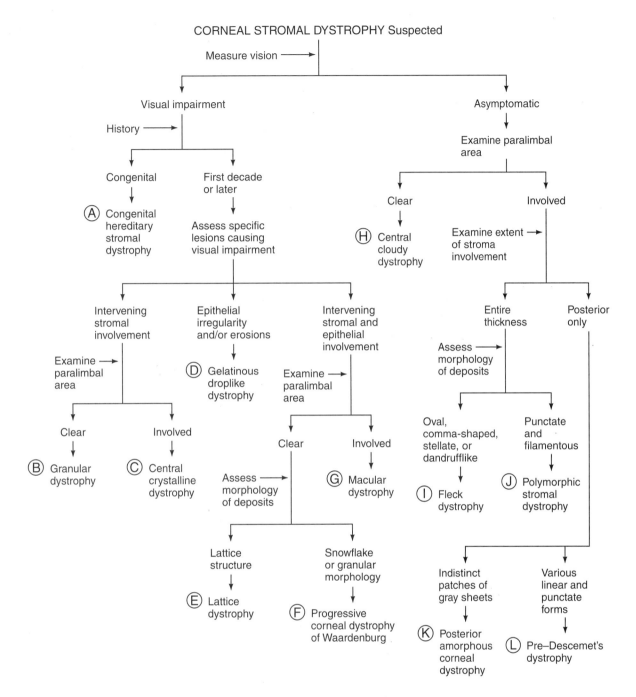

CORNEAL STROMAL DYSTROPHY Suspected

Measure vision

Visual impairment

History

Congenital
Ⓐ Congenital hereditary stromal dystrophy

First decade or later
Assess specific lesions causing visual impairment

Intervening stromal involvement
Examine paralimbal area
Clear
Ⓑ Granular dystrophy
Involved
Ⓒ Central crystalline dystrophy

Epithelial irregularity and/or erosions
Ⓓ Gelatinous droplike dystrophy

Intervening stromal and epithelial involvement
Examine paralimbal area
Clear
Assess morphology of deposits
Lattice structure
Ⓔ Lattice dystrophy
Snowflake or granular morphology
Ⓕ Progressive corneal dystrophy of Waardenburg
Involved
Ⓖ Macular dystrophy

Asymptomatic
Examine paralimbal area
Clear
Ⓗ Central cloudy dystrophy
Involved
Examine extent of stroma involvement
Entire thickness
Assess morphology of deposits
Oval, comma-shaped, stellate, or dandrufflike
Ⓘ Fleck dystrophy
Punctate and filamentous
Ⓙ Polymorphic stromal dystrophy
Indistinct patches of gray sheets
Ⓚ Posterior amorphous corneal dystrophy
Various linear and punctate forms
Ⓛ Pre–Descemet's dystrophy
Posterior only

K. In posterior amorphous dystrophy, gray, patchy, sheet-like opacifications are present at various levels of the posterior stroma and involve the entire width of the cornea. The opacities are noted during the first decade and may be congenital. This dystrophy is associated with corneal thinning and anterior iris abnormalities, yet it rarely impairs visual acuity significantly. Descemet's membrane is variably involved.

L. Pre–Descemet's dystrophy is thought to represent a degenerative process, which includes four clinical types. Onset occurs between the fourth and seventh decades of life. Focal, gray opacities are located in the deep stroma and may have various shapes and distributions. Visual acuity is not affected.

References

Hida T, Tsubota K, Kigasawa K, et al. Clinical features of a newly recognized type of lattice corneal dystrophy. Am J Ophthalmol 1987; 104:241–248.

Miller CA, Krachmer JH. Epithelial and stromal dystrophies. In: Kaufman HE, ed. The cornea. New York: Churchill Livingstone, 1988: 383–424.

Smolin G, Thoft RA. The cornea: Scientific foundations and clinical practice. 2nd ed. Boston: Little, Brown, 1987: 111.

Stock EL, Deder RS, O'Grady RB, et al. Lattice corneal dystrophy type IIIA. Clinical and histopathology correlations. Arch Ophthalmol 1991; 109:354–358.

Waring GO, Rodrigues MM, Laibson PR. Corneal dystrophies. J Surv Ophthalmol 1978; 23:71–112.

CORNEAL HYPESTHESIA

Elmer Y. Tu, M.D.
Mark L. McDermott, M.D.

Sensory innervation of the cornea is provided by the ophthalmic division of the trigeminal nerve (V1). This division splits into three branches: the lacrimal, innervating the lacrimal gland; the frontal, supplying sensation to the superior conjunctiva, upper eyelid, and forehead; and the nasociliary. The nasociliary branch divides, providing sensory innervation of the cornea, iris, and ciliary body, as well as motor innervation of the iris via the long and short posterior ciliary nerves. Other portions of the nasociliary branch provide sensation to the conjunctiva, lacrimal drainage system, and skin of the nose. Sensory innervation enters the cornea radially from a circumferential network at the corneoscleral limbus through large trunks that arborize and demyelinate as they reach midperipheral stroma. Branches travel centrally into the corneal stroma and superficially into the epithelium.

Adequate innervation of the cornea is critical in its maintenance and repair. The neurotrophic cornea is at risk for both infectious and noninfectious keratitis, as well as chronic epithelial defects and stromal lysis. Various chemotactic factors have been implicated, but supplementation of these factors has yielded varying results. Corneal hypesthesia has many systemic and local causes, making a detailed systemic and ophthalmic history critical in the diagnosis.

A. Central corneal sensation is known to decrease, in the absence of other disease, with age. Exacerbating factors may include long-term environmental exposures to sun, wind, fumes, and other ocular irritants, which may contribute to desensitizing the cornea and ocular surface. Corneal hypesthesia from age or long-term exposure uncommonly leads to clinical disease and should be considered only when other causes have been excluded.

B. Herpetic disease is usually, but not exclusively, unilateral. The herpes viruses are neurotrophic, with most studies localizing their latency and reactivation to the trigeminal ganglion. Herpes simplex has the ability to manifest in many different forms. Initial infection commonly presents as a nonspecific conjunctivitis, with recurrences producing more profound symptoms of visual loss, pain, and keratitis. The loss of sensation in herpes simplex is characteristically more focal than with herpes zoster and may result in metaherpetic or trophic ulcers. Herpes zoster virus (HZV) infection is more evident with involvement and scarring of adjacent structures supplied by the trigeminal ganglion in an acute setting. HZV corneal disease may precede, coincide with, or follow acute dermatologic disease by several weeks. Hypesthesia is often global, rather than focal, and may be severe resulting in chronic epithelial defects and visual loss.

C. Acute infectious keratitis, chronic keratitis, and local trauma may result in the focal loss of corneal sensation in the resultant scar secondary to local nerve damage. *Acanthamoeba* infection may present early with corneal hypesthesia. Ocular cicatricial pemphigoid and conjunctival inflammatory disorders may lead to loss of corneal sensitivity. Chronic or recurrent corneal erosions may result in loss of corneal sensation from local trauma. Patients predisposed to abnormal basement membrane deposition such as Reis-Bückler's, lattice dystrophy, and some forms of chronic bullous keratopathy will have painful erosions and paradoxically decreased corneal sensations. Keratoconus will exhibit decreased sensation in areas of greatest thinning.

D. Any type of ocular surgery that interrupts the radial flow of sensory information from the cornea to the nasociliary nerve can result in corneal hypesthesia. Circumferential incision in cataract surgery results in a loss of sensation extending radially from the incision site toward the central cornea for >1 year in some studies. Small incision surgery should theoretically decrease the area of hypesthesia. Damage to the long ciliary nerves in panretinal photocoagulation may decrease corneal sensation. Keratoplasty, both penetrating and lamellar, results in early hypesthesia, with partial restoration of sensation after several years. Excimer photoablation and astigmatic keratotomy have been shown to reduce central corneal sensation, whereas radial incisions appear to preserve sensation. Sensation after LASIK keratorefractive surgery appears to be greater than that after standard photorefractive keratectomy.

E. Both soft and gas permeable contact lens wear are known to decrease corneal sensitivity. Numerous ocular medications have been implicated in loss of corneal sensation. β Blockers impair corneal sensation by direct anesthetic action on corneal nerves. Topical anesthetic use may lead to corneal hypesthesia or ulceration and may mimic the appearance of infectious keratitis with infiltration and a chronic epithelial defect.

F. Selective involvement of portions of the trigeminal nerve will lead to isolated hypesthesia in patients with multiple sclerosis or myasthenia gravis. Peripheral neuropathy correlates well with the presence of corneal neuropathy in diabetic patients.

G. Corneal hypesthesia may be the presenting sign in patients with compressive lesions of the trigeminal nerve. A thorough evaluation is required to rule out CNS aneurysm or tumor. Involvement of other cranial nerves or other localizing signs may be useful in the diagnosis. A thorough evaluation, including imaging of the cerebellopontine angle and cavernous sinus, is required. Brainstem cerebrovascular accidents (CVAs) may also manifest with decreased corneal sensation, as can intracranial surgery or radiation therapy of the head.

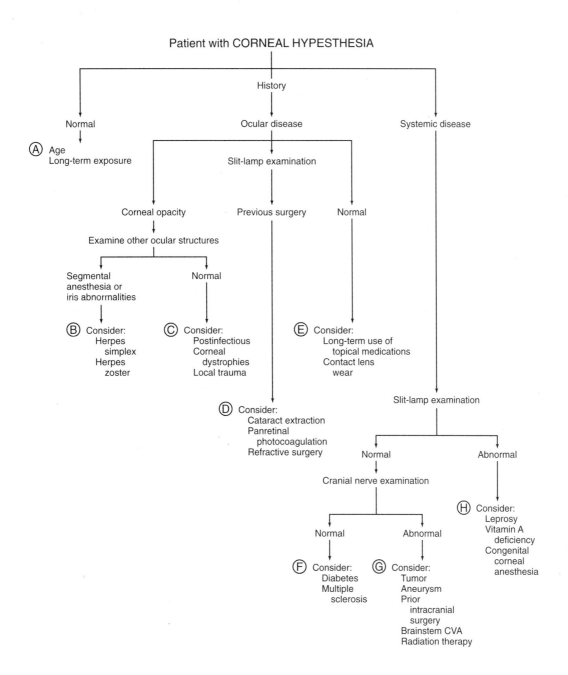

Patient with CORNEAL HYPESTHESIA

History

Normal | Ocular disease | Systemic disease

Ⓐ Age
Long-term exposure

Slit-lamp examination

Corneal opacity | Previous surgery | Normal

Examine other ocular structures

Segmental anesthesia or iris abnormalities | Normal

Ⓑ Consider:
Herpes simplex
Herpes zoster

Ⓒ Consider:
Postinfectious
Corneal dystrophies
Local trauma

Ⓔ Consider:
Long-term use of topical medications
Contact lens wear

Ⓓ Consider:
Cataract extraction
Panretinal photocoagulation
Refractive surgery

Slit-lamp examination

Normal | Abnormal

Cranial nerve examination

Ⓗ Consider:
Leprosy
Vitamin A deficiency
Congenital corneal anesthesia

Normal | Abnormal

Ⓕ Consider:
Diabetes
Multiple sclerosis

Ⓖ Consider:
Tumor
Aneurysm
Prior intracranial surgery
Brainstem CVA
Radiation therapy

H. Many systemic diseases may include corneal hypesthesia with ocular involvement. Vitamin A deficiency may lead to keratoconjunctivitis sicca, conjunctival and corneal keratinization, epithelial defect, and stromal lysis. Leprosy results in large corneal nerves, scarring of the ocular adnexa, keratinization of the ocular surface, exposure, and corneal hypesthesia. A rare syndrome with signs and symptoms of corneal hypesthesia can be found at birth.

References

Ben Osman N, Jeddi A, Sebai L, et al. The cornea of diabetics. J Fran Ophthal 1995; 18:120–123.

Campos M, Hertzog L, Garbus JJ, McDonnell PJ. Corneal sensitivity after photorefractive keratectomy. Am J Ophthal 1992; 114:51–54.

Krachmer JH, Mannis M, Palay DA. Cornea. St Louis: Mosby, 1996.

Lyne A. Corneal sensitivity after surgery. Trans Ophthal Soc UK 1982; 102:302–305.

Martin XY, Safran AB. Corneal hypoesthesia. Surv Ophthal 1998; 33:28–40.

Miller NR. Walsh and Hoyt's clinical neuro-ophthalmology. 4th ed. Vol. 2. Baltimore: Williams & Wilkins, 1985: 1056.

Myles WM, LaRoche GR. Congenital corneal anesthesia. Am J Ophthal 1994; 118:818–820.

Smolin G, Thoft RA, eds. The cornea. New York: Little, Brown, 1994: 183–208, 490–492.

Van Buskirk EM. Corneal anesthesia after timolol maleate therapy. Am J Ophthalmol 1979; 88:739–743.

GLAUCOMA AND INTRAOCULAR PRESSURE PROBLEMS

DIAGNOSIS OF GLAUCOMA

Scott D. Smith, M.D., M.P.H.

The diagnosis of glaucoma requires the identification of damage to the optic nerve in a characteristic, nerve fiber bundle pattern. If optic disc cupping and/or nerve fiber layer atrophy are moderate or advanced, corresponding visual field defects are present and the diagnosis can be made with certainty. When the disease is less advanced, definitive diagnosis on a single examination is difficult because of the variability of the optic nerve appearance and intraocular pressure (IOP) in the normal population.

A. During the history and ophthalmic examination, identify factors that increase an individual's risk of having glaucomatous optic nerve damage. A family history of primary open-angle glaucoma (POAG), particularly in first-degree relatives, is associated with an increased risk of developing the disease. The prevalence of both POAG and primary narrow-angle glaucoma (PNAG) increases with age. POAG is about four times more common in individuals of African descent than in Caucasians. PNAG appears to be more common in individuals of Asian descent. Diabetes and myopia appear to be associated with a greater risk of POAG. Episodic eye pain, redness, blurred vision, and/or seeing halos around lights should alert the clinician to possible intermittent angle closure. Check the angle for the presence of peripheral anterior synechiae (PAS).

B. Measurement of IOP is a poor method of glaucoma screening. Based on a single reading, as many as one third of individuals with glaucoma have normal IOP, and many glaucoma patients consistently fall within the normal range. Furthermore, a substantial proportion of those with statistically elevated IOP may never experience optic nerve injury. Because of the variability in IOP over time within an individual and differences in susceptibility to pressure-related optic nerve damage within the population, a comprehensive ophthalmic examination is required to properly diagnose glaucoma. Although glaucoma may occur at any level of IOP, it plays a role in the classification of glaucoma subtypes and is the primary target of current medical and surgical treatments (see p 236 for the management of elevated IOP).

C. When the anterior chamber angle is open and the IOP is normal, glaucoma may be suspected on the basis of the optic nerve appearance. Glaucomatous loss of nerve fibers leads to thinning of the neuroretinal rim, with a resultant increased size of the optic cup. Because normal eyes with small optic nerves tend to have a smaller cup/disc ratio, consider optic disc cupping in conjunction with the optic nerve size. In nor-

mally sized nerves, a cup/disc ratio of about 0.6 or greater may arouse suspicion of early glaucomatous damage. In eyes with small discs, glaucoma may be present with a much smaller cup/disc ratio. Examination of the retinal nerve fiber layer may provide important clues to the presence of glaucomatous optic disc damage before changes in the optic disc or visual field are evident. Although damage from glaucoma may be diffuse, it is often asymmetric both with respect to the upper and lower hemiretina within an eye, and with respect to the contralateral eye. Therefore the identification of vertical and/or contralateral asymmetry of the optic nerve and nerve fiber layer is important in evaluating cases of suspected glaucoma.

D. When glaucomatous optic nerve damage with visual field loss is present and the IOP is normal, consider intermittent IOP elevation as part of the diagnostic evaluation for low-tension glaucoma. Visual field loss that does not correlate with glaucomatous optic nerve injury should prompt consideration of alternative diagnoses (p 374).

E. In the absence of definitive optic nerve or visual field abnormality, periodic clinical evaluation with serial stereo disc photographs and visual field tests are required to confirm stability. Consider evidence of change in the optic disc appearance, the development of a visual field defect, or a rise in IOP in determining the need for treatment. Base the frequency of follow-up visits on the level of suspicion for glaucoma. When multiple risk factors are present or when there is a risk of secondary open-angle glaucoma from pseudoexfoliation or pigment dispersion (p 72), closer follow-up may be advisable.

References

Airaksinen PJ, Tuulonen A, Werner EB. Clinical evaluation of the optic disc and retinal nerve fiber layer. In: Ritch R, Shields MB, Krupin T, eds. The glaucomas. St Louis: Mosby, 1996: 617–657.

Tielsch JM, Katz J, Sommer A, et al. Family history and risk of primary open-angle glaucoma: The Baltimore Eye Survey. Arch Ophthalmol 1994; 112:69–73.

Tielsch JM, Sommer A, Katz J, et al. Racial variations in the prevalence of POAG: The Baltimore Eye Survey. JAMA 1991; 266:369–374.

Wilson MR, Martone JF. Epidemiology of chronic open-angle glaucoma. In: Ritch R, Shields MB, Krupin T, eds. The glaucomas. St Louis: Mosby, 1996: 753–768.

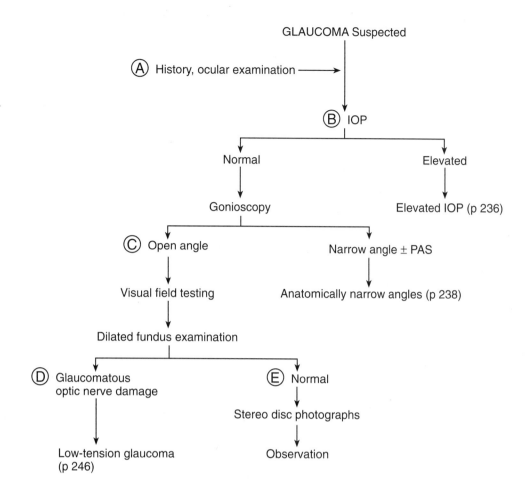

GLAUCOMA Suspected

(A) History, ocular examination ⟶

(B) IOP

Normal   Elevated

Gonioscopy   Elevated IOP (p 236)

(C) Open angle   Narrow angle ± PAS

Visual field testing   Anatomically narrow angles (p 238)

Dilated fundus examination

(D) Glaucomatous   (E) Normal
optic nerve damage

Stereo disc photographs

Low-tension glaucoma   Observation
(p 246)

ELEVATED INTRAOCULAR PRESSURE

Scott D. Smith, M.D., M.P.H.

Elevated intraocular pressure (IOP) is an important risk factor for the development of glaucomatous optic nerve damage. Therefore all patients with elevated IOP, traditionally defined as IOP ≥22 mm Hg, require careful evaluation to determine the mechanism of IOP elevation and the presence and extent of optic nerve injury.

A. The first step in determining the mechanism of IOP elevation is a thorough history and slit-lamp examination. Patients may neglect to report a distant history of ocular trauma or inflammation unless specifically questioned. Slit-lamp findings that provide evidence for secondary IOP elevation may be very subtle and require careful observation by the clinician.

B. Primary open-angle glaucoma (POAG) is the most common form of glaucoma in the United States. In addition to the presence of an open anterior chamber angle on gonioscopy, the diagnosis of POAG requires the exclusion of any identifiable underlying cause for elevation of IOP greater than that which an individual can safely tolerate. Asymmetry of IOP can be suggestive of the presence of a secondary form of glaucoma. However, unilateral or highly asymmetric IOP is occasionally seen in POAG and bilateral, symmetric secondary open-angle glaucoma is not uncommon. Therefore evaluation for secondary OAG should be equally thorough in all patients regardless of the IOP symmetry.

C. In primary narrow-angle glaucoma (PNAG), a narrow or closed approach into the anterior chamber angle may make visualization of peripheral anterior synechiae (PAS) impossible until compression gonioscopy is performed. Before the diagnosis of PNAG can be made, a different set of secondary causes of IOP elevation must be considered. Iridocyclitis and neovascular glaucoma can cause secondary open-angle or angle-closure glaucoma, depending on whether PAS have developed. In these cases a wide approach into the anterior chamber angle may be present with a tented appearance to the PAS. Asymmetry of the angle approach in comparison with the contralateral eye can be suggestive of a posterior segment pathologic condition such as choroidal effusion (e.g., after panretinal photocoagulation) or tumor.

D. When pupillary block results in a narrow or closed anterior chamber angle, laser peripheral iridotomy is indicated. This procedure is required in all cases of PNAG. Repeat gonioscopy after laser treatment confirms the efficacy in opening the anterior chamber angle and permits the diagnosis of plateau iris syndrome (p 238). Laser iridotomy is also helpful when secondary pupillary block causes IOP elevation, such as in phacomorphic glaucoma or when iridocyclitis leads to pupillary seclusion and iris bombé. If second-

ary pupillary block is present, however, treatment must also be directed at the causative factor. For phacomorphic glaucoma, cataract extraction with or without combined filtration surgery is the definitive treatment. In uveitic glaucoma, treatment of the underlying inflammatory process is necessary.

E. Visual field testing and dilated fundus examination are required to determine whether IOP elevation has resulted in damage to the optic nerve. In cases of primary angle closure, dilated fundus examination must not be performed until after laser iridotomy has been completed to prevent possible acute exacerbation of the increased IOP.

F. If no evidence of optic nerve damage is present, consider the level of IOP and the presence of risk factors for the future development of damage in determining the need for medical treatment. Because the risk of developing glaucoma increases dramatically when IOP exceeds 30 mm Hg, initiate medical treatment in such cases. Initial glaucoma therapy usually consists of a topical β blocker regardless of the underlying mechanism. When the IOP is <30 mm Hg, observation without treatment may be reasonable, especially when risk factors for progression to glaucoma are absent. Factors to consider include a strong family history of glaucoma (especially blindness resulting from glaucoma) and the degree of suspicion of disc damage based on the cup/disc ratio and disc asymmetry. Social factors such as the patient's level of apprehension regarding untreated ocular hypertension and the likelihood of reliable follow-up must also be assessed. Elevated IOP from pseudoexfoliation or pigment dispersion may have an aggressive course with dramatic changes in IOP over a short time. Greater caution should be taken in following these patients without treatment.

G. Patients with glaucomatous optic nerve damage require medical therapy to lower the IOP to a level that is unlikely to lead to further damage. The level of IOP before initiation of therapy should be used to help determine a target pressure below which further damage is unlikely. Advanced damage may lower the target pressure level even further in that extensively damaged optic nerves may be more susceptible to injury. A significant reduction in IOP may follow laser iridotomy in patients with PNAG, particularly when PAS formation has not been extensive. However, most patients will require the addition of medical therapy to reach an appropriate target pressure.

H. If the target IOP is attained, visual fields and optic nerve status must be carefully monitored to rule out ongoing damage. If progressive damage occurs, a new, lower target pressure must be chosen and therapy adjusted accordingly. The medical treatment of PNAG

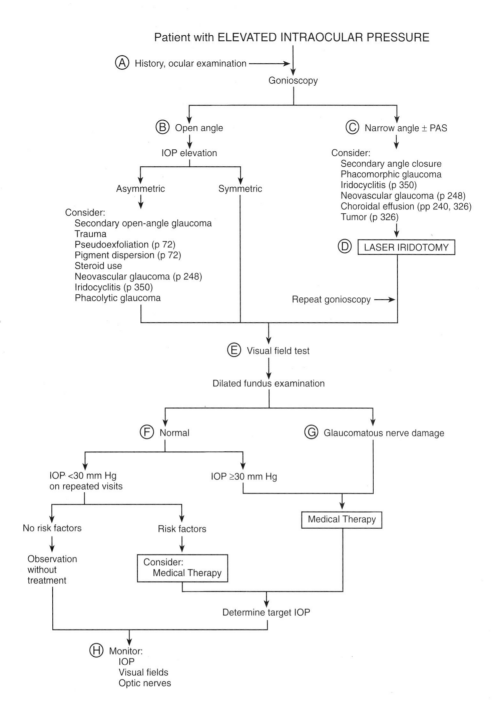

Patient with ELEVATED INTRAOCULAR PRESSURE

(A) History, ocular examination

Gonioscopy

(B) Open angle

IOP elevation

Asymmetric

Consider:
  Secondary open-angle glaucoma
  Trauma
  Pseudoexfoliation (p 72)
  Pigment dispersion (p 72)
  Steroid use
  Neovascular glaucoma (p 248)
  Iridocyclitis (p 350)
  Phacolytic glaucoma

Symmetric

(C) Narrow angle ± PAS

Consider:
  Secondary angle closure
  Phacomorphic glaucoma
  Iridocyclitis (p 350)
  Neovascular glaucoma (p 248)
  Choroidal effusion (pp 240, 326)
  Tumor (p 326)

(D) LASER IRIDOTOMY

Repeat gonioscopy

(E) Visual field test

Dilated fundus examination

(F) Normal

IOP <30 mm Hg
on repeated visits

No risk factors

Observation
without
treatment

Risk factors

Consider:
  Medical Therapy

(G) Glaucomatous nerve damage

IOP ≥30 mm Hg

Medical Therapy

Determine target IOP

(H) Monitor:
  IOP
  Visual fields
  Optic nerves

differs from that of POAG in that medications that act by increasing outflow facility (e.g., pilocarpine) are ineffective when extensive PAS are present. As a result, options for medical treatment of PNAG with extensive PAS are generally limited to aqueous suppressants, including β blockers, α₂ agonists, and carbonic anhydrase inhibitors. For details of the management of POAG, see p 244.

References

McGalliard JN, Wishart PK. The effect of Nd:YAG iridotomy on IOP in hypertensive eyes with shallow anterior chambers. Eye 1990; 4:823–829.

Pohjanpelto P. Influence of exfoliation syndrome on prognosis in ocular hypertension ≥25 mm: a long-term follow-up. Acta Ophthalmol (Copenh) 1986; 64:39–44.

Quigley HA, Enger C, Katz J, et al. Risk factors for the development of glaucomatous visual field loss in ocular hypertension. Arch Ophthalmol 1994; 112:644–649.

Ritch R, Liebmann JM. Laser iridotomy and peripheral iridoplasty. In: Ritch R, Shields MB, Krupin T, eds. The glaucomas. St Louis: Mosby, 1996: 1549–1573.

ANATOMICALLY NARROW ANGLES

John M. Parkinson, M.D.
J. Kevin McKinney, M.D.

Relative pupillary block is the most common cause of anatomically narrow angles. Laser peripheral iridotomy (LPI) has been shown to be safe and effective for preventing angle-closure glaucoma caused by pupillary block. Because the visual sequelae of acute angle closure can be devastating and the risk of LPI is small, eyes with angles narrow enough to raise clinical suspicion of potential angle closure should receive a prophylactic LPI.

A. Attention to detail and experience in gonioscopy are necessary to accurately evaluate the angle configuration and thereby assess the potential for future angle closure. With proper training and practice, a general ophthalmologist should be able to perform gonioscopy with accuracy and skill. A four-mirror lens, such as a Zeiss or Posner lens, is best suited for evaluating the angle in this setting. During gonioscopy, the lens is held lightly against the cornea. Excessive pressure artificially widens the angle and is indicated by corneal striae. The room should be dark, and the light beam should be narrow and small, avoiding direct illumination of the pupil, which would open the angle via pupillary miosis. If significant iris bombé (iris convexity indicative of relative pupillary block) is present, the mirror is rotated toward the observed angle or the patient is asked to look toward the mirror, allowing one to "look over the hill" into the angle. The ability to accurately identify the trabecular meshwork (TM) in the presence of varying amounts of pigmentation is essential (e.g., pigment at Schwalbe's line may mimic the TM in a closed angle).

B. If the peripheral iris lies in direct contact with the posterior TM, appositional closure is present. Indentation gonioscopy with a four-mirror lens can often differentiate appositional closure from synechial angle closure. Peripheral anterior synechiae can result from prolonged or intermittent appositional contact and may progress to extensive, irreversible angle closure. The presence of either apposition or synechiae implies the need for LPI.

C. An angle is imminently occludable if the angular separation between the TM and peripheral iris is <10 degrees. Pharmacologic dilation of such eyes may precipitate acute angle closure and is usually deferred until an iridotomy has been performed.

D. Angles that are possibly occludable have a 10- to 20-degree angle of separation between the peripheral iris and the TM. In this case the decision to perform LPI is based on the presence of symptoms consistent with intermittent episodes of angle closure (e.g., colored halos around lights, blurred or misty vision, ocular redness and discomfort), as well as the individual's social situation (e.g., the ability to identify and report symptoms of angle closure and to readily access medical care). Other relative indications for iridotomy include individuals with possibly occludable angles who require frequent dilation (e.g., diabetic patients) or who take systemic medications that might provoke acute angle closure (e.g., tricyclic antidepressants, some cold preparations).

E. An iridotomy is proven to be patent by direct visualization of lens capsule or a black void posterior to the iris plane. Transillumination alone is insufficient to prove patency. Gonioscopy should be repeated after laser iridotomy to determine the effectiveness of treatment. If the narrow angle configuration was caused by relative pupillary block and the LPI is of adequate size and patency, a relatively flat iris configuration and an open angle should be found.

F. Up to one third of angles without PAS remain narrow after LPI, because of either plateau iris configuration or a relatively crowded anterior segment (e.g., a large lens). With plateau iris, anteriorly located ciliary processes hold the peripheral iris forward, creating a narrow angle in the face of a flat iris configuration. With a crowded anterior segment, the iris assumes a convex configuration as it drapes over the lens curvature. Once an appropriate plan has been instituted (i.e., observation, miotics, or iridoplasty), gonioscopy should be repeated after pharmacologic dilation to rule out appositional angle closure.

G. Because narrow angles tend to become narrower with age (as a result of increasing lens size), continued gonioscopy is indicated if iridotomy is deferred or if the angle remains narrow after iridotomy. Eyes with coexistent pseudoexfoliation are especially prone to this phenomenon.

H. In the absence of other indications for LPI, some specialists would recommend provocative testing to further determine susceptibility to angle closure. Although such tests may be reassuring to the patient and physician, their sensitivity, specificity, and predictive power are uncertain. If such a test is performed, gonioscopic evidence of angle closure must accompany a rise in intraocular pressure before the test can be considered positive.

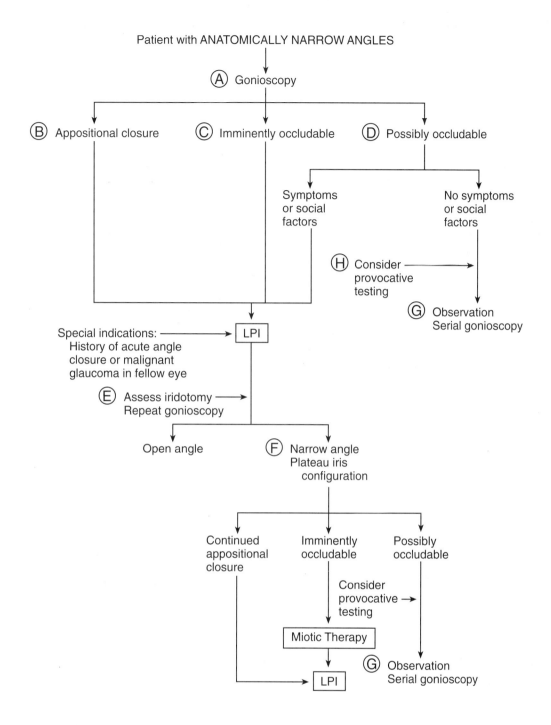

Patient with ANATOMICALLY NARROW ANGLES

(A) Gonioscopy

(B) Appositional closure   (C) Imminently occludable   (D) Possibly occludable

Symptoms or social factors   No symptoms or social factors

(H) Consider provocative testing

(G) Observation Serial gonioscopy

Special indications: ——→ LPI
History of acute angle closure or malignant glaucoma in fellow eye

(E) Assess iridotomy ——→
Repeat gonioscopy

Open angle   (F) Narrow angle Plateau iris configuration

Continued appositional closure   Imminently occludable   Possibly occludable

Consider provocative testing →

Miotic Therapy

LPI   (G) Observation Serial gonioscopy

References

Alward WLM. Color atlas of gonioscopy. London: Wolfe, 1994.

Moster MR, Schwartz LW, Spaeth GL, et al. Laser iridectomy: A controlled study comparing argon and neodymium:YAG. Ophthalmology 1986; 93:20–24.

Ritch R, Lowe RF. Angle closure glaucoma: Clinical types. In: Ritch R, Shields MB, Krupin T, eds. The glaucomas. St Louis: Mosby, 1996: 821–840.

Ritch R, Lowe RF. Angle closure glaucoma: Therapeutic overview. In: Ritch R, Shields MB, Krupin T, eds. The glaucomas. St Louis: Mosby, 1996: 1521–1531.

ACUTELY ELEVATED INTRAOCULAR PRESSURE

John M. Parkinson, M.D.
Scott D. Smith, M.D., M.P.H.

A. A complete medical and ocular history may provide clues about the cause of acutely elevated intraocular pressure (IOP). Give special attention to a history of ocular trauma, inflammation, and previous episodes of elevated IOP. History of systemic vascular disease such as diabetes mellitus that might result in anterior segment neovascularization should be determined. The nature and timing of the current ophthalmic condition should be described, including any symptoms of visual loss, blurred or boggy vision, colored haloes around lights, pain, redness, or photophobia.

B. When secondary corneal edema is present, slit-lamp examination and gonioscopy are facilitated by the application of topical glycerin. If gonioscopy is limited even with the use of glycerin, a narrow angle in the opposite eye helps confirm angle closure caused by pupillary block in the affected eye. Asymmetry in anterior chamber angles should suggest another cause of angle closure. Careful examination of the iris and anterior chamber angle for the presence of iris neovascularization is required to distinguish neovascular glaucoma from other causes of acute elevation of IOP. IOP elevation caused by neovascular glaucoma is generally accompanied by partial or complete synechial angle closure and requires prompt management of the cause of the anterior segment neovascularization (p 248).

C. Perform a dilated fundus examination in cases of open-angle glaucoma to identify abnormalities of the posterior segment and to evaluate the optic nerve. Although more commonly associated with chronic, asymptomatic elevation of IOP, acute IOP elevation may occur in pigmentary or pseudoexfoliation glaucoma.

D. Glaucomatocyclitic crisis occurs in young to middle-aged adults with symptoms of mild uniocular irritation and blurred vision. IOP in the range of 40–60 mm Hg is usually associated with mild ocular inflammation (ciliary injection with trace anterior chamber cells and flare, and fine keratic precipitates). Posterior and peripheral anterior synechiae are notably absent in this syndrome. Episodes are self-limited (lasting several hours to several weeks) and variably recurrent.

E. Trauma may result in acutely elevated IOP by direct damage to outflow structures or by occlusion of these structures with erythrocytes, inflammatory cells, pigment, fibrin, and other debris. In cases of hyphema in African-Americans, obtain a sickle cell preparation to identify patients at risk for prolonged pressure elevation because of obstruction of outflow by sickled erythrocytes.

F. Elevated IOP in uveitis results from direct inflammatory involvement of the trabecular meshwork and obstruction of outflow by inflammatory cells and fibrin. Progressive synechial angle closure caused by contraction of inflammatory membranes or precipitates in the angle may also occur.

G. Medical therapy in each condition is directed primarily at aqueous humor suppression. Effective medications include topical β blockers, α_2 agonists, and carbonic anhydrase inhibitors (CAIs). Systemic CAIs may be more effective in treating acute IOP elevation than topical dorzolamide, but they are contraindicated in patients with sickle cell disease. Hyperosmotic agents can also be used for temporary control of IOP when the initial response to other medications is inadequate. Parasympathomimetic agents and latanoprost may increase ocular inflammation and should be avoided. Topical steroids are used in all three conditions to reduce ocular inflammation, but prolonged use may be associated with a subsequent steroid-induced rise in IOP. Short-acting cycloplegic agents help relieve symptoms of ciliary spasm and may help prevent posterior synechiae by ensuring pupillary mobility. Long-acting cycloplegic agents may help reduce rebleeding in traumatic hyphema by immobilizing the iris.

H. Most cases of acutely elevated IOP resulting from these conditions can be successfully managed medically. When necessary, traditional filtration surgery is most successful after acute inflammation is medically controlled. In cases of imminent corneal blood staining, previous optic nerve damage, or impending retinal vascular occlusion, early surgical intervention may be necessary. Adjunctive mitomycin-C or 5-fluorouracil can improve the success of trabeculectomy in patients with inflammatory glaucoma. Glaucoma drainage implant surgery may be required when conjunctival scarring is present or when previous trabeculectomy with an adjunctive antimetabolite has failed.

I. Ultrasonography effectively rules out uncommon secondary causes of acute angle-closure glaucoma. If ultrasonography is not available, an anatomically narrow angle in the fellow eye supports the diagnosis of simple pupillary block as the mechanism of angle closure. Perform a dilated fundus examination after the angle closure is adequately treated to rule out abnormalities of the posterior segment.

J. The presence of high IOP with a shallow axial anterior chamber, particularly in patients with a history of prior ocular surgery or peripheral iridotomy, suggests aqueous misdirection (p 254). An extremely narrow anterior chamber angle in the presence of mature cataract and a normal posterior segment on ultrasound suggests phacomorphic glaucoma. Definitive therapy requires cataract extraction with or without combined trabeculectomy, depending on the chronicity of IOP elevation. Before surgery, medical therapy is required to attempt to lower IOP and reduce ocular inflammation. Laser iridotomy can relieve angle closure before definitive surgery is performed because an element of pupillary block may also be present.

K. In the absence of choroidal abnormality, medical therapy is directed at reducing IOP, corneal edema, and iris ischemia. Aqueous humor suppressants, including β blockers, CAIs, and α₂ agonists, are used initially. Hyperosmotic agents are often necessary in patients with extremely high IOP or when the initial response to other medications is inadequate. In phakic eyes, several doses of 1% or 2% pilocarpine may effectively break an attack of angle-closure glaucoma but may be more effective after aqueous suppression has begun to lower IOP and iris ischemia has decreased. In aphakic or pseudophakic eyes without an iridectomy, pupillary block may be relieved by pupillary dilation and cycloplegia.

L. When acute IOP elevation is caused by pupillary block, perform laser peripheral iridotomy. If possible, this should be delayed until medical treatment has reduced the IOP and corneal edema has cleared. In cases refractory to medical treatment, topical glycerin may be helpful in clearing the cornea long enough to permit laser iridotomy. Emergent filtration surgery is rarely required in the treatment of primary angle-closure glaucoma.

M. Recurrent acute angle closure after laser iridotomy suggests the presence of plateau iris syndrome, which can be confirmed by gonioscopy. Such patients should be continued on 1% or 2% pilocarpine to reduce the risk of recurrent episodes. See p 238 for additional therapeutic considerations.

N. Choroidal elevation or thickening on ultrasonography suggests choroidal effusion, choroidal hemorrhage, or tumor. Choroidal effusion may be primary (idiopathic) or secondary to posterior scleritis, central retinal vein occlusion, scleral buckling procedures, or panretinal photocoagulation. Appropriate management of these patients usually includes vitreoretinal consultation.

O. Medical therapy consists of aqueous humor suppression with maximal cycloplegia to allow posterior rotation of the ciliary body, lens, and iris.

P. Surgical intervention is indicated in cases of persistently flat anterior chamber, corneal decompensation, refractory pressure elevation, or "kissing choroidals." When some degree of pupillary block also exists, a laser iridotomy may re-establish anterior aqueous flow. Drainage of choroidal effusion or blood (in the absence of intraocular tumor) is definitive therapy.

References

Hoskins HD Jr, Kass MA. Becker-Shaffer's diagnosis and therapy of the glaucomas. 6th ed. St Louis: Mosby, 1989: 308–335.

Maus TL, Larsson L, McLaren JW, Brubaker RF. Comparison of dorzolamide and acetazolamide as suppressors of aqueous humor flow in humans. Arch Ophthalmol 1997; 115:45–49.

Raitta C, Vannas A. Glaucomatocyclitic crisis. Arch Ophthalmol 1977; 95:608–612.

Ritch R, Lowe RF. Angle closure glaucoma: Clinical types. In: Ritch R, Shields MB, Krupin T, eds. The glaucomas. St Louis: Mosby, 1996: 821–840.

Walsh JB, Muldoon TO. Glaucoma associated with retinal and vitreoretinal disorders. In: Ritch R, Shields MB, Krupin T, eds. The glaucomas. St Louis: Mosby, 1996: 1055–1071.

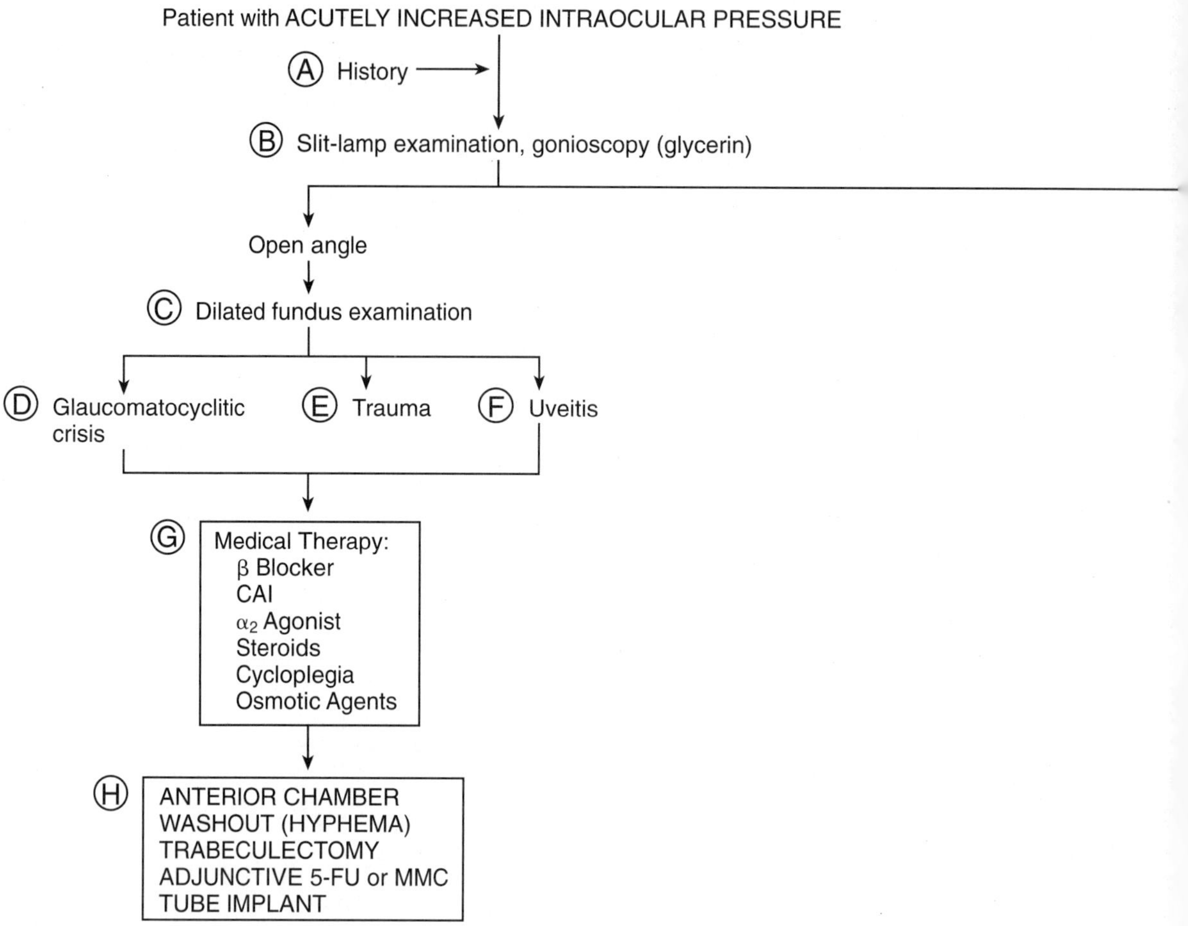

Patient with ACUTELY INCREASED INTRAOCULAR PRESSURE

(A) History →

(B) Slit-lamp examination, gonioscopy (glycerin)

Open angle

(C) Dilated fundus examination

(D) Glaucomatocyclitic crisis   (E) Trauma   (F) Uveitis

(G) Medical Therapy:
  β Blocker
  CAI
  α_2 Agonist
  Steroids
  Cycloplegia
  Osmotic Agents

(H) ANTERIOR CHAMBER
WASHOUT (HYPHEMA)
TRABECULECTOMY
ADJUNCTIVE 5-FU or MMC
TUBE IMPLANT

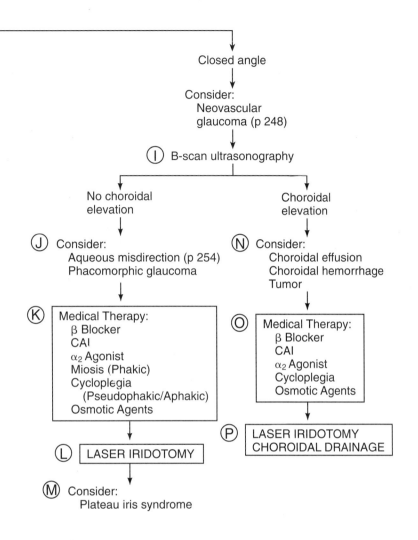

Closed angle

Consider:
Neovascular
glaucoma (p 248)

Ⓘ B-scan ultrasonography

No choroidal
elevation

Choroidal
elevation

Ⓙ Consider:
Aqueous misdirection (p 254)
Phacomorphic glaucoma

Ⓝ Consider:
Choroidal effusion
Choroidal hemorrhage
Tumor

Ⓚ Medical Therapy:
β Blocker
CAI
α₂ Agonist
Miosis (Phakic)
Cycloplegia
(Pseudophakic/Aphakic)
Osmotic Agents

Ⓞ Medical Therapy:
β Blocker
CAI
α₂ Agonist
Cycloplegia
Osmotic Agents

Ⓛ LASER IRIDOTOMY

Ⓟ LASER IRIDOTOMY
CHOROIDAL DRAINAGE

Ⓜ Consider:
Plateau iris syndrome

PRIMARY OPEN-ANGLE GLAUCOMA

Scott D. Smith, M.D., M.P.H.
Roy Whitaker Jr., M.D.

After the diagnosis of primary open-angle glaucoma (POAG) is established, medical therapy should be instituted to prevent progressive visual loss. The lowest dosage that achieves an intraocular pressure (IOP) level that prevents progressive damage to the optic nerve and nerve fiber layer is desirable because lower dosages are less likely to cause medication side effects. All medications used to treat glaucoma are potentially harmful; therefore the practitioner treating glaucoma should fully understand the pharmacology and side effects of these medications.

Several lines of therapy are necessary because the effect of a given treatment may dissipate with loss of the drug's effect or worsening of the disease. Different medications or medical combinations work for different patients; therefore therapy must be individualized.

A. The level of IOP before initiation of therapy should be used to help determine a target pressure below which further damage is unlikely. Advanced damage may lower the target pressure level even further in that extensively damaged optic nerves may be more susceptible to injury.

B. The accumulation of data from long-term studies coupled with the clinical experience of ophthalmologists has made the use of topical β blockers common as initial therapy for POAG. Several nonselective β blockers are available in the United States. These drugs are contraindicated in patients with greater than first-degree heart block and bronchospastic disorders and should be used cautiously in patients with diabetes and congestive heart failure. Because of its intrinsic sympathomimetic activity, carteolol appears to be less likely to cause bradycardia and has a less detrimental effect on serum lipid profiles than other β blockers. Betaxolol, a selective β_1-adrenergic antagonist, is associated with fewer pulmonary side effects than the nonselective β blockers but should still be avoided in patients with bronchospastic disorders.

    Because of the fluctuation of IOP, the efficacy of treatment of POAG with β blockers or other drugs can be difficult to determine if treatment is initiated bilaterally. The use of a one-eyed treatment trial when beginning a new drug can improve the clinician's ability to assess the efficacy of treatment. Ineffective drugs can be discontinued in favor of alternative treatments, thereby avoiding potential adverse effects from unnecessary medications.

C. Recent advances in glaucoma therapy have led to a greater number of therapeutic options for patients in whom β blockers are ineffective or contraindicated. When β blockers are effective but the IOP reduction is insufficient to reach the target IOP, combinations of medications may be used to treat the patient successfully.

Latanoprost is a prostaglandin $F_{2\alpha}$ analog that has been shown to be at least as effective as timolol in IOP reduction in patients with POAG and ocular hypertension. Its effectiveness in IOP reduction in individuals with other forms of glaucoma has not yet been evaluated. Latanoprost reduces IOP by increasing uveoscleral outflow, a mechanism that differs from any other class of glaucoma medication. Conjunctival irritation and increased iris pigmentation may limit its usefulness in some patients.

Although oral carbonic anhydrase inhibitors (CAIs) are effective in reducing IOP, systemic side effects often limit their usefulness in the treatment of glaucoma. The recently introduced CAI dorzolamide, which is effective by topical administration and appears to have minimal systemic effects, has largely replaced its oral counterparts for long-term treatment.

D. Argon laser trabeculoplasty (ALT) has traditionally been reserved for the treatment of medically uncontrolled open-angle glaucoma. Studies evaluating ALT as an alternative to medical therapy as initial treatment for newly diagnosed POAG have shown it to be nearly 50% effective in controlling IOP without the need for medications for at least 2 years. Although most clinicians continue to use medications as first-line therapy for POAG, many are considering ALT earlier in the course of the disease, particularly for individuals with significant medication side effects or when compliance is inadequate.

E. α_2-Adrenergic agonists such as apraclonidine are most commonly used as prophylactic treatment against postlaser IOP spikes. However, these drugs have also been shown to be effective in some individuals with uncontrolled IOP despite multiple medications. Their long-term usefulness can be limited by allergy in a significant proportion of subjects.

Pilocarpine and other parasympathomimetic agents reduce IOP by increasing trabecular outflow. Miosis, induced accommodation, and ciliary spasm are responsible for significant side effects in many individuals. In particular, young people and individuals with early or moderate cataract tend to tolerate this class of medication poorly. Epinephrine is ineffective in many individuals and is often associated with significant side effects, including ocular surface irritation, blepharoconjunctivitis, and cystoid macular edema in aphakic and pseudophakic patients. Dipivefrin, a prodrug converted to epinephrine inside the eye, causes less ocular surface irritation but is still prone to many of the same side effects as its parent compound. As newer glaucoma medications with fewer side effects and/or greater efficacy have been introduced, these drugs are less commonly used in the treatment of POAG. Nevertheless, these agents still have a role

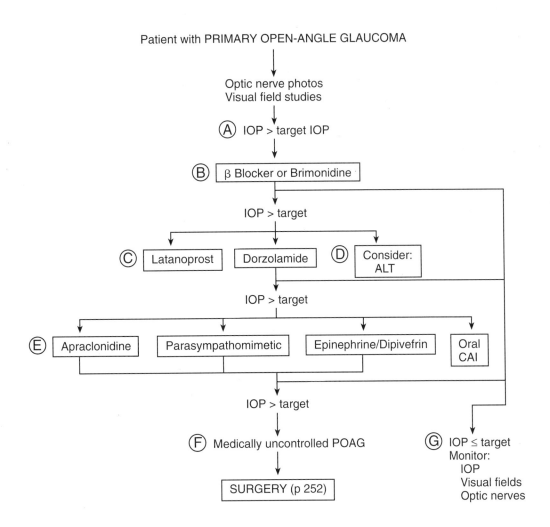

Patient with PRIMARY OPEN-ANGLE GLAUCOMA

↓

Optic nerve photos
Visual field studies

↓

(A) IOP > target IOP

↓

(B) β Blocker or Brimonidine

↓

IOP > target

(C) Latanoprost   Dorzolamide   (D) Consider: ALT

↓

IOP > target

(E) Apraclonidine   Parasympathomimetic   Epinephrine/Dipivefrin   Oral CAI

↓

IOP > target

(F) Medically uncontrolled POAG

↓

SURGERY (p 252)

(G) IOP ≤ target
Monitor:
IOP
Visual fields
Optic nerves

---

when others are ineffective and/or poorly tolerated before proceeding to filtering surgery.

F. When glaucoma is progressive despite the use of maximally tolerated medical therapy and ALT, invasive glaucoma surgery is indicated. Trabeculectomy has traditionally been delayed because its complications may lead to significant ocular morbidity. Current research is evaluating the potential risks and benefits of early glaucoma surgery as an alternative to medical and laser treatment. Until these risks are more clearly understood, surgery should be reserved for patients who respond poorly to standard initial treatment.

G. If the target IOP is attained, visual fields and optic nerve status must be carefully monitored to rule out ongoing damage. If progressive damage occurs, a new, lower target pressure must be chosen and therapy adjusted accordingly.

References

Freedman SF, Freedman NJ, Shields MB, et al. Effects of ocular carteolol and timolol on plasma high-density lipoprotein cholesterol level. Am J Ophthalmol 1993; 116:600–611.

Glaucoma Laser Trial Research Group. The Glaucoma Laser Trial (GLT): 2. Results of argon laser trabeculoplasty versus topical medicines. Ophthalmology 1990; 97:1403–1413.

Mishima HK, Masuda K, Kitazawa Y, et al. A comparison of latanoprost and timolol in primary open-angle glaucoma and ocular hypertension. Arch Ophthalmol 1996; 114: 929–932.

Netland PA, Weiss HS, Stewart WC, et al. Cardiovascular effects of topical carteolol hydrochloride and timolol maleate in patients with ocular hypertension and primary open-angle glaucoma. Am J Ophthalmol 1997; 123:465–477.

Robin AL, Ritch R, Shin DH, et al. Short-term efficacy of apraclonidine hydrochloride added to maximum tolerated medical therapy for glaucoma. Am J Ophthalmol 1995; 120:423–432.

Strahlman E, Tipping R, Vogel R. A six-week dose-response study of the ocular hypotensive effect of dorzolamide with a one-year extension. Am J Ophthalmol 1996; 122:183–194.

LOW-TENSION GLAUCOMA

Peter A. Netland, M.D., Ph.D.
Roy Whitaker Jr., M.D.

Low-tension glaucoma is characterized by glaucomatous optic nerve cupping, visual field defects, open anterior chamber angles, and the absence of elevated intraocular pressure (IOP). The absence of elevated IOP usually is defined as IOP <22 mm Hg for all recorded measurements of IOP. The diagnosis is less certain in the absence of demonstrable progressive optic nerve changes or visual field loss over time. Low-tension glaucoma occurs primarily in the elderly, with onset usually in the sixth or seventh decade of life. This entity is relatively common, present in one fifth to one half of all patients with open-angle glaucoma.

A. Low-tension glaucoma is a diagnosis of exclusion based on the history and the clinical findings. The evaluation of a patient with low-tension glaucoma should include a careful history and a complete ophthalmic examination, including IOP determination, gonioscopy, visual fields, dilated funduscopic examination, and disc photographs. The history should include inquiries about migraine, Raynaud's, cancer, toxic exposures such as methanol or ethambutol, hemodynamic crisis, or abnormalities of blood pressure. The past and present medication list is also relevant because systemic β blockers and calcium channel blockers may mask elevated IOP. In select patients, a general physical examination may be performed to evaluate for systemic diseases, including neurologic and vascular abnormalities (including carotid artery abnormalities). In the ocular examination, note the finding of optic disc hemorrhage. A higher prevalence of optic disc hemorrhages has been reported in patients with low-tension glaucoma compared with those with open-angle glaucoma.

B. IOP measurements <22 mm Hg have been considered normal, but intermittent elevations of IOP may not be detected or glaucoma may be "in remission." Some nonglaucoma conditions, such as congenital abnormalities and compressive lesions of the optic nerve, may also resemble low-tension glaucoma. Patients with IOP <22 mm Hg should have pressure measurements on more than one occasion and at different times of the day in an attempt to detect IOP fluctuation. Diurnal variations of IOP can occur, and these may be exaggerated in glaucoma patients. Transient elevations of IOP may be found in intermittent angle-closure glaucoma, glaucomatocyclitic crisis, and glaucoma associated with uveitis. Previous elevations of IOP may occur in glaucoma associated with corticosteroid use, uveitis, or trauma. If repeated measurements of the IOP are always in the normal range, continue the evaluation for low-tension glaucoma.

C. Observe patients with a normal visual field, normal IOP, and an optic disc that appears suspicious for glaucoma. Because glaucoma may develop in the future, stereo disc photographs are useful to document progressive changes of optic nerve head contour. Repeat visual field tests at regular intervals. Such patients can be observed without treatment.

D. If visual field testing reveals glaucomatous loss, the diagnosis is most likely glaucoma. However, laboratory and imaging studies may be useful to identify other causes of visual field loss and optic nerve damage. Although not recommended for patients with typical clinical findings of low-tension glaucoma, CT scanning can identify patients with compressive lesions of the optic nerve. Patients suspected of having low-tension glaucoma who are <50 years old with optic nerve atrophy and normal IOP should be considered for a CT scan. Also, obtain a CT scan in any patient with significant asymmetry of the optic nerve heads, optic nerve head pallor, pain, or dyschromatopsia. Visual field results that are not characteristic for glaucoma, such as temporal field loss or field loss respecting the vertical meridian, should prompt neurologic evaluation (p 374).

E. Treat patients with low-tension glaucoma who have progressive visual field loss to lower the IOP to a level that prevents progression. This may require medical, laser, or surgical therapy. The use of therapy in low-tension glaucoma is controversial, but most treatment strategies for low-tension glaucoma center around the assumption that IOP should be as low as possible. Surgical treatment of low-tension glaucoma is usually reserved for patients in whom progression of their disease is well documented despite conventional medical and even laser therapy. Trabeculectomy with antifibrosis agents has become a popular surgical therapy for progressive low-tension glaucoma because this procedure achieves low mean IOP and has a low complication rate. Despite conventional medical and surgical therapy, patients with low-tension glaucoma may continue to demonstrate intractable progression of their disease.

References

Drance SM. Low-tension glaucoma, enigma and opportunity. Arch Ophthalmol 1985; 103:1131–1133.

Epstein DL. Low tension glaucoma. In: Epstein DL, Allingham RR, Schuman JS, eds. Chandler and Grant's glaucoma. 4th ed. Baltimore: Williams & Wilkins, 1997: 199–211.

Grosskreutz CL, Netland PA. Low-tension glaucoma. Int Ophthalmol Clinics 1994; 34:173–185.

Netland PA. Low-tension glaucoma. Mediguide Ophthalmol 1997; 7:1–6.

Werner EB. Normal-tension glaucoma. In: Ritch R, Shields MB, Krupin T, eds. The glaucomas. 2nd ed. St Louis: Mosby, 1996: 769–797.

Patient with OPTIC NERVE CUPPING OR VISUAL FIELD LOSS

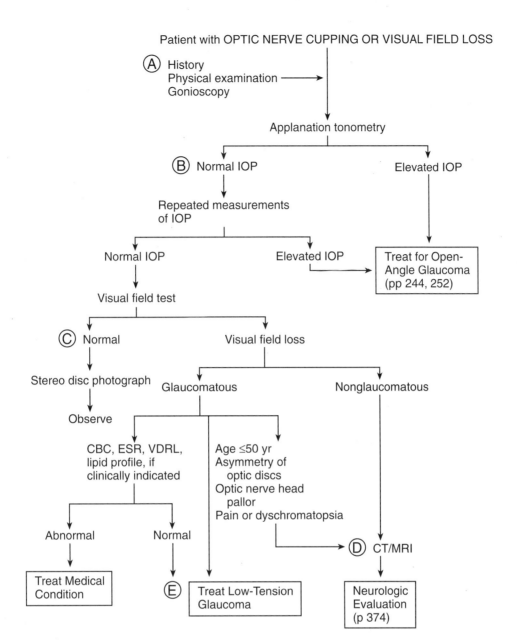

NEOVASCULARIZATION OF THE IRIS

Scott D. Smith, M.D., M.P.H.
Roy Whitaker Jr., M.D.
W.A.J. van Heuven, M.D.

The presence of abnormal vessels on or within the iris is called *neovascularization of the iris (NVI)* or *rubeosis iridis.* In lightly pigmented irides, normal iris vessels are sometimes visible and can be clearly distinguished from iris neovascularization because normal vessels radiate out from the pupillary margin and do not extend into the anterior chamber angle. With iris fluorescein angiography, normal vessels do not leak. Because NVI is generally caused by ocular ischemia, local and systemic conditions that may result in ischemia should be sought.

A. When NVI is present, gonioscopy is required to determine whether the neovascularization involves the anterior chamber angle. A dilated fundus examination after gonioscopy often identifies causes of ocular ischemia. Once the cause of ocular ischemia is identified, appropriate treatment can be instituted.

B. If the fundus examination is normal, consider extraocular causes of ischemia and evaluate the carotid arteries and heart. The presence of a carotid bruit is an important clue to the presence of carotid stenosis. However, the absence of a bruit does not rule out carotid stenosis because the low flow state of high-grade stenosis may not produce an audible bruit. Therefore obtain appropriate referral for carotid noninvasive studies regardless of the results of carotid auscultation. Laboratory studies are needed to rule out diabetes, hyperviscosity syndromes, and other hematologic disorders.

C. The fundus examination is important to rule out retinal detachment, malignant melanoma or other intraocular tumors, and retinal vascular disease such as central or branch retinal vein occlusion (CRVO, BRVO). Central and branch retinal artery occlusion (CRAO, BRAO) rarely cause NVI because they tend to produce tissue anoxia rather than hypoxia.

D. When bilateral NVI is present, suspect systemic causes. However, symmetric involvement of the eyes can be often seen, and unilateral involvement is often seen even when a systemic cause is present. If a patient has no known systemic disease that can account for the ocular findings, order the appropriate laboratory tests. When common conditions such as diabetes have been ruled out, obtain further tests such as a CBC, serum lipid studies, and hemoglobin and protein electrophoresis.

E. When gonioscopy shows an open angle with no vessels, the results of dilated fundus examination determine the appropriate treatment. In diabetic patients without retinopathy or with mild nonproliferative retinopathy, fluorescein angiography may reveal areas of retinal ischemia not visualized clinically. If no retinal ischemia is present, consider other potential causes of NVI. Careful observation with an initial follow-up after several weeks is needed to prevent undetected progression to neovascular glaucoma. When proliferative diabetic retinopathy or retinal vascular occlusion are present, prompt panretinal photocoagulation (PRP) is required. Regression of NVI on follow-up examination confirms that photocoagulation has been adequate.

F. When gonioscopy shows an open angle with neovascularization, urgent PRP is indicated in an effort to prevent progressive synechial angle closure. Goniophotocoagulation (GPC) of the angle vessels may be considered to reduce the risk of synechiae formation while awaiting a response to PRP. If the intraocular pressure (IOP) is elevated, medical treatment with drugs that suppress aqueous production may be required. Effective medications include topical β blockers, α$_2$-adrenergic agents, and topical or systemic carbonic anhydrase inhibitors (CAIs).

G. When synechial angle closure has already developed, the IOP is usually elevated and corneal edema is often present, which limits the ability to perform adequate PRP. Medical therapy, including β blockers, α$_2$ agonists, CAIs, topical steroids, and cycloplegia, is often effective. However, hyperosmotic agents are often needed to adequately reduce the IOP and improve corneal clarity. Perform PRP promptly after medical therapy. If persistent corneal opacity or vitreous hemorrhage is present, PRP may not be possible and peripheral retinal cryopexy may be necessary. Because neovascular glaucoma can often be refractory to medical treatment, surgical intervention is often necessary. The choice of an appropriate procedure is influenced by the potential for recovery of useful vision, based on optic nerve and retinal examination. When visual potential is limited, laser cyclophotocoagulation may be preferable to filtration surgery. The success of trabeculectomy for neovascular glaucoma is substantially lower than that for most other glaucoma subtypes. As a result, adjunctive mitomycin-C is often necessary to increase the probability of a successful outcome. Because of the substantial risk of hyphema after surgery and the limited success even when antimetabolites are used, some specialists prefer tube implant surgery when active NVI is present. With either procedure, the risk of choroidal effusion and shallow anterior chamber are higher than usual when PRP has been recently performed or when ocular inflammation is present at the time of surgery. As a result, it is preferable to delay surgery for up to 3–4 weeks unless unacceptable IOP elevation persists despite medical therapy. When vitreous hemorrhage is present, vitrectomy with endolaser to the retina and ciliary processes can be effective in aphakic or pseudophakic eyes. Early recognition of NVI is important so that the development of neovascular glaucoma can be prevented.

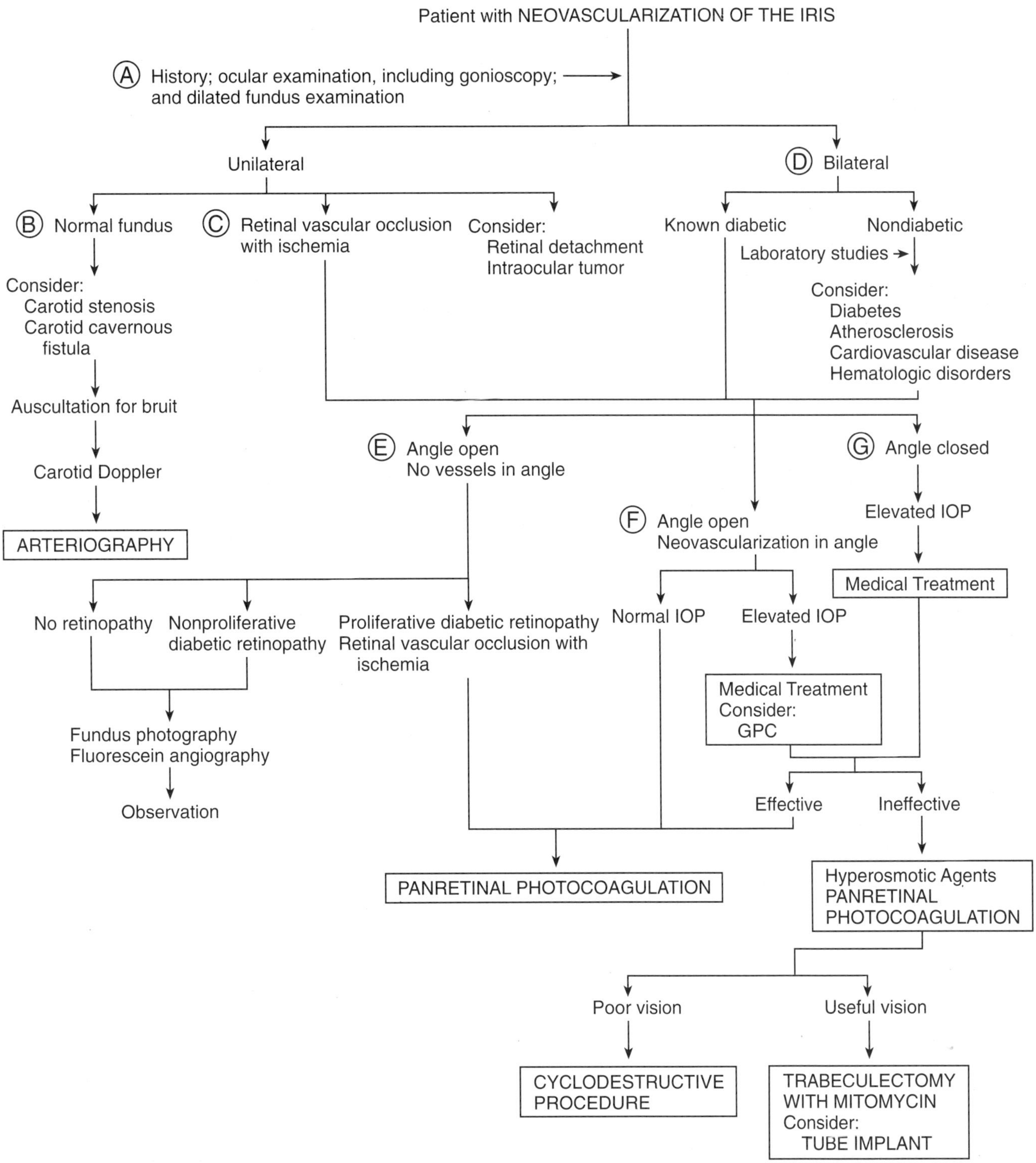

Patient with NEOVASCULARIZATION OF THE IRIS

(A) History; ocular examination, including gonioscopy; and dilated fundus examination

Unilateral

(D) Bilateral

(B) Normal fundus

(C) Retinal vascular occlusion with ischemia

Consider:
Retinal detachment
Intraocular tumor

Known diabetic

Nondiabetic

Laboratory studies →

Consider:
Carotid stenosis
Carotid cavernous
fistula

Consider:
Diabetes
Atherosclerosis
Cardiovascular disease
Hematologic disorders

Auscultation for bruit

Carotid Doppler

(E) Angle open
No vessels in angle

(G) Angle closed

Elevated IOP

ARTERIOGRAPHY

(F) Angle open
Neovascularization in angle

Medical Treatment

No retinopathy Nonproliferative diabetic retinopathy

Proliferative diabetic retinopathy
Retinal vascular occlusion with ischemia

Normal IOP Elevated IOP

Fundus photography
Fluorescein angiography

Medical Treatment
Consider:
GPC

Observation

Effective Ineffective

PANRETINAL PHOTOCOAGULATION

Hyperosmotic Agents
PANRETINAL
PHOTOCOAGULATION

Poor vision Useful vision

CYCLODESTRUCTIVE
PROCEDURE

TRABECULECTOMY
WITH MITOMYCIN
Consider:
TUBE IMPLANT

References

Diabetic Retinopathy Study Research Group. Photocoagulation treatment of proliferative diabetic retinopathy: The second report of the Diabetic Retinopathy Study findings. Am J Ophthalmol 1978; 85:82–106.

Laatikainen L. Development and classification of rubeosis iridis in diabetic eye disease. Br J Ophthalmol 1979; 63:150–156.

Ward M. Neovascular glaucoma. In: Ritch R, Shields MB, Krupin T, eds. The glaucomas. St Louis: Mosby, 1996:1073–1129.

Ward M, Dueker DR, Aiello LM, Grant WM. Effects of panretinal photocoagulation on rubeosis iridis, angle neovascularization and neovascular glaucoma. Am J Ophthalmol 1978; 86:332–339.

ENLARGED EPISCLERAL VEINS

J. Kevin McKinney, M.D.
Roy Whitaker Jr., M.D.

Enlarged episcleral veins may result from a variety of ocular and nonocular conditions, many involving venous obstruction or an abnormal arteriovenous connection. These cases can present diagnostic challenges and a detailed evaluation is often necessary to elucidate the underlying disorder. The ophthalmologist should be familiar with the spectrum of these conditions because many are associated with significant morbidity and may require comanagement with an internist, oncologist, neuroradiologist, or neurosurgeon.

A. Careful examination should differentiate between superficial and deep vascular engorgement. Conjunctival vessels are freely moveable with a cotton-tipped applicator and will blanch with topical phenylephrine, whereas deeper episcleral vessels have neither of these characteristics.

B. Elevated episcleral venous pressure (EVP) can occur in most of the conditions listed and is usually associated with dilated and tortuous episcleral veins and elevated intraocular pressure (IOP). Measurement of the EVP can be confirmatory, but the diagnosis is usually made based on clinical suspicion in the proper clinical setting, especially if blood is noted in Schlemm's canal on gonioscopy. A commercial venomanometer is available for measuring EVP but is not in widespread use. The normal EVP is from 9–12 mm Hg.

C. Elevated EVP decreases aqueous outflow, elevating the IOP and most commonly causing an open-angle glaucoma. Standard medical therapy may be beneficial, although it is unlikely to lower IOP below the level of EVP. Surgical therapy is more definitive but carries increased risk of intraoperative hemorrhage and choroidal effusions (prophylactic sclerotomies may prevent effusions). Indirect effects of elevated EVP may cause other forms of glaucoma. If elevated EVP involves the vortex vein system, resultant choroidal congestion and detachment may cause angle closure (best managed with cycloplegia and hyperosmotic agents). Venous obstruction may lead to ocular ischemia or a central retinal vein occlusion with subsequent neovascular glaucoma. If severe, orbital congestion may raise the IOP through compression of the globe.

D. Glaucoma accompanies Sturge-Weber syndrome 30% of the time. The adult glaucoma is often associated with elevated EVP, whereas the infantile form more likely results from an angle malformation. Pseudoproptosis may occur in the infantile form as a result of unilateral globe enlargement (buphthalmos).

E. Idiopathic elevated EVP is a diagnosis of exclusion to be considered only after ruling out more serious causes of elevated EVP. It occurs in sporadic and familial forms.

F. A classification based on the presence, laterality, and chronicity of proptosis cannot be followed rigidly given the variability of biologic systems. For example, carotid-cavernous fistulas are almost exclusively unilateral but may cause bilateral proptosis. Conversely, thyroid ophthalmopathy is usually bilateral but may manifest very asymmetrically. With regard to chronicity, an orbital varix typically causes intermittent proptosis but may present acutely with thrombosis. Clinical suspicion must remain high in the appropriate clinical setting.

G. Unilateral or significantly asymmetric proptosis with enlarged episcleral veins commonly results from abnormal arteriovenous connections. Carotid cavernous fistulas tend to follow severe head trauma, usually in young adults. This direct, high-flow arteriovenous fistula results in pulsatile proptosis, chemosis, restricted motility, ocular or temporal bruits, elevated IOP, and ocular ischemia. Visual loss occurs in up to 50% of patients. In contrast, dural shunts are characterized by spontaneous, low-flow fistulas in middle-aged to elderly individuals. The proptosis is mild and nonpulsatile, although the ocular pulse amplitude is often increased as measured by pneumotonometry or Goldmann applanation tonometry. These shunts may close spontaneously or after angiography, with a resultant decrease in IOP. Orbital varices may be congenital or acquired. Intermittent proptosis occurs with any maneuver increasing venous pressure, such as sneezing and the Valsalva maneuver, and may be associated with blurred vision and pain. A small proportion of individuals lose vision permanently because of repeated optic nerve damage.

H. Bilateral proptosis with enlarged episcleral veins most commonly indicates venous obstruction associated with a systemic condition. Cavernous sinus thrombosis is a life-threatening emergency that requires immediate IV antibiotics. Superior vena cava syndrome may also present acutely and suggests the presence of a mediastinal malignancy. Thyroid ophthalmopathy (Graves' disease) may cause glaucoma by elevated EVP or by progressive restriction of the extraocular muscles and orbital congestion. Obtain the appropriate consultations to assist in the systemic evaluation and management of these conditions.

I. The finding of proptosis mandates a careful search for its cause. Although thyroid ophthalmopathy is a clinical diagnosis, a thyroid panel may be confirmatory and will provide information for managing a dysthyroid state. Orbital ultrasound, CT, and MRI may demonstrate mass lesions, as well as enlargement of orbital vessels, extraocular muscles, and the cavernous sinus. Color Doppler imaging is a noninvasive technique to

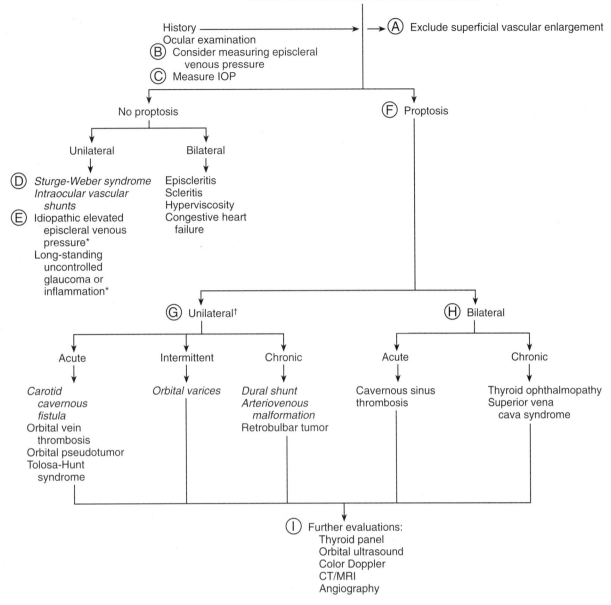

Patient with ENLARGED EPISCLERAL VEINS

History ──────────────────→ (A) Exclude superficial vascular enlargement
Ocular examination
(B) Consider measuring episcleral
    venous pressure
(C) Measure IOP

No proptosis   (F) Proptosis

Unilateral   Bilateral

(D) *Sturge-Weber syndrome*   Episcleritis
    Intraocular vascular   Scleritis
    shunts   Hyperviscosity
(E) Idiopathic elevated   Congestive heart
    episcleral venous   failure
    pressure*
    Long-standing
    uncontrolled
    glaucoma or
    inflammation*

(G) Unilateral†   (H) Bilateral

Acute   Intermittent   Chronic   Acute   Chronic

Carotid   *Orbital varices* *Dural shunt*   Cavernous sinus   Thyroid ophthalmopathy
cavernous   *Arteriovenous* thrombosis   Superior vena
fistula   *malformation*   cava syndrome
Orbital vein   Retrobulbar tumor
   thrombosis
Orbital pseudotumor
Tolosa-Hunt
   syndrome

(I) Further evaluations:
    Thyroid panel
    Orbital ultrasound
    Color Doppler
    CT/MRI
    Angiography

*With the exception of these entities, the following apply: *Italicized type*, abnormal arteriovenous
 connections; normal type, venous obstruction.
†Includes significantly asymmetric proptosis.

evaluate the direction and speed of blood flow, but high-resolution angiography is still the gold standard for evaluation of possible arteriovenous malformations and fistulas.

References

Fiore PM, Latina MA, Shingleton BJ, et al. The dural shunt syndrome: I. Management of glaucoma. Ophthalmology 1990; 97:56–62.

Higginbotham EJ. Glaucoma associated with increased episcleral venous pressure. In: Albert DM, Jakobiec FA, eds. Principles and practice of ophthalmology. Philadelphia: WB Saunders, 1994: 1467–1479.

Watson P. Diseases of the sclera and episclera. In: Tasman W, Jaeger EA, eds. Duane's clinical ophthalmology. Philadelphia: Lippincott-Raven, 1995; 4:1–45.

Weinreb RN, Karwatowski WSS. Glaucoma associated with elevated episcleral venous pressure. In: Ritch R, Shields MB, Krupin T, eds. The glaucomas. St Louis: Mosby: 1996: 1143–1155.

Zeimer RC, Gieser DK, Wilensky JT, et al. A practical venomanometer: Measurement of episcleral venous pressure and assessment of the normal range. Arch Ophthalmol 1983; 101:1447–1449.

SURGICAL TREATMENT OF MEDICALLY UNCONTROLLED PRIMARY OPEN-ANGLE GLAUCOMA

Scott D. Smith, M.D., M.P.H.
John M. Parkinson, M.D.

A. Primary open-angle glaucoma is considered medically uncontrolled when, despite maximum tolerated medical therapy, progressive damage occurs (documented by changes in serial disc photographs and/or visual fields) or is likely to occur (based on the clinical experience of the physician). Examination of the optic nerve by biomicroscopy and serial photography must include contour changes, as well as changes in vessel position and disc color. Progressive visual field deterioration must be differentiated from change from other causes (e.g., cataract, retinal degeneration) and from intertest variability. SWAP (short-wave automatic perimetry/blue-yellow perimetry) may detect field loss or progression several years before standard perimetry.

B. Knowledge of intraocular pressure (IOP) levels before initiation of therapy (pressure levels at which damage presumably occurred) helps determine a target pressure (30%–50% reduction) below which further damage is unlikely. The target pressure should be adjusted lower in view of a younger patient's age, degree of glaucomatous damage, or signs of ongoing damage (disc changes, hemorrhage, or progressive field loss).

C. Because of its low complication rate compared with traditional filtering surgery, argon laser trabeculoplasty should usually be attempted as a first step in surgical therapy. After treatment, monitor the IOP to determine the efficacy of treatment in achieving the target pressure. The maximal treatment effect may not be observed for 4–6 weeks after the procedure. Topical α agonists can be used before and immediately after laser trabeculoplasty to reduce the incidence of postlaser IOP spikes. In cases in which the IOP is extremely elevated and an urgent threat to vision is present or when an extremely low target IOP is required because of advanced disc damage, it may be appropriate to proceed directly to filtering surgery.

D. The decision to use adjunctive mitomycin-C is based on the risk of failure of standard filtering surgery and on the desired target pressure. When conjunctival scarring is present from previous ocular surgery, when trabeculectomy without an adjunctive antimetabolite has already failed, or when a postoperative IOP <10–12 mm Hg is desired, adjunctive mitomycin-C may be required. Careful consideration of the potential benefit of mitomycin-C is necessary for each patient, given the evidence of an increased risk of persistent hypotony, cataract, and late bleb leak, particularly when higher dosages are used. Lower concentrations of mitomycin-C (0.2–0.25 mg/ml) and shorter application times (1–3 minutes) have reduced the incidence of postoperative complications. Adjunctive 5-fluorouracil may not be as effective as mitomycin-C, requires multiple postoperative injections, and can lead to corneal epithelial toxicity. However, the dosage can be tailored to the individual patient based on the postoperative inflammatory response, and the risks of hypotony and other complications may be less than with mitomycin.

E. Procedures to reduce elevated IOP after glaucoma filtration surgery are most effective if performed within the first few weeks of surgery. Slit-lamp examination and gonioscopy help determine the cause of diminished outflow. Internal obstruction of the sclerostomy with pigment or membranes can be treated with the argon or YAG laser. If outflow is restricted externally, laser lysis of trabeculectomy flap sutures combined with digital pressure, steroids, or adjunctive 5-FU can be beneficial. If elevated IOP persists, resumption of medical therapy is required.

F. Encapsulation of the filtering bleb often responds to conservative treatment, including aqueous suppression and digital massage. Steroid use is controversial; some authors advocate continuation, and others their discontinuation. When these measures fail to result in an adequate level of IOP control, bleb needling to incise the tissue surrounding the trabeculectomy flap may give good long-term results. Adjunctive 5-FU after bleb needling may increase the probability of success. Surgical revision of an encapsulated bleb is occasionally necessary when the IOP remains uncontrolled or in cases of secondary dellen unresponsive to medical therapy.

G. If a scarred, flat bleb results from primary surgery, perform a second filtering operation in an unoperated quadrant using adjunctive mitomycin-C. When remaining free conjunctiva is limited, a glaucoma drainage implant may be necessary. Because of complications of visual loss and phthisis, ciliodestructive procedures such as cyclocryotherapy have traditionally been reserved for end-stage cases without potential for central vision. Laser transscleral cyclophotocoagulation appears to be safer than cyclocryotherapy and may be a reasonable alternative for the treatment of eyes with refractory glaucoma with or without central vision.

H. If the target IOP is attained after surgical intervention, visual fields and optic nerve status must be carefully monitored to rule out ongoing damage. If progressive damage occurs, a new, lower target pressure must be chosen and therapy adjusted accordingly.

Patient with MEDICALLY UNCONTROLLED PRIMARY OPEN-ANGLE GLAUCOMA

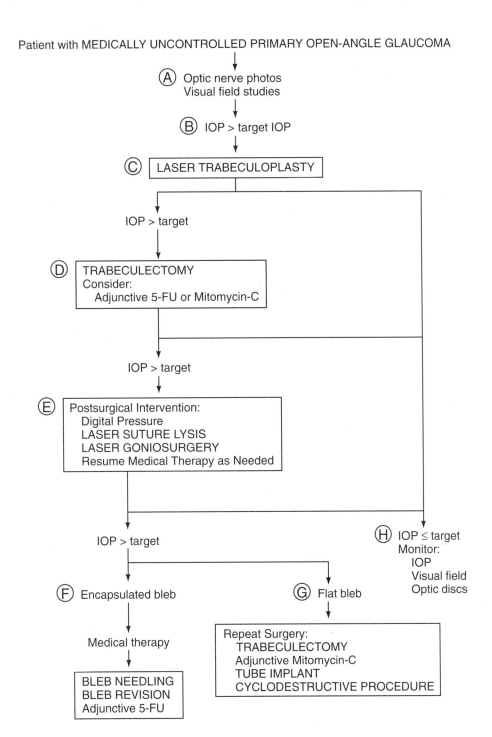

References

Hoskins HD Jr, Kass MA. Becker-Shaffer's diagnosis and therapy of the glaucomas. 6th ed. St Louis: Mosby, 1989: 288–301.

Kosoko O, Gaasterland DE, Pollack IP, Enger CL. Long-term outcome of initial ciliary ablation with contact diode laser transscleral cyclophotocoagulation for severe glaucoma. Ophthalmology 1996; 103:1294–1302.

Pederson JE, Smigh SG. Surgical management of encapsulated filtering blebs. Ophthalmology 1985; 92:956–958.

Price FW, Wellemeyer M. Long-term results of Molteno implants. Ophthalmic Surg 1995; 26:130–135.

Robin AL, Ramakrishnan R, Bhatnagar R, et al. A long-term dose-response study of mitomycin in glaucoma filtration surgery. Arch Ophthalmol 1997; 115:969–974.

Scott DR, Quigley HA. Medical management of the high bleb phase after trabeculectomy. Ophthalmology 1988; 95: 1169–1173.

Shingleton BJ, Richter CU, Dharma SK. Long-term efficacy of argon laser trabeculoplasty: A 10 year follow-up study. Ophthalmology 1993; 100:1324–1329.

SHALLOW ANTERIOR CHAMBER AFTER GLAUCOMA SURGERY

J. Kevin McKinney, M.D.
Roy Whitaker Jr., M.D.

Glaucoma filtration surgery is designed to lower the intraocular pressure (IOP) to a level that prevents progressive visual loss by creating an alternate drainage pathway for the escape of aqueous humor from the anterior chamber (AC). A shallow or flat AC in the early postoperative course implies either excessive escape of aqueous from overfiltration or a wound leak, or posterior pressure on the lens-iris diaphragm from pupillary block, aqueous misdirection, or choroidal hemorrhage. Postoperative shallow chambers after trabeculectomy are less common with the use of adjunctive antimetabolites such as 5-fluorouracil (5-FU) and mitomycin-C because a tighter scleral flap closure is necessary to prevent postoperative hypotony. Recognition of the cause underlying a shallow AC and timely institution of appropriate management are essential to preserving postoperative IOP control and visual function.

A. The AC depth may be unstable for several days after filtration surgery. Both the patient and examiner must avoid excessive pressure on the globe to prevent flattening of the AC. IOP measurement is critical in determining the cause of a shallow AC but must be performed and interpreted with caution. In a very soft eye, applanation IOP is notoriously difficult to measure but can be obtained with accuracy if performed gently with the applanation dial initially set to <10 mm Hg. Folds in Descemet's membrane are a useful slit-lamp indicator of a potentially low IOP. With a flat AC, IOP measurements may be spurious as a result of applanation of the lens or intraocular lens (IOL). Cautious tactile assessment of the IOP is useful in this situation. A careful ocular examination should be performed daily until intraocular conditions stabilize.

B. Iris bombé with a relatively deeper central AC in the absence of a patent iridectomy implies the presence of pupillary block. The AC tends to be diffusely shallow with choroidal hemorrhage and aqueous misdirection (see p 256 for details of evaluation and management of elevated IOP with a shallow AC).

C. When a shallow AC and a low IOP are present, a wound or bleb leak should be excluded by application of topical fluorescein (moistened strip or 2% solution) to the wound and bleb under illumination with a cobalt blue light (Seidel test). A stream of bright yellow-green fluid against the dark background indicates a leak. Such leaks are more common if adjunctive antimetabolites have been used (see p 260 for management of wound leaks).

D. With a low IOP, careful funduscopy and/or B-scan ultrasonography should be used to determine the presence, extent, and nature of choroidal detachment. Although serous choroidal detachment most often results from hypotony, it may also perpetuate hypotony and AC shallowing because of detachment of the ciliary body with aqueous hyposecretion.

E. With a low IOP and no evidence for a wound leak, overfiltration, with or without choroidal detachment, is the most likely cause for a shallow AC. A shallow chamber from overfiltration may be diagnosed by placing a pressure patch for 10–20 minutes or by applying gentle pressure over the scleral flap with a moistened cotton-tipped applicator for 1–2 minutes: deepening of the AC indicates overfiltration. Management varies with the central depth of the AC and the presence or absence of lens-cornea touch.

F. Although prolonged iris-cornea touch may cause some endothelial cell loss and peripheral anterior synechiae (PAS) formation, if the AC depth is greater than or equal to one corneal thickness over the lens, conservative measures are usually adequate until spontaneous deepening occurs. Inflammation should be suppressed with frequent steroids and adequate cycloplegia (atropine) should be maintained to encourage posterior rotation of the ciliary body and hinder PAS formation.

G. A central AC depth of less than one corneal thickness runs the risk of intermittent lens-cornea touch and therefore warrants additional efforts to deepen the AC. Maximal cycloplegia (atropine) and mydriasis (phenylephrine) are indicated and may be initiated as a "burst" of one drop every 5 minutes for three doses. If the AC deepens to one corneal thickness or greater, careful observation is continued. If no effect is observed, various methods of tamponading filtration may be tried. A properly applied pressure patch (particularly a "torpedo" patch) is usually sufficient to deepen the chamber. If the AC shallows again with observation, the patch may be replaced daily for several days until the AC remains deep spontaneously. An oversized soft contact lens may provide sufficient tamponade in some eyes, whereas others may require placement of a Simmons glaucoma shell or symblepharon ring. These devices should be used only by those with skill and experience in their proper placement and management because significant side effects (discomfort, corneal epithelial defects, corneal edema) may occur with their use. Some specialists would recommend use of a hyperosmotic to shrink the vitreous at this point. Caution should be used because these agents carry some risk of potentiating the hypotony and its attendant complications. If the AC remains so shallow that the lens almost touches the cornea, proceed to the measures outlined for lens-cornea touch.

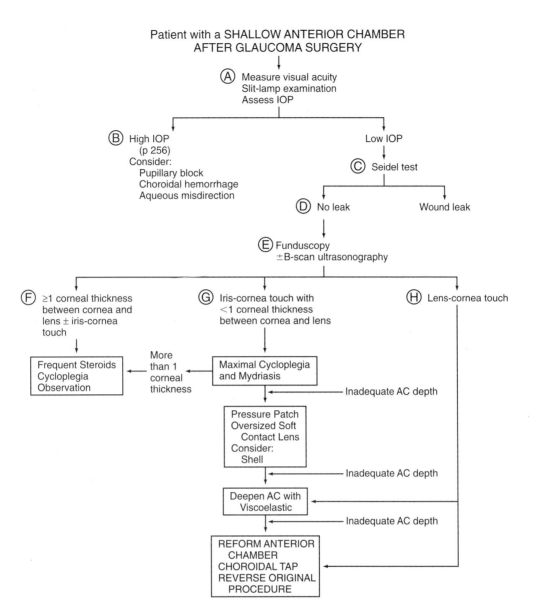

Patient with a SHALLOW ANTERIOR CHAMBER
AFTER GLAUCOMA SURGERY

(A) Measure visual acuity
Slit-lamp examination
Assess IOP

(B) High IOP
(p 256)
Consider:
Pupillary block
Choroidal hemorrhage
Aqueous misdirection

Low IOP

(C) Seidel test

(D) No leak   Wound leak

(E) Funduscopy
±B-scan ultrasonography

(F) ≥1 corneal thickness
between cornea and
lens ± iris-cornea
touch

(G) Iris-cornea touch with
<1 corneal thickness
between cornea and lens

(H) Lens-cornea touch

More
than 1
corneal
thickness

Frequent Steroids
Cycloplegia
Observation

Maximal Cycloplegia
and Mydriasis

Inadequate AC depth

Pressure Patch
Oversized Soft
Contact Lens
Consider:
Shell

Inadequate AC depth

Deepen AC with
Viscoelastic

Inadequate AC depth

REFORM ANTERIOR
CHAMBER
CHOROIDAL TAP
REVERSE ORIGINAL
PROCEDURE

H. Lens-cornea touch mandates immediate intervention because of the high risk of corneal decompensation and cataract formation. A cycloplegic/mydriatic "burst" may be given followed by a temporary pressure patch for a few hours, but continued conservative management is indicated only if the chamber deepens to one corneal thickness or greater. A completely flat chamber after a glaucoma drainage tube implant is a special situation that also may damage the cornea and lens, seldom responds to conservative measures, and usually requires surgical intervention. Deepening of the AC with viscoelastic through a pre-existing or new paracentesis track can cause permanent deepening but may require repeated injections. This may be performed at the slit lamp with instillation of appropriate broad-spectrum antibiotics or 5% povidone iodine drops before the injection. For a more definitive approach, the patient is returned to the operating room so that the AC can be reformed with saline or viscoelastic and so that choroidals can be drained. Occasionally, this procedure must be repeated. If all of the aforementioned measures fail, the original procedure may need to be revised with resuturing of a scleral flap or ligation of a drainage implant tube (using an absorbable suture). Cycloplegia and patching may still prove useful for persistent or recurrent AC shallowing after these procedures.

References

Cioffi GA. Postoperative flat anterior chamber. In: Roy FH, ed. Master techniques in ophthalmic surgery. Baltimore: Williams & Wilkins, 1995: 37–45.

Fourman S. Management of lens-cornea touch after filtering surgery for glaucoma. Ophthalmology 1990; 97:424–428.

Liebermann JM, Ritch R. Complications of glaucoma filtering surgery. In: Ritch R, Shields MB, Krupin T, eds. The glaucomas. St Louis: Mosby, 1996: 1703–1736.

Simmons RJ, Kimbrough RL. Shell tamponade in filtering surgery for glaucoma. Ophthalmic Surg 1979; 10:17–34.

Stewart WC, Shields MD. Management of anterior chamber depth after trabeculectomy. Am J Ophthalmol 1988; 106:41–44.

HIGH INTRAOCULAR PRESSURE AFTER GLAUCOMA FILTRATION SURGERY

John M. Parkinson, M.D.
J. Kevin McKinney, M.D.

A. Careful slit-lamp examination is essential in differentiating causes of elevated intraocular pressure (IOP) after glaucoma filtration surgery. Most commonly, elevated postoperative pressure is associated with a deep anterior chamber (AC) and only mild to moderate discomfort. Bleb appearance can be helpful but must be interpreted in light of other findings. A flat bleb indicates internal or external obstruction of filtration, but an elevated bleb does not rule out partial obstruction.

B. Despite open angles by gonioscopy, the internal sclerostomy may be occluded by iris, iris pigment epithelium, blood, fibrin, or viscoelastic or transparent membranes (inflammatory, proliferative, or residual Descemet's membrane). The argon or YAG laser can be used to reopen the internal sclerostomy. Blood and fibrin clots that occlude the internal sclerostomy often resorb spontaneously. If available, fibrinolytic agents such as tissue plasminogen activator (tPA) or streptokinase may be injected intracamerally to dissolve the clot.

C. In the presence of a patent internal sclerostomy, external factors are responsible for elevated pressure. Within the first few postoperative days, ocular digital pressure may break fibrinous adhesions between the scleral bed and trabeculectomy flap to restore adequate outflow. If elevated IOP persists, serial laser suture lysis (argon, krypton, or diode) of trabeculectomy flap sutures can be performed using a handheld contact lens to compress overlying conjunctiva. If significant external scarring is likely, consider supplemental injections of 5-fluorouracil (5-FU).

D. In the early postoperative period, encapsulation of the filtering bleb (a Tenon's "cyst") may respond to the measures outlined in section C. Failing this, pharmacologic aqueous suppression and intermittent digital massage will often soften the cyst. Refractory IOP elevation may require needling of the cyst or revision of the bleb. A well-defined cyst and supplemental 5-FU enhance the success of these procedures.

E. In the presence of a shallow AC, use funduscopy and B-scan ultrasonography to determine the presence, extent, and nature (serous or hemorrhagic) of choroidal elevation.

F. The presence of choroidal elevation in the face of elevated IOP and shallow or flat anterior chamber usually implies a hemorrhagic cause. In such cases, a history of sudden, severe eye pain is usually obtained.

G. Initial treatment includes maximum cycloplegia (atropine), frequent topical and possibly systemic steroids, and aqueous suppression if the IOP is elevated (β blocker, carbonic anhydrase inhibitor, and/or α agonist). Treat underlying systemic problems (uncontrolled hypertension or bleeding diatheses).

H. After consultation with a vitreoretinal subspecialist, surgical drainage may be performed after waiting 7–10 days to allow the clot to liquefy. Indications for surgical drainage include massive choroidal detachment with decreased visual acuity, corneal decompensation, persistently flat AC, and elevated IOP unresponsive to medical therapy.

I. In the absence of choroidal separation, rule out pupillary block by ensuring the patency of the peripheral iridectomy (PI). In aphakic and pseudophakic eyes, posterior loculation of aqueous may occur despite a patent iridectomy, and another laser PI in the affected quadrant(s) may be curative.

J. A centrally shallow or flat AC in the presence of a patent iridectomy and elevated or normal IOP implies posterior misdirection of aqueous into the vitreous (malignant glaucoma). This may occur as a result of ciliary-lenticular apposition (ciliary block) or may represent misdirection of aqueous behind an intact anterior vitreous face.

K. Medical therapy includes maximal cycloplegia (atropine) and pupillary dilation (phenylephrine), aqueous suppressant therapy (see section F), and hyperosmotic therapy (glycerin, mannitol, or isosorbide). Approximately 50% of cases resolve within 3–5 days with medical therapy. Monitor the patient for electrolyte imbalance and dehydration. Indications for earlier surgical intervention include a persistently flat AC, corneal decompensation, cataract development in phakic eyes, and uncontrolled IOP (depending on the optic nerve status).

L. In patients who do not respond to medical therapy, laser treatment is often effective. In phakic eyes, the argon laser can be applied gonioscopically through the PI or pupil to shrink visible ciliary processes, thus breaking ciliolenticular block. Because of its high success rate in aphakic and pseudophakic eyes, laser treatment may be attempted before a trial of medical therapy in such eyes. In aphakic eyes, YAG laser disruption of the anterior hyaloid face may promote normal anterior flow of aqueous. YAG capsulotomy/hyaloidotomy is often successful in pseudophakic eyes

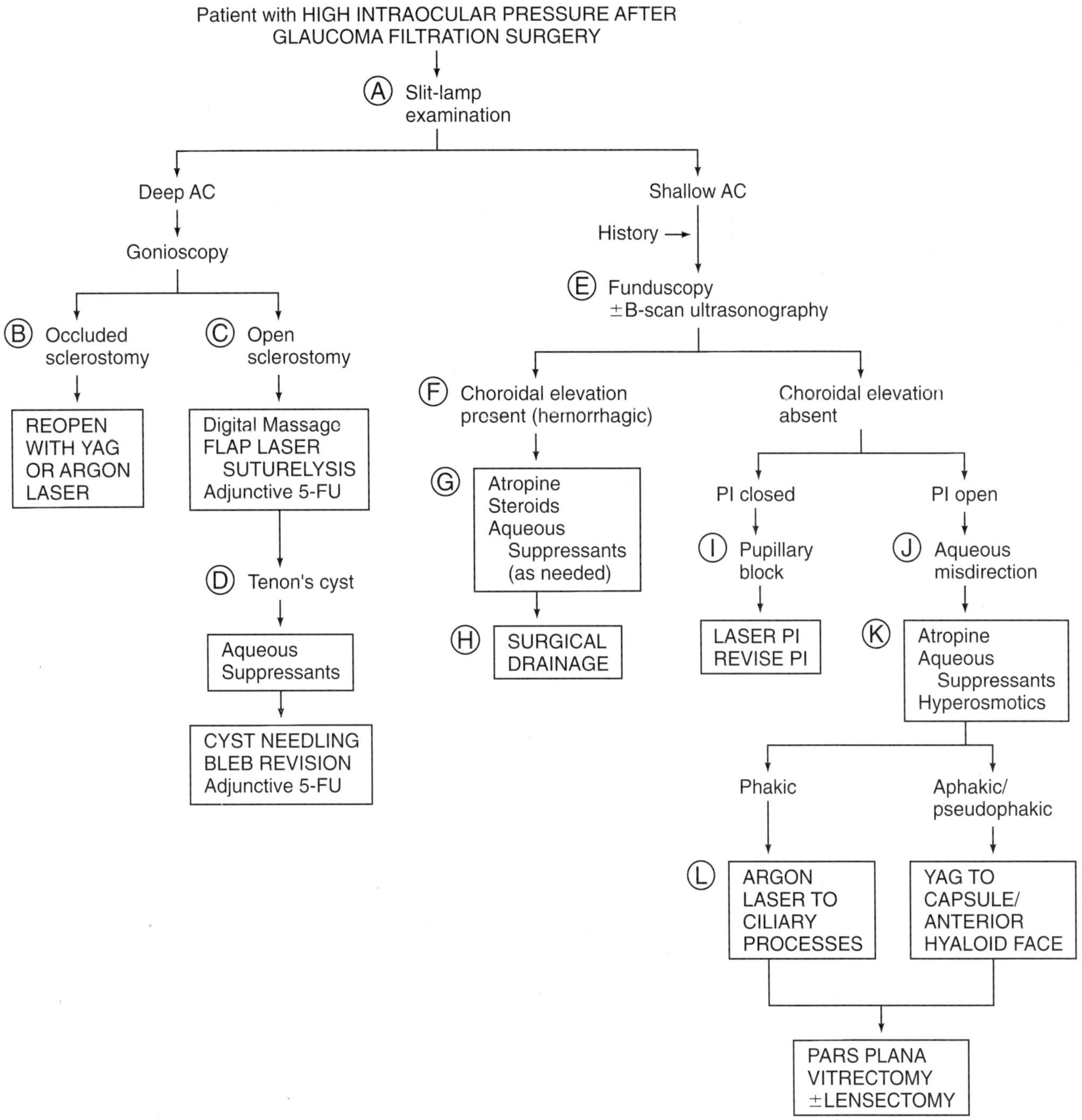

Patient with HIGH INTRAOCULAR PRESSURE AFTER GLAUCOMA FILTRATION SURGERY

Ⓐ Slit-lamp examination

Deep AC

Gonioscopy

Ⓑ Occluded sclerostomy
→ REOPEN WITH YAG OR ARGON LASER

Ⓒ Open sclerostomy
→ Digital Massage FLAP LASER SUTURELYSIS Adjunctive 5-FU

Ⓓ Tenon's cyst
→ Aqueous Suppressants
→ CYST NEEDLING BLEB REVISION Adjunctive 5-FU

Shallow AC

History →

Ⓔ Funduscopy ±B-scan ultrasonography

Ⓕ Choroidal elevation present (hemorrhagic)

Ⓖ Atropine Steroids Aqueous Suppressants (as needed)

Ⓗ SURGICAL DRAINAGE

Choroidal elevation absent

PI closed

Ⓘ Pupillary block
→ LASER PI REVISE PI

PI open

Ⓙ Aqueous misdirection

Ⓚ Atropine Aqueous Suppressants Hyperosmotics

Phakic
Ⓛ ARGON LASER TO CILIARY PROCESSES

Aphakic/ pseudophakic
→ YAG TO CAPSULE/ ANTERIOR HYALOID FACE

→ PARS PLANA VITRECTOMY ±LENSECTOMY

and is best performed beyond the edge of the optic. In refractory cases, pars plana vitrectomy with disruption of the anterior hyaloid is indicated and lensectomy may be necessary in phakic eyes.

References

Lundy DC, Sidoti P, Winarko T, et al. Intracameral tissue plasminogen activator after glaucoma surgery. Ophthalmology 1996; 103:274–282.

Pederson JE, Smith SG. Surgical management of encapsulated filtering blebs. Ophthalmology 1985; 92:955–958.

Simmons RJ, Maestre FA. Malignant glaucoma. In: Ritch R, Shields MB, Krupin T, eds. The glaucomas. St Louis: Mosby, 1996: 841–855.

Stamper RL. Elevated intraocular pressure after filtering surgery. In: Roy FH, ed. Master techniques in ophthalmic surgery. Baltimore: Williams & Wilkins, 1995: 629–638.

THE GLAUCOMA PATIENT WITH CATARACT

Peter A. Netland, M.D., Ph.D.

Both cataract and glaucoma may coexist in the same individual, especially in older patients. Management of the glaucoma patient often requires consideration of surgical treatment of cataract. In patients with well-controlled intraocular pressure (IOP) or early glaucoma, cataract surgery alone may be effective. In patients with advanced glaucoma or poor control of IOP, combining trabeculectomy with cataract extraction and intraocular lens implantation in one operation may be the preferred option.

A. The evaluation of a patient with glaucoma and cataract should include a careful history and a complete ophthalmic examination. The history includes questions about the onset and time course of visual loss, current medications, previous eye history, and any systemic illnesses. Examination includes assessment of the best corrected vision, with optimal refraction. Visual acuity testing in high- and low-contrast settings may be performed, as well as potential acuity testing. IOP measurement and visual field analysis are obtained. The surgeon's view into the eye should correspond to the patient's symptoms. In patients in whom media opacity caused by cataract precludes examination of the fundus, ultrasonography may be required. Assessment of the pupil size after dilation may help the surgeon plan for intraoperative management of small pupil.

B. In the glaucoma patient with a cataractous lens, there are several indications for surgical cataract extraction. First, cataract surgery is indicated when decreased visual acuity causes limitation of the patient's ability to function in daily activities, including employment, reading, writing, driving, or recreation. Second, surgery may benefit the patient when cataract precludes diagnosis and/or treatment of other eye disease, such as diabetic retinopathy. Third, cataract extraction is necessary when there are actual or impending complications of lens-induced ocular disease, such as phacolytic and phacomorphic glaucoma.

C. In patients who require cataract surgery who have had successful filtration surgery in the past, cataract surgery may be performed from the side or below, away from the filtration site. Phacoemulsification with small incisions is well suited to this procedure because there is minimal damage to the conjunctiva. Clear cornea incisions may be helpful in altogether avoiding conjunctival incisions.

D. Glaucoma filtering surgery is indicated in patients with glaucoma that is not adequately controlled by medications. Glaucoma patients with cataract and with a history of borderline or difficult glaucoma may also benefit from filtration surgery performed at the time of cataract surgery. This is a poorly delineated category, which some surgeons define on the basis of the number of medications required for control of IOP. According to this approach, a filter is performed in patients requiring two or more medications for control of glaucoma. Patients with low-tension glaucoma may require several medications to maintain a low target IOP and may benefit from filtration surgery performed at the time of cataract extraction. In other glaucoma patients with cataract, the IOP may be controlled with medications, but the patient may have moderate to advanced glaucomatous cupping and/or visual field loss. In these patients, in addition to the potential for long-term control of IOP, filtration surgery may avoid the risk of an early postoperative increase in IOP. Postoperative elevation of IOP may occur after cataract extraction alone and may further damage the already compromised optic nerve in patients with moderate to advanced glaucoma.

E. Combined cataract extraction and filtering surgery may benefit patients with significant cataract and moderate to advanced glaucoma and/or IOP that is poorly controlled or uncontrolled by medications. When there is an urgent need to reduce the IOP, some surgeons advocate a two-stage approach, with filtration surgery performed first, followed later by cataract extraction. However, the two-stage approach is rarely necessary because of the improvements of techniques for combined surgery. Small-incision phacoemulsification combined with trabeculectomy theoretically minimizes astigmatism and conjunctival scarring and may reduce the frequency and duration of wound leaks. With foldable lenses, the entire combined procedure can be carried out through the standard trabeculectomy flap. Antifibrosis agents may improve the success of combined cataract and filtration surgery. Mitomycin C may be administered as a single intraoperative dose, or 5-fluorouracil may be administered postoperatively.

Small pupils are commonly encountered in glaucoma patients and may be surgically enlarged during cataract surgery. Adequate pupil size enhances visualization and reduces the incidence of intraoperative complications during cataract extraction. Synechialysis and stretch pupilloplasty, to gently stretch the iris sphincter, will often yield a suitable pupillary aperture. Sector or keyhole iridectomy is not optimal for several reasons: the pupil is cosmetically deformed, aspiration of the cut ends of iris may interfere with phacoemulsification, and visualization often remains poor in the area away from the sector iridectomy. Small iris sphincterotomies with subsequent stretching of the sphincter is a useful option. Various elegant iris suturing techniques have been described, but these often require considerable effort and operating time. Iris hook retractors can be helpful, particularly in enlarging very small pupils to an adequate size to perform phacoemulsification. The protective iris expander ring

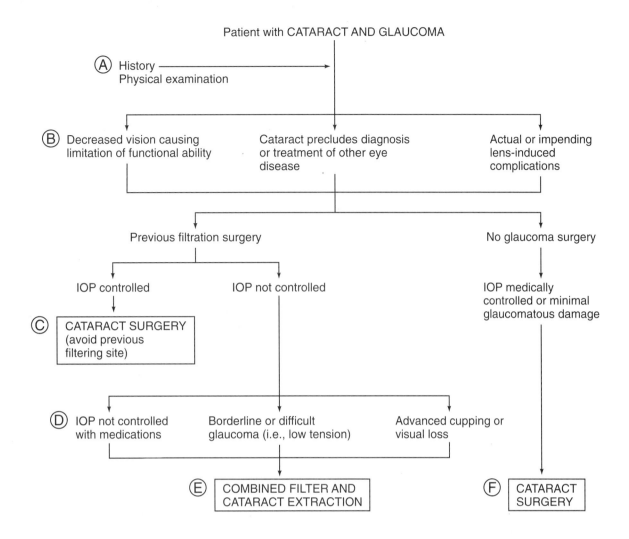

Patient with CATARACT AND GLAUCOMA

Ⓐ History ——————————→
Physical examination

Ⓑ Decreased vision causing
limitation of functional ability

Cataract precludes diagnosis
or treatment of other eye
disease

Actual or impending
lens-induced
complications

Previous filtration surgery

No glaucoma surgery

IOP controlled

IOP not controlled

IOP medically
controlled or minimal
glaucomatous damage

Ⓒ CATARACT SURGERY
(avoid previous
filtering site)

Ⓓ IOP not controlled
with medications

Borderline or difficult
glaucoma (i.e., low tension)

Advanced cupping or
visual loss

Ⓔ COMBINED FILTER AND
CATARACT EXTRACTION

Ⓕ CATARACT
SURGERY

is an appliance that can be placed in the eye during surgery to expand the pupil.

F. Eyes with cataract and glaucoma with mild disc damage and control of IOP with one or two medications can be considered for cataract extraction alone. Cataract surgery alone is technically simpler and is associated with fewer complications than combined cataract extraction and glaucoma filtration procedures. In patients who do not require trabeculectomy, clear cornea incisions are useful because they preserve the conjunctiva for later filtration surgery, if necessary. When limbal peritomy is performed, incisions should ideally be restricted to one quadrant to preserve areas for possible subsequent filtration surgery. Scar formation is minimized, and thus filtration surgery at a later date is facilitated following small incision phacoemulsification compared with extracapsular cataract extraction. In patients with dense cataracts, intraoperative assessment of the optic nerve may be necessary to determine whether the eye has minimal optic nerve damage and may be treated with cataract surgery alone or whether it has extensive optic nerve damage and should be treated with combined cataract and filtration surgery.

References

Cashwell LF, Shields MB. Surgical management of coexisting cataract and glaucoma. In: Ritch R, Shields MB, Krupin T, eds. The glaucomas. 2nd ed. St Louis: Mosby, 1996: 1745–1759.

Cohen JS, Greff LJ, Novack GD, Wind BE. A placebo-controlled, double-masked evaluation of mitomycin C in combined glaucoma and cataract procedures. Ophthalmology 1996; 103:1934–1942.

Nelson DB, Donnenfeld ED. Small-pupil phacoemulsification and trabeculectomy. Int Ophthalmol Clin 1994; 34:131–144.

Schuman JS. The management of coexisting cataract and glaucoma. In: Epstein DL, Allingham RR, Schuman JS, eds. Chandler and Grant's glaucoma. 4th ed. Baltimore: Williams & Wilkins, 1997: 551–564.

Shields MB. Another reevaluation of combined cataract and glaucoma surgery. Am J Ophthalmol 1993; 115:806–811.

OCULAR HYPOTONY

John M. Parkinson, M.D.
J. Kevin McKinney, M.D., M.P.H.

An intraocular pressure (IOP) <6.5 mm Hg is statistically defined as ocular hypotony. However, visually significant sequelae are most common with an IOP <4 mm Hg. These sequelae include corneal folds, serous ciliochoroidal detachment, optic disc swelling, hypotony maculopathy, cataract, and phthisis bulbi. Timely diagnosis and treatment of ocular hypotony is critical to restoration and preservation of vision.

A. A detailed history is essential in determining the cause and proper treatment of ocular hypotony. Most cases of persistent hypotony follow ocular trauma or intraocular surgery. Ocular medications used for the affected or fellow eye may cause or potentiate hypotony (especially systemic carbonic anhydrase inhibitors and topical β blockers). Symptoms of uveitis (decreased vision, photophobia, discomfort) and retinal detachment (flashing lights, curtain or veil-like field loss) should be sought.

B. Uveitis may lead to hypotony through decreased aqueous production and increased uveoscleral outflow. The hypotony is usually mild in acute anterior uveitis, but chronic inflammation with a cyclitic membrane may result in profound and intractable hypotony. Treatment of the hypotony is aimed at control of inflammation with topical steroids and occasionally periocular and systemic steroids. Cycloplegic agents reduce discomfort from ciliary spasm and decrease formation of posterior synechiae.

C. Wound leaks may occur after any form of intraocular surgery or penetrating ocular trauma. The source of the leakage is best identified by the application of fluorescein dye to the wound (Seidel's test, using a moist fluorescein strip) under illumination with cobalt blue light. Light ocular digital pressure may be required to demonstrate leakage in profoundly hypotonous eyes. A wound leak beneath intact conjunctiva may produce an inadvertent filtering bleb, suggested by subconjunctival fluid and conjunctival "microcysts." Posterior wounds such as scleral rupture from blunt ocular trauma and inadvertent scleral perforation from retrobulbar needles and bridle sutures should be kept in mind as less obvious causes of hypotony.

D. Depending on the size and location of the leak, aqueous suppression (β blocker, carbonic anhydrase inhibitor, and/or α₂ agonist), and pressure patching may be adequate. Decreasing the frequency of topical anti-inflammatory medications may promote healing of the wound. Tamponade with a soft contact lens or scleral shell and gluing with a tissue adhesive (cyanoacrylate or fibrin) often work when conservative measures fail. A subconjunctival injection of autologous blood may promote closure of an inadvertent bleb. Large or persistent leaks are most effectively repaired surgically. Wound leaks and conjunctival buttonholes seen after glaucoma filtration surgery often require direct suture closure, especially if antimetabolites (5-fluorouracil [5-FU] or mitomycin C) were used. Significant elevation of IOP may follow closure of the leak, but the IOP usually normalizes as the trabecular meshwork recovers function.

E. Cyclodialysis clefts most commonly occur as a result of trauma or iris manipulation during intraocular surgery. The size of the cleft does not correlate with the degree of hypotony. Diagnosis is made after careful gonioscopy, although ultrasound biomicroscopy is a new alternative technique that allows precise, noninvasive localization of clefts. When gonioscopy is difficult because of hypotony and chronic corneal changes, the diagnosis is often presumed after other causes of hypotony have been excluded. Cycloplegic agents alone may close the cleft, but persistent cases require laser photocoagulation of the cleft or cryotherapy applied over the cleft. In refractory cases, direct suturing (cyclopexy) of the cleft is often successful. Closure of the cleft may be associated with a dramatic increase in IOP that lasts days to weeks.

F. Retinal detachment must be excluded in any case of unexplained ocular hypotony. The exact mechanism of decreased IOP is undetermined but may involve one or more of the following: reduced aqueous production, increased uveoscleral outflow, or posterior flow of fluid through the retinal break and across the retinal pigment epithelium. The extent of the detachment does not correlate with the degree of hypotony. Surgical repair is indicated.

G. Many "idiopathic" cases of chronic hypotony are caused by occult cyclodialysis clefts. These may be obscured by peripheral anterior synechiae. Detection of the cleft can be improved by gonioscopy after deepening of the anterior chamber with a viscoelastic agent (photocoagulation can be applied at the same time). After injection of fluorescein into the anterior chamber, recovery of fluorescein-stained fluid from a sclerostomy over the ciliary body confirms the diagnosis of an occult cleft. If no cleft is identified, drainage of suprachoroidal fluid may lead to improvement in "idiopathic" hypotony.

References

Dreyer EB, Aquino MA. Cyclodialysis cleft in anterior chamber area. In: Roy FH, ed. Master techniques in ophthalmic surgery. Baltimore: Williams & Wilkins, 1995: 3–8.

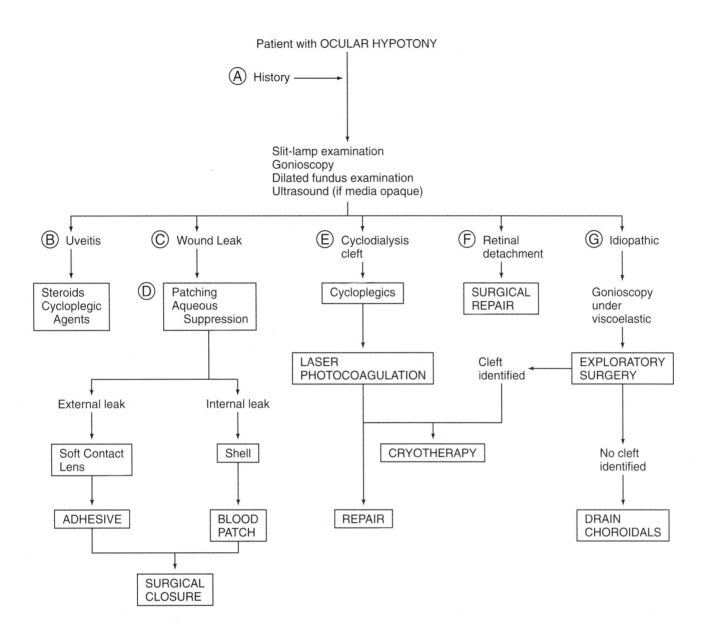

Patient with OCULAR HYPOTONY

(A) History ⟶

Slit-lamp examination
Gonioscopy
Dilated fundus examination
Ultrasound (if media opaque)

(B) Uveitis

(C) Wound Leak

(E) Cyclodialysis cleft

(F) Retinal detachment

(G) Idiopathic

Steroids
Cycloplegic
Agents

(D) Patching
Aqueous
Suppression

Cycloplegics

SURGICAL
REPAIR

Gonioscopy
under
viscoelastic

External leak

Internal leak

LASER
PHOTOCOAGULATION

Cleft
identified

EXPLORATORY
SURGERY

Soft Contact
Lens

Shell

CRYOTHERAPY

No cleft
identified

ADHESIVE

BLOOD
PATCH

REPAIR

DRAIN
CHOROIDALS

SURGICAL
CLOSURE

Gentile RC, Pavlin CJ, Liebmann JM, et al. Diagnosis of traumatic cyclodialysis by ultrasound biomicroscopy. Ophthalmic Surg Lasers 1996; 27:97–105.

Pederson JE. Ocular hypotony. In: Ritch R, Shields MB, Krupin T, eds. The glaucomas. St Louis: Mosby, 1996: 385–395.

Schuman JS, Zaltas MM. Management of the leaking bleb. In: Ritch R, Shields MB, Krupin T, eds. The glaucomas. St Louis: Mosby, 1996: 1737–1744.

Smith PD, Belcher CD, Thomas JV. Anterior chamber deepening with intraoperative gonioscopy. In: Thomas JV, Belcher CD, Simmons RJ, eds. Glaucoma surgery. St Louis: Mosby, 1992: 215–221.

Wise J. Treatment of chronic postfiltration hypotony by intrableb injection of autologous blood. Arch Ophthalmol 1993; 11:827–830.

CHOICE OF GLAUCOMA MEDICATIONS

Johan Zwaan, M.D., Ph.D.

Up to 20 years ago, only three major glaucoma medications were available: oral carbonic anhydrase inhibitors, miotics (topical cholinergic agonists and cholinesterase inhibitors), and sympathomimetics (topical epinephrine). Since then they have largely been replaced by four new groups of drugs: β blockers, α-adrenergic agonists, topical carbonic anhydrase inhibitors (CAIs), and prostaglandins. In addition, two uncommonly used groups remain available: hyperosmotic agents, used only in an acute setting, and anticholinesterase agents, which are rarely used. This plethora of drugs has made the choice of therapy for a given patient more difficult and by no means has a consensus been reached among practitioners about the best choices. Certain principles apply for rational choices. The drug should be effective and side effects should be minimal or avoided altogether. Cost is a consideration. The drug regimen should be as simple as possible; many studies have shown a direct correlation between simplicity and compliance. Comfort and influence on lifestyle also relate to compliance.

The decision tree proposed here is only one of many possible scenarios and for each patient the choice of treatment should be individualized.

A. The proposed treatment is applicable to open-angle glaucoma. Although much of it applies to other types of glaucoma, other considerations become important. For instance, in a patient with pigmentary glaucoma, the practitioner may elect to use pilocarpine as (one of) the medication(s). The resulting miosis reduces the rubbing of the iris epithelium against the lenticular zonules and hence fewer pigment granules are released. Congenital glaucoma is primarily a surgical disease, and drugs are used only as a holding action.

B. It is imperative to do complete examinations on all glaucoma patients. Records should be organized to allow easy comparison of the results of subsequent visits so that progression of the disease is detected early.

C. Depending on the findings of the initial examination, a goal should be set for lowering the intraocular pressure (IOP). The IOP to be achieved depends on the patient's initial status, such as the extent of glaucomatous damage already done and the IOP at presentation. The goal should be considered a flexible endpoint and may be adjusted if visual field loss progresses despite the goal IOP being maintained.

D. It is best to start a new therapy on one eye only. This allows the other eye to be used as a control, making it easier to judge the effect of the new medication. This trial should be relatively short, 3–4 weeks, and if the desired goal is not reached, switch to another medication or add a second medication.

E. Most practitioners prefer to start treatment of new glaucoma patients with one of the β blockers, which are still the most effective suppressors of aqueous flow. They are the only class of drugs approved by the FDA as a first-line therapy. They have no ocular side effects with the possible exception of metipranolol, which in one study was associated with granulomatous uveitis, although this was not confirmed in a later publication. The lowest possible dosage should be used. If patients are taught properly how to occlude the lacrimal drainage system when applying the drop, 0.25% of timolol once daily is adequate for many patients. The cost of β blockers is relatively low, and generic equivalents are available. The main disadvantages of the β blockers are potential systemic side effects. They can trigger bronchospasm and respiratory failure in patients with asthma or obstructive pulmonary disease. They also may cause bradycardia and hypotension and, uncommonly, cardiac arrhythmia up to cardiac block, and congestive heart failure. For patients with asthma or with cardiovascular disease, another first medication should be chosen, such as brimonidine or latanoprost.

Other possible side effects include depression, fatigue, and impotence. Ask patients about the occurrence of these, and if the effects are significant, switch to another medication.

Within the β blockers, timolol is still the most widely used drug. Betaxolol is preferred by some because it has fewer cardiopulmonary side effects. Both betaxolol and carteolol increase systemic cholesterol levels less than other β blockers and may be of advantage for older males and for postmenopausal women who are not receiving hormone replacement therapy. However, they have a smaller IOP lowering effect than timolol.

F. If IOP is lowered inadequately, a second medication may be added. Because the action of latanoprost is entirely different from β blockers (it increases uveoscleral outflow), it has a significant additive effect on IOP. There are no known systemic side effects, but ocular ones are common. Iris pigmentation tends to become darker, and the drug stimulates eyelash growth, leading to longer and darker lashes. There is some evidence that latanoprost may cause uveitis and increase the risk for cystoid macular edema (CME). Most practitioners avoid latanoprost in patients at risk for CME, such as those with aphakia or pseudophakia with a compromised capsule and in patients with (a history of) chronic inflammatory eye disease. Alternative choices are brimonidine or a topical carbonic anhydrase inhibitor. If the latter is chosen, a convenient combination preparation of timolol and dorzolamide is available.

For most patients the use of timolol as a drop or in gel form in the morning and latanoprost at night is an effective regimen that is easy to follow and thus gives better compliance.

G. An attempt may be made to omit the β blocker and use latanoprost alone. The simpler the prescribed treatment is, the better the compliance will be and the lower the cost will be. For these reasons, switching drugs is often preferable over adding a second, third, or even more medications. If a switch is made, it should be to a drug of another class. Switching within a class (i.e., from one β blocker to another) rarely makes sense.

H. If the combination of a β blocker and Xalatan or a topical carbonic anhydrase inhibitor does not lower the IOP adequately, a third medication may be added. Neither brimonidine nor a topical carbonic anhydrase inhibitor by itself is as efficacious as timolol or latanoprost, but they do have an additive effect. Some physicians prefer not to add a third medication because with increased treatment complexity, cost goes up and compliance decreases. Instead, they recommend argon laser trabeculoplasty (ALT) at this stage.

I. If IOP control is still unacceptable (even with three medications), if compliance is poor, or if intolerance for any of the drugs develops, ALT is advisable. If properly done this is a highly effective treatment modality, giving adequate IOP control in most patients for several (up to 5) years, without any medications.

J. In patients in whom ALT does not lower IOP enough or in whom the IOP creeps up again after initial good control, medications should be started again. The regimen advocated here can be followed or an alternative pathway may be preferred.

K. Filtration surgery should be done only in patients with open-angle glaucoma in whom the IOP is uncontrollable by other means. In general, the surgery consists of a trabeculectomy. The use of cytostatic agents, such as mitomycin C, as an adjunct during surgery has increased its success rate, particularly in cases with a high failure risk, but has also increased the incidence of complications such as hypotony-associated maculopathy, "blebitis," and endophthalmitis.

L. Open-angle glaucoma is a chronic disease, and continuity of care is imperative. If good IOP control has been achieved with stable vision, visual fields, and optic nerve, follow-up visits every 3 months with measurement of IOP and inspection of the disc are adequate. Visual fields should be done at least annually. Gonioscopy, although less essential in open-angle glaucoma, should be done when indicated. Serial photographs of the disc facilitate comparison from one visit to the next. If control is not acceptable, more frequent examinations and adjustments of therapy are needed. If a patient misses appointments or is "lost to follow up," every attempt should be made to contact the patient and to ensure that continued care has been obtained. "Return receipt requested" postcards are advisable. For medicolegal reasons, these attempts should be documented fully in the chart.

In some older patients, in whom the optic nerve can reasonably be expected to outlive the patient even in the presence of increased IOP, some physicians may withhold glaucoma treatment when it is not thought to improve the patient's quality of life. The reasons for nontreatment should be documented.

References

Al-Hazmi A, Zwaan J, Awad A, et al. Effectiveness and complications of mitomycin C use during pediatric glaucoma surgery. Ophthalmology 1998; 105:1915–1920.

Freedman S, Freedman M, Shields MB, et al. Effects of carteolol and timolol on plasma high-density lipoprotein cholesterol level. Am J Ophthalmol 1993; 116:600–610.

Gottfredsdottir MS, Allingham RR, Shields MB. Physicians' guide to interactions between glaucoma and systemic medications. J Glaucoma 1997; 6:377–383.

LeBlanc RP. Twelve-month results of an ongoing randomized trial comparing brimonidine tartrate 0.2% and timolol 0.5% given twice daily in patients with glaucoma or ocular hypertension. Ophthalmology 1998; 105:1960–1967.

Rowe J, Herman D, Hattenhauer M. Adverse side effects associated with latanoprost. Am J Ophthalmol 1997; 124:683–688.

Schuman JS, Horwitz B, Choplin NT, et al. A 1-year study of brimonidine twice daily in glaucoma and ocular hypertension. A controlled, randomized, multicenter clinical trial. Arch Ophthalmol 1997; 115:847–852.

Strohmaier K, Snyder E, DuBiner H, et al. The efficacy and safety of the dorzolamide-timolol combination versus the concomitant administration of its components. Ophthalmology 1998; 105:1936–1944.

Warwar RE, Bullock JD, Ballal D. CME and anterior uveitis associated with latanoprost use: Experience and incidence in a retrospective study of 94 patients. Ophthalmology 1998; 105:263–267.

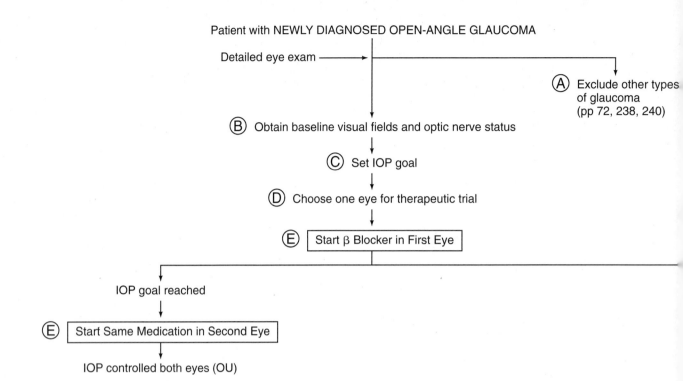

Patient with NEWLY DIAGNOSED OPEN-ANGLE GLAUCOMA

Detailed eye exam

(A) Exclude other types of glaucoma (pp 72, 238, 240)

(B) Obtain baseline visual fields and optic nerve status

(C) Set IOP goal

(D) Choose one eye for therapeutic trial

(E) Start β Blocker in First Eye

IOP goal reached

(E) Start Same Medication in Second Eye

IOP controlled both eyes (OU)

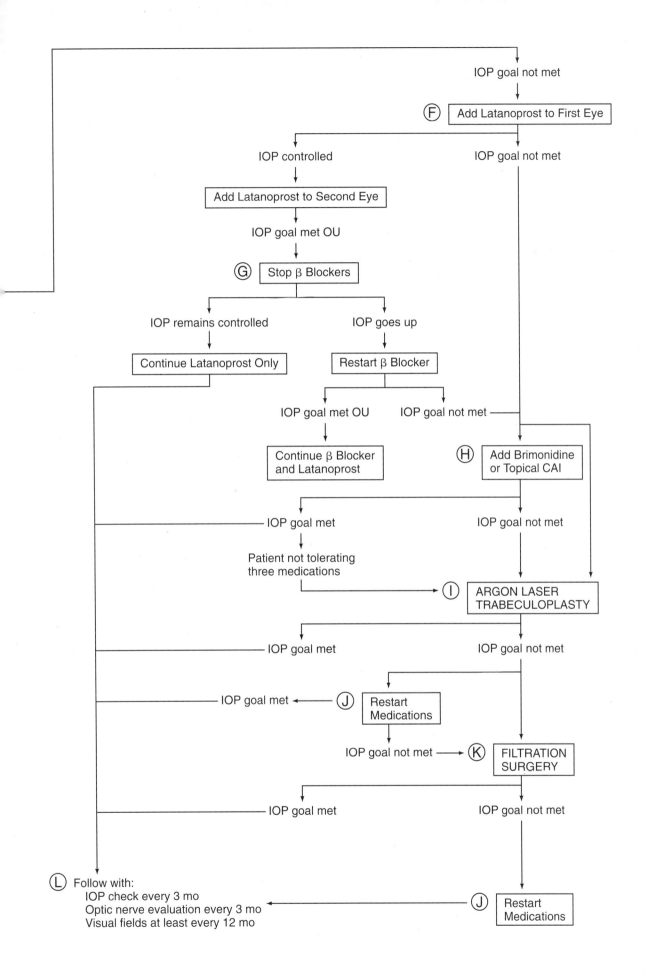

IOP goal not met

Ⓕ Add Latanoprost to First Eye

IOP controlled   IOP goal not met

Add Latanoprost to Second Eye

IOP goal met OU

Ⓖ Stop β Blockers

IOP remains controlled   IOP goes up

Continue Latanoprost Only   Restart β Blocker

IOP goal met OU   IOP goal not met

Continue β Blocker and Latanoprost   Ⓗ Add Brimonidine or Topical CAI

IOP goal met   IOP goal not met

Patient not tolerating three medications

Ⓘ ARGON LASER TRABECULOPLASTY

IOP goal met   IOP goal not met

IOP goal met ← Ⓙ Restart Medications

IOP goal not met → Ⓚ FILTRATION SURGERY

IOP goal met   IOP goal not met

Ⓛ Follow with:
   IOP check every 3 mo
   Optic nerve evaluation every 3 mo
   Visual fields at least every 12 mo

Ⓙ Restart Medications

265

LENS DISORDERS

OPACITIES ON THE LENS SURFACE

Johan Zwaan, M.D., Ph.D.

Opacities associated with the anterior lens surface may be caused by abnormalities of the lens capsule and epithelium, by irregularities in the most superficial anterior cortex, or by abnormal deposits on the anterior lens capsule. Visual acuity is affected less than in posterior lens opacities because the lesions are farther removed from the macula and generally are smaller and lead to less irregularity of the lens surface.

A. White, flaky material is found on the lens capsule, iris, trabecular meshwork, lens zonules, and anterior vitreous face in pseudoexfoliation syndrome. Typically, the material is best seen as a disc of dandrufflike material on the anterior lens capsule after the pupil has been dilated. The disc is surrounded by a clear zone, which is followed by fibrillar white material on the peripheral lens surface and the zonules. The syndrome is rarely seen before the age of 50 years and doubles in prevalence for every decade after this. The nature of the white material and its origin are unclear (p 72).

B. True exfoliation of the lens capsule is rare and is usually caused by infrared irradiation. It was commonly seen in glass blowers. It is caused by delamination of the anterior lens capsule, resulting in a very thin membrane with a free edge floating in the aqueous.

C. Pigmentary dispersion syndrome results from the release of melanosomes from the posterior iris epithelium, which rubs against the lens zonules when the iris has a concave configuration within a deep anterior chamber (AC). Thus the syndrome is primarily seen under conditions leading to a concave iris (i.e., myopia, male sex). Both of these factors lead to a deep AC. The pigment granules accumulate in the trabecular meshwork, increasing the risk for glaucoma, and on the corneal endothelium and lens capsule (p 72).

D. Posterior synechiae may be the first indication for the presence of juvenile rheumatoid arthritis (JRA). Asymptomatic, chronic, nongranulomatous iridocyclitis may precede the onset of arthritis. Acute febrile and polyarticular forms of arthritis are generally not associated with eye findings. However, the pauciarticular types carry a much higher risk for the development of iritis, up to 20%. Because the onset is insidious, significant ocular damage may be done before the disease is diagnosed. In addition to pigment deposits on the lens capsule and posterior synechiae, band keratopathy and cataracts are common complications.

E. Epicapsular stars are minimal remnants of the embryonic pupillary membrane. These stellate clusters of epithelial cells in the shape of bird tracks have no clinical significance.

F. Remnants of the pupillary membrane are commonly adherent to the anterior capsule in small areas. At the adhesion site a small anterior lens opacity is often present. Neither the cataract nor the membrane is progressive, and unless they are in the visual axis, they do not interfere with vision.

G. In some inherited syndromes or after localized trauma to the epithelium, groups of anterior lens epithelial cells take on a fibroblast-like configuration. They become arranged in whorls and produce abnormal amounts of capsular materials, interspersed between and around the cells. Sometimes, the lens capsule becomes duplicate or the plaques may protrude from the anterior lens surface. These plaques are an example of true metaplasia of lens epithelial cells into myofibroblasts.

H. Trisomy 21 may be associated with cataract formation, which usually develops later in childhood rather than in infancy. The capsule is often thickened and shows the anomalies discussed in section G.

I. Children with Lowe's syndrome often have cataracts, in which the lens is reduced to a relatively thin disc with epithelial cells both anteriorly and posteriorly. Anterior plaques are usually present. The face has a characteristic appearance with frontal bossing and chubby cheeks. The syndrome is associated with mental retardation, hypotonia, and aminoaciduria. Glaucoma and anterior segment dysgenesis are common. Inheritance is X-linked, and carriers may be detected by the presence of punctate lens opacities in the peripheral cortex.

J. Pyramidal cataracts are small pyramids of lens tissue protruding into the AC. They are considered remnants of the embryonic lens stalk, which connected the lens rudiment with the surface epithelium. Anterior polar cataracts are small and located in the center of the anterior capsule and may have a similar origin as the pyramidal cataracts. Either type is generally not progressive and causes little visual disturbance. There are exceptions to this, and in some reports, as many as 30% of patients developed amblyopia or other visual problems. Periodic follow-up is therefore recommended.

K. Alport's syndrome is a nephropathy with progressive hematuria and is often associated with sensorineural deafness and anterior lenticonus. It is usually an X-linked dominant trait but in some cases appears to be autosomal recessive. The molecular defect in the X-linked form has been identified as an abnormality of the common subunit of collagen IV (COL4A5), which is found in the glomerular basement membrane.

L. In the most severe forms of Peters' anomaly, the lens can be broadly adherent to the cornea. More commonly, a stalk-shaped adhesion is present or a pyramidal cataract is found as a remnant of the corneolenticular connection. Although the lens anomalies are variable, Peters' syndrome always has a central corneal leukoma with abnormal or absent endothelium and adhesions between the edge of the leukoma and the peripupillary iris.

M. An inherited absence or low level of the copper-transporting serum protein ceruloplasmin (Wilson's disease) leads to high tissue levels of copper. The effects of the abnormal copper levels become manifest in young adults. Basal ganglia degeneration in the CNS causes tremors and choreoathetosis. Liver cirrhosis occurs, and renal involvement results in aminoaciduria. Brownish green copper deposits may be seen in the peripheral Descemet's membrane, particularly at 6 and 12 o'clock (Kayser-Fleischer ring). The subcapsular sunflower cataract is highly characteristic but not always present.

N. Localized trauma to the anterior lens epithelium may lead to a localized repair process, which results in plaque formation at the lens surface (see section G).

O. A variety of drug exposures may lead to opacities in the anterior superficial lens cortex. Best known for this complication are chlorpromazine and anticholinesterases.

P. Periods of elevation of intraocular pressure by acute angle closure may cause focal necrosis of lens epithelial cells. These form irregular subcapsular lens opacities first consisting of necrotic epithelium and later of fibroblast-like repair tissue. These "Glaukom Flecken" can be subtle and require careful slit-lamp examination of the anterior lens. Their presence necessitates a work-up for occludable AC angles.

References

Cashwell LF Jr, Holleman IL, Weaver RG, van Rens GH. Idiopathic true exfoliation of the lens capsule. Ophthalmology 1989; 96:348–350.

Cibis GW, Waeltermann JM, Whitcraft CT, et al. Lenticular opacities in carriers of Lowe's syndrome. Ophthalmology 1986; 93:1041–1045.

Foster CS, Barrett F. Cataract development and cataract surgery in patients with juvenile rheumatoid arthritis-associated iridocyclitis. Ophthalmology 1993; 100:809–817.

Jaafar MS, Robb RM. Congenital anterior polar cataracts: A review of 63 cases. Ophthalmology 1984; 91:249–254.

Knebelmann B, Breillat C, Forestier L, et al. Spectrum of mutations in the COL4A5 collagen gene in X-linked Alport syndrome. Am J Hum Genet 1996; 59:1221–1232.

Lipman RM, Tripathi BJ, Tripathi RC. Cataracts induced by microwave and ionizing radiation. Surv Ophthalmol 1988; 33:200–210.

Richter CU, Richardson TM, Grant WM. Pigmentary dispersion syndrome and pigmentary glaucoma: A prospective study of the natural history. Arch Ophthalmol 1986; 104:211–217.

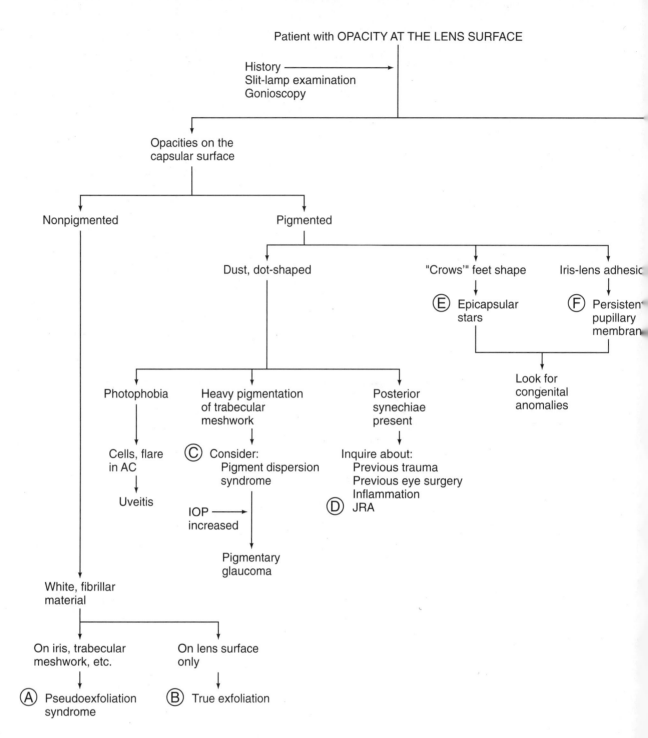

Patient with OPACITY AT THE LENS SURFACE

History
Slit-lamp examination
Gonioscopy

Opacities on the
capsular surface

Nonpigmented

Pigmented

Dust, dot-shaped

"Crows'" feet shape

Iris-lens adhesic

Ⓔ Epicapsular
stars

Ⓕ Persisten
pupillary
membran

Photophobia

Heavy pigmentation
of trabecular
meshwork

Posterior
synechiae
present

Look for
congenital
anomalies

Cells, flare
in AC

Ⓒ Consider:
Pigment dispersion
syndrome

Inquire about:
Previous trauma
Previous eye surgery
Inflammation

Ⓓ JRA

Uveitis

IOP ⟶
increased

Pigmentary
glaucoma

White, fibrillar
material

On iris, trabecular
meshwork, etc.

On lens surface
only

Ⓐ Pseudoexfoliation
syndrome

Ⓑ True exfoliation

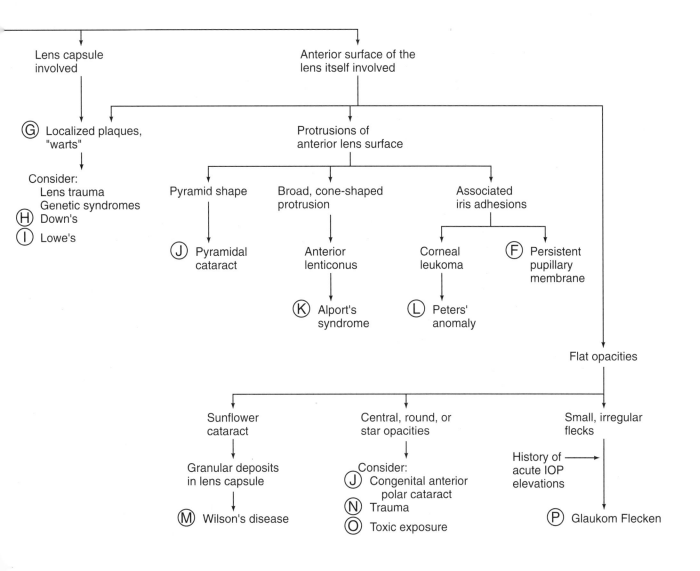

Lens capsule
involved

Anterior surface of the
lens itself involved

(G) Localized plaques,
"warts"

Consider:
Lens trauma
Genetic syndromes
(H) Down's
(I) Lowe's

Protrusions of
anterior lens surface

Pyramid shape

(J) Pyramidal
cataract

Broad, cone-shaped
protrusion

Anterior
lenticonus

(K) Alport's
syndrome

Associated
iris adhesions

Corneal
leukoma

(L) Peters'
anomaly

(F) Persistent
pupillary
membrane

Flat opacities

Sunflower
cataract

Granular deposits
in lens capsule

(M) Wilson's disease

Central, round, or
star opacities

Consider:
(J) Congenital anterior
polar cataract
(N) Trauma
(O) Toxic exposure

Small, irregular
flecks

History of
acute IOP
elevations

(P) Glaukom Flecken

SUBLUXATED AND DISLOCATED LENSES

Johan Zwaan, M.D., Ph.D.

In many patients, eye complaints are the presenting symptoms of ectopia lentis. This obligates the ophthalmologist not only to evaluate and treat the ectopia lentis by itself but also to initiate the work-up or make the necessary referrals to diagnose the systemic disease underlying the ocular manifestation. In a small group of patients the dislocation of the lens is secondary to eye abnormalities or to systemic diseases that are severe enough to allow a diagnosis well before the ectopia lentis is discovered. The emphasis in this chapter is on patients whose presenting problem is ectopia lentis.

A. Reduced vision is the presenting symptom in many patients for several reasons. Fluctuations in refraction may be caused by small changes in lens position or by image formation through different parts of the lens. Myopic astigmatism is the rule in patients with moderately subluxated lenses, whereas an aphakic correction is needed when the lens is (almost) totally dislocated. Particularly challenging are the lenses, which are halfway dislocated, thus bringing the edge close to the visual axis. Changes from aphakia to high myopia may occur, and monocular diplopia is not uncommon. In a child this situation is highly amblyopiogenic, another cause for reduced vision. Finally, accommodation is hampered, disturbing the switch from distance to near vision.

B. Slit-lamp examination is the best way to diagnose ectopia lentis. A subluxated lens, although not in its normal position, remains within the pupillary space. A dislocated lens is away from the pupillary space. The lens may be dislocated anteriorly, which carries the risk of acute glaucoma and corneal decompensation, or posteriorly into the vitreous.

C. Bilaterally dislocated lenses almost always indicate a genetic disorder or a congenital eye abnormality. They often are congenital but may be acquired and progressive. Most present in children.

D. A unilateral dislocated lens usually indicates an acquired problem and may occur at any age.

E. Although tallness and arachnodactyly are thought to be typical for Marfan's syndrome, they are also present in homocystinuria.

F. Marfan's syndrome is the most common cause for pediatric ectopia lentis. High myopia, a tendency for retinal detachments, and cataracts may also be found. Cardiac anomalies are the most important systemic findings (i.e., a dilated aortic root, aortic aneurysms, mitral valve prolapse). Thus always obtain cardiologic consultation. Kyphoscoliosis and chest deformities are typical. There is a wide variation in expression, and the diagnosis is not always easy. Inheritance is autosomal dominant, and Marfan's syndrome may be genetically heterogeneous. Mutations in the fibrillin gene are responsible for the various manifestations of Marfan's syndrome. The variations in patients with different severity of phenotype may result from differences in the mutations or in the level of mutant protein being expressed. Autosomal-dominant ectopia lentis has also been linked to a fibrillin abnormality. The dislocation of the lens in these syndromes is probably congenital and is stable in >90% of patients.

G. Homocystinuria, an autosomal-recessive disease, is often not diagnosed until later in childhood, when psychomotor retardation and failure to thrive are present. Dislocation of the lens may not be present early and is typically progressive. A urine nitroprussid test is a good screening test, although it can be falsely negative. If a diagnosis of homocystinuria is suspected, serum and urinary aminoacids (homocystine levels) should be studied, ideally after a loading dose of methionine. The underlying cause in most patients is a deficiency of cystathione-β-synthetase. Pyridoxine is a cofactor of this enzyme, and about half of patients benefit from large doses of this vitamin B_6. Patients are at risk for thromboembolic episodes, which can be lethal and can be provoked by surgery. Thus eye surgery should not be undertaken lightly.

H. Patients with Weill-Marchesani's syndrome have a spherical lens, which tends to dislocate anteriorly, giving pupillary block glaucoma and acute severe pain.

I. Isolated ectopia lentis is a diagnosis of exclusion, which should be made only after a systemic work-up. A work-up should be performed in all patients with ectopia lentis.

J. Ectopia lentis et pupillae is characterized by dislocation of lens and pupil in opposite directions. The corectopia may be absent or hardly noticeable. In my experience these patients almost always have remnants of persistent pupillary membranes, which may

TABLE 1 Disorders Sometimes Associated with Ectopia Lentis

Ocular disorders	Systemic disorders
Megalocornea	Hyperlysinemia
Congenital glaucoma	Sulfite oxidase deficiency
Aniridia	Scleroderma
Rieger's syndrome	Sturge-Weber's syndrome
Retinitis pigmentosa	Ehlers-Danlos syndrome
	Craniofacial disorders

play a role in the pathogenesis of the dislocation. Myopia is not only lenticular but also axial. The cornea may be enlarged and the iris translucent. Inheritance is autosomal recessive.

K. Several rare disorders and some ocular anomalies can be associated with ectopia lentis. The primary diagnosis is usually well established, and the ectopia lentis is a secondary finding in most of these patients. Several disorders are listed in Table 1.

L. Unilateral lens dislocation in a child almost always results from trauma. Even in bilateral cases, trauma may be the cause. Consider the possibility of child abuse, most certainly when there is evidence for other unusual trauma (e.g., many bruises, burns, multiple fractures). Up to 40% of nonaccidental injuries in children may involve the eyes.

M. The position of the lens gives some indication about the cause of ectopia lentis but is not pathognomonic. Usually, the lens is displaced upward and temporally in Marfan's syndrome, downward in homocystinuria. A position in the anterior chamber is typical for homocystinuria and Weill-Marchesani's syndrome, but not exclusively so.

N. If the lens is anteriorly dislocated, attempt first to reposition it posteriorly by dilating the pupil, placing the patient in a supine position, and pressing on the cornea. Even if this is successful, consider lensectomy to prevent further episodes. Alternatively, long-term treatment with miotics is useful.

O. The decision to remove a dislocated lens must be individualized; it may often be unnecessary. Minor subluxations and complete dislocations can be treated with refractive corrections. A posteriorly dislocated lens needs to be removed only if it causes complications, such as lens-induced uveitis. Surgery should be undertaken in the children with fluctuating refraction, who are at risk for amblyopia. Closed lensectomy and anterior vitrectomy with vitreous cutting instruments, either through the limbus or through the pars plana/plicata, is the technique of choice. Occasionally, intracapsular delivery, extracapsular methods, or aspiration can be appropriate, but be prepared to deal with the vitreous loss that almost always accompanies these methods.

P. Frequent follow-up is essential in all children with ectopia lentis to adjust refractive corrections, provide amblyopia therapy as required, and check for the many possible complications.

Q. Glaucoma, lens-induced uveitis, cystic retinal degeneration, peripheral retinal tears, retinal dialysis, and retinal detachment can all accompany ectopia lentis, whether lens removal has taken place or not. They need to be diagnosed and treated promptly.

References

Goldberg MF. Clinical manifestations of ectopia lentis et pupillae in 16 patients. Ophthalmology 1988; 95:1080–1088.

Gray JR, Davies SJ. Marfan syndrome. J Med Genet 1996; 33:403–408.

Halpert M, BenEzra D. Surgery of the hereditary subluxated lens in children. Ophthalmology 1996; 103:681–686.

Michalski A, Leonard J, Taylor D. The eye and inherited metabolic disease. J R Soc Med 1988; 81:286–290.

Nelson LB, Maumenee IH. Ectopia lentis. In: Rennie WA, ed. Goldberg's genetic and metabolic eye diseases. Boston: Little, Brown, 1986.

Tongue AC. The ophthalmologist's role in diagnosing child abuse. Ophthalmology 1991; 98:1009–1010.

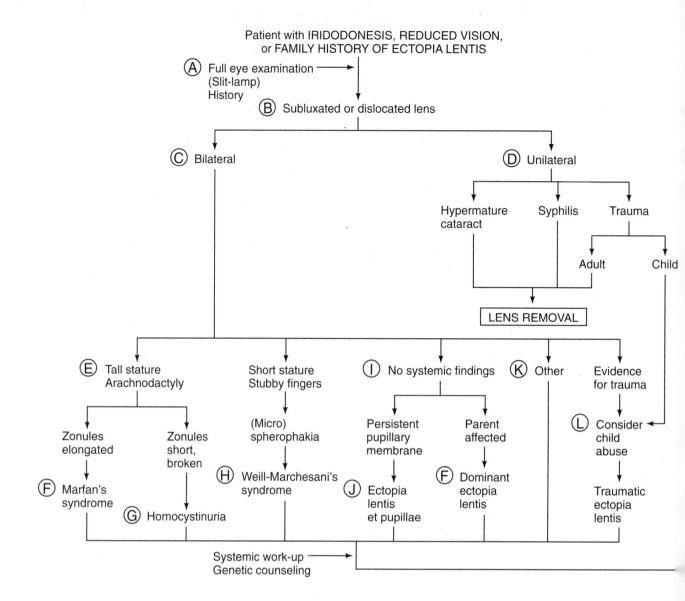

Patient with IRIDODONESIS, REDUCED VISION,
or FAMILY HISTORY OF ECTOPIA LENTIS

(A) Full eye examination
(Slit-lamp)
History

(B) Subluxated or dislocated lens

(C) Bilateral

(D) Unilateral

Hypermature cataract   Syphilis   Trauma

Adult   Child

LENS REMOVAL

(E) Tall stature
Arachnodactyly

Short stature
Stubby fingers

(I) No systemic findings

(K) Other

Evidence for trauma

Zonules elongated

Zonules short, broken

(Micro) spherophakia

Persistent pupillary membrane

Parent affected

(L) Consider child abuse

(F) Marfan's syndrome

(G) Homocystinuria

(H) Weill-Marchesani's syndrome

(J) Ectopia lentis et pupillae

(F) Dominant ectopia lentis

Traumatic ectopia lentis

Systemic work-up
Genetic counseling

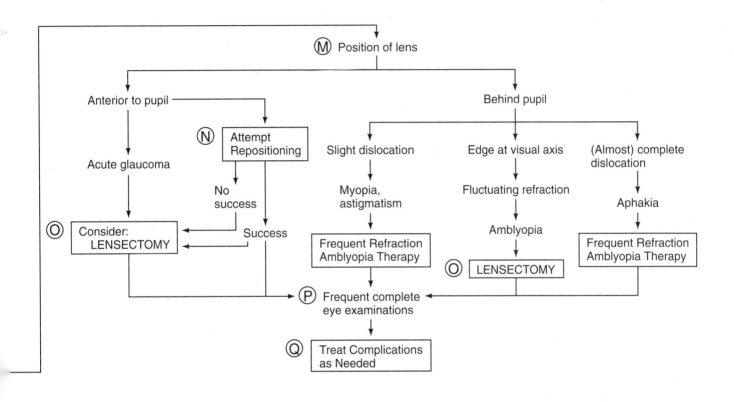

PAIN AFTER CATARACT SURGERY

Kristin Story Held, M.D.

Pain after cataract surgery can be produced by a broad spectrum of causes—some obvious, easily cured, and benign; others obscure, difficult to manage, and potentially devastating. The conjunctiva, cornea, and iris are exquisitely sensitive to pain. The extraocular muscles, sclera, choroid, and optic nerve sheath require a stronger stimulus to produce pain, and the optic nerve itself and the retina are pain free. The eye is innervated by the nasociliary branch of the ophthalmic nerve. Before entering the orbit, the ophthalmic nerve gives off several recurrent meningeal branches, which innervate the dura of the tentorium and falx and segments of the blood vessels at the base of the brain. Consequently, eye pain may be referred pain from intracranial abnormality. Patient history, pupillary response, visual fields, and associated neurologic signs and symptoms are important in differentiating local ocular disease from nonocular causes. Thorough, systematic patient history and physical examination are key in identifying the source of ocular discomfort and allowing one to institute appropriate therapy.

A. The patient history must be detailed and specifically address associated systemic conditions, all systemic and topical medications used, and the character and course of the pain. Underlying systemic conditions such as diabetes mellitus, rheumatoid arthritis, or alcohol abuse might predispose the patient to poor healing or delayed postoperative complications. Specifically ask about ocular trauma. Any topical preparations used, including preserved topical steroid preparations, which are so commonly used, are potential offenders and should not be overlooked. Review the nature of the pain in detail. A foreign body sensation present immediately postoperatively might suggest an exposed suture or other foreign body, whereas a relatively asymptomatic postoperative course followed by the development of pain, photophobia, and redness might suggest epithelial downgrowth or delayed-onset endophthalmitis.

B. A complete systematic examination begins with examination of the lids and ocular adnexa for structural or functional abnormalities, which can then be medically or surgically treated. A thorough slit-lamp examination and funduscopic examination follow.

C. Thoroughly inspect the conjunctiva, including upper lid eversion, to look for giant papillae associated with suture reactions. Rose bengal staining suggests keratitis sicca or toxic conjunctivitis.

D. The surgical wound can be a great source of persistent ocular discomfort after cataract surgery. Carefully inspect the incision for loose or exposed sutures; suture-induced inflammation; a rolled, mobile conjunctival lip; wound leak; inadvertent bleb; and tissue incarceration. Suture-induced inflammation is characterized by infiltrates around loose sutures or inflammation around the suture. The symptoms range from none to severe and can result in wound slippage. The inflammation is treated by increasing the topical steroids.

E. The cornea is very sensitive to pain. Use fluorescein and rose bengal dye to look for epithelial abnormalities, which are particularly problematic in patients with underlying epithelial disease, such as corneal epithelial dystrophy, keratitis sicca, blepharitis, and systemic disorders, such as diabetes mellitus. Preparations used preoperatively, intraoperatively, and postoperatively, especially gentamicin and any preserved preparations such as topical steroids, can result in corneal epithelial toxicity. Corneal edema may occur in patients with preexisting corneal endothelial disease such as Fuchs' dystrophy, prior intraocular surgery, or angle-closure glaucoma. Corneal edema may also be a result of surgical insult by either direct mechanical trauma, such as Descemet's detachment, or endothelial touch with surgical instruments or the intraocular lens (IOL), or may be a result of toxic agents injected into the eye, including miotics and viscoelastics, particularly if reusable cannulas are cleaned with detergents. Pseudophakic bullous keratopathy is occasionally seen and is a leading cause of penetrating keratoplasty in the United States. Corneal edema may be secondary to or exacerbated by increased intraocular pressure (IOP). Late corneal edema may be from epithelial downgrowth.

F. Chronic uveitis can result in persistent ocular discomfort and may be secondary to microbial agents, retained lens material, the IOL, incarcerated iris or vitreous, or toxic substances such as IOL polishing compounds and viscoelastics. Phacoanaphylactic endophthalmitis has been well described after extracapsular cataract extraction and may present days to months after surgery. It is clinically similar to delayed-onset endophthalmitis, which must be excluded when this diagnosis is entertained. When suspected, acute endophthalmitis requires immediate diagnostic aqueous and vitreous cultures and intravitreal injection of an antibiotic and steroid combination. Obtain cultures on aerobic and anaerobic media and hold for 14 days. Topical, periocular, and systemic antibiotics are used as well. Vitrectomy and repeat intravitreal antibiotic injections may be needed in more severe cases. Delayed-onset postoperative endophthalmitis is caused by less virulent organisms, especially *Propionibacterium* species, *Staphylococcus epidermidis*, and fungi. It has a more favorable prognosis than acute-onset endophthalmitis; however, aggressive diagnostic and therapeutic measures are essential. Obtain vitreous cultures in all cases, preferably by pars plana vitrectomy, with concurrent injection of vancomycin hydrochloride, 1.0 mg. Intravitreal corticosteroids are used in severely inflamed eyes. Fungal cases require intravitreal amphotericin B, 5 μg. Refractory cases may require repeat vitrectomy, intravitreal antibiotics, removal of capsular remnants, and IOL removal or exchange. The role of periocular and systemic antibiotics is unclear.

G. Problems related to the type, size, and position of the IOL may lead to ocular pain. Rigid anterior chamber IOLs cause ocular pain that increases with pressure applied to the eye, especially if vertically oriented or oversized. Rough, sharp edges on the lenses may lead to chafing of the iris and uveitis-glaucoma-hyphema (UGH) syndrome. Pupillary block may occur, as well as iris tuck from a poorly positioned lens. Evaluate the IOL position with the patient's head in various positions to look for movement and contact with corneal endothelium or iris. Macular edema and corneal edema may occur even months or years postoperatively, especially in patients with iris-plane or closed-loop IOLs. Consider IOL repositioning or exchange in these cases.

H. Increased IOP indicates a potential source of pain. Glaucoma is common in the postoperative course and is responsible for the largest number of eyes enucleated after cataract surgery. Consider all causes of secondary glaucoma, including pupillary block, malignant glaucoma, peripheral anterior synechiae formation, epithelial or fibrous downgrowth, hemolytic glaucoma, inflammatory glaucoma, and pseudophakic glaucoma. In acute cases the IOP may be elevated by retained sodium hyaluronate, α-chymotrypsin, or excessively tight wound closure. Lower IOP suggests wound leak, cyclodialysis cleft, or choroidal folds.

I. A pale or swollen nerve on funduscopic examination suggests optic neuritis. Temporal arteritis must be excluded in the elderly population with cataracts. Patients may complain of pain with movement and photophobia and exhibit blurred vision, decreased color vision, afferent pupillary defect, and visual field abnormalities. An ESR must be obtained and the patient treated accordingly.

J. Finally, once one has excluded an ocular cause of the pain as well as nonocular causes, such as intracranial disease, palpate important trigger points to rule out oc-cipital or supraorbital neuralgia. Occipital neuralgia or neuritis is referred pain from the occipital region and is diagnosed by reproducing the pain with palpation of the greater occipital nerve in the region of the posterior insertion of the sternocleidomastoid on the mastoid process or at the base of the skull midway between the occipital protuberance and the mastoid process. Similarly, some patients experience pain with palpation over the supraorbital notch. Treatment initially includes warm compresses and aspirin or NSAIDs. Local injection of lidocaine or steroids into the trigger point is dramatically effective. Recurrence of symptoms is common.

References

Brady SE, Cohen FJ, Fischer DH. Diagnosis and treatment of chronic postoperative bacterial endophthalmitis. Ophthalmic Surg 1988; 19:580–584.

Endophthalmitis Vitrectomy Study Group. Results of the endophthalmitis vitrectomy. Arch Ophthalmol 1995; 113:1479–1496.

Fastenberg DM, Schwartz PL, Golub BM. Management of dislocated nuclear fragments after phacoemulsification. Am J Ophthalmol 1991; 112:535–539.

Fong DS, Topping TM. Postoperative endophthalmitis. In: Steinert RF, ed. Cataract surgery: Technique, complications, & management. Philadelphia: WB Saunders, 1995: 426–433.

Fox GM, Joondeph BC, Flynn HW, et al. Delayed-onset pseudophakic endophthalmitis. Am J Ophthalmol 1991; 112:163–173.

Jaffe NS, Jaffe MS, Jaffe GF. Cataract surgery and its complications. 6th ed. St Louis: Mosby, 1997.

Kohrman SD, Warfield CA. Eye pain: Ocular and nonocular causes. Hosp Pract (Off) 1987; 11:33–50.

Meisler DM, Mandelbaum S. Propionibacterium-associated endophthalmitis after extracapsular cataract extraction. Review of reported cases. Ophthalmology 1989; 96:59–61.

Olk RI, Bohigian GM. The management of endophthalmitis: Diagnostic and therapeutic guidelines including the use of vitrectomy. Ophthalmic Surg 1987; 18:262–267.

Stern GA, Engel HM, Driebe WT. The treatment of postoperative endophthalmitis: Results of differing approaches to treatment. Ophthalmology 1989; 96:62–66.

Zambrano W, Flynn HW, Pflugfelder SC, et al. Management options for *Propionibacterium acnes* endophthalmitis. Ophthalmology 1989; 96:1100–1105.

Patient with PAIN AFTER CATARACT SURGERY

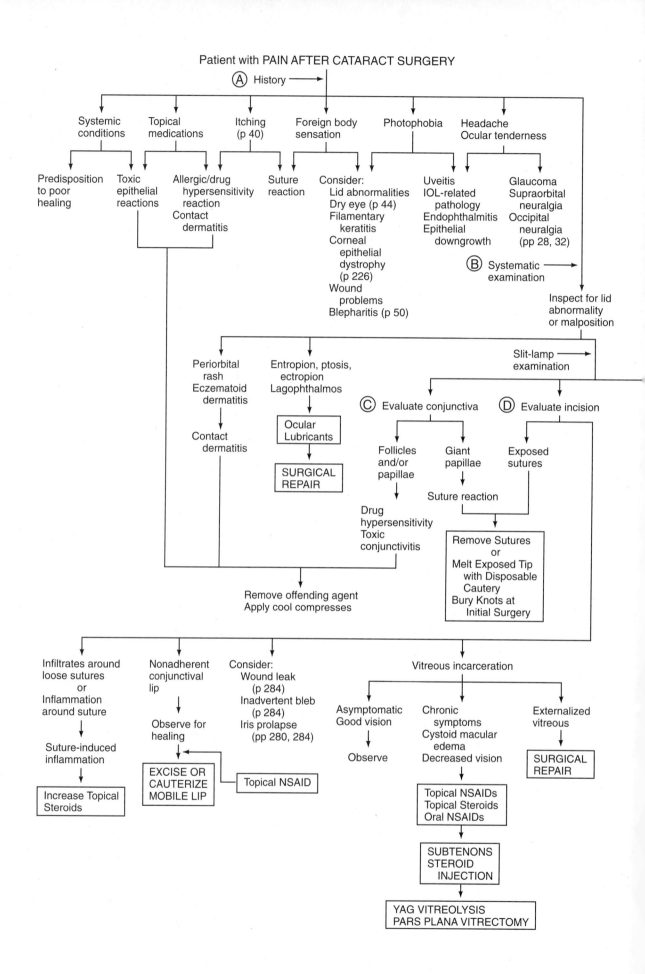

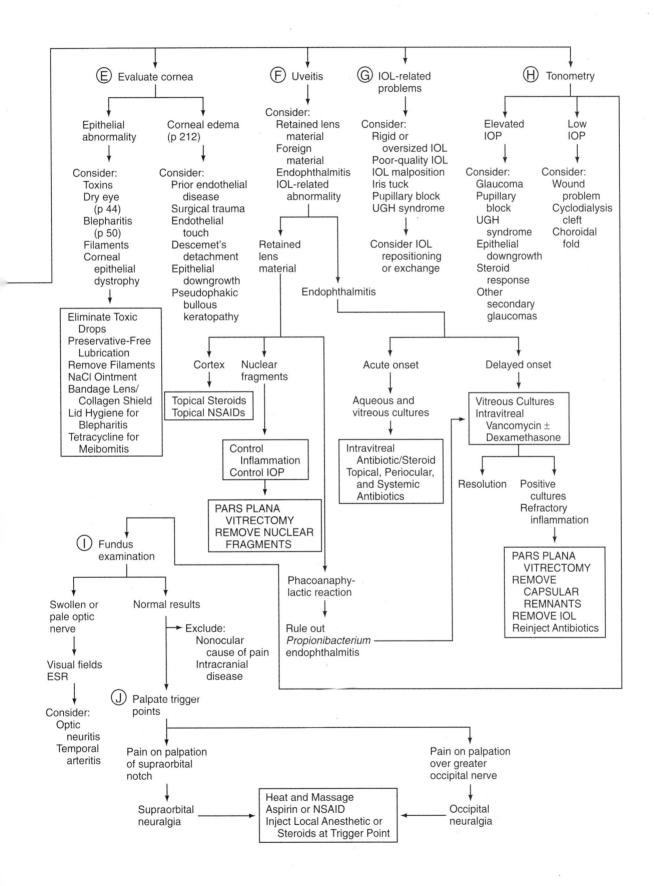

E Evaluate cornea

Epithelial abnormality

Consider:
Toxins
Dry eye (p 44)
Blepharitis (p 50)
Filaments
Corneal epithelial dystrophy

Eliminate Toxic Drops
Preservative-Free Lubrication
Remove Filaments
NaCl Ointment
Bandage Lens/ Collagen Shield
Lid Hygiene for Blepharitis
Tetracycline for Meibomitis

Corneal edema (p 212)

Consider:
Prior endothelial disease
Surgical trauma
Endothelial touch
Descemet's detachment
Epithelial downgrowth
Pseudophakic bullous keratopathy

F Uveitis

Consider:
Retained lens material
Foreign material
Endophthalmitis
IOL-related abnormality

Retained lens material

Cortex   Nuclear fragments

Topical Steroids
Topical NSAIDs

Control Inflammation
Control IOP

PARS PLANA VITRECTOMY
REMOVE NUCLEAR FRAGMENTS

G IOL-related problems

Consider:
Rigid or oversized IOL
Poor-quality IOL
IOL malposition
Iris tuck
Pupillary block
UGH syndrome

Consider IOL repositioning or exchange

Endophthalmitis

Acute onset

Aqueous and vitreous cultures

Intravitreal Antibiotic/Steroid
Topical, Periocular, and Systemic Antibiotics

H Tonometry

Elevated IOP

Consider:
Glaucoma
Pupillary block
UGH syndrome
Epithelial downgrowth
Steroid response
Other secondary glaucomas

Low IOP

Consider:
Wound problem
Cyclodialysis cleft
Choroidal fold

Delayed onset

Vitreous Cultures
Intravitreal Vancomycin ± Dexamethasone

Resolution   Positive cultures
              Refractory inflammation

PARS PLANA VITRECTOMY
REMOVE CAPSULAR REMNANTS
REMOVE IOL
Reinject Antibiotics

I Fundus examination

Swollen or pale optic nerve

Visual fields
ESR

Consider:
Optic neuritis
Temporal arteritis

Normal results

Exclude:
Nonocular cause of pain
Intracranial disease

Phacoanaphy-lactic reaction

Rule out Propionibacterium endophthalmitis

J Palpate trigger points

Pain on palpation of supraorbital notch

Supraorbital neuralgia

Pain on palpation over greater occipital nerve

Occipital neuralgia

Heat and Massage
Aspirin or NSAID
Inject Local Anesthetic or Steroids at Trigger Point

279

POOR VISION AFTER CATARACT SURGERY

Kristin Story Held, M.D.

Poor vision after cataract surgery is a source of great disappointment and frustration for the patient and cataract surgeon alike. The key to avoiding this problem is to obtain a detailed preoperative history and to perform a thorough physical examination so that coexisting ocular abnormalities are recognized and the patient can be properly counseled about realistic expectations for postoperative vision. Especially important is a history of amblyopia, previous ocular diagnoses, diabetes, and other systemic disorders; the use of potentially toxic drugs; sudden visual loss; scotoma; metamorphopsia; and other symptoms suggestive of eye disease other than cataracts. One must always look closely at the fellow eye for clues to bilateral ocular disease. Ultrasonography should be performed if there is no view of the fundus. A Marcus Gunn pupil in the cataractous eye portends a poor visual prognosis, and electrophysiology should be considered. Each patient should be counseled about his or her expected visual potential to avoid undue postoperative disappointment and unwanted surprises. When confronted with the patient with unexpected poor vision after uncomplicated cataract surgery, the surgeon must expediently and effectively pursue a definitive diagnosis so that treatable conditions can be managed early and appropriately and untreatable conditions will not be subjected to fruitless therapeutic endeavors.

A. A detailed history of the visual loss provides clues to the diagnosis. Old photographs may show strabismus in a patient whose visual loss suggests amblyopia. A four-base-out prism test or Worth-4-dot test might be useful. Characterization of the chronology and pattern of the visual loss provides clues to the diagnosis as well. A thorough ocular examination should follow.

B. A thorough ocular examination begins with the swinging flashlight test to detect a Marcus Gunn pupil. This is most commonly seen with optic nerve lesions. Retinal lesions occasionally produce this finding, but it is much less marked; that is, an eye with 20/40 vision because of optic neuritis is likely to show a more pronounced afferent pupillary defect than an eye with 20/400 vision from a retinal lesion. In the presence of a Marcus Gunn pupil, obtain bilateral formal visual fields and carefully evaluate the optic nerve and macula. In the absence of a Marcus Gunn pupil, the decreased vision could be caused by a refractive error, cloudy media, macular abnormality, a chiasmal lesion, amblyopia, or functional visual loss.

C. Keratometry or corneal topography is extremely useful in revealing irregular astigmatism, which is caused by ocular surface or corneal abnormalities, and high astigmatism, which is important in determining the proper refraction. They are helpful in determining when the refraction is stable, allowing one to assess one's wound closure technique and to detect wound healing problems; for example, a sudden shift from 2 diopters of cylinder at 90 degrees to 2 diopters at 180 degrees indicates alteration of the wound, possibly from suture breakage or ocular trauma. One should then evaluate the wound for leakage or an inadvertent bleb and perform gonioscopy. Keratometry readings help one fine-tune the axis and amount of cylinder. Disparity between keratometry readings and retinoscopy indicates intraocular lens (IOL) tilt or decentration. A hard contact lens is useful in evaluating decreased vision from irregular astigmatism. Combining keratometry, topography, and retinoscopy allows one to solve most refractive problems.

D. Retinoscopy provides crucial information about the cause of decreased vision. An abnormal "scissoring" streak indicates an astigmatic or corneal problem, whereas a dull streak indicates a media problem anterior to the retina. A normal crisp streak in the face of poor vision indicates a problem with the retina, optic nerve, or central visual pathways.

E. A media opacity is an abnormality that impairs transmission of light to the retina. The abnormality is easily identified by slit-lamp examination. The cornea is a common source of poor vision after cataract surgery. Careful preoperative evaluation of the cornea is essential. Specular microscopy in select cases is important in developing a surgical strategy. Intraoperatively, take great care to avoid damaging the cornea both mechanically and with injection of substances such as viscoelastics and miotics. Postoperatively, vitreous, lens capsule, nuclear fragments, or foreign bodies adherent to the back of the cornea may need to be removed. Control intraocular pressure (IOP) to minimize stress on the endothelial cells. Minimize topical medications in the face of epithelial erosion, especially in diabetic patients and in patients with underlying problems such as corneal epithelial dystrophy or dry eye syndrome. Maintain a high index of suspicion for acute endophthalmitis if there is a hypopyon or vitreous opacity and for sequestered postoperative endophthalmitis in cases of persistent uveitis. The key to effective therapy is rapid intervention with vitreous culture and injection of intravitreal antibiotics.

F. Biomicroscopic examination of the posterior pole with a fundus contact lens is essential. Many retinal causes of decreased vision can be diagnosed by characteristic clinical appearance. Patients with macular abnormality complain of central scotoma and metamorphopsia, and Amsler grid testing is useful. Cystoid macular edema (CME) is the most common alteration of the posterior pole after cataract surgery. The vision is good immediately postoperatively but then blurs 6–10 weeks later. CME is more common after surgical complications, including vitreous incarceration

(Irvine-Gass syndrome), iris prolapse, and vitreous loss.

Examination reveals a classic honeycombed lesion with one or more large cystic spaces centrally and smaller oval spaces surrounding it. Small perifoveal hemorrhages can be seen. If the history suggests CME but the classic clinical findings are not obvious, fluorescein angiography is indicated and is diagnostic. CME occurs angiographically in 5%–16% of patients and clinically in 0.8%–3.5% after extracapsular cataract extraction (ECCE) and posterior chamber IOL implantation with an intact posterior capsule. Many cases resolve spontaneously within 6 months. However, treat clinically apparent cases that cause decreased vision. Rule out vitreous incarceration, IOL chafing, and persistent uveitis. The first line of treatment is topical steroids and cycloplegics and oral NSAIDs. Topical NSAIDs appear to be effective as well. If these are ineffective, consider subtenon's or systemic steroids. Acetazolamide may also help. If these measures fail, YAG laser vitreolysis or vitrectomy for vitreous incarceration or IOL repositioning or exchange may be needed.

"Dry" age-related macular degeneration (AMD) is characterized by drusen, pigment clumping, and geographic atrophy. This may be poorly seen preoperatively, but postoperatively it is usually obvious. Fluorescein angiography shows characteristic transmission defects. "Wet" AMD has additional features of hemorrhage, exudates, retinal elevation, or a grayish subretinal neovascular membrane. Fluorescein angiography makes the diagnosis and localizes the source of leakage to guide laser treatment.

Macular pucker is commonly seen in people >50 years old and is one of the more common causes of failure to achieve good vision after cataract surgery. The membrane may be surgically removed if the vision is worse than 20/50.

Photic maculopathy is more common than expected and may be seen in up to 7% of patients after ECCE with posterior chamber IOL implantation. Patients may report an oval-shaped central scotoma that correlates with a macular lesion that is the shape of the filament from the operating microscope. Minimize exposure intraoperatively, using a microscope filter and "pupil paper."

G. Like macular lesions, many retinal vascular diseases can be diagnosed on clinical appearance and history. However, fluorescein angiography is useful in more subtle cases.

H. The appearance of the optic nerve is key in diagnosis. Decreased vision and visual field defects (nerve fiber bundle defects) result from optic nerve damage. If optic atrophy is present, check the visual field in the other eye. Postoperative anterior ischemic optic neuropathy can present with disc edema and hemorrhage or atrophy. In one study 47% had the same problem in the second eye. An ESR is used to exclude temporal arteritis. CT scanning and MRI may be indicated.

References

Cionni RJ, Osher RH. Intraoperative complications of phacoemulsification surgery. In: Steinert RF, ed. Cataract surgery: Technique, complications, & management. Philadelphia: WB Saunders, 1995: 325–439.

Jaffe NS, Jaffe MS, Jaffe GF. Cataract surgery and its complications. 6th ed. St Louis: Mosby, 1997.

Ruiz RS, Saatci OA. Visual outcome in pseudophakic eyes with clinical cystoid macular edema. Ophthal Surg 1991; 22:190–195.

Stark WJ, Terry AC, Maunenee AE. Anterior segment surgery: IOLs, lasers, and refractive keratoplasty. Baltimore: Williams & Wilkins, 1987.

Patients with POOR VISION AFTER CATARACT SURGERY

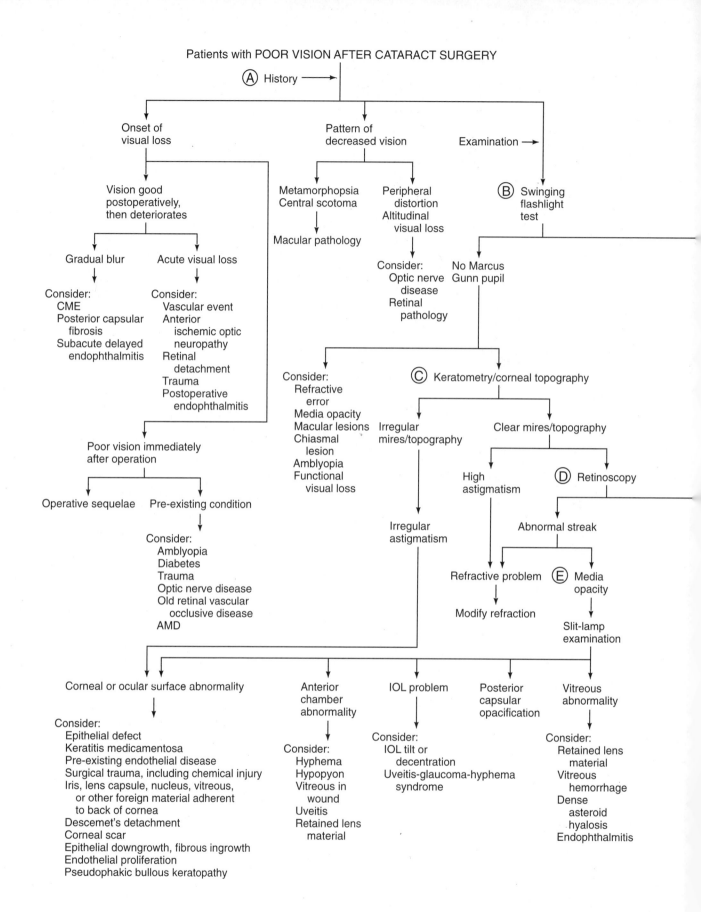

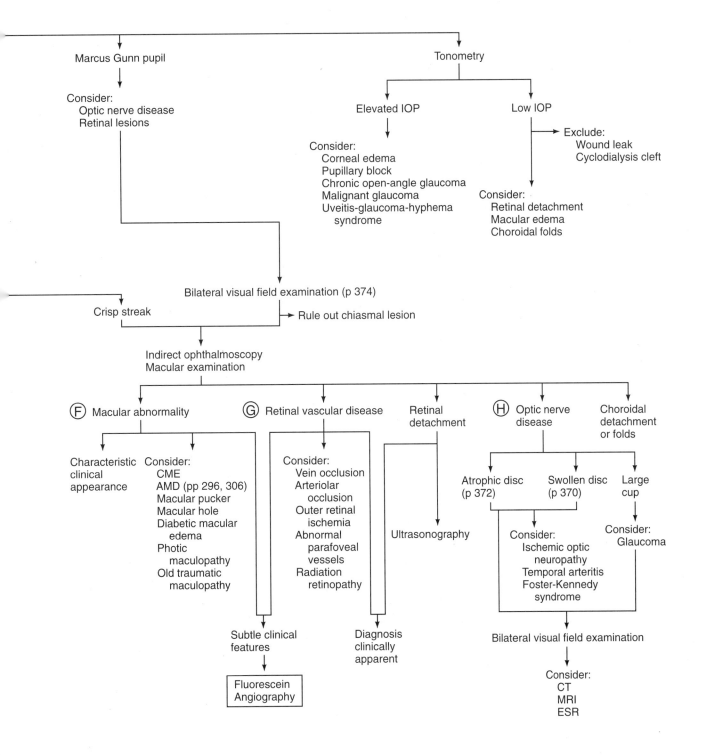

Marcus Gunn pupil

Consider:
  Optic nerve disease
  Retinal lesions

Tonometry

Elevated IOP

Low IOP

Consider:
  Corneal edema
  Pupillary block
  Chronic open-angle glaucoma
  Malignant glaucoma
  Uveitis-glaucoma-hyphema
    syndrome

Exclude:
  Wound leak
  Cyclodialysis cleft

Consider:
  Retinal detachment
  Macular edema
  Choroidal folds

Bilateral visual field examination (p 374)

Crisp streak

Rule out chiasmal lesion

Indirect ophthalmoscopy
Macular examination

F Macular abnormality

G Retinal vascular disease

Retinal detachment

H Optic nerve disease

Choroidal detachment or folds

Characteristic clinical appearance

Consider:
  CME
  AMD (pp 296, 306)
  Macular pucker
  Macular hole
  Diabetic macular edema
  Photic maculopathy
  Old traumatic maculopathy

Consider:
  Vein occlusion
  Arteriolar occlusion
  Outer retinal ischemia
  Abnormal parafoveal vessels
  Radiation retinopathy

Ultrasonography

Atrophic disc (p 372)

Swollen disc (p 370)

Large cup

Consider:
  Ischemic optic neuropathy
  Temporal arteritis
  Foster-Kennedy syndrome

Consider:
  Glaucoma

Subtle clinical features

Fluorescein Angiography

Diagnosis clinically apparent

Bilateral visual field examination

Consider:
  CT
  MRI
  ESR

SHALLOW ANTERIOR CHAMBER AFTER CATARACT SURGERY

Kristin Story Held, M.D.

A flat or shallow anterior chamber (AC) after cataract surgery is a major cause of poor visual outcome. Fortunately, this complication occurs much less often since the use of the operating microscope, 10-0 nylon suture, extracapsular and phacoemulsification techniques, and intraocular lens (IOL) implantation. It is most commonly seen in patients with diabetes mellitus, progressive open-angle glaucoma, and narrow-angle glaucoma. The most common causes are wound leak, pupillary block, or a combination of the two. Serous choroidal detachment may occur simultaneously, either causally or secondary to the low intraocular pressure (IOP) from a wound leak. Most cases occur within the first 3 weeks postoperatively. Proper diagnosis and treatment are imperative because permanent pathologic sequelae occur after 5–7 days of a shallow AC. Complications include glaucoma secondary to peripheral anterior synechia or pupillary block, hypotony from choroidal detachment, inflammation, or keratopathy. Fortunately, the AC usually reforms spontaneously after medical treatment, and surgery is rarely needed. A shallow AC late in the postoperative period is usually secondary to epithelial or fibrous invasion.

A. A flat AC in the presence of an IOL, particularly an AC IOL, is a surgical emergency that requires immediate correction to minimize the corneal damage.

B. Seidel's test is used to reveal an area of wound leak. Place 2% fluorescein sodium solution over the wound while observing the area with a slit lamp and a cobalt blue filter. The dark orange fluorescein turns bright green and fluoresces if it is diluted by leaking aqueous. If the AC is completely flat, there may not be enough aqueous to leak. In this situation, cautiously apply external pressure to provoke the leak. If a flat AC persists, it may be reformed with balanced salt solution (BSS) in the operating room, where Seidel's test may be repeated and definitive repair undertaken.

C. Pupillary block results when there is an adhesion between the iris and the vitreous face, capsular tags, retained lens material, or IOL. The normal flow of aqueous from the posterior chamber through the pupil is somehow obstructed, so the aqueous does not reach the AC and shallowing results. The IOP is high if no leak is present but normal or low if a leak is present. In some cases the wound leak is the inciting event for shallowing of the AC; subsequently, inflammation, adhesions, and occlusion of the pupil and peripheral synechiae occur. In other cases the pupillary block occurs first, and the wound leak develops in the setting of a fresh incision and significantly elevated IOP. Initial treatment includes vigorous pupillary dilation with 2.5% phenylephrine and 1% cyclopentolate. Topical corticosteroids are used to decrease the associated inflammation and prevent adhesions. Osmotic agents may dehydrate the vitreous and retract the anterior hyaloid face from the iris. If these measures fail, a peripheral iridectomy (PI) is performed. The argon or YAG laser is used to create the PI if the chamber is adequately deep. If the laser PI is unsuccessful or if the AC is too shallow (risk of corneal endothelial damage with laser), a surgical PI is created. Resolution of the pupillary block results in immediate deepening of the AC. Occasionally, a localized occlusion of the pupil and PI may be present with pockets of aqueous in the posterior chamber. Additional PIs may be placed in these regions. If the AC fails to deepen immediately after creation of a PI, consider the diagnosis of malignant glaucoma.

D. Malignant glaucoma is a rare but disastrous complication after cataract surgery. The aqueous is diverted from its normal course and accumulates posterior to the vitreous, forcing the anterior vitreous forward and resulting in a flat AC and high IOP. The response to mydriatics is limited, and the AC fails to reform after PI. Medical treatment, including cycloplegics, aqueous suppressants, and osmotic agents, may abort the posterior aqueous diversion. If medical treatment fails, proceed surgically. The anterior hyaloid face may be incised with the YAG laser or surgically. If this is not successful, an anterior vitrectomy is performed and is curative.

E. Wound leak, the most common cause of a flat AC, is caused by poor wound apposition secondary to incarceration of vitreous, capsule, or iris in the wound; excess cautery; poor wound closure; or postoperative trauma, emesis, or increased IOP. Most cases occur within 3 weeks postoperatively and resolve with conservative measures. Throughout the observation period topical antibiotics must be applied. Wound leak is best prevented by using sharp beveled incisions, proper placement of 10-0 nylon suture, avoidance of excess cautery and incarceration of tissue into the wound, a postoperative shield, and control of IOP and nausea.

F. Iris prolapse is clear evidence of a wound leak. Iris incarceration may result in poor wound healing, excess astigmatism, epithelial or fibrous ingrowth, striate keratopathy, iridocyclitis, cystoid macular edema, sympathetic ophthalmia, or endophthalmitis. If the iris is externalized and the prolapse is progressive or associated with excess astigmatism, it must be repaired promptly. A prolapsed iris rapidly becomes necrotic and strongly adherent to the wound, Tenon's capsule, and conjunctiva. Osmotics are given preoperatively to decrease the incidence of operative complications. If prolapse is recognized early (<48 hours), the iris may be swept from the wound and repositioned. Otherwise, the tissue must be dissected from the conjunctiva and wound edge and excised before wound revision. A small area of prolapse (<1.5 clock hours) well covered with conjunctiva may be treated with transconjunctival cryopexy or photocoagulation to induce necrosis of the iris and subsequent healing of the wound beneath.

G. After 5–7 days of medical management, the shallow AC must be definitively surgically repaired. Because wound leak, pupillary block, and choroidal detachment may occur together, adequate surgical repair of an aphakic or pseudophakic flat AC eliminates all possible causes. General anesthesia is preferred, and mannitol is given preoperatively to decrease the risk of vitreous loss. A corneal paracentesis site is created. Viscoelastics may be helpful. An additional iridectomy is created. The AC is filled with BSS, and any areas of possible leak are identified and resutured. Incarcerated tissue must be removed by appropriate means (e.g., anterior vitrectomy). Large choroidal detachments are drained, and the AC is reformed. Rarely, the anterior hyaloid face must be incised and/or anterior vitrectomy performed in the face of malignant glaucoma.

H. A shallow AC in the late postoperative period is usually related to epithelial or fibrous invasion. Careful examination, including biomicroscopy, Seidel's test, gonioscopy, fundus examination, and ultrasonography, identify the cause in most cases. Consider epithelial ingrowth in all cases. If Seidel's test is positive, the wound leak must be definitively repaired with great care to treat any fistula or incarcerated tissue.

I. If a filtering bleb is present but Seidel's test is negative, the patient may be observed for 6 months while using topical antibiotic coverage. Of inadvertent filtering blebs, 80% spontaneously disappear within 4 months. Beyond 6 months the bleb should be closed to prevent endophthalmitis, particularly if the bleb is thin walled or a contact lens is to be worn. Laser photocoagulation or cryotherapy may be applied to the bleb to initiate an inflammatory response with subsequent bleb closure 1–8 weeks later. Chemical cauterization with a 50% solution of trichloroacetic acid may be tried. Finally, the bleb may be surgically closed.

J. A delayed choroidal detachment presenting in the absence of a wound leak may occasionally present a problem with a differential diagnosis that includes retinal detachment and intraocular tumor. Clinical examination and ultrasonography aid in the diagnosis. Medical treatment is similar to that used for other forms of shallow AC. In addition, systemic corticosteroids may result in more rapid resolution of the choroidal detachment by decreasing the associated ocular inflammation.

K. If a wound leak or filtering bleb is not detected on examination in the setting of persistent ocular hypotony, perform gonioscopy to rule out a cyclodialysis cleft. If the chamber is not deep enough, reform the AC and repeat gonioscopy. A suspected cleft may also be diagnosed after injecting fluorescein solution into the AC and retrieving this fluorescein in the suprachoroidal fluid. Attempt to close the cleft using either laser photocoagulation, cryotherapy, partial-thickness diathermy, or through-and-through sutures to secure the detached ciliary body to the overlying sclera.

L. Epithelial inclusion cysts may occur secondary to faulty wound healing. The cyst may lie dormant for years, and unsuccessful attempts at removal may convert them to true ingrowths. Observe the cyst, and treat only if it is definitively growing or the eye is irritated. True epithelial ingrowth carries a guarded prognosis. The patient complains of tearing, photophobia, and pain after a relatively normal immediate postoperative course. Epithelium may be seen on the back of the cornea as an irregularly shaped advancing line. Photocoagulation of the epithelium on the iris turns it into a fluffy white material. Specular microscopy may be useful. Treatment is usually unsuccessful and must be radical. This complication is best avoided by achieving meticulous wound closure, correct placement of suture depth, and minimal corneal endothelial trauma. Fibrous ingrowth tends to be self-limited. The leading edge looks frayed in contrast to that of epithelial downgrowth. The treatment involves treating only the sequelae, such as glaucoma or keratic precipitates.

References

Bauer B. Argon laser photocoagulation of cyclodialysis clefts after cataract surgery. Acta Ophthalmol Scand 1995; 73:283–284.

Cionni RJ, Osher RH. Intraoperative complications of phacoemulsification surgery. In: Steinert RF, ed. Cataract surgery: Technique, complications, & management. Philadelphia: WB Saunders, 1995: 325–439.

Jaffe NS, Jaffe MS, Jaffe GF. Cataract surgery and its complications. 6th ed. St Louis: Mosby, 1997.

Menapace, R. Delayed iris prolapse with unsutured 5.1 mm clear corneal incisions. J Cataract Refract Surg 1995; 21:353–357.

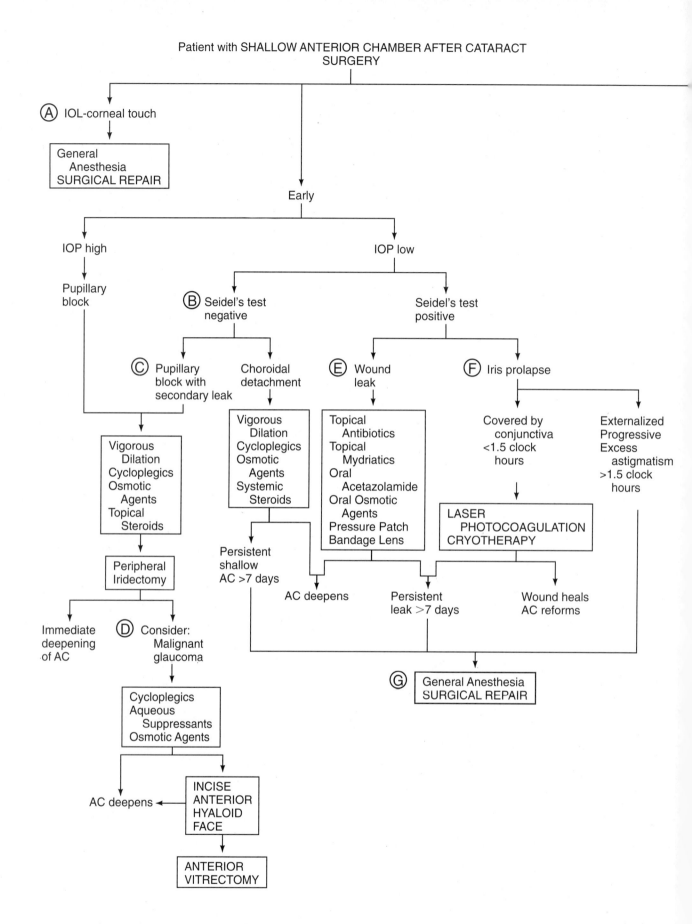

Patient with SHALLOW ANTERIOR CHAMBER AFTER CATARACT SURGERY

Ⓐ IOL-corneal touch

General
Anesthesia
SURGICAL REPAIR

Early

IOP high

Pupillary
block

IOP low

Ⓑ Seidel's test
negative

Seidel's test
positive

Ⓒ Pupillary
block with
secondary leak

Choroidal
detachment

Ⓔ Wound
leak

Ⓕ Iris prolapse

Vigorous
Dilation
Cycloplegics
Osmotic
Agents
Topical
Steroids

Vigorous
Dilation
Cycloplegics
Osmotic
Agents
Systemic
Steroids

Topical
Antibiotics
Topical
Mydriatics
Oral
Acetazolamide
Oral Osmotic
Agents
Pressure Patch
Bandage Lens

Covered by
conjunctiva
<1.5 clock
hours

Externalized
Progressive
Excess
astigmatism
>1.5 clock
hours

Peripheral
Iridectomy

Persistent
shallow
AC >7 days

LASER
PHOTOCOAGULATION
CRYOTHERAPY

Immediate
deepening
of AC

Ⓓ Consider:
Malignant
glaucoma

AC deepens

Persistent
leak >7 days

Wound heals
AC reforms

Cycloplegics
Aqueous
Suppressants
Osmotic Agents

Ⓖ General Anesthesia
SURGICAL REPAIR

AC deepens

INCISE
ANTERIOR
HYALOID
FACE

ANTERIOR
VITRECTOMY

286

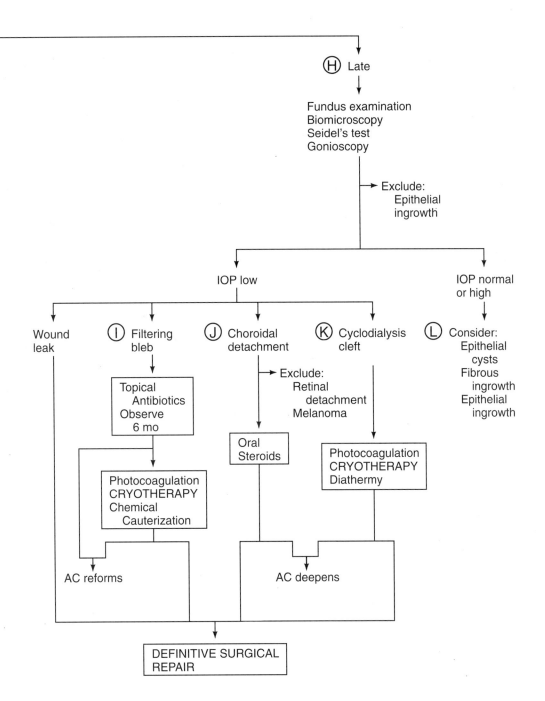

H Late

Fundus examination
Biomicroscopy
Seidel's test
Gonioscopy

→ Exclude:
     Epithelial
     ingrowth

IOP low

IOP normal
or high

Wound
leak

I Filtering
  bleb

J Choroidal
  detachment

K Cyclodialysis
  cleft

L Consider:
  Epithelial
     cysts
  Fibrous
     ingrowth
  Epithelial
     ingrowth

Topical
Antibiotics
Observe
6 mo

→ Exclude:
     Retinal
       detachment
     Melanoma

Oral
Steroids

Photocoagulation
CRYOTHERAPY
Diathermy

Photocoagulation
CRYOTHERAPY
Chemical
Cauterization

AC reforms

AC deepens

DEFINITIVE SURGICAL
REPAIR

RETINAL AND VITREOUS DISORDERS

MACULAR BULL'S EYE

Joseph M. Harrison, Ph.D.

A. A macular bull's eye is an ophthalmoscopic pattern of a more pigmented area in the center of the fovea surrounded by a partial or full ring of depigmented retinal pigment epithelium (RPE), which is seen as a transmission defect with fluorescein angiography. Complaints of blurry vision, difficulty in reading (because of paracentrally decreased sensitivity), or decreased visual acuity generally precedes discovery of the bull's eye lesion. The history and physical examination should determine whether the following are present: CNS symptoms, extra digits on hands or feet, history of medication by synthetic antimalarials, acquired nystagmus, photophobia, or problems with night or color vision.

B. Chloroquine and other synthetic antimalarials bind to melanin in the RPE and choroid. A paracentral scotoma demonstrable with red test objects and increased macular dazzle occur early in the toxicity but are not signs of irreversible dysfunction. Later, there may be complaints of blurred and decreased vision as the lesion spreads inward. A frequent later manifestation is a type 3 (blue-yellow or tritan) color vision defect on the Farnsworth-Munsell 100-hue (FM 100-hue) test of color vision. The bull's eye lesion is also a later development. There is a cumulative effect, which sometimes leads to deterioration despite discontinuation because chloroquine is excreted very slowly. Rare advanced retinopathy can cause a tapetoretinal fundus appearance with constricted visual fields and equal loss of the cone and rod electroretinogram (ERG), ending in an unrecordable ERG and flat electrooculogram (EOG). Even so, the final dark-adapted threshold tends to be normal. Clofazimine, a phenazine dye used to treat dapsone-resistant leprosy and inflammation in other diseases, has also been reported to cause a bull's eye lesion.

C. Cone or cone-rod degeneration is a photoreceptor degeneration, presenting with photophobia, decreased vision, acquired nystagmus, poor color vision (even though visual acuity may be only 20/40 to 20/60), normal peripheral visual fields, decreased cone ERG and preserved rod ERG, elevated or absent cone threshold, and normal final rod threshold during dark adaptation. The color vision defect is usually type 1 (red-green or protan-deutan) on the FM 100-hue test. Fluorescein angiography often shows bull's eye lesions not visible ophthalmoscopically, with widespread RPE defects. In the more common autosomal-dominant form, the bull's eye pattern remains stable, with later development of pigment clumping and midperipheral and peripheral pigmentation. The autosomal-recessive form may have a paramacular "crown" of Stargardt-like flecks. Often, there is a small central atrophic spot in the foveolar pigmented island, which progresses peripherally to complete foveolar atrophy. Vision is usually decreased. If foveal function is retained, color vision may be normal or there may be a type 3 defect that progresses to a type 2 defect (red-green and blue-yellow defect, p 8) with loss of the preserved central island and occasionally to complete achromatopsia. Night vision is normal in the early stages. The cone ERG is almost always abnormal, but the rod ERG is normal in the early stages. This ERG pattern is diagnostic and is the defining characteristic of cone degeneration. With progression, there is a slightly elevated final dark-adapted threshold (less than a factor of 100) and depressed or absent rod ERG.

D. In Stargardt's fundus flavimaculatus, there is a widespread retinal pigment epitheliopathy with engorgement of cells by a lipofuscin-like substance. It is usually autosomal recessive, causing a central maculopathy with early complaints of decreased vision. Classically, there is a type 1 color vision defect (red-green), some loss of cone and rod ERG amplitude, a prolonged cone-rod break on dark adaptation, and central visual field defects. Early, there is macular mottling and broadening of the foveal reflex. Often, a small region of atrophy develops in the center of the central pigmented island. This may progress to the atrophic "beaten bronze" macula. One form is without flecks (feathery soft yellow or gray deposits in the RPE), although flecks are a part of the classic description. These generally develop after the central maculopathy and may be seen as a crown surrounding the macula or may be more widespread in the posterior pole beyond the arcades and nasal to the disc. Unlike drusen, the fresh flecks do not fluoresce. With time, the RPE cells die, leaving window defects. Fluorescein angiography may show a faint bull's eye or the dark choroid sign because of RPE blocking (vermilion fundus on ophthalmoscopy), which occurs in 50%–80% of the cases early in the disease, even though ophthalmoscopically, the defect appears limited to the posterior pole. There can be a reticular pattern of flecks and atrophic pigment patches or even "bone spicule" pigmentation and localized "punched-out" areas. A type 1 color vision defect is a classic finding seen in 50% of the cases with macular involvement. In about 8% of the cases, there is a type 3 color vision defect, when foveolar fixation is preserved. In 37%, there is no or only a mild color vision defect. The final dark-adapted threshold is normal or slightly elevated.

E. In the original description of benign concentric annular macular dystrophy with bull's eye lesions (autosomal dominant), there was unusually good visual acuity (20/25 or better), even in the oldest patients. With 10 years follow-up, some of these patients complained of deterioration of day vision, night vision, and color vision. The fundus abnormalities progressed with involvement of the periphery, including bone spicule pigmentation in some. Rod and cone ERGs were equally involved.

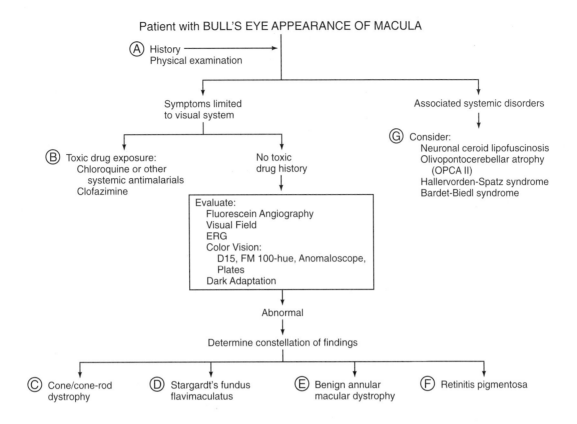

Patient with BULL'S EYE APPEARANCE OF MACULA

(A) History
Physical examination

Symptoms limited to visual system

Associated systemic disorders

(B) Toxic drug exposure:
Chloroquine or other systemic antimalarials
Clofazimine

No toxic drug history

(G) Consider:
Neuronal ceroid lipofuscinosis
Olivopontocerebellar atrophy (OPCA II)
Hallervorden-Spatz syndrome
Bardet-Biedl syndrome

Evaluate:
Fluorescein Angiography
Visual Field
ERG
Color Vision:
D15, FM 100-hue, Anomaloscope, Plates
Dark Adaptation

Abnormal

Determine constellation of findings

(C) Cone/cone-rod dystrophy

(D) Stargardt's fundus flavimaculatus

(E) Benign annular macular dystrophy

(F) Retinitis pigmentosa

F. Bull's eye lesions are also seen in 30%–40% of patients with retinitis pigmentosa, a rod-cone photoreceptor degeneration, which is sporadic in about half the cases or inherited by any of the genetic patterns. Patients complain of problems with night vision and have an elevated final dark-adapted threshold (greater than a factor of 100). They also have constricted visual fields or an expanding midperipheral ring scotoma, photophobia, selectively more decreased rod ERG, a delayed cone ERG, and a type 3 color vision defect. The ERG is absent or too small to be recorded by standard techniques in 70% of patients. Classically, there are attenuated arterioles, midperipheral pigment clumping and depigmentation, bone spicule pigmentation, and waxy-appearing discs. In the early stages of the disease, the fundus signs may only be a blond or mottled appearance.

G. Bull's eye lesions are also seen in syndromes—neuronal ceroid lipofuscinosis (Jansky-Bielchowsky and Vogt-Spielmeyer), olivopontocerebellar atrophy with retinal dystrophy (OPCA II) (autosomal dominant), Hallervorden-Spatz, and Bardet-Biedl—and rarely in fucosidosis and methylmalonic aciduria. The latter two are diagnosed by enzyme assays and urinalysis, respectively. Fucosidosis is rare and includes prominent facial and skeletal abnormalities. In neuronal storage diseases associated with bull's eye lesions (Jansky-Bielchowsky, Vogt-Spielmeyer, fucosidosis and methylmalonic aciduria and Bardet-Biedl syndrome—all autosomal recessive), the ERG is either unrecordable or very subnormal in children. Bardet-Biedl syndrome also includes polydactyly, obesity, and renal disorders. Neuronal ceroid lipofuscinosis can be dis-

tinguished from the other conditions with CNS symptoms by the finding of curvilinear or fingerprint inclusion bodies in ultrastructural examination of conjunctival biopsies and peripheral blood lymphocytes. OPCA II involves cerebellar symptoms, such as ataxia, whereas Hallervorden-Spatz syndrome includes deterioration of voluntary movements and increased involuntary movements and muscle rigidity. The macula is hyperpigmented in Hallervorden-Spatz syndrome and may have a fine granular pigmentation in OPCA II.

References

Batemen JR, Lange GE, Maumenee IH. Genetic metabolic disorders associated with retinal dystrophies. In: Ryan SJ, ed. Retina. Vol. 1. St Louis: Mosby, 1989: 421–445.

Blacharski PA. Fundus flavimaculatus. In: Newsome DA, ed. Retinal dystrophies and degenerations. New York: Raven, 1988: 135–139.

Deutman AF. Macular dystrophies. In: Ryan SJ, ed. Retina. Vol. 2. St Louis: Mosby, 1989: 243–298.

Gass JDM. Stereoscopic atlas of macular diseases: Diagnosis and treatment. 3rd ed. Vols. 1 and 2. St Louis: Mosby, 1987.

Krill AE. Hereditary retinal and choroidal diseases. Vol.2. Clinical characteristics. Philadelphia: Harper & Row, 1977.

Weleber RG. Retinitis pigmentosa and allied disorders. In: Ryan SJ, ed. Retina. Vol. 1. St Louis: Mosby, 1989: 299–420.

Weleber RG, Eisner A. Cone degeneration (Bull's-eye dystrophies) and color vision defects. In: Newsome DA, ed. Retinal dystrophies and degenerations. New York: Raven, 1988: 233–256.

MACULAR STAR

G. Robert Hampton, M.D.
Peter B. Hay, B.A.
Bailey L. Lee, M.D.

A macular star is formed when lipid-rich exudate accumulates in the outer plexiform layer of Henle. The lipids precipitate in a stellate pattern, following the anatomy of that layer, as the serous component of capillary leakage is absorbed (Figure 1).

A. The earliest ophthalmoscopic manifestation of hypertension is narrowing and irregularity of the arterioles. More severe signs of hypertensive retinopathy include hemorrhage, cotton-wool spots, exudate, edema, and papilledema. The exudates may align to form a macular star. Visual disturbance depends on the coincidental involvement of the central macula.

B. Capillary angiomas have the initial ophthalmoscopic appearance of a red or grayish dot. As the tumor grows, associated enlargement of afferent and efferent vessels progresses. The incompetent capillary walls of the shunt vessels lead to progressive exudation and formation of circinate rings with subsequent exudative retinal detachment. If the peripheral retina is not carefully examined in a patient with posterior circinate retinopathy, it is possible to miss the peripheral angioma and feeder vessels. Fluorescein angiography demonstrates rapid flow through an incompetent highly vascular network. Prognosis is excellent for small tumors treated with laser and/or cryopexy. Von Hippel-Lindau disease is the association with hemangioblastoma of the cerebellum, brainstem, or spinal cord, with retinal cell carcinoma, or with pheochromocytoma.

C. Macular neuroretinitis (Leber's idiopathic stellate retinopathy) typically occurs in children or young adults with a recent history of febrile illness. Within the first week, a macular star is usually associated with optic nerve swelling and leakage on angiography. Visual acuity may range from 20/20 to 20/200. No treatment is indicated. The visual acuity usually spontaneously improves over 3–12 weeks, and the macular star resolves over several months. Visual dysfunction results from the optic nerve abnormality. No angiographic abnormality is seen in the macula.

Cat-scratch disease has been implicated as cause of neuroretinitis. *Bartonella henselae* (formerly *Rochalimaea henselae*) is now recognized as the causative agent for cat-scratch disease. A history of cat exposure, prodrome or febrile illness, or lymphadenopathy may be elicited. Laboratory test of indirect immunofluorescent antibody (IFA) for *B. henselae* may help establish the diagnosis. Early antibiotic therapy with rifampin and doxycycline may shorten the course of infection and hasten visual recovery.

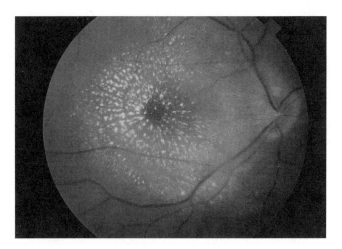

Figure 1 Lipid exudates forming a macular star.

D. Papillitis usually presents with variable reduction of visual acuity and an afferent pupillary defect (APD). There may be associated pain in or behind the globe and typically a central or paracentral scotoma. There is usually swelling of the optic nerve with obliteration of the cup. Leakage of this small vessel on the nerve may lead to a macular star.

E. A macular star may be associated with papilledema, although the other signs of papilledema should be obvious. Typically, there is hyperemia and obscuration of the disc margin with venous congestion. Flame-shaped hemorrhages and cotton-wool spots may surround the nerve, and in contrast to papillitis, there is no associated loss of vision and no afferent pupillary defect.

References

Annesley WH, Leonard BC, Shields JA, Tasman WS. Fifteen year review of treated cases of retinal angiomatosis. Trans Am Acad Ophthalmol Otolaryngol 1977; 832:446–453.

Francois J, Verriest G, DeLaey J. Leber's idiopathic stellate retinopathy. Am J Ophthalmol 1969; 68:340–345.

Gass JD, Braunstein R: Sessile and exophytic capillary angiomas of the juxtapapillary retina and optic nerve head, Arch Ophthalmol 1980; 98:1790–1797.

Hardwig P, Robertson DM. Von Hippel-Lindau disease: A familial, often lethal, multi-system phakomatosis. Ophthalmology 1984; 91:263–270.

Reed JB, Scales DK, Wong MT, et al. *Bartonella hanselae* neuroretinitis in cat scratch disease. Diagnosis, management, and sequelae. Ophthalmology 1998; 105:459–466.

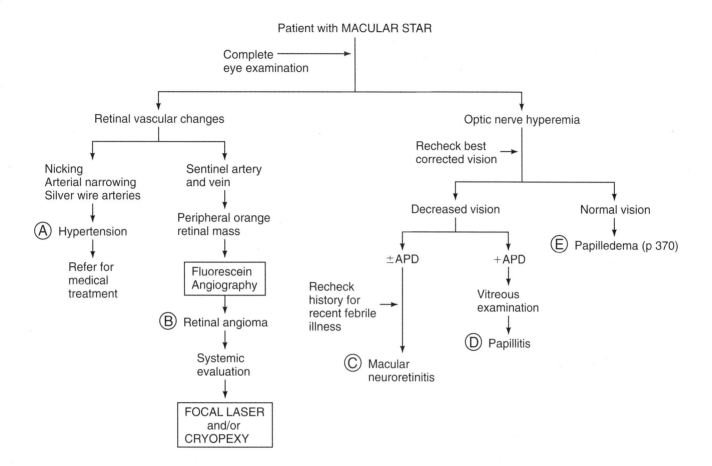

Patient with MACULAR STAR

Complete eye examination

Retinal vascular changes

Nicking
Arterial narrowing
Silver wire arteries

(A) Hypertension

Refer for medical treatment

Sentinel artery and vein

Peripheral orange retinal mass

Fluorescein Angiography

(B) Retinal angioma

Systemic evaluation

FOCAL LASER and/or CRYOPEXY

Optic nerve hyperemia

Recheck best corrected vision

Decreased vision

±APD

Recheck history for recent febrile illness

(C) Macular neuroretinitis

+APD

Vitreous examination

(D) Papillitis

Normal vision

(E) Papilledema (p 370)

MACULAR CHERRY-RED SPOT

G. Robert Hampton, M.D.
Peter B. Hay, B.A.

A. Central retinal artery occlusion (CRAO) typically is the most common cause of acute cherry-red spot of the macula. On presentation the posterior edematous retina is a pale, opaque white, except for the foveolar cherry-red spot, and an afferent pupillary defect is present. The central red spot represents normal, nonedematous, thin retina in the fovea, most of which is supplied by the posterior retinal (choroidal) circulation, which is not occluded. CRAO presents typically as painless loss of vision occurring over seconds. The patient often can date the onset to the minute. The mean age at presentation is the early sixties. CRAO is more common in men than in women. Fluorescein angiography can show a delay in retinal filling, but the most common finding is delay in retinal arteriovenous transit time. The choroidal filling is normal, although there may be some blockage as a result of retina edema. There is usually rapid reopening of the arteries, and soon after the occlusion, the angiogram may appear normal. The most common causes of CRAO are emboli, vasculitis, intraluminal thrombosis, spasm, and dissecting aneurysm.

B. Macular hole may mimic a cherry-red spot as a result of the clear view of the pigment epithelium and choroid through the absent central retina. In contrast to a true cherry-red spot, the surrounding retina and vasculature appear normal. On slit-lamp examination, the central defect is more obvious as the light "falls" into the central hole, and there may be a small cuff of surrounding retinal detachment. The patient may note a discontinuity in the slit-lamp beam as it passes over the hole. In contrast to a CRAO, it is often difficult for the patient to note the exact time of the hole's occurrence, typically noting a gradual, rather than sudden, loss of vision. Fluorescein angiography demonstrates a window defect of hyperfluorescence throughout the angiogram that does not leak and gradually fades. There may be partial blockage of fluorescence on the borders of the hole because of surrounding retinal elevation. The cause of most holes is unknown.

C. Berlin's edema (commotio retinae) is the result of blunt injury to the globe. It is most common in the posterior pole and may be the result of paralytic vasodilation. It appears as variable white edema with a cherry-red spot of the fovea (see section A). Variable retinal hemorrhage, also caused by the trauma, may be present. Visual acuity is usually decreased. The edema often increases over the first 24 hours and then gradually subsides. Prognosis for visual recovery depends on the degree of initial damage, and visual recovery may be complete. Pigmentary disturbance, macular hole, and macular cyst, when present, are reasons for visual impairment.

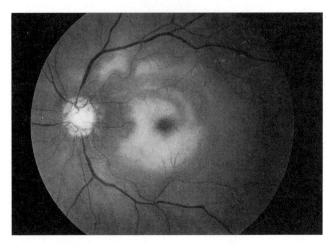

Figure 1   A cherry-red spot in the macula caused by central retinal artery occlusion.

D. Typically in immunocompromised individuals, varicella-zoster virus has been shown to be the cause of a distinctive form of retinopathy, called *progressive outer retinal necrosis syndrome.* It is characterized by multifocal, deep retinal opaque lesions that quickly coalesce to involve the entire retina. Parafoveal lesions may be the first manifestation and can cause the appearance of a "cherry-red spot." The retina can become completely necrotic over a few days to a couple of weeks. Acute retinal necrosis (ARN) is most commonly reported in otherwise healthy individuals. ARN is characterized by prominent vitreous and anterior-chamber inflammatory reactions, although it does not typically have macular involvement. Occlusive vasculopathy is usually a prominent clinical feature.

E. Clinical features of *Niemann-Pick disease* are related to accumulation of sphingomyelin and cholesterol. During the first 6 months, hepatosplenomegaly, jaundice, mental retardation, seizures, and failure to thrive develop in the infant. The macular cherry-red spot is the major ocular manifestation of type A, and it is caused by accumulation of sphingomyelin in the ganglion cells surrounding the fovea. *Tay-Sachs disease* is the most common gangliosidosis. At birth, children show no abnormality, but signs develop over the first few months of life and progress to death by age 3. Symptoms are caused by ganglioside accumulation in ganglion cells of the nervous system, producing progressive deafness, blindness, and macrocephaly. *Sandhoff's disease* is a phenotypic variant of Tay-Sachs disease characterized by storage of excess lipids in the viscera. The clinical and pathologic features are otherwise almost identical to those of Tay-Sachs. *General-*

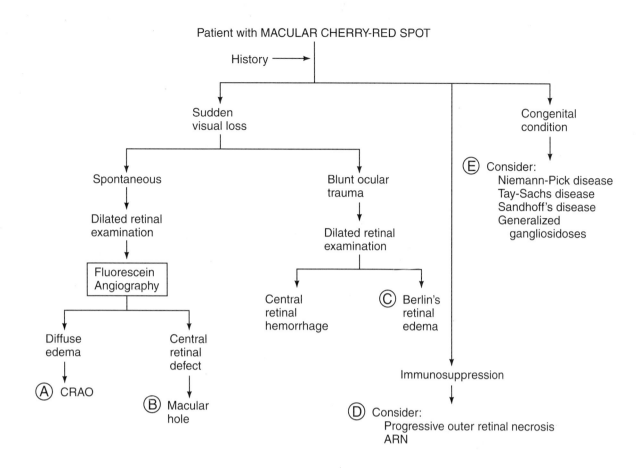

Patient with MACULAR CHERRY-RED SPOT

ized gangliosidosis (GM, gangliosidosis type 1) is characterized by abnormal storage of ganglioside GM, in the brain and viscera and a mucopolysaccharide in the viscera, with severe bony abnormalities resembling those of Hurler's syndrome. Symptoms are present at birth, and there is rapid onset of severe cerebral degeneration and hepatosplenomegaly (Figure 1).

References

Brown GC, Magargal LE. Central retinal artery obstruction and visual acuity. Ophthalmology 1982; 89:14–19.

Brown GC, Magargal LE, Sergott R. Acute obstruction of the retinal and choroidal circulations. Ophthalmology 1986; 93:1373–1382.

Cogan DG. Ocular correlates of inborn metabolic defects. Can Med Assoc J 1966; 95:1055.

Cogan DG, Kuwabara T. The sphingolipidoses and the eye. Arch Ophthalmol 1968; 79:437.

Forster DJ, Dugal PU, Frangieh JT, et al. Rapidly progressive outer retinal necrosis in the acquired immunodeficiency syndrome. Am J Ophthalmol 1990; 110:341.

Gass JDM. Idiopathic senile macular hole: Its early stages and pathogenesis. Arch Ophthalmol 1988; 106:629.

Johnson RN, Gass JDM. Idiopathic macular holes: Observations, stages of formation and implications for surgical intervention. Ophthalmology 1988; 95:917–924.

Morgan Schatz H. Idiopathic macular holes. Am J Ophthalmol 1985; 99:437–444.

Sternberg P Jr, Knox DL, Finkelstein D, et al. Acute retinal necrosis syndrome. Retina 1982; 2:145.

SUBRETINAL NEOVASCULAR MEMBRANES

Lina M. Marouf, M.D.
Bailey L. Lee, M.D.

Subretinal neovascular membrane (SRNVM) refers to the growth of choroidal vessels through Bruch's membrane into the subretinal pigment epithelial space or the subretinal space. Any disease process that affects the integrity of the retinal pigment epithelium—Bruch's membrane—choriocapillaris complex can be associated with an SRNVM. Patients with SRNVMs usually present with sudden onset of painless decrease in central vision and metamorphopsia.

A. Visual field testing is important in assessing a patient with metamorphopsia and decreased central vision. The central 20 degrees of the visual field can be assessed with an Amsler grid. A central scotoma may denote macular, optic nerve, or cortical abnormality; however, metamorphopsia indicates macular disease.

B. A detailed dilated fundus examination is performed with contact lens biomicroscopy and indirect ophthalmoscopy. Signs of subretinal neovascular proliferation include macular hemorrhages, serous macular detachment, serous or hemorrhagic retinal pigment epithelial detachment (RPED), and macular exudates. Funduscopic findings in the same or fellow eye may help establish the cause of an SRNVM.

C. Age-related macular degeneration (ARMD) is the leading cause of central visual loss in the United States in people >60 years of age. Signs of ARMD include macular drusen, retinal pigment epithelial changes, atrophic changes, serous and hemorrhagic RPEDs, choroidal neovascularization (SRNVM), subretinal fibrosis, and disciform scars. The disease presents in two forms. The nonexudative or dry form affects most patients; the exudative form is responsible for severe visual loss in affected eyes. There is no known therapy for the atrophic form of ARMD.

D. SRNVM secondary to presumed ocular histoplasmosis syndrome (POHS) usually occurs in healthy persons 20–50 years old. The classically described triad of the disease includes peripheral punched-out atrophic lesions (histo spots), peripapillary chorioretinal scarring, and macular scars.

E. Angioid streaks are linear dehiscences in Bruch's membrane. Clinically, they are irregular, jagged lines that vary from reddish orange to dark red. They typically extend from the peripapillary area to the peripheral fundus. The disease is usually bilateral. Choroidal vessels may grow through breaks in Bruch's membrane into the subretinal pigment epithelial space, resulting in serous and hemorrhagic RPED. The visual prognosis in such eyes is usually poor. Of patients with angioid streaks, 50% have associated systemic abnormalities, the most common being Paget's disease, sickle cell hemoglobinopathy, Ehlers-Danlos syndrome, and pseudoxanthoma elasticum.

F. Trauma to the eye can rupture Bruch's membrane and the choroidal layers. This is known clinically as choroidal rupture. SRNVM may arise at the site of rupture months to years after the injury, resulting in decreased vision.

G. The progressive thinning of the choroidal and retinal layers in pathologic myopia can result in pen papillary chorioretinal atrophy, geographic areas of chorioretinal atrophy, and linear breaks in Bruch's membrane called *lacquer cracks*. SRNVM can grow through these foci, resulting in decreased central vision.

H. Several hereditary macular dystrophies and inflammatory retinal diseases are associated with SRNVMs. Each exhibits a characteristic funduscopic lesion in the fellow eye, denoting the cause of the SRNVM.

I. In the absence of drusen and chorioretinal abnormalities, young patients with SRNVM are classified as having idiopathic SRNVM.

J. Posterior segment uveitis can lead to choroidal inflammation and the development of SRNVM. Examples include multifocal choroiditis, punctate inner choroidopathy, toxoplasmosis retinochoroiditis, multiple evanescent white dot syndrome, and serpiginous choroiditis.

K. Before laser photocoagulation of an SRNVM, fluorescein angiography performed within the previous 72 hours should be available. Fluorescein angiography can help define the margins of an SRNVM and its proximity to the foveal avascular zone (FAZ). Choroidal neovascularization (CN) is accordingly categorized into well-defined or poorly defined extrafoveal (200–2500 μ from the center of the fovea), juxtafoveal (<199 μ), or subfoveal SRNVM. A characteristic angiographic finding of a well-defined SRNVM is early hyperfluorescence in the area of CN with late leakage.

L. The value of laser photocoagulation in patients with subfoveal SRNVM secondary to ARMD and in those with well-defined extrafoveal and juxtafoveal neovascularization secondary to ARMD, POHS, and idiopathic SRNVM has been demonstrated. Its value in those with SRNVMs and RPEDs is unknown. One should be careful in treating SRNVMs adjacent to an RPED because of the risk of inducing a rip or tear in the retinal pigment epithelium. Patients with extrafoveal SRNVM secondary to angioid streaks or trauma should undergo laser treatment. Laser therapy for SRNVM in pathologic myopia is controversial. After laser therapy patients should be re-examined at frequent intervals. Fluorescein angiography should be performed at approximately 2 and 6 weeks and 3, 6, 9, and 12 months after treatment to confirm complete

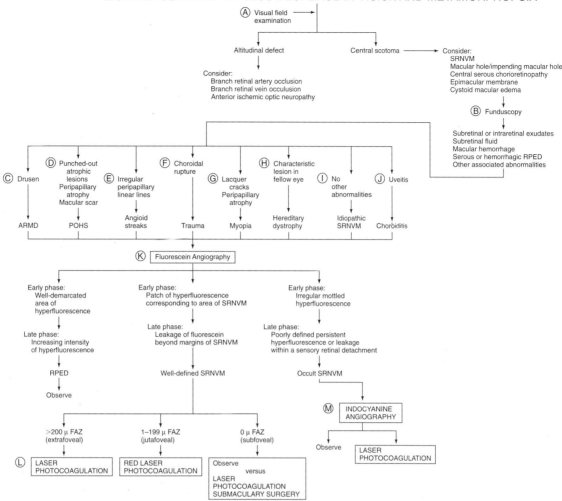

Patient with CENTRAL PAINLESS DECREASE IN VISION AND METAMORPHOPSIA

occlusion of the SRNVM and to detect recurrence. Initial enthusiasm for submacular surgery in treating subfoveal SRNVM has been tempered by the poor visual results in patients with ARMD. Better visual outcomes are seen in younger patients with POHS or idiopathic SRNVMs. This may be because of the location of the SRNVM (primarily sub-RPE versus subretinal) and the status of the retinal epithelium (older patients in ARMD versus younger patients in POHS). Even with submacular surgery, there is a risk of recurrence comparable with laser photocoagulation. Currently, there is the ongoing observation in patients with POHS and idiopathic SRNVM. All patients at risk for SRNVM should be taught to monitor their vision with an Amsler grid and to see an ophthalmologist as soon as new symptoms develop. Low-vision rehabilitation for patients with bilateral visual loss is essential.

M. Indocyanine green angiography (ICG) can be a useful adjunct in visualizing SRNVMs that are occult by fluorescein angiography or those SRNVMs with overlying hemorrhage. Focal areas of leakage or well-defined plaques visualized with ICG have been treated with involution of the SRNVM.

References

Macular Photocoagulation Study Group. Krypton laser photocoagulation for neovascular lesions of ocular histoplasmosis: Results of a randomized clinical trial. Arch Ophthalmol 1987; 105:1499–1507.

Macular Photocoagulation Study Group. Krypton laser photocoagulation for idiopathic neovascular lesions: Results of a randomized clinical trial. Arch Ophthalmol 1990; 108:832–837.

Macular Photocoagulation Study Group. Krypton laser photocoagulation for neovascular lesions of age-related macular degeneration: Results of a randomized clinical trial. Arch Ophthalmol 1990; 108:816–824.

Macular Photocoagulation Study Group. Argon laser photocoagulation for neovascular maculopathy: Five-year results from randomized clinical trials. Arch Ophthalmol 1991; 109:1109–1114.

Macular Photocoagulation Study Group. Laser photocoagulation of subfoveal neovascular lesions in age-related macular degeneration: Results of a randomized clinical trial. Arch Ophthalmol 1991; 109:1220–1231.

Thomas MA, Dickinson JD, Melberg NS, et al. Visual results after surgical removal of subfoveal choroidal neovascular membranes. Ophthalmology 1994; 101:1384–1396.

JUXTAPAPILLARY LESION

G. Robert Hampton, M.D.
Peter B. Hay, B.A.

Juxtapapillary lesions can be broadly classified on the basis of appearance: atrophic, tumorous, and edematous.

A. Pigmented or nonpigmented scleral crescent is a common developmental variation in which the retinal pigment epithelium (RPE) or pigmented choroid does not fully reach the optic nerve, thereby permitting a view of the choroid or underlying sclera (Figure 1). Coloboma results from incomplete closure of the embryonic fissure, appearing as sharply demarcated loss of Bruch's membrane with overlying retinal atrophy (Figure 2). Pits appear as dark gray depressions, usually in the temporal aspect of the optic nerve. Serous macular detachments may be associated in 40%–50% of cases (Figure 3).

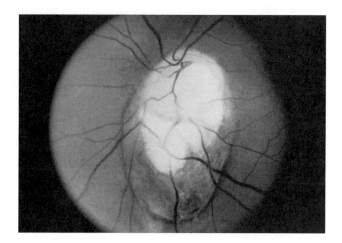

Figure 2 Coloboma.

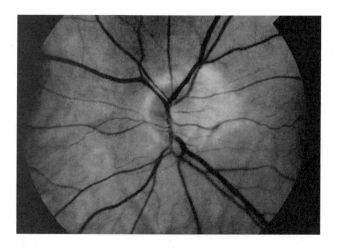

Figure 1 Scleral crescent.

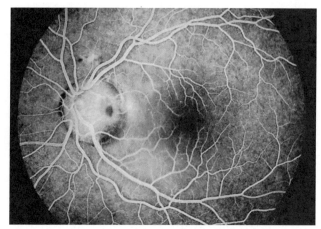

Figure 3 Optic pit.

B. Inflammatory conditions of the optic nerve often resolve to leave an atrophic crescent on the border. Presumed ocular histoplasmosis (POHS) is also associated with scattered midperipheral "punched-out" chorioretinal scars (p 304). Serpiginous choroiditis is a focal recurring inflammatory process that affects primarily the choriocapillaris and pigment epithelium. It begins in the peripapillary region and spreads over months to years in a serpiginous fashion outward to involve the peripheral retina and macula.

C. Myopic lacunar atrophy may be present both surrounding the optic nerve and in isolated patches involving the posterior pole. When surrounding the optic nerve, it is usually broader than a simple scleral crescent. Angioid streaks are lacunar cracklike dehiscences radiating outward from the optic nerve, developing in Bruch's membrane. Near the optic nerve they may be interconnected circumferentially. Choroidal osteoma appears as a yellow-white choroidal lesion typically in the juxtapapillary region. Variability in color occurs secondary to thinning, depigmentation, or hyperplasia of the RPE. The tumor is usually oval with well-defined scalloped margins. The retinal vasculature and the optic nerve are unaffected. Ocular echography is most helpful in making the diagnosis because of the bony content, which causes acoustic shadowing.

D. Melanocytoma is a benign pigmented tumor that appears as a jet-black lesion with fibrillated margins adjacent to or over the optic nerve (Figure 4). Choroidal melanomas arising in the peripapillary region may extend anteriorly over the optic nerve head but are generally mottled gray or yellow-white and do not insinuate into the nerve fiber layer.

E. Melanoma may arise in the peripapillary region. Classic ophthalmoscopic findings are a pigmented "collar button" tumor with exudative detachment. There is often intrinsic pigmentation with orange lipofuscin. Fluorescein angiography reveals hot spots and an intrinsic circulation, but this is not diagnostic. Echography typically demonstrates solid consistency (inability to indent), medium to low reflectivity, and internal blood flow (pp 326 and 330). Astrocytic hamartoma typically occurs at or near the optic nerve, appearing as a yellow-gray or pink-gray mulberry. Fluorescein angiography demonstrates a diffuse capillary network. Capillary hemangioma may arise on the border of the optic nerve. When located elsewhere in the retina, it may be associated with feeder vessels. A variably sized net of fine vasculature with or without exudation is typically present, demonstrating diffuse leakage on fluorescein angiography. Drusen of the optic nerve are 70% bilateral and appear as opalescent autofluorescent "rocks" within the optic cup. When deep within the nerve, they are best seen with the slit lamp in retroillumination (Figure 5). Hyperplasia of the RPE is black but is usually associated with other signs of prior inflammation, whereas congenital hypertrophy of the RPE is flat, has a distinct margin, and does not occur within the optic disc.

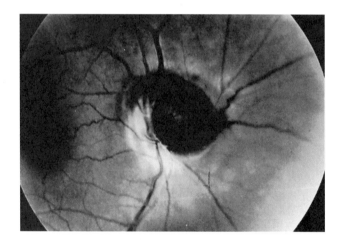

Figure 4 Melanocytoma.

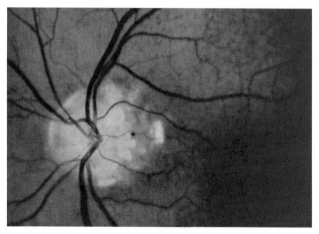

Figure 5 Disc drusen.

F. Myelinated nerve fibers may be mistaken for edema and may look like a glossy white patch within the nerve fiber layer, feathering out peripherally like the end of a paintbrush (Figure 6). Combined hamartomas have proliferation of pigment epithelial, glial, and vascular elements of the sensory retina. The vascular components may create an angiomatous appearance in the lesion, and glial components create traction on the internal limiting membrane.

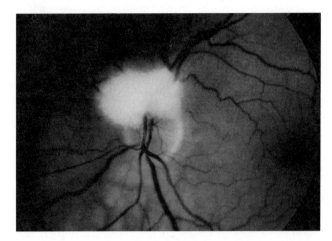

Figure 6 Myelinated nerves.

References

Brown GC, Shields JA, Goldberg RE. Congenital pits of the optic nerve head. Clinical studies in humans. Ophthalmology 1980; 87:51–65.

Char DH, Stone RD. Irvine AR, et al. Diagnostic modalities in choroidal melanoma. Am J Ophthalmol 1980; 89:223–230.

Federman JL, Shields JA, Tomer TH. Angioid streaks. Arch Ophthalmol 1975; 93:951–962.

Friedman AH, Gartner S, Modi SS. Drusen of the optic disc. Br J Ophthalmol 1975; 59:413–421.

Hamilton AM, Bird AC. Geographical choroidopathy. Br J Ophthalmol 1974; 58:784–797.

Hogan MJ, Alvarado JA, Weddell JE. Histology of the human eye: An atlas and textbook. Philadelphia: WB Saunders 1971: 525–526, 537–571.

Joffe L, Shields JA, Osher RH, Gass JDM: Clinical and follow up studies of melanocytomas of the optic disc. Ophthalmology 1979; 86:1067–1078.

Reidy JJ, Apple DJ, Steimnetz RL, et al. Melanocytoma: Nomenclature, pathogenesis, natural history and treatment. Surv Ophthalmol 1985; 29:319–327.

Shields JA, Augsburger JJ. Current approaches to the diagnosis and management of retinoblastoma. Surv Ophthalmol 1981; 25:347–371.

Teich SA, Walsh YB. Choroidal osteoma, Ophthalmology 1981; 88:696–698.

Williams R, Taylor D. Tuberous sclerosis. Surv Ophthalmol 1985; 30:143–153.

Patient with JUXTAPAPILLARY LESION

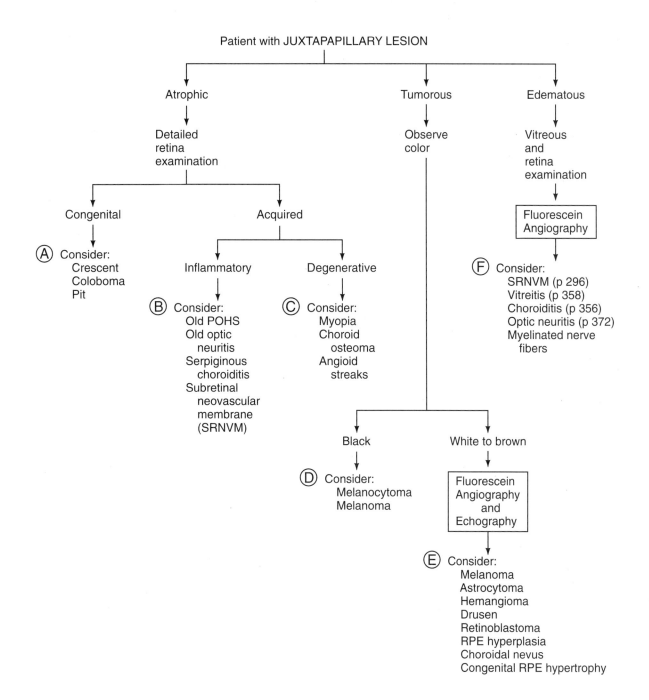

Atrophic

Detailed
retina
examination

Congenital

Ⓐ Consider:
Crescent
Coloboma
Pit

Acquired

Inflammatory

Ⓑ Consider:
Old POHS
Old optic
neuritis
Serpiginous
choroiditis
Subretinal
neovascular
membrane
(SRNVM)

Degenerative

Ⓒ Consider:
Myopia
Choroid
osteoma
Angioid
streaks

Tumorous

Observe
color

Black

Ⓓ Consider:
Melanocytoma
Melanoma

White to brown

Fluorescein
Angiography
and
Echography

Ⓔ Consider:
Melanoma
Astrocytoma
Hemangioma
Drusen
Retinoblastoma
RPE hyperplasia
Choroidal nevus
Congenital RPE hypertrophy

Edematous

Vitreous
and
retina
examination

Fluorescein
Angiography

Ⓕ Consider:
SRNVM (p 296)
Vitreitis (p 358)
Choroiditis (p 356)
Optic neuritis (p 372)
Myelinated nerve
fibers

CHOROIDAL FOLDS

W.A.J. van Heuven, M.D.
Peter B. Hay, B.A.

Choroidal folds, sometimes called *chorioretinal folds* or *choroidal striae,* are usually caused by pressure that deforms the eye and can cause choriocapillaris congestion, so they are often seen in cases of orbital tumors and other causes of proptosis. The exact mechanism of formation of these folds is not understood because the presence of folds seems unrelated to the degree of exophthalmos present. In addition, choroidal folds can be seen with no exophthalmos or orbital lesions present at all.

The clinical appearance is distinct ophthalmoscopically and with fluorescein angiography. The folds appear as alternating light and dark, roughly parallel lines, usually horizontal, which make the fundus appear corrugated (Figure 1). The elevated portions of the folds are the lighter, yellowish stripes, and the valleys are the darker stripes. On fluorescein angiography, the elevated lines transmit fluorescence, as if the pigment epithelium is less dense, and the valleys block fluorescence. There is no leakage. Histopathologically, the pigment epithelium and Bruch's membrane have wavelike folds, and the choriocapillaris is congested. The overlying sensory retina may also participate in the folding.

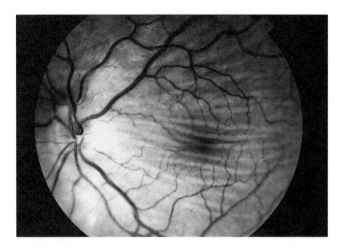

Figure 1 Choroidal folds in a patient with proptosis caused by an orbital tumor.

A. The history is important because recent trauma or eye surgery would suggest the causes of ocular or orbital edema, choroidal detachments, or hypotony. Although folds may produce no symptoms, the recent onset of blurring, distortion, or hyperopia may suggest an active pathologic process rather than idiopathic congenital folds of the choroid.

B. The association of high hyperopia and choroidal folds is interesting in that it may shed light on the pathogenesis. Small eyes may be subject to increased choroidal congestion, which may cause the folding of the choroid in these cases.

C. Choroidal folds are usually in the posterior pole and rarely anterior to the equator. Therefore they must be differentiated from other macular lesions, which may also cause folding. Whether the folding is choroidal or purely retinal must be determined. Retinal folding may occur in several vitreoretinal diseases that cause swelling of the retina, tangential traction on the retina, or puckering of the retina, such as papilledema, chorioretinal and vitreoretinal scars, preretinal fibrosis, and disciform macular degeneration.

D. Anything that causes hypotony of the eye can cause choroidal edema and congestion, which can produce choroidal folds.

E. Any moderately severe ocular inflammation can cause choroidal congestion, which can cause choroidal folds. In addition, inflammation may be associated with poor aqueous production, causing additional hypotony.

F. Orbital tumors are probably the most common known causes of choroidal folds. These tumors include hemangioma (the most common orbital tumor), meningioma, and tumors arising from any tissues within the orbit, as well as metastatic tumors. Orbital infections, including those arising from the sinuses, and scleritis can also cause secondary congestion of the choroid, producing folds. Pseudotumor and thyroid exophthalmos are also secondary to orbital tissue swelling. The latter is the most common cause of bilateral as well as unilateral exophthalmos in an adult and has been reported to cause choroidal folds. Most patients with thyroid exophthalmos are euthyroid when the exophthalmos is diagnosed. Thus orbital examination with ultrasonography and radiologic techniques must be done to establish the specific diagnosis. Measurement of the extraocular muscles, which are enlarged in thyroid disease, is especially accurate with standardized A-scan echography.

References

Kalina RE, Mills RP. Acquired hyperopia with choroidal folds. Ophthalmology 1980; 87:44–50.

Kroll AJ, Norton EWD. Regression of choroidal folds. Am Acad Ophthalmol Otolaryngol 1970; 74:515–525.

Newell FW. Choroidal folds. Am J Ophthalmol 1975; 75:930–942.

Patient with CHOROIDAL FOLDS

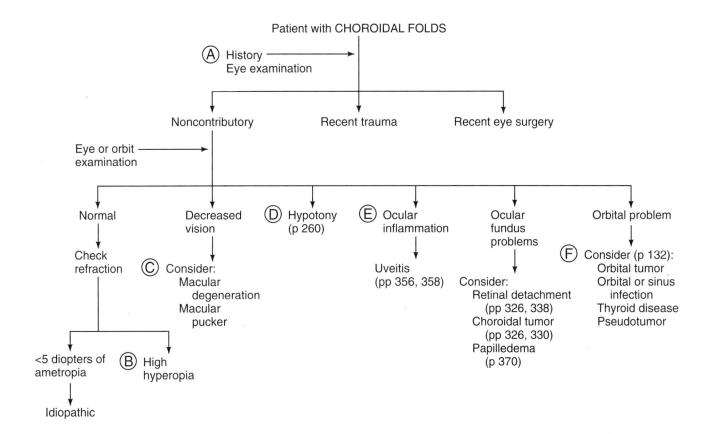

A History
Eye examination

Noncontributory

Recent trauma

Recent eye surgery

Eye or orbit examination

Normal

Check refraction

<5 diopters of ametropia

Idiopathic

B High hyperopia

Decreased vision

C Consider:
Macular degeneration
Macular pucker

D Hypotony (p 260)

E Ocular inflammation

Uveitis (pp 356, 358)

Ocular fundus problems

Consider:
Retinal detachment (pp 326, 338)
Choroidal tumor (pp 326, 330)
Papilledema (p 370)

Orbital problem

F Consider (p 132):
Orbital tumor
Orbital or sinus infection
Thyroid disease
Pseudotumor

WHITE SPOTS IN THE FUNDUS

G. Robert Hampton, M.D.

A. Tamoxifen in excess of 90 g for treatment of breast carcinoma may produce white refractile deposits of the inner retinal layers with loss of central vision and macular edema. Deposition of calcium oxalate in oxalosis may be limited to the eye or part of a diffuse process. Yellow-white crystalline deposits are found in the posterior pole and midperiphery. Long-term use of oral canthaxanthine as a tanning aide may lead to symmetric distribution of yellow flecks in the macula.

B. The exudate along retinal vessels associated with posterior uveitis may appear initially as white focal spots. Choroiditis, such as caused by histoplasmosis, may also leave white "punched-out" lesions throughout the fundus.

C. Myelinated nerve fibers may appear as a discrete fan-shaped spot. Although usually about 1 disc diameter, they may be large enough to cover an entire quadrant. The peripheral edge appears like the end of a paintbrush.

D. Astrocytic hamartoma typically presents as a large white calcified mulberry mass or flat translucent noncalcified lesion. Most occur at or near the optic nerve. Fluorescein angiography demonstrates a rich capillary network. It is typically associated with tuberous sclerosis or neurofibromatosis.

E. Birdshot retinochoroidopathy typically presents bilaterally in white women aged 40–50. Eyes have a quiet anterior chamber with vitreal inflammation without pars planitis. Deep, circular cream-colored lesions are present in the posterior pole. Fluorescein angiography is helpful in delineating the degree of retinal vascular leakage and associated macular edema.

F. Acute posterior multifocal placoid pigment epitheliopathy (APMPPE) is a syndrome of multiple plaque-like lesions, posterior to the equator, at the level of the retinal pigment epithelium (RPE) associated with temporary visual loss. APMPPE typically presents as sudden visual blurring in a man or woman <30, often with a history of recent viral illness. Fluorescein angiography demonstrates initial blockage at the lesions with late staining. There is usually spontaneous improvement, with visual acuity returning to normal and residual RPE stippling in areas of previous lesions.

G. Multiple evanescent white dot syndrome (MEWDS) typically presents as a unilateral sudden drop in visual acuity, predominantly in young women. Multiple small discrete white dots at the level of the RPE are present in the posterior pole to the midperiphery with a "grainy" macular appearance. There is an average 7-week course to regain 20/20 to 20/40 acuity, when the lesions gradually fade. Fluorescein angiography reveals early hyperfluorescence with late staining. The cause is unknown.

H. Fundus flavimaculatus, or Stargardt's disease, is a bilateral, progressive RPE disorder typically presenting in the second or third decade; it causes blurring of vision. Retinal findings range from diffuse soft yellow-gray pigment epithelial flecks without macular findings to atrophic macular findings without flecks. The electroretinogram (ERG) is typically mildly reduced, and electroculographic (EOG) ratios are abnormal in 75%–80% of patients. Fluorescein angiography is extremely helpful in making the diagnosis as a result of the typical blocked choroidal fluorescence or "dark choroid."

I. Dominant drusen appear as round, discrete, sharply defined yellow lesions in clusters predominating in the posterior pole. They appear rounder, whiter, and more sharply defined than fundus flavimaculatus. Fluorescein angiography demonstrates sharply defined round spots that brightly fluoresce, often revealing more spots than visible on ophthalmoscopy.

J. Fundus albipunctatus is a recessive stationary night-blinding condition with small, discrete, raised, uniform white dots ranging from the posterior pole to the entire retina. The dots do not appear in clusters, and fluorescein angiography shows a mottled pattern to the pigment epithelium. In contrast to drusen, the dots do not hyperfluorescence with time. The visual acuity is typically minimally affected.

K. Best's vitelliform is an autosomal-dominant dystrophy of the RPE initially presenting with a distinctive "egg yolk" appearance in the macula between ages 4 and 10. More than 75% of patients maintain better than 20/40 acuity. Only Best's vitelliform and butterfly dystrophy share the trait of a normal ERG with an abnormal EOG light-to-dark ratio.

References

Carr RE. Fundus flavimaculatus. Arch Ophthalmol 1965; 74:163–168.

Cleasby GW, Fung WE, Shelker WB. Astrocytoma of the retina. Am J Ophthalmol 1967; 64:633–637.

Cortin P, Corriveau LA, Rousseau A, et al. Canthaxanthine retinopathy. J Ophthalmic Photogr 1983; 6:68.

Damato BE, Nanjiani M, Foulds WS. Acute posterior multifocal placoid pigment epitheliopathy. A follow-up study. Trans Ophthalmol Soc UK 1983; 103:517–522.

Deutman AF, Jansen LMAA. Dominantly inherited drusen of Bruch's membrane. Br J Ophthalmol 1970; 54:373–382.

Fuerst DI, Tessler HH, Fishman GA. Birdshot retinochoroidopathy. Arch Ophthalmol 1984; 102:214–219.

Patient with WHITE SPOTS IN FUNDUS

Examine for location →

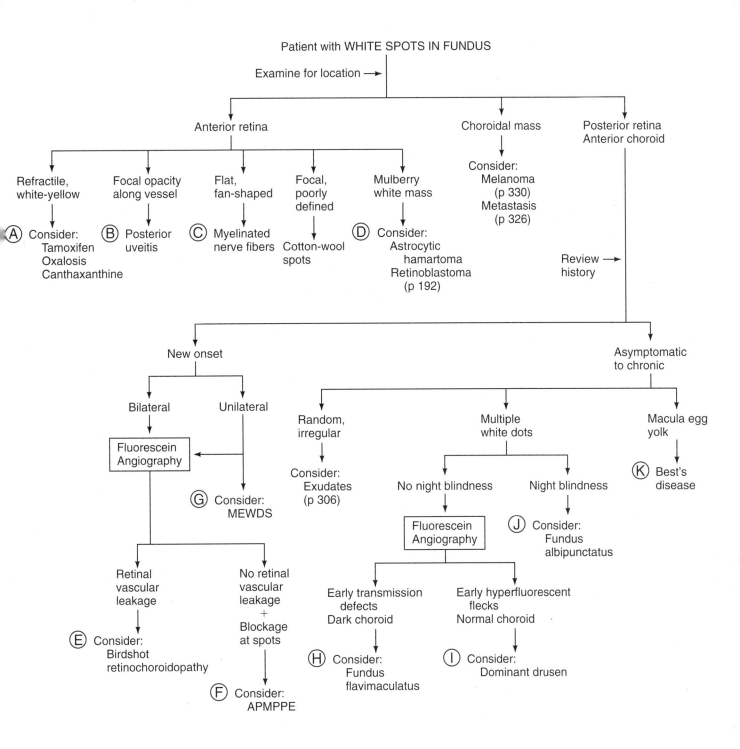

Gass JDNI. Acute posterior multifocal placoid pigment epitheliopathy. Arch Ophthalmol 1968; 80:177–185.

Kaiser-Kupfer MI, Kupfer C, Rodrigues MM. Tamoxifen retinopathy: A clinicopathologic report. Ophthalmology 1981; 88:89–93.

Meredith TA, Wright JD, Gammon JA, et al. Ocular involvement in primary hyperoxaluria. Arch Ophthalmol 1984; 102:584–587.

Mohler CW, Fine SL. Long term evaluation of patients with Best's disease vitelliform dystrophy. Ophthalmology 1981; 88:688–692.

Newsome DA, ed. Retinal dystrophies and degeneration. New York: Raven, 1988.

Ryan SI, Maumenee AE. Birdshot retinochoroidopathy. Am J Ophthalmol 1980; 89:31–45.

HARD EXUDATES IN THE FUNDUS

G. Robert Hampton, M.D.
Peter B. Hay, B.A.

True exudates present ophthalmoscopically as punctate yellowish or white spots scattered throughout the fundus (Figure 1). Sometimes called *hard, waxy,* or *fatty exudates,* they are most prevalent in the posterior pole. They occur nonspecifically in any retinal vasculopathy that produces leaky vessels. The exudate may erupt posteriorly into the subretinal space to form yellowish contiguous masses. Histologically, the exudate consists of serum confined initially to the outer reticular layer of the retina. The vertical orientation of Mueller's fibers and of neurons restrains the lateral spread of the exudate and accounts for the punctate appearance seen on clinical examination.

A. Peripapillary subretinal neovascularization (SRNVM) can threaten the macula from serous exudation, hard exudate, or subretinal hemorrhage. When the neovascular process is located on the temporal, superior, or inferior border of the optic nerve, laser photocoagulation is indicated. Carefully observe patients with peripapillary hemorrhage because recurrence of SRNVM is common.

B. Macular edema is the most common cause of visual loss among patients with diabetic retinopathy. Several clinical trials have demonstrated the efficacy of laser photocoagulation in treatment of clinically significant macular edema. Laser treatment tends to reduce the rate of visual loss, but relatively few eyes show substantial visual improvement. One arm of the Early Treatment Diabetic Retinopathy Study (ETDRS) studied laser treatment for hard exudate close to the fovea with thickening of adjacent retina. For this group, at 3 years' follow-up, 12% of the immediately treated eyes compared with 24% of the deferred treated eyes had significant loss of visual acuity.

C. A resolving branch retinal vein occlusion (BRVO) may present with signs of inner retinal hard exudate. In this presentation the original hemorrhage and soft exudates have resolved to leave shunt vessels and persistent or slowly resolving hard exudates. The collaborative BRVO Study demonstrated that photocoagulation with the argon laser is useful for reducing visual loss from macular edema in patients who meet the study criteria.

D. Retinal macroaneurysms are acquired fusiform or round dilations of the retinal arterioles, often at an arteriovenous (AV) crossing or bifurcation, usually unrelated to any other retinal disease. Typically, the lesion thromboses and undergoes spontaneous involution. However, when a hard exudate threatens the fovea, focal laser may be of benefit. No clear indications have been established for treatment, and beneficial effects have not been proved.

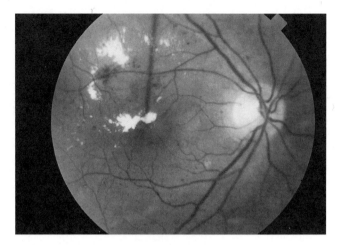

Figure 1 Hard exudates in a ring (circinate) pattern indicate leakage in the center of the circle.

E. Parafoveal telangiectasia is a condition of microaneurysmal and saccular dilation of the parafoveal capillaries. Visual decline may be secondary to serous edema accompanied by hard exudates. In those who demonstrate significant visual loss or in whom hard exudate threatens the fovea, focal laser may be of benefit. Because no controlled trials have been completed, the true value of laser for this condition is speculative.

F. Coats' disease is an idiopathic occurrence of telangiectasia and aneurysmal retinal vessels associated with massive subretinal exudation. The exudative process may be limited to the periphery or may extend to the posterior pole, even with no posterior focal vascular leakage. When the hard exudate threatens the fovea, laser photocoagulation of the leaking areas in the periphery, guided by fluorescein angiography, is indicated.

G. Hard exudates may be associated with radiation retinopathy after treatment of intraocular tumors. They occur more often after radioactive cobalt plaques (brachytherapy) as compared with external beam irradiation.

References

Branch Vein Occlusion Study Group. Argon laser photocoagulation for macular edema in branch vein occlusion. Am J Ophthalmol 1984; 98:271–282.

Brown GO, Shields JA, Sanborn G, et al. Radiation retinopathy. Ophthalmology 1982; 89:1494–1501.

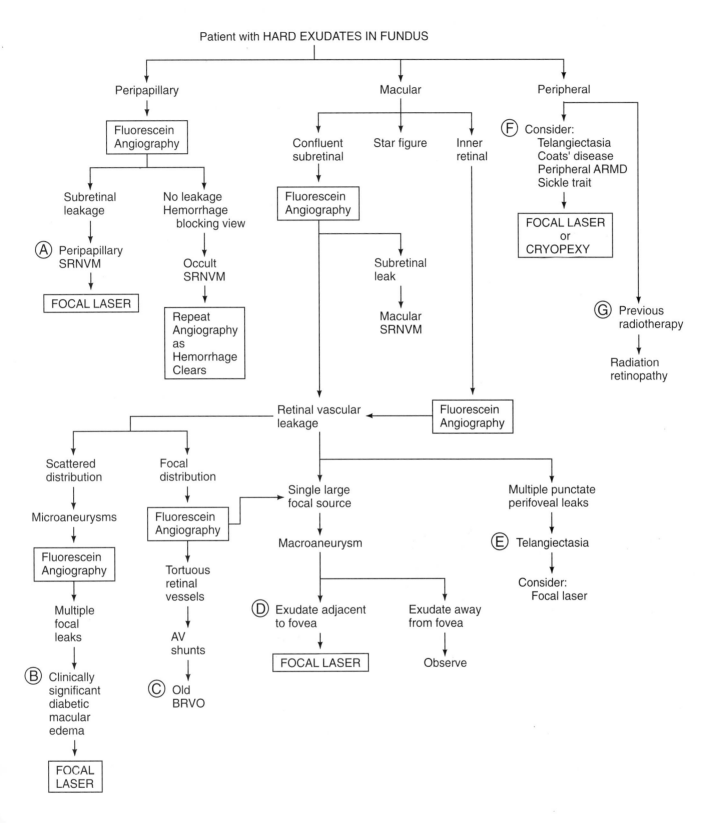

Patient with HARD EXUDATES IN FUNDUS

Peripapillary

Fluorescein Angiography

Subretinal leakage

Ⓐ Peripapillary SRNVM

FOCAL LASER

No leakage Hemorrhage blocking view

Occult SRNVM

Repeat Angiography as Hemorrhage Clears

Macular

Confluent subretinal

Star figure

Inner retinal

Fluorescein Angiography

Subretinal leak

Macular SRNVM

Peripheral

Ⓕ Consider: Telangiectasia Coats' disease Peripheral ARMD Sickle trait

FOCAL LASER or CRYOPEXY

Ⓖ Previous radiotherapy

Radiation retinopathy

Fluorescein Angiography

Retinal vascular leakage

Scattered distribution

Microaneurysms

Fluorescein Angiography

Multiple focal leaks

Ⓑ Clinically significant diabetic macular edema

FOCAL LASER

Focal distribution

Fluorescein Angiography

Tortuous retinal vessels

AV shunts

Ⓒ Old BRVO

Single large focal source

Macroaneurysm

Ⓓ Exudate adjacent to fovea

FOCAL LASER

Exudate away from fovea

Observe

Multiple punctate perifoveal leaks

Ⓔ Telangiectasia

Consider: Focal laser

Chopdar A. Retinal telangiectasia in adults: Fluorescein angiographic findings and treatment by argon laser. Br J Ophthalmol 1978; 62:243–250.

Early Treatment Diabetic Retinopathy Study Research Group. Photocoagulation for diabetic macular edema: Early Treatment Diabetic Retinopathy Study report number 1. Arch Ophthalmol 1985; 103:1796–1806.

Ridley ME, Shields JA, Brown GO, Tasman W. Coats' disease: Evaluation of management. Ophthalmology 1982; 89: 1381–1387.

BLACK SPOTS IN THE FUNDUS

G. Robert Hampton, M.D.
Peter B. Hay, B.A.

A. Nevus of Ota is a type of blue nevus of the skin around the orbit, brow, and conjunctiva, including a diffuse nevus of the choroid. It occurs in African-Americans and Asians and is rare in whites. It is potentially malignant, only when occurring in whites.

B. Congenital melanocytosis is best considered a diffuse blue nevus of the conjunctiva. Generally unilateral in African-Americans and Asians, it is associated with a diffuse uveal nevus that causes heterochromia of the iris. Involvement may be segmental and, when present in whites, is potentially malignant.

C. Fuchs' spot is commonly considered any dark spot in the macula of a patient with high myopia. It appears that the pigmented lesion of Fuchs and the hemorrhagic lesion of Foerster represent different stages of subretinal neovascularization development in myopia (Figure 1).

D. Retinal pigment epithelial (RPE) hypertrophy (CHRPE) presents as a focal, jet-black, often mottled, slightly raised area of pigment epithelium with a halo of depigmentation. RPE hypertrophy has no malignant potential. However, because it can enlarge, it has been mistaken for malignant melanoma. When RPE hypertrophy is present in multiple locations, the association with Gardner's syndrome should be investigated (Figure 2).

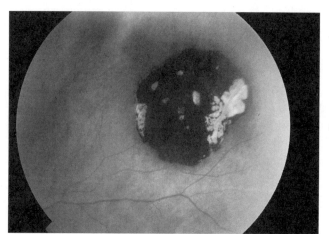

A

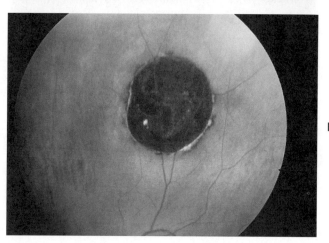

B

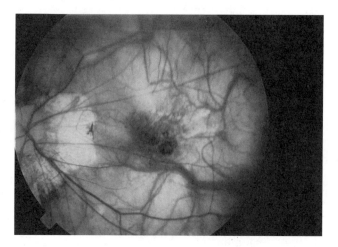

Figure 1 Fuchs' spot with myopic atrophy around disc.

Figure 2 **A** and **B,** Congenital hypertrophy of the retinal pigment epithelium.

E. The retinal pigment epithelium is a very reactive tissue that may undergo hyperplasia after an inflammation, producing alternating areas of hyperplasia and atrophy.

F. Clumping of pigment over a sclerosed choroidal vessel, usually associated with severe hypertension, often forms a linear streak (Siegrist's streak).

G. Pigmented paravenous retinochoroidal atrophy (PPRCA) is a pigmentary retinopathy that may represent an acquired response pattern to an infectious or inflammatory disease rather than a genetic dystrophy. The pigmentary changes follow the distribution of retinal veins, and in most cases the electroretinogram is mildly or moderately abnormal, if at all, and the electroculographic (EOG) ratio is usually abnormal.

H. Grouped pigmentation of the retina, also called *bear tracks,* is a benign condition presenting as round, irregularly shaped lesions representing RPE hypertrophy scattered through out the fundus. Retinal function and electrophysiology are normal (Figure 3).

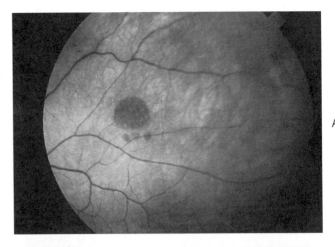

A

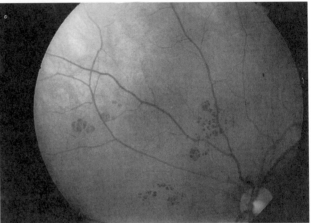

B

Figure 3 **A** and **B,** Group pigmentation of the retina: "bear tracks."

I. Retinitis pigmentosa (RP) is a group of inherited disorders characterized by progressive dysfunction involving photoreceptors and, progressively, other cell layers. Visual impairment is usually manifested as night blindness, peripheral field loss, and in some cases, central field loss. The classic appearance includes mottling and granularity of the RPE, migration of pigment to form clumps and "bone spicules," attenuation of retinal vessels, and optic nerve pallor. Electrophysiology demonstrates reduced or absent rod and cone amplitudes (Figure 4).

J. Many syndromes involve either typical RP or a similar retinal dystrophy. The most common is Usher's syndrome, defined as congenital deafness plus RP.

K. Diffuse granular pigment clumping can occur as a reactive response of the RPE to a variety of inflammatory insults. Diffuse unilateral subacute neuroretinitis (DUSN) is probably what has been referred to as *unilateral RP*. DUSN results from the diffuse retinal degeneration that occurs in eyes infected by any of several possible worms. Careful examination may reveal the presence of a living nematode.

L. Severe blinding retinal toxicity has been linked only to one phenothiazine: thioridazine. Phenothiazines bind to melanin and presumably concentrate in the RPE. Thioridazine can cause a pigmentary retinopathy that, early on, can be confused with RP. The typical appearance of advanced chloroquine toxicity is bull's eye maculopathy, although pigmentary changes with bone spicule formation can occur in the periphery.

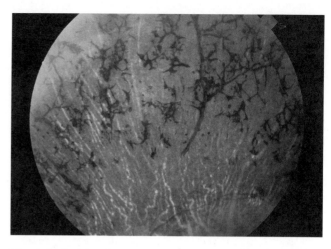

Figure 4 Retinitis pigmentosa with bone spicule-like pigmentation.

References

Buettner H. Congenital hypertrophy of the retinal pigment epithelium. Am J Ophthalmol 1975; 79:177–189.

Foxman SG, Heckenlively JR, Sinclair SH. Rubeola retinopathy and pigmented paravenous retinochoroidal atrophy. Am J Ophthalmol 1985; 99:605–606.

Gass JDM, Braunstein RA. Further observations concerning the diffuse unilateral subacute neuroretinitis syndrome. Arch Ophthalmol 1983; 101:1689–1697.

Hampton GR, Kohen D, Bird AC. Visual prognosis of disciform degeneration in myopia. Ophthalmology 1983; 90:923–926.

Lewis RA, Crowder WE, Eierman LA, et al. The Gardner's syndrome: Significance of ocular features. Ophthalmology 1984; 91:916–925.

Meredith TA, Aaberg TM, Wilkerson WD. Progressive chorioretinopathy after receiving thioridazine. Arch Ophthalmol 1978; 96:1172–1176.

Newsome DA. Retinitis pigmentosa, Usher's syndrome, and other pigmentary retinopathies. In: Newsome DA, ed. Retinal dystrophies and degeneration. New York: Raven, 1983: 1–94.

Noble KG, Carr RE. Pigmented paravenous chorioretinal atrophy. Am J Ophthalmol 1983; 96:338–344.

Tobin DR, Krohel GB, Rynes RI. Hydroxychloroquine: Seven-year experience. Arch Ophthalmol 1982; 100:81–83.

Traboulsi EJ, Maumenee IH, Krush AJ, et al. Congenital hypertrophy of the retinal pigment epithelium predicts colorectal polyposis in Gardner's syndrome. Arch Ophthalmol 1990; 108:525–526.

Weleber RG. Syndromes associated with retinitis pigmentosa. In: Ryan SI, ed. Retina. St Louis: Mosby, 1989: 379–381.

Zimmerman LE. Melanocyte, melanocytic nevi, and melanocytomas. Invest Ophthalmol 1965; 4:11–41.

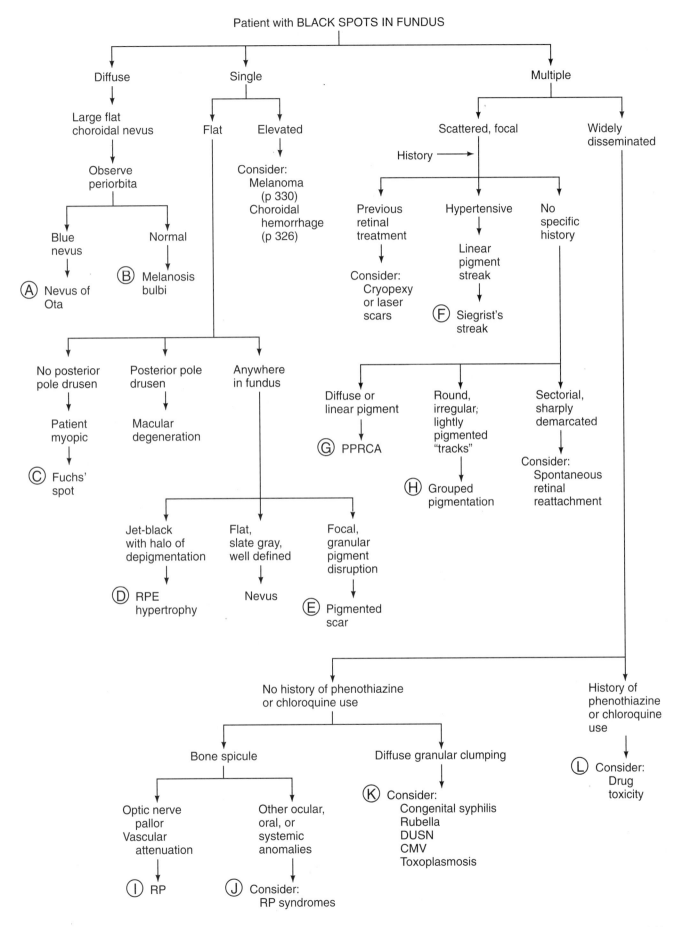

Patient with BLACK SPOTS IN FUNDUS

Diffuse

Large flat
choroidal nevus

Observe
periorbita

Blue
nevus

(A) Nevus of
Ota

Normal

(B) Melanosis
bulbi

Single

Flat

Elevated

Consider:
Melanoma
(p 330)
Choroidal
hemorrhage
(p 326)

No posterior
pole drusen

Patient
myopic

(C) Fuchs'
spot

Posterior pole
drusen

Macular
degeneration

Anywhere
in fundus

Jet-black
with halo of
depigmentation

(D) RPE
hypertrophy

Flat,
slate gray,
well defined

Nevus

Focal,
granular
pigment
disruption

(E) Pigmented
scar

Multiple

Scattered, focal

History

Previous
retinal
treatment

Consider:
Cryopexy
or laser
scars

Hypertensive

Linear
pigment
streak

(F) Siegrist's
streak

No
specific
history

Diffuse or
linear pigment

(G) PPRCA

Round,
irregular;
lightly
pigmented
"tracks"

(H) Grouped
pigmentation

Widely
disseminated

Sectorial,
sharply
demarcated

Consider:
Spontaneous
retinal
reattachment

No history of phenothiazine
or chloroquine use

Bone spicule

Optic nerve
pallor
Vascular
attenuation

(I) RP

Other ocular,
oral, or
systemic
anomalies

(J) Consider:
RP syndromes

Diffuse granular clumping

(K) Consider:
Congenital syphilis
Rubella
DUSN
CMV
Toxoplasmosis

History of
phenothiazine
or chloroquine
use

(L) Consider:
Drug
toxicity

HEMORRHAGES IN THE FUNDUS

G. Robert Hampton, M.D.
Peter B. Hay, B.A.

Hemorrhage of the fundus may present as flame-shaped, punctate, subretinal, preretinal, or intraretinal.

A. Flame-shaped hemorrhages are superficial and owe their configuration to the nerve fiber layer. They are most suggestive of diffuse vascular disease and predominate in hypertension. With papilledema they radiate from the swollen, congested optic disc. Venous occlusion produces extensive flame hemorrhage, the extent depending on the location of occlusion (Figure 1).

B. The Collaborative Branch Vein Occlusion Study demonstrated that argon laser photocoagulation is useful for reducing visual loss from persistent macular edema in patients who meet the study criteria.

C. Central retinal vein occlusion (CRVO) presents with retinal hemorrhage in all four quadrants, and there is a dilated retinal venous system. Clinical appearance may vary from scattered retinal hemorrhages with a few cotton-wool spots to massive flame hemorrhages. Central vision is almost always affected by macular involvement; secondary neovascular glaucoma may result in severe vision loss. CRVO may be subdivided into ischemic and nonischemic types. Fluorescein angiography demonstrates prominent retinal capillary nonperfusion throughout the posterior fundus in the ischemic CRVO. There is a significant risk of neovascular glaucoma in eyes with >10 disc areas of capillary nonperfusion. The Central Vein Occlusion Study Group recommends careful observation with frequent follow-up examinations in the early months after CRVO and prompt panretinal photocoagulation (PRP) of eyes in which iris or angle neovascularization develops. Grid laser photocoagulation for macular edema associated with CRVO does not appear to be of benefit.

D. Punctate hemorrhages are deeper in the retina, and the configuration results from the lateral restraint afforded by the inner and outer nuclear layers and the outer plexiform layer of the retina (Figure 2).

E. The occurrence of ocular symptoms and signs secondary to severe carotid artery obstruction is called the *ocular ischemic syndrome*. Other findings may include neovascularization of the retina and iris, glaucoma, pain, vision loss, and cotton-wool spots.

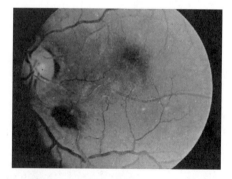

Figure 1   Flame hemorrhage along inferior temporal arcade.

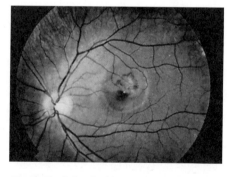

Figure 3   Subretinal hemorrhage of macula.

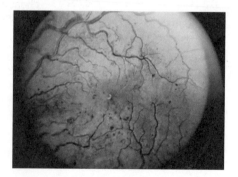

Figure 2   Diffuse punctate retinal hemorrhages.

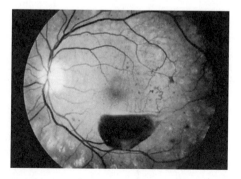

Figure 4   Subhyaloid hemorrhage inferior to macula associated with diabetic retinopathy.

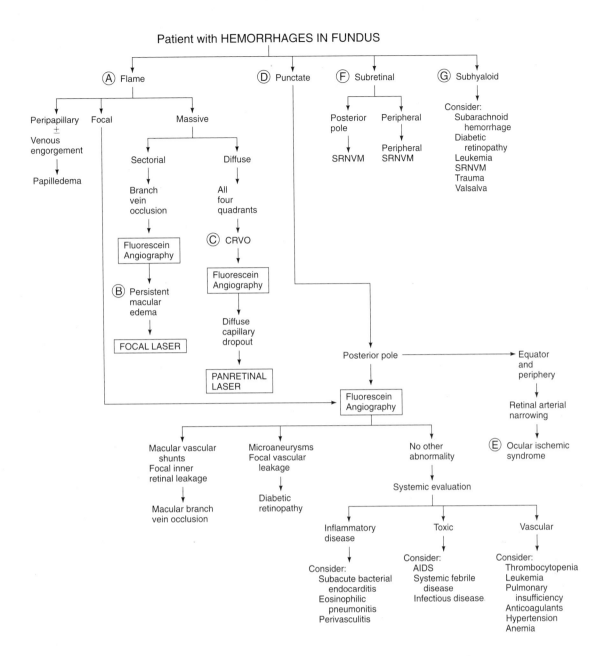

Patient with HEMORRHAGES IN FUNDUS

(A) Flame
- Peripapillary ± Venous engorgement → Papilledema
- Focal
- Massive
  - Sectorial → Branch vein occlusion → Fluorescein Angiography → (B) Persistent macular edema → FOCAL LASER
  - Diffuse → All four quadrants → (C) CRVO → Fluorescein Angiography → Diffuse capillary dropout → PANRETINAL LASER

(D) Punctate

(F) Subretinal
- Posterior pole → SRNVM
- Peripheral → Peripheral SRNVM

(G) Subhyaloid
- Consider: Subarachnoid hemorrhage, Diabetic retinopathy, Leukemia, SRNVM, Trauma, Valsalva

Posterior pole → Fluorescein Angiography → Equator and periphery → Retinal arterial narrowing → (E) Ocular ischemic syndrome

Fluorescein Angiography:
- Macular vascular shunts / Focal inner retinal leakage → Macular branch vein occlusion
- Microaneurysms / Focal vascular leakage → Diabetic retinopathy
- No other abnormality → Systemic evaluation
  - Inflammatory disease → Consider: Subacute bacterial endocarditis, Eosinophilic pneumonitis, Perivasculitis
  - Toxic → Consider: AIDS, Systemic febrile disease, Infectious disease
  - Vascular → Consider: Thrombocytopenia, Leukemia, Pulmonary insufficiency, Anticoagulants, Hypertension, Anemia

F. Subretinal hemorrhage is dark red to black. It may be punctate or large enough to produce measurable retinal elevation. Subretinal hemorrhage is liable to phagocytosis and lipid metamorphosis, producing yellowish white masses. The most common cause of subretinal hemorrhage is subretinal neovascularization (SRNVM). However, it may arise from retinal vascular hemorrhage, gaining access to the subretinal space by direct extension through the external limiting membrane (Figure 3).

G. Subhyaloid hemorrhage may be located behind the internal limiting membrane of the retina, in which case the hemorrhage emanates from the superficial capillaries of the retina. True preretinal hemorrhages are located anterior to the internal limiting membrane and have a more indistinct border. Both may form a fluid level. Most preretinal hemorrhages arise from proliferating preretinal neovascular tissue (Figure 4).

References

Bresnick GH. Diabetic macular edema: A review. Ophthalmology 1986; 93:989–997.

Kahn M, Green WR, Knox DL, Miller NR. Ocular features of carotid artery disease. Retina 1986; 6:239–252.

Macular edema in branch vein occlusion. Am J Ophthalmol 1984; 98:271–282.

Magargal LE, Donoso LA, Sanbom GA. Retinal ischemia and risk of neovascularization following central retinal vein occlusion. Ophthalmology 1982; 89:1241–1245.

Merimee TJ. Diabetic retinopathy. A synthesis of perspectives. N Engl J Med 1990; 322:978–983.

The Central Vein Occlusion Study Group. A randomized clinical trial of early panretinal photocoagulation for ischemic central vein occlusion. Ophthalmology 1995; 102:1434–1444.

The Central Vein Occlusion Study Group. Evaluation of grid pattern photocoagulation for macular edema in central vein occlusion. Ophthalmology 1995; 102:1425–1433.

COTTON-WOOL SPOTS IN THE FUNDUS

G. Robert Hampton, M.D.
Peter B. Hay, B.A.

Cotton-wool spots appear as focal areas of ischemic whitening of the retina and represent a microinfarct in the nerve fiber layer. The finding of even a single cotton-wool spot in a nondiabetic patient with an otherwise normal fundus necessitates a systemic work-up for possible causes. In approximately 95% of cases, a serious underlying systemic disorder can be found. In addition to the conditions discussed here, other disease entities associated with cotton-wool spots include radiation retinopathy, partial retinal arterial obstruction, trauma, papillitis, papilledema, septicemia, dysproteinemias, acute blood loss, severe anemia, metastatic carcinoma, high-altitude retinopathy, Rocky Mountain spotted fever, leptospirosis, acute pancreatitis, and aortic arch syndrome.

A. Cotton-wool spots are easily identified by their white color and superficial position in the retina, often covering a retinal vessel, and by their almost exclusive position in the posterior retina (Figure 1). They vary in size but are rarely bigger than half the disc diameter. Cotton-wool spots are not associated with vitreous cells, inflammation, or vascular leakage. Typically, with fluorescein angiography, the lesion appears as a nonfluorescent area, surrounded by a rim of dilated capillaries, sometimes showing multiple beadlike microaneurysmal changes. On light microscopy a cystoid body is identified as a cellular-appearing structure with a pseudonucleus within the nerve fiber layer. On electron microscopy the cytoid body is seen to be largely mitochondria with a major lipid component.

B. Ischemic vein occlusion is manifested by tortuous veins with dark deoxygenated blood, indicating stagnation and increased intravascular pressure. Hemor-

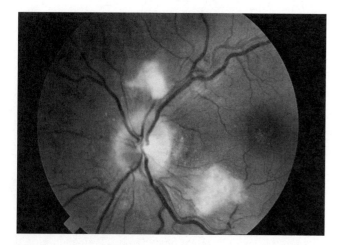

Figure 1 Two microinfarcts in the retinal superficial nerve fiber layer; also called *cotton-wool spots.*

rhages are extensive, and in some cases the intravascular pressure is sufficiently high to impair arterial inflow, resulting in cotton-wool spots.

C. *Ocular ischemic syndrome* refers to the symptoms and signs relating to severe carotid artery obstruction. Of patients, 5% usually have cotton-wool spots in the posterior pole. The syndrome is associated with a significant risk of rubeosis of the iris, and patients should be observed with gonioscopy.

D. Diabetes is the most common cause of cotton-wool spots, with an overall 32%–44% incidence. Cotton-wool spots tend to last longer in diabetic patients than in nondiabetic patients (half-life in patients <40 years old is 8 months, >40 years old, 1–7 months). The presence of more than eight cotton-wool spots has been correlated with a higher risk of proliferative diabetic retinopathy.

E. Systemic hypertension, defined as diastolic pressure >90 mm Hg, had a 50% incidence in a group of patients presenting with cotton-wool spots.

F. Macular epiretinal membranes may exhibit cotton-wool spots or fluffy, whitish opacities of the inner retina. The more fluffy appearance probably relates to blockage of axoplasmic transport and is not a true cotton-wool spot.

G. Cotton-wool spots and hemorrhages, the most common ocular manifestations of infection with HIV, are observed in more than half of the patients with established AIDS. They correlate with a low ratio of T-helper to suppressor cells and thus may be an important clinical sign of the severity of HIV-related disease.

H. Cardiac valvular disease, including mitral valve prolapse, rheumatic heart disease, and endocarditis, may produce cotton-wool spots as a result of microembolic phenomena of the retina. Cotton-wool spots associated with leukemia may be caused by local factors, such as an abnormally large cell or cluster of cells occluding retinal arterioles, and may not be related to the overall peripheral blood composition. Cotton-wool spots and retinal hemorrhages related to anemia or thrombocytopenia are also common in patients with non-Hodgkin's lymphoma.

I. The most common retinal vascular manifestations in systemic lupus erythematosus (SLE) includes cotton-wool spots with or without intraretinal hemorrhages. The retinal vascular changes occur independently of hypertension and are thought to be related to the underlying microangiopathy of SLE.

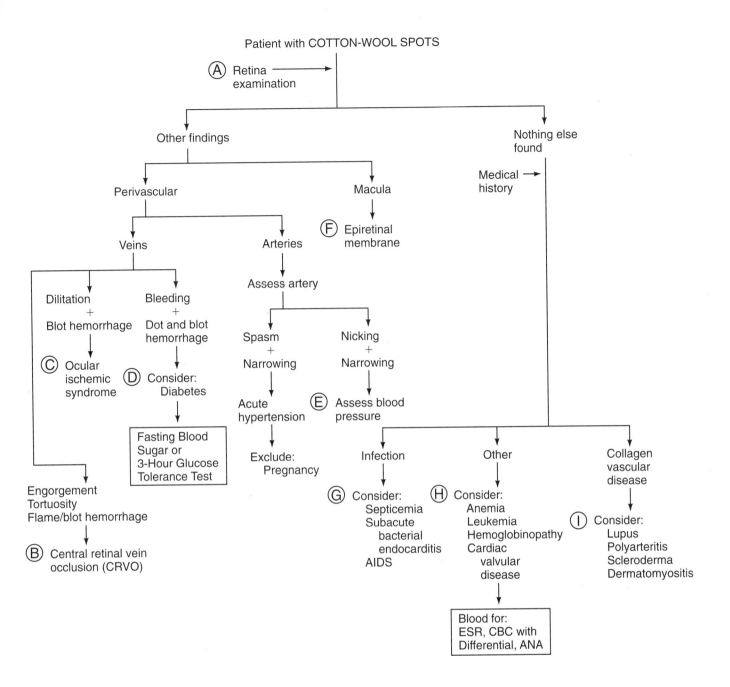

Patient with COTTON-WOOL SPOTS

(A) Retina examination

Other findings → Perivascular → Veins → Dilitation + Blot hemorrhage → (C) Ocular ischemic syndrome

Veins → Bleeding + Dot and blot hemorrhage → (D) Consider: Diabetes → Fasting Blood Sugar or 3-Hour Glucose Tolerance Test

Engorgement Tortuosity Flame/blot hemorrhage → (B) Central retinal vein occlusion (CRVO)

Arteries → Assess artery → Spasm + Narrowing → Acute hypertension → Exclude: Pregnancy

Assess artery → Nicking + Narrowing → (E) Assess blood pressure

Macula → (F) Epiretinal membrane

Nothing else found → Medical history

Infection → (G) Consider: Septicemia Subacute bacterial endocarditis AIDS

Other → (H) Consider: Anemia Leukemia Hemoglobinopathy Cardiac valvular disease → Blood for: ESR, CBC with Differential, ANA

Collagen vascular disease → (I) Consider: Lupus Polyarteritis Scleroderma Dermatomyositis

References

Ashton N. Pathological and ultrastructural aspects of the cotton-wool spot. Proc R Soc Med 1969; 62:1271–1275.

Brown GC, Brown MM, Hiller T, et al. Cotton-wool spots. Retina 1985; 5:206–214.

Gold DH, Morris DA, Henkind P. Ocular findings in systemic lupus erythematosus. Br J Ophthalmol 1972; 56:800–804.

Gutman FA. Evaluation of a patient with central retinal vein occlusion. Ophthalmology 1983; 90:481–483.

Hayreh SS, Servais G, Virdi PS. Cotton-wool spots (inner retinal ischemic spots) in malignant arterial hypertension. Ophthalmologica 1989; 198:197–215.

Kohner EM, Dollery CT, Bulpitt CJ. Cotton-wool spots in diabetic retinopathy. Diabetes 1969; 18:691–704.

Roy MS, Rick ME, Higgins KE, McCulloch JC. Retinal cotton-wool spots: An early finding in diabetic retinopathy? Br J Ophthalmol 1986; 70:772–778.

Schachat AP, Markowitz JA, Guyer DR, et al. Ophthalmic manifestations of leukemia. Arch Ophthalmol 1989; 107:697–700.

RETINAL VASCULAR ANOMALIES

G. Robert Hampton, M.D.
Peter B. Hay, B.A.

Retinal vascular anomalies encompass a wide variety of conditions that can be subdivided by the vessel system primarily affected: arterial, venous, arteriovenous (AV), capillary, or neovascular.

A. It is best to estimate arterial narrowing as a function of other landmarks in the fundus because the actual viewed size of a vessel varies with the refractive status. However, pathologic narrowing of retinal arteries is usually obvious when it is moderate or severe.

B. Retinal veins are approximately one and a half to twice the size of corresponding arteries. With congestion, they may exceed this difference by several times. The corresponding blood column appears darker. Ancillary signs of venous congestion are tortuosity and accentuation of AV crossings. Sheathing of veins is caused by infiltration of their walls or cellular changes in the walls secondary to venous stasis. Extreme sheathing occurs with venous occlusion, producing a white, bloodless column.

C. Retinal arteries generally cross superficial to the veins, and the two are bound in a common adventitia. This predisposes the veins to occlusion with either sclerosis of the artery or congestion of the veins. The veins at the AV crossing have more right-ankle branching, banking of blood, and occasionally dilation of collaterals (Figures 1 through 4).

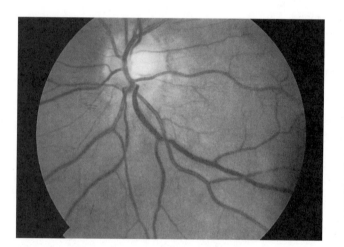

Figure 1 AV nicking in hypertension.

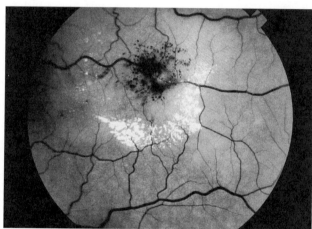

Figure 3 Macroaneurysm in hypertension surrounded by blood (black) and exudates (white).

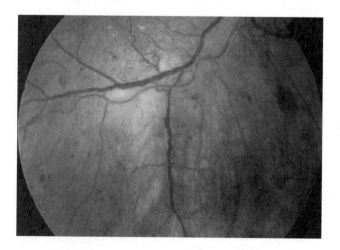

Figure 2 Venous beading in diabetic retinopathy.

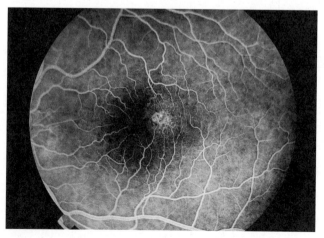

Figure 4 Angiogram of telangiectasia of the retina near the jovea.

D. Neovascularization grows from the retina into the vitreous to lie on the surface of the retina or grow onto the gel. The new vessels have fragile walls permeable to fluorescein and serum and are at risk of hemorrhage (Figure 5).

E. Vascular tumors of the retina are distinctive. Von Hippel tumors (Figure 6) are angiomatous hamartomas of the retina and optic nerve that, when congenital, are inherited in an incomplete autosomal-dominant pattern with variable penetrance. A parent with a von Hippel tumor has a 50% chance of having a child with such a tumor as well. Of patients with angiomatosis of the retina, 25% have CNS tumors as well as tumors elsewhere (von Hippel-Lindau disease). The most typical manifestation of von Hippel-Lindau disease is a cerebellar hemangioblastoma, although tumors or cysts may also occur in the spinal cord, viscera, lung, and thyroid gland. Renal cell carcinoma and pheochromocytoma may rarely be associated. Periodically evaluate patients with von Hippel-Lindau tumors with CT or MRI as well as with intravenous pyelography. The angioblastoma may occur on the nerve or in the retina anywhere and may be multiple. Each tumor is supplied and drained by characteristic "sentinel" dilated vessels between the disc and tumor. Extravasation from the tumors may cause retinal edema, exudation, and vitreous hemorrhage. There may be secondary vitreoretinal changes, including vitreous traction and retinal detachment. Treatment of retinal angiomas is with photocoagulation or cryotherapy. Racemose angioma of the retina is a congenital AV communication and not a true angioma. It is usually found incidentally in young adults without visual complaints. Cerebrovascular malformations may be associated with the ocular malformation (Wyburn-Mason syndrome). CT or MRI may be indicated to identify cerebral involvement. These lesions are prominent in the eye and consist of either a dilated vascular loop or a set of dilated vessels with a capillary plexus between them. When extensive, cerebral involvement may be associated with visual loss in the area of the anomaly and the fundus can look like a bag of worms. Although intraretinal hemorrhage, retinal vascular occlusions, vitreous hemorrhage, and neovascular glaucoma can occur, many patients do not have these complications and require no treatment.

A
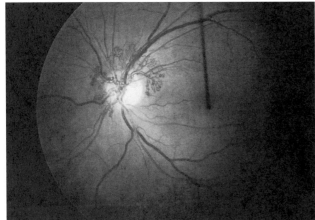

B
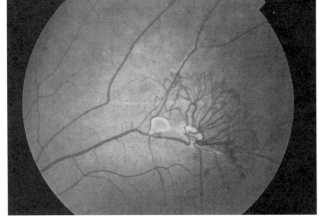

Figure 5 **A,** Neovascularization of the disc (NVD). **B,** Neovascularization elsewhere in the retina (NVE).

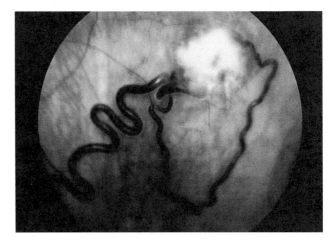

Figure 6 Von Hippel retinal angioma with large feeding artery and draining vein.

317

References

Archer DB, Deutman A, Ernest T, Krill AE. Arteriovenous communications of the retina. Am J Ophthalmol 1973; 75:224–241.

Cohen SB, Goldberg MF, Fletcher ME, Jednock NJ. Diagnosis and management of ocular complications of sickle hemoglobinopathies, part I. Ophthalmic Surg 1986; 17:57–59.

Committee for the Classification of Retinopathy of Prematurity. An international classification of retinopathy of prematurity. Arch Ophthalmol 1984; 102:1130–1134.

Egerer I, Tasman W, Tomer TL. Coats' disease. Arch Ophthalmol 1974; 92:109–112.

Ehlers N, Jenses VA. Hereditary central retinal angiopathy. Acta Ophthalmol 1973; 51:171–178.

Grennan DM, Forrester J. Involvement of the eye in SLE and scleroderma. Ann Rheum Dis 1977; 36:152–156.

Hayreh SS. Classification of central retinal vein occlusion. Ophthalmology 1983; 90:458–474.

Lavin MJ, Marsh RJ, Peart S, Rehman A. Retinal arterial macroaneurysms: A retrospective study of 40 patients. Br J Ophthalmol 1987; 71:817–825.

Merimee TJ. Diabetic retinopathy. A synthesis of perspectives, N Engl J Med 1990; 322:978–983.

Orth DH, Patz A. Retinal branch vein occlusion. Surv Ophthalmol 1978; 22:357–376.

Tso MOM, Jampol LM. Pathophysiology of hypertensive retinopathy. Ophthalmology 1982; 89:1132–1145.

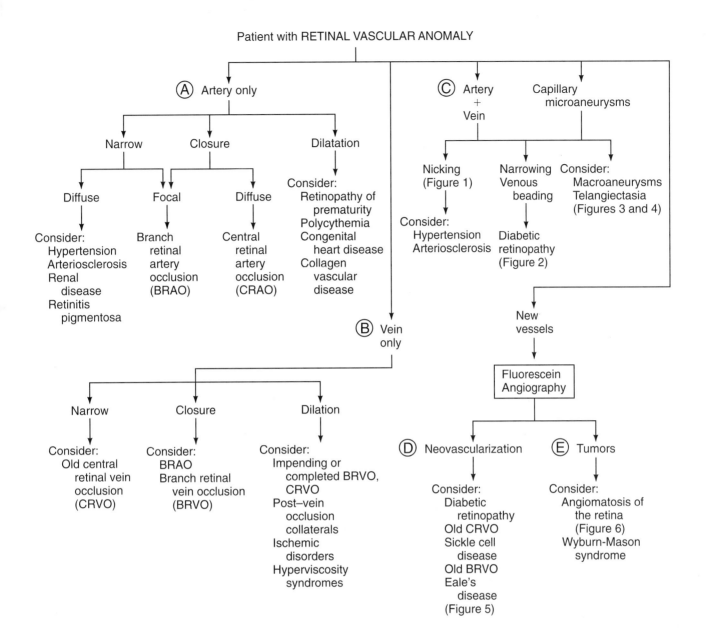

Patient with RETINAL VASCULAR ANOMALY

Ⓐ Artery only

Narrow

Diffuse

Consider:
Hypertension
Arteriosclerosis
Renal
  disease
Retinitis
  pigmentosa

Closure

Focal

Branch
retinal
artery
occlusion
(BRAO)

Diffuse

Central
retinal
artery
occlusion
(CRAO)

Dilatation

Consider:
Retinopathy of
  prematurity
Polycythemia
Congenital
  heart disease
Collagen
  vascular
  disease

Ⓒ Artery
  +
  Vein

Capillary
microaneurysms

Nicking
(Figure 1)

Consider:
Hypertension
Arteriosclerosis

Narrowing
Venous
beading

Diabetic
retinopathy
(Figure 2)

Consider:
Macroaneurysms
Telangiectasia
(Figures 3 and 4)

Ⓑ Vein
  only

New
vessels

Fluorescein
Angiography

Narrow

Consider:
Old central
  retinal vein
  occlusion
  (CRVO)

Closure

Consider:
BRAO
Branch retinal
  vein occlusion
  (BRVO)

Dilation

Consider:
Impending or
  completed BRVO,
  CRVO
Post–vein
  occlusion
  collaterals
Ischemic
  disorders
Hyperviscosity
  syndromes

Ⓓ Neovascularization

Consider:
Diabetic
  retinopathy
Old CRVO
Sickle cell
  disease
Old BRVO
Eale's
  disease
(Figure 5)

Ⓔ Tumors

Consider:
Angiomatosis of
  the retina
(Figure 6)
Wyburn-Mason
  syndrome

SHEATHING OF RETINAL VESSELS

Lanny Odin, M.D.
Lina M. Marouf, M.D.
Bailey L. Lee, M.D.

The retinal vascular walls are usually transparent and invisible. What one sees clinically is the blood column within the vascular lumen. *Vascular sheathing* is a general term used to describe clinically visible whitening of the vessel wall. Complete occlusion of a retinal vessel, resulting in obliteration of the funduscopically visible blood column, results in a ghost vessel rather than vascular sheathing. Sheathing comprises several pathologic changes that can involve the arteries and/or veins. It may be primarily occlusive, with secondary exudation of the vascular elements, or it may be inflammatory in origin, with or without altered blood flow in the affected vessel. Infiltration of a retinal vessel (vein) with lymphocytes, as seen in leukemia, is an example of occlusive vascular sheathing. Sheathing secondary to retinal phlebitis or arteritis, as seen in sarcoidosis and syphilis, presents as white, fuzzy, irregular cuffing of the retinal vasculature associated with other signs of anterior uveitis, vitreitis, or chorioretinitis and is an example of inflammatory sheathing. Aging, retinal vascular occlusive disease, hypertension, and diabetes can also result in thickening of the retinal vascular wall and obscuration of the blood column, giving the vessel wall a whitish sheathed appearance.

Patients with retinal vascular sheathing may be asymptomatic or present with decreased visual acuity, visual field defects, pain, floaters, photophobia, and redness. They may also have systemic symptoms, including fever, myalgia, arthralgia, skin rash, and gastrointestinal or respiratory problems. Ocular examination helps in determining the site and extent of vascular sheathing. Many disorders associated with retinal vascular sheathing are likely to affect other ocular structures, and uveitis is also commonly seen. General medical history and examination often help in narrowing the differential diagnosis. Neurologic disease (multiple sclerosis and optic neuropathies), metabolic disease (diabetes mellitus and hypercholesterolemia), collagen vascular disease (SLE and periarteritis nodosa), infectious diseases (bacterial, helminthic, mycobacterial, mycotic, protozoan, rickettsial, spirochetal, and viral), vascular occlusive disease (embolic and arteriosclerotic), hematologic disease (sickle cell and leukemia), hemostatic disease (retinal metastasis and lymphocytic lymphoma), and idiopathic disease (idiopathic uveitis, Behçet's disease, Eales' disease, and sarcoidosis) all may display retinal vascular sheathing.

A. White sheathing of disc vessels and immediate peripapillary venules or arterioles is a developmental anomaly. The sheathing is smooth and is densest over the disc. It is most easily diagnosed when associated with papillary membranes or Bergmeister's papilla.

B. Sheathing of disc and retinal vessels also may occur after papillitis and optic disc edema. Unlike in congenital vascular sheathing, the vascular whitening is less uniform and is often associated with abnormalities of the optic nerve and retina (e.g., pallor, atrophy, filled-in physiologic cup, retinal folds, and loss of nerve fiber layer).

C. Various inflammatory and infectious diseases can result in retinal venous sheathing. Consider diagnostic stains and cultures from appropriate sources. In candidal endophthalmitis, diagnostic vitrectomy may be indicated. Other tests to be considered are CBC (leukemia), VDRL and FTA-ABS (syphilis), chest film and ACE (sarcoidosis), and hemoglobin electrophoresis (sickle cell disease).

D. Infectious diseases are best treated by specific antimicrobial agents. Steroid therapy may be needed to treat Behçet's disease and sarcoidosis. Chemotherapeutic drugs are used to treat myelogenous leukemia and at times Behçet's disease.

E. Many disorders associated with periarteritis retinalis can also cause inflammation of the conjunctiva, cornea, sclera, vitreous, and/or uvea. The differential diagnosis is influenced by the site and presence or absence of ocular inflammation.

F. In the absence of ocular inflammatory disease, fluorescein angiography may demonstrate vascular occlusion. Retinal emboli should alert one to look for a source (i.e., carotid or cardiac). Blood pressure, blood sugar, and serum cholesterol determination may lead to the cause of vascular sheathing. Retinal angiomas can represent isolated ocular abnormalities or can be associated with systemic abnormalities; therefore CT scanning of the head, upper cervical spine, and abdomen may be indicated.

G. Specific medication may be indicated to treat the underlying disorder (i.e., antihypertensives, hypoglycemic agents, cholesterol-lowering drugs, and antiplatelet medications). More invasive intervention could be indicated in carotid artery disease and angiomatosis of the retina.

H. When both retinal arterial sheathing and ocular inflammation are present, a thorough medical work-up is indicated to look for evidence of collagen vascular disease and/or infection. Biopsy may assist in diagnosing sarcoidosis and tuberculosis.

I. Intravenous followed by oral acyclovir is the treatment for acute retinal necrosis. Also oral acyclovir may reduce the incidence and severity of herpes zoster ophthalmicus. Antimicrobial medications are useful in treating syphilis and tuberculosis. Prednisone may be indicated in the treatment of SLE, periarteritis nodosa, temporal arteritis, and sarcoidosis.

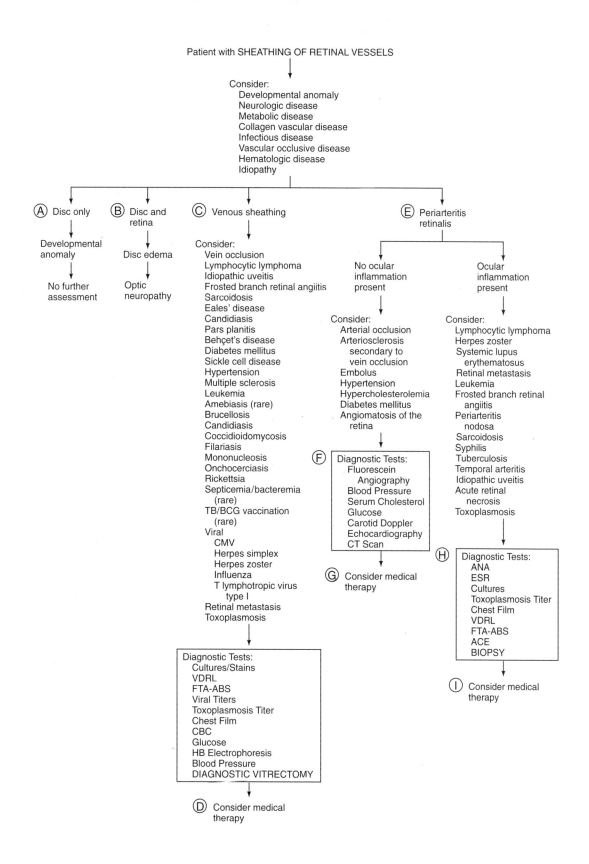

Patient with SHEATHING OF RETINAL VESSELS

Consider:
- Developmental anomaly
- Neurologic disease
- Metabolic disease
- Collagen vascular disease
- Infectious disease
- Vascular occlusive disease
- Hematologic disease
- Idiopathy

(A) Disc only

Developmental anomaly

No further assessment

(B) Disc and retina

Disc edema

Optic neuropathy

(C) Venous sheathing

Consider:
- Vein occlusion
- Lymphocytic lymphoma
- Idiopathic uveitis
- Frosted branch retinal angiitis
- Sarcoidosis
- Eales' disease
- Candidiasis
- Pars planitis
- Behçet's disease
- Diabetes mellitus
- Sickle cell disease
- Hypertension
- Multiple sclerosis
- Leukemia
- Amebiasis (rare)
- Brucellosis
- Candidiasis
- Coccidioidomycosis
- Filariasis
- Mononucleosis
- Onchocerciasis
- Rickettsia
- Septicemia/bacteremia (rare)
- TB/BCG vaccination (rare)
- Viral
  - CMV
  - Herpes simplex
  - Herpes zoster
  - Influenza
  - T lymphotropic virus type I
- Retinal metastasis
- Toxoplasmosis

Diagnostic Tests:
- Cultures/Stains
- VDRL
- FTA-ABS
- Viral Titers
- Toxoplasmosis Titer
- Chest Film
- CBC
- Glucose
- HB Electrophoresis
- Blood Pressure
- DIAGNOSTIC VITRECTOMY

(D) Consider medical therapy

(E) Periarteritis retinalis

No ocular inflammation present

Consider:
- Arterial occlusion
- Arteriosclerosis secondary to vein occlusion
- Embolus
- Hypertension
- Hypercholesterolemia
- Diabetes mellitus
- Angiomatosis of the retina

(F) Diagnostic Tests:
- Fluorescein Angiography
- Blood Pressure
- Serum Cholesterol
- Glucose
- Carotid Doppler
- Echocardiography
- CT Scan

(G) Consider medical therapy

Ocular inflammation present

Consider:
- Lymphocytic lymphoma
- Herpes zoster
- Systemic lupus erythematosus
- Retinal metastasis
- Leukemia
- Frosted branch retinal angiitis
- Periarteritis nodosa
- Sarcoidosis
- Syphilis
- Tuberculosis
- Temporal arteritis
- Idiopathic uveitis
- Acute retinal necrosis
- Toxoplasmosis

(H) Diagnostic Tests:
- ANA
- ESR
- Cultures
- Toxoplasmosis Titer
- Chest Film
- VDRL
- FTA-ABS
- ACE
- BIOPSY

(I) Consider medical therapy

References

Gass JDM. Stereoscopic atlas of macular diseases diagnosis and treatment. 4th ed. St Louis: Mosby, 1997.

Roy FH. Ocular differential diagnosis. Baltimore: Williams & Wilkins, 1997.

Ryan SJ, ed. Retina. 2nd ed. Vol 2. St Louis: Mosby, 1994.

RETINAL ARTERIAL OCCLUSIVE DISEASE

Lina M. Marouf, M.D.
Bailey L. Lee, M.D.

Central retinal artery occlusion (CRAO) has been reported to occur in 1 in 10,000 outpatient visits. It involves men and women >60 years of age with an equal frequency. Unilateral involvement is the rule in 98% of patients.

A. Of patients, 90% present with sudden onset of decreased vision in the finger-counting to light-perception range. The absence of light perception should raise the suspicion of ophthalmic artery occlusion or optic nerve disease. The presence of a cilioretinal artery in 25% of the population accounts for sparing of central vision in the remaining 10% of patients. An afferent pupillary defect can be detected within seconds of visual symptoms.

B. The site of vascular occlusion determines the type of visual field defect produced. An altitudinal or nerve fiber bundle field defect occurs in branch retinal artery occlusion (BRAO), and complete loss of the central and peripheral visual fields occurs in CRAO.

C. Funduscopic examination reveals retinal opacification in the area of vascular occlusion. Emboli have been detected in 20%–60% of eyes. "Boxcarring" of the blood column may be present in both retinal arterioles and venules. A cherry-red spot is present in the macula.

D. Although ancillary studies such as fluorescein angiography and electroretinography may be helpful in confirming the diagnosis, careful funduscopic examination alone should establish the diagnosis of a retinal arterial occlusion. On fluorescein angiography there is delayed perfusion of the involved artery (normal retinal arterial filling time is approximately 12 seconds). There may be retrograde filling of the obstructed branch by neighboring collateral vessels in a BRAO. In a CRAO, filling of the optic nerve capillaries by way of the central retinal artery and vein. As a result of inner retinal ischemia, the electroretinogram reveals diminution of the B wave.

E. Although studies in primates have suggested that irreversible damage occurs to the retina after 90 minutes in a complete CRAO, it is still considered an ocular emergency in patients who present within 24 hours of onset of symptoms. As soon as the diagnosis is established, attempt to dislodge the embolus to a more distal arteriole in cases that are caused by embolic phenomena. Dislodgement may be accomplished by inducing retinal vasodilation. Intermittent ocular massage and inspiration of a mixture of 95% oxygen and 5% carbon dioxide can result in increased retinal vascular caliber. Reduce the intraocular pressure by performing an anterior chamber paracentesis and instituting IV acetazolamide.

Patients with retinal embolic phenomena have a 10% risk of stroke during the first year and an additional 6% risk per year subsequently. Patients with retinal artery occlusive disease have a higher risk of death because of cardiac or cerebrovascular disease and therefore should undergo a thorough medical evaluation. Of patients with retinal arterial occlusive disease, 90% have associated medical abnormalities, the most common of which are hypertension (66%), carotid atherosclerosis (45%), diabetes mellitus (25%), cardiac valvular disease (25%), and giant cell arteritis (2%). Retinal vascular occlusive disease in the young may occur secondary to migraine, coagulation abnormalities, ocular anomalies, trauma, IV drug abuse, pregnancy, use of oral contraceptives, DIC, and the antiphospholipid antibody syndrome. Tests should include CBC, platelets, ESR, lipid profile, coagulation profile, lupus anticoagulant antibody, ANA, serum complement, protein electrophoresis, echocardiography, and duplex carotid ultrasonography.

Patients should be observed closely during the first 3 months for the development of rubeosis iridis and neovascular glaucoma, which have been reported to occur in 18.2% and 15.2% of patients, respectively, in one prospective study. A retrospective uncontrolled study by Duker and Brown has demonstrated the beneficial effects of panretinal photocoagulation in inducing regression of the rubeosis in 89% of patients and preventing the occurrence of neovascular glaucoma in all patients when performed early in the course of rubeosis iridis after CRAO.

References

Atebara NH, Brown GC, Cater J. Efficacy of anterior chamber paracentesis and carbogen in treating acute nonarteritic central retinal artery occlusion. Ophthalmology 1995; 102:2029–2034.

Duker SJ, Brown GC. The efficacy of panretinal photocoagulation for neovascularization of the iris after central retinal artery obstruction. Ophthalmology 1989; 96:92–95.

Duker SJ, Sivalingam A, Brown GC, Reber R. A prospective study of acute central retinal artery obstruction. The incidence of secondary ocular neovascularization. Arch Ophthalmol 1991; 10:339–342.

Hayreh SS, Kolder HE, Weingeist TA. Central retinal artery occlusion and retinal tolerance time. Ophthalmology 1980; 87:75–78.

Wiznia A, Pearson WN. Use of transesophageal echocardiography for detection of a likely source of embolization to the central retinal artery. Am J Ophthalmol 1991; 111:104–105.

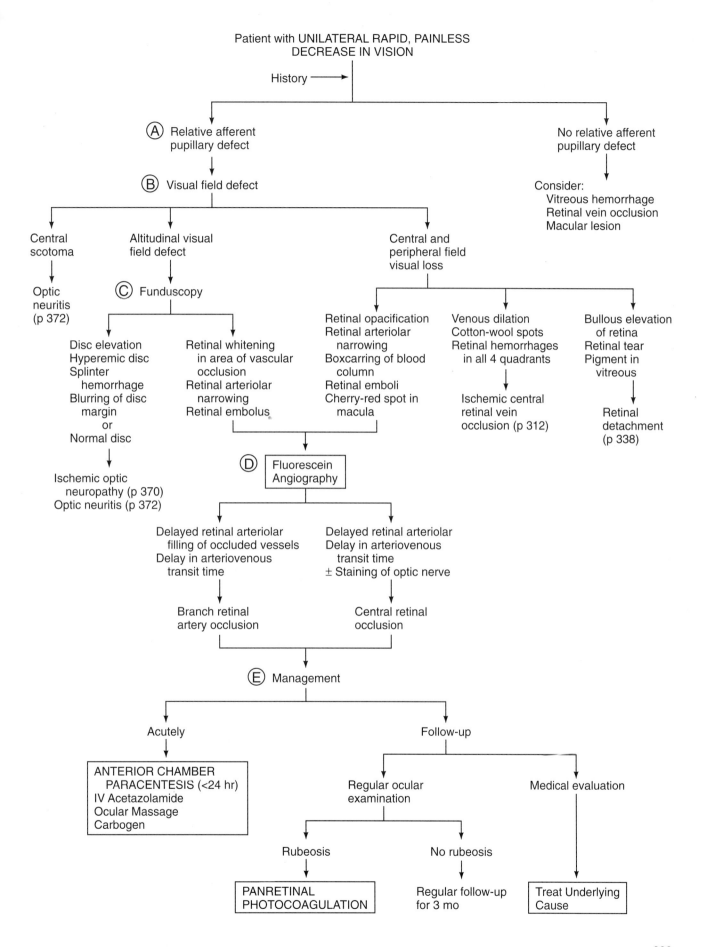

Patient with UNILATERAL RAPID, PAINLESS DECREASE IN VISION

History →

Ⓐ Relative afferent pupillary defect

No relative afferent pupillary defect

Consider:
  Vitreous hemorrhage
  Retinal vein occlusion
  Macular lesion

Ⓑ Visual field defect

Central scotoma

Altitudinal visual field defect

Central and peripheral field visual loss

Optic neuritis (p 372)

Ⓒ Funduscopy

Disc elevation
Hyperemic disc
Splinter hemorrhage
Blurring of disc margin
or
Normal disc

Retinal whitening in area of vascular occlusion
Retinal arteriolar narrowing
Retinal embolus

Retinal opacification
Retinal arteriolar narrowing
Boxcarring of blood column
Retinal emboli
Cherry-red spot in macula

Venous dilation
Cotton-wool spots
Retinal hemorrhages in all 4 quadrants

Bullous elevation of retina
Retinal tear
Pigment in vitreous

Ischemic optic neuropathy (p 370)
Optic neuritis (p 372)

Ischemic central retinal vein occlusion (p 312)

Retinal detachment (p 338)

Ⓓ Fluorescein Angiography

Delayed retinal arteriolar filling of occluded vessels
Delay in arteriovenous transit time

Delayed retinal arteriolar
Delay in arteriovenous transit time
± Staining of optic nerve

Branch retinal artery occlusion

Central retinal occlusion

Ⓔ Management

Acutely

Follow-up

ANTERIOR CHAMBER PARACENTESIS (<24 hr)
IV Acetazolamide
Ocular Massage
Carbogen

Regular ocular examination

Medical evaluation

Rubeosis

No rubeosis

PANRETINAL PHOTOCOAGULATION

Regular follow-up for 3 mo

Treat Underlying Cause

RETINAL VEIN OCCLUSION

Lina M. Marouf, M.D.
Bailey L. Lee, M.D.

Branch and central retinal vein occlusions are the second and third most common retinal vascular diseases, respectively. They occur in the 50- to 70-year-old age group. Ocular involvement is unilateral in 90% of cases. Diabetic retinopathy predisposes to the patient to the development of bilateral disease. The histopathologic change in venous occlusive disease is a thrombus at the site of occlusion. In branch retinal vein occlusion (BRVO), there is usually sclerosis of the corresponding branch retinal artery. A mechanical factor is proposed in the development of the BRVO. Occlusion usually occurs at the site of an arteriovenous crossing. The artery has been reported to lie anterior to the vein at the site of crossing in 100% of patients with vein occlusion as compared with 65% of controls. Atherosclerotic arteriolar changes plus the presence of a common perivascular adventitial sheath result in narrowing of the venular lumen, turbulent blood flow, intimal damage, and initiation of the clotting mechanism. Patients usually present with sudden onset of painless decrease in vision associated with a visual field defect.

A. Patients with BRVO or central retinal vein occlusion (CRVO) should undergo a thorough ocular examination. Glaucoma or increased intraocular pressure, trauma, and optic disc drusen may be present in 23%–69%, 14%, and 7% of patients with CRVO, respectively. Pupillary testing is helpful in differentiating optic nerve and widespread retinal disease from localized retinal abnormalities. This is particularly important in the presence of opaque media. Retinal findings in CRVO include disc edema, macular edema, dilated retinal veins, and retinal hemorrhages with or without cotton-wool spots in all four quadrants of the retina. Funduscopic findings for BRVO in the acute phase of the disease include intraretinal hemorrhages, retinal edema, and retinal venous dilation in the involved quadrant. Later in the course of the disease collateral vessel formation, microaneurysms, and retinal neovascularization (RNV) may be observed.

B. Fluorescein angiography may not be helpful acutely because there will be hypofluorescence from blockage as a result of the intraretinal hemorrhage. As the hemorrhage clears, it is important to photograph the peripheral retina as well as the posterior hole if one is trying to quantitate the amount of retinal ischemia. In patients with either CRVO or BRVO, decreased vision can result from hemorrhage in the fovea, macular edema, or ischemias. If there is still decreased vision after the hemorrhage clears, fluorescein angiography can be helpful in determining whether there is significant component of macular ischemia or edema.

C. CRVO has two forms: ischemic and nonischemic, with each requiring different management and bearing different prognoses. Ocular neovascularization attributable to CRVO is the major complication of the ischemic CRVO. Earlier studies have shown that rubeosis developed in 60% of patients, angle neovascularization in 47%, and neovascular glaucoma in 33%. The Central Vein Occlusion Study (CVOS) showed that 34% of nonischemic CRVO converted to ischemic CRVO. An abnormal electroretinogram (ERG) with subnormal B-wave amplitude, reduction of oscillatory potentials, B-A–wave amplitude ratio >1, decrease in ERG sensitivity, and delay in ERG implicit time are indicative of an ischemic CRVO. Poor visual acuity, a relative afferent pupillary defect 0.7 log units, and retinal nonperfusion >10 disc areas by fluorescein angiogram are also indicative of ischemic CRVO.

D. Several medical conditions have been reported in association with CRVO: cardiovascular disease (70%), platelet function abnormalities (73%), elevation of serum lipids (30%–60%), hyperviscosity (53%), elevated blood glucose (15%–34%), and chronic obstructive pulmonary disease (20%). Hypertension and arteriosclerosis are the most common medical problems associated with BRVO.

E. Several earlier studies have shown the benefit of panretinal photocoagulation in preventing neovascular glaucoma and rubeosis iridis in ischemic CRVO. The CVOS showed that prophylactic panretinal photocoagulation did not prevent neovascularization of the iris (NVI) or neovascularization of the angle (NVA) in ischemic CRVO and one could wait for the development of NVI or NVA before trying panretinal photocoagulation. The CVOS also showed the lack of benefit of macular grid photocoagulation in patients with CRVO. Other investigators have noted improvement with laser-induced chorioretinal venous anastomosis for treatment of patients with nonischemic CRVO.

Recommendations for management of patients with BRVO based on the Branch Retinal Vein Occlusion Study are as follows: (1) Patients with decreased vision approximately 20/40 secondary to macular edema of 6 months should undergo macular grid laser photocoagulation. (2) Patients with retinal nonperfusion defined as 5 disc diameters should be every 4 months observed for the development of RNV, at which time they should receive scatter laser photocoagulation to the involved quadrant.

References

The Branch Vein Occlusion Study Group. Argon photocoagulation for macular edema in branch vein occlusion. Am Ophthalmol 1984; 98:271–282.

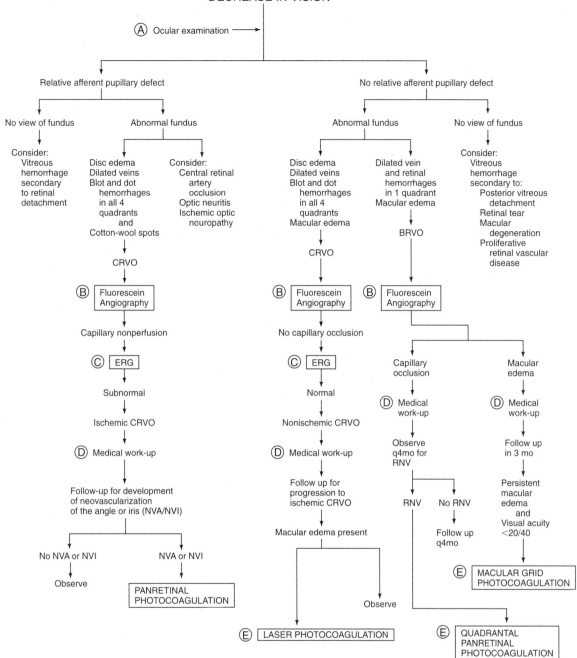

Patient with SUDDEN, PERSISTENT, PAINLESS DECREASE IN VISION

Ⓐ Ocular examination

Relative afferent pupillary defect

No view of fundus

Consider:
Vitreous
hemorrhage
secondary
to retinal
detachment

Abnormal fundus

Disc edema
Dilated veins
Blot and dot
hemorrhages
in all 4
quadrants
and
Cotton-wool spots

CRVO

Ⓑ Fluorescein Angiography

Capillary nonperfusion

Ⓒ ERG

Subnormal

Ischemic CRVO

Ⓓ Medical work-up

Follow-up for development
of neovascularization
of the angle or iris (NVA/NVI)

No NVA or NVI

Observe

NVA or NVI

PANRETINAL PHOTOCOAGULATION

Consider:
Central retinal
artery
occlusion
Optic neuritis
Ischemic optic
neuropathy

No relative afferent pupillary defect

Abnormal fundus

Disc edema
Dilated veins
Blot and dot
hemorrhages
in all 4
quadrants
Macular edema

CRVO

Ⓑ Fluorescein Angiography

No capillary occlusion

Ⓒ ERG

Normal

Nonischemic CRVO

Ⓓ Medical work-up

Follow up for
progression to
ischemic CRVO

Macular edema present

Ⓔ LASER PHOTOCOAGULATION

Observe

Dilated vein
and retinal
hemorrhages
in 1 quadrant
Macular edema

BRVO

Ⓑ Fluorescein Angiography

Capillary
occlusion

Ⓓ Medical
work-up

Observe
q4mo for
RNV

RNV

No RNV

Follow up
q4mo

Macular
edema

Ⓓ Medical
work-up

Follow up
in 3 mo

Persistent
macular
edema
and
Visual acuity
<20/40

Ⓔ MACULAR GRID PHOTOCOAGULATION

Ⓔ QUADRANTAL PANRETINAL PHOTOCOAGULATION

No view of fundus

Consider:
Vitreous
hemorrhage
secondary to:
Posterior vitreous
detachment
Retinal tear
Macular
degeneration
Proliferative
retinal vascular
disease

The Branch Vein Occlusion Study Group. Argon photocoagulation for prevention of neovascularization and vitreous hemorrhage in branch vein occlusion. Arch Ophthalmol 1986; 104:34–41.

The Central Vein Occlusion Study Group. A randomized clinical trial of early panretinal photocoagulation for ischemic central vein occlusion. The Cental Vein Occlusion Study Group—Report. Ophthalmology 1995; 102:1434–1444.

The Central Vein Occlusion Study Group. Evaluation of grid pattern photocoagulation for macular edema in central vein occlusion. The Central Vein Occlusion Study Group—Report. Ophthalmology 1995; 102:1425–1433.

Hayreh SS, Klugman MR, Podhajsky P, Kolder HE. Electroretinography in central retinal vein occlusion, correlation of the electroretinographic changes with pupillary abnormalities. Graefe's Arch Clin Exp Ophthalmol 1989; 227:549–561.

Hayreh SS, Rojas P, Podhajsky P, et al. Ocular neovascularization with retinal vascular occlusion-III. Incidence of ocular neovascularization with retinal vein occlusion. Ophthalmology 1983; 90:488–506.

McAllister IL, Constable IJ. Laser-induced chorioretinal venous anastomosis for treatment of nonischemic central retina vein occlusion. Arch Ophthalmol 1995; 113:456–462.

RETINAL ELEVATION

W.A.J. van Heuven, M.D.

Large, highly elevated lesions in the fundus are most easily seen by using indirect ophthalmoscopy. Their characteristics and size can be further determined using scleral depression when the lesions are peripherally located. Posteriorly located retinal elevations, especially minimal elevations, are more easily characterized by using the slit lamp and a precorneal lens.

A. Because many fundus elevations are found incidentally, there may not be a chief complaint. However, if the patient has symptoms, the rapidity of onset may give clues about the natural history of the process (e.g., tumors grow slowly, hemorrhages occur rapidly). Peripheral visual field defects are more likely to be retinal detachments than purely central defects. The association with flashes of light and floaters suggests rhegmatogenous (caused by a retinal tear) retinal detachment. Bilaterality suggests a systemic cause. An ocular or family history of retinal detachment, especially with high myopia, also suggests retinal detachment. A medical history of severe systemic disease can also be helpful. However, the true nature of the fundus elevation is determined by the eye examination.

B. Because the retina has a dual circulation, with the inner retina nourished by the retinal circulation and the outer retina nourished by the choroid, and because tissues separated from their blood supply become edematous, interference with two different circulations can produce retinal edema. When the total retina is detached from the pigment epithelium, the space between the posterior retina and the choroidal vasculature interferes with proper retinal nutrition. When the retina is highly detached, the posterior retinal layers become edematous and opaque. However, if the retinal elevation is only minimal, there appears to be enough choroidal nutrition traversing the subretinal space to keep the retina transparent. Also, if the retinal detachment shifts so that it is present in one location only momentarily, the retina has no time to become edematous. In addition, if only the inner retinal layers are elevated (retinoschisis), there is no circulatory interference because the inner retinal circulation is still within the inner retina, which it supplies.

C. The more common "senile" retinoschisis is generally peripheral and predominantly in the inferotemporal quadrant. It may be marginally present in all quadrants and can also extend into the posterior pole. It is congenital and rarely progressive. Occasionally, it has associated ovoid retinal breaks in the outer layer, which can lead to retinal detachment. As a result, some ophthalmologists recommend prophylactic cryotherapy of the breaks.

D. Secondary retinal detachments are transparent, have rapidly shifting fluid to the dependent part of the retina, rarely extend to the ora serrata, and have a smooth surface because of lack of traction. In addition, secondary implies that no retinal hole or tear has caused the detachment.

E. Any condition that breaks down the inner (tight endothelial junctions in retinal vessels) or outer (pigment epithelial tight junctions) retinal barrier or interferes with the pigment epithelial pump can produce accumulation of fluid under the retina. Systemic diseases include severe hypertension, toxemia, renal disease, dysproteinemias, and hematologic disorders. Orbital diseases include inflammations such as scleritis or episcleritis from any cause. Ocular diseases include inflammations, neoplasms, and drug toxicity.

F. A retinal detachment caused by a retinal hole or tear, which permits liquid vitreous and aqueous to enter the subretinal space, is called *rhegmatogenous*. Its typical characteristics are an opaque retina, nonshifting fluid, extension to the ora serrata, a bullous appearance with retinal folds (traction), and the presence of a retinal hole. Occasionally, all of these characteristics are present, but the retinal hole cannot be found. In that case, assume that the detachment is rhegmatogenous and treat it as such.

G. Two specific conditions associated with opaque subretinal fluid and exudates are Coats' disease and familial exudative vitreoretinopathy (Criswick-Schepens syndrome). Retinal vascular abnormalities are the cause of Coats' disease and can be treated with cryotherapy or laser.

H. Ophthalmic ultrasonography, especially standardized A-scan, is important in differentiating elevated lesions of the fundus. Initially, it can differentiate a solid mass from an elevation of choroid and retina with subchoroidal fluid. If the lesion is truly solid, it cannot be further differentiated if it is <2 mm high. Even if a choroidal melanoma is suspected, it is customary to observe the lesion for growth as long as it is <2 mm high. If it is higher than 2 mm, standardized A-scan can determine the internal reflectivity, which is typically low to medium in melanomas and high in other tumors. The regularity of the internal echoes can further differentiate hemangioma (regular) and metastatic tumors (irregular).

I. Most choroidal detachments occur after surgery and are associated with ocular hypotony. They can also occur in ocular and orbital inflammatory conditions and in nanophthalmos. The uveal effusion syndrome is a rare condition, sometimes associated with hyperopia, dilation of large conjunctival veins, and cells in the vitreous cavity. The cause is unknown. Trauma may also cause choroidal detachments.

J. Tractional retinal detachments are tentlike and concave, unlike rhegmatogenous or secondary detachments, which are convex toward the observer. Although indirect ophthalmoscopy with scleral indentation can give an overview of the fundus I changes, the tractional aspects can be best appreciated with slit-lamp and contact lens examination of the vitreoretinal relationships. Proliferative vitreoretinopathy (PVR) is proliferation of fibrous tissue on both surfaces of the retina after trauma, eye surgery, or rhegmatogenous retinal detachment. The presence of a retinal hole must therefore be ruled out. After blunt or penetrating ocular trauma, the choroid, retina, and vitreous may have scars that can contract and produce retinal tears and detachment. They can also produce traction on the retina that can distort the macula, resulting in decreased vision. Vitreoretinal surgery may then be indicated. Diabetes and other diseases in which proliferations occur between the retinal surface and the vitreous gel can also cause tractional retinal detachments, which at times can become rhegmatogenous. These tractional detachments are classically slowly progressive and should be observed until vision is threatened.

K. Inflammation of the retina, such as toxoplasmosis or *Toxocara canis* infection, often also involves the vitreous gel and may cause vitreous shrinkage with traction on the retina.

L. Occasionally, retinal elevation is misdiagnosed when the retina is thickened or the presence of preretinal tissue makes the retina appear elevated. Central retinal artery occlusion, which produces acute retinal edema, has been mistaken for a tumor. Preretinal fibrosis from any cause, particularly overlying the macula, may have a defect within it overlying the fovea, which appears like a retinal hole. Vitreous opacities, particularly new or old vitreous hemorrhage on the surface of a detached vitreous gel, can also mimic retinal detachment.

References

Machemer R. The importance of fluid absorption, traction, intraocular currents, and chorioretinal scars in the therapy of rhegmatogenous retinal detachments. Am J Ophthalmol 1984; 98:681–693.

Wilkinson CP, Rice TA. Michels retinal detachment. 2nd ed. St Louis: Mosby, 1997.

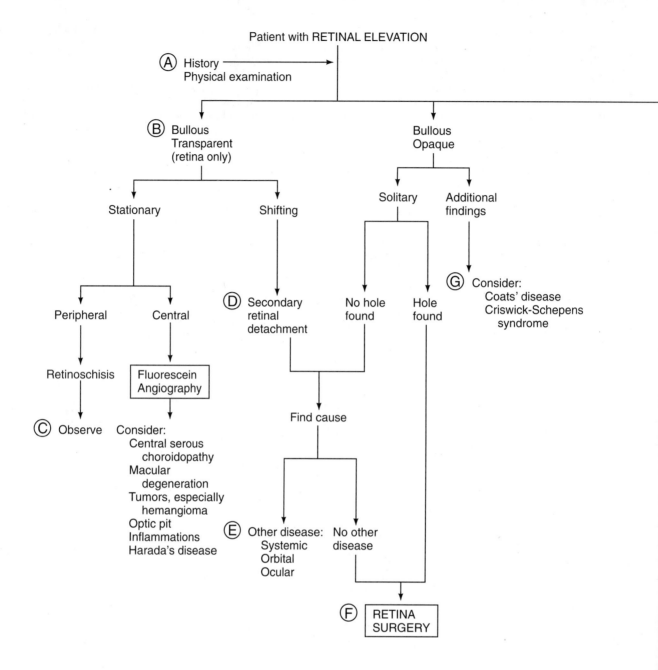

Patient with RETINAL ELEVATION

Ⓐ History
Physical examination

Ⓑ Bullous
Transparent
(retina only)

Bullous
Opaque

Stationary

Shifting

Solitary

Additional
findings

Peripheral

Central

Ⓓ Secondary
retinal
detachment

No hole
found

Hole
found

Ⓖ Consider:
Coats' disease
Criswick-Schepens
syndrome

Retinoschisis

Fluorescein
Angiography

Ⓒ Observe

Consider:
Central serous
choroidopathy
Macular
degeneration
Tumors, especially
hemangioma
Optic pit
Inflammations
Harada's disease

Find cause

Ⓔ Other disease:
Systemic
Orbital
Ocular

No other
disease

Ⓕ RETINA
SURGERY

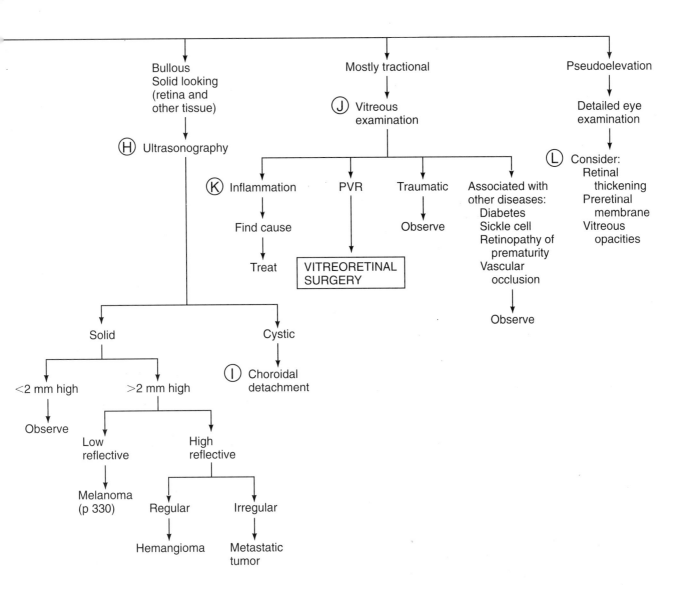

Bullous
Solid looking
(retina and
other tissue)

Ⓗ Ultrasonography

Solid

<2 mm high   >2 mm high

Observe   Low   High
                 reflective   reflective

                 Melanoma   Regular   Irregular
                 (p 330)

                                  Hemangioma   Metastatic
                                               tumor

Cystic

Ⓘ Choroidal
   detachment

Mostly tractional

Ⓙ Vitreous
   examination

Ⓚ Inflammation   PVR   Traumatic   Associated with
                                              other diseases:
Find cause   Observe   Diabetes
                                              Sickle cell
Treat   VITREORETINAL   Retinopathy of
               SURGERY   prematurity
                                              Vascular
                                                 occlusion

                                              Observe

Pseudoelevation

Detailed eye
examination

Ⓛ Consider:
   Retinal
      thickening
   Preretinal
      membrane
   Vitreous
      opacities

MALIGNANT MELANOMA OF THE CHOROID

Frank W. Scribbick, M.D.
W.A.J. van Heuven, M.D.

Choroidal melanoma, the primary intraocular malignancy in adults, is most often diagnosed in the sixth decade of life. Unlike other melanocytic tumors, the incidence of choroidal melanoma has remained relatively stable. Choroidal melanomas become symptomatic when they involve the fovea or cause an exudative retinal detachment. They are often discovered during routine ophthalmoscopy. Definitive therapy for choroidal melanoma is controversial, a debate which the Collaborative Ocular Melanoma Study (COMS) is attempting to resolve.

A. A thorough examination of a patient who presents with a choroidal mass begins with a complete medical history and eye examination. Melanomas are rare before age 50 or in African-Americans. They are usually unilateral and single and may be located anywhere in the fundus. A tumor under the macula in an elderly patient with age-related macular degeneration (ARMD) in the other eye might suggest bilateral ARMD. Dermal or scleral pigmentation may suggest oculodermal syndromes. Multiple iris nevi may accompany choroidal melanoma. Melanomas may be pigmented or not and are usually dome-shaped or mushroom-shaped (not pathognomonic), although they may be flat and diffuse. Nevi or melanomas may have drusen or lipofuscin deposits on their surface, the latter being more suggestive of malignancy or growth, as is the presence of subretinal fluid. Binocular indirect ophthalmoscopy by an experienced observer is 95% accurate in diagnosis.

B. Standardized A-scan diagnostic ultrasound is the best method of narrowing the diagnosis. In the COMS, it provided >99% accuracy in tumors >2 mm in height. Typical echographic findings in melanoma are low internal reflectivity, regular structure, solid consistency, and the presence of detectable blood flow. In contrast, metastatic tumors are more highly reflective and irregular.

C. Quantitative A-scan is accurate within 0.1 mm in measuring height of intraocular tumors. Tumors <2 mm high should usually be observed, whereas patients with tumors >3 mm high do better with some form of treatment.

D. Nevi and minimally elevated masses are followed with stereo fundus photographs and dilated fundus examinations, at first every 3–6 months and later every 12 months. If growth is suspected or if subretinal fluid appears, repeat ultrasound is indicated for confirmation. Treatment can then be considered after a thorough medical examination to rule out metastases, including abdominal imaging and liver function tests.

E. The liver, the primary site for metastasis, is the focus of the metastatic work-up, which includes liver function tests that, if abnormal, should prompt abdominal imaging. An examination by an oncologist is recommended, with special attention to subcutaneous tissues.

F. If no metastases are found, the exact dimensions and location of the tumor dictate the treatment. Traditionally, enucleation had been the treatment of choice. However, during the last decade, multiple globe and sight therapies have become popular. Yet, for tumors <10 mm high or 16 mm across, no specific therapy has proven to be superior, although it is generally accepted that treatment is better than none. The usual methods of treatment are enucleation or I^{125} plaque radiation, which are being studied in the COMS. So far, no results of this prospective randomized NIH sponsored trial have been published. Local excision, external beam therapy (EBT), and transpupillary thermotherapy (TTT) have also been tried. EBT is the use of charged particle radiation, using either protons or helium ions. The external beam is usually given in five or six divided doses of 1000–1500 cGy/dose. The therapy can be used before or after enucleation and also as an eye-sparing procedure. Side effects from collateral damage are common. Access to a cyclotron limits the widespread availability of the procedure, and there is no proof that it is any better than plaque irradiation. TTT is an externally applied 810-nm diode laser to relatively small uveal melanomas. The purpose is to increase the temperature of the tumor to a tumorcidal level. The advantages include an external approach, absence of surgical intervention, and relative widespread availability. These last three modalities have not yet been studied prospectively in large enough clinical studies to determine their precise indications and efficacy.

G. According to a recent COMS report, no survival difference attributable to pre-enucleation radiation of large choroidal melanomas has been demonstrated to date (1998).

H. If the metastatic work-up is positive, the prognosis for survival is generally <18 months. Palliative and systemic chemotherapy may be offered.

References

Byron SF, Green RL. Ultrasound of the eye and orbit. St Louis: Mosby, 1992: 134–187.

COMS Group. Radiation treatment for eye cancer does not change patients' five year survival. Am J Ophthalmol 1998; 125:779–796.

Finger PT. Radiation Therapy for Choroidal Melanoma. Surv Ophthalmol 1997; 42:215–232.

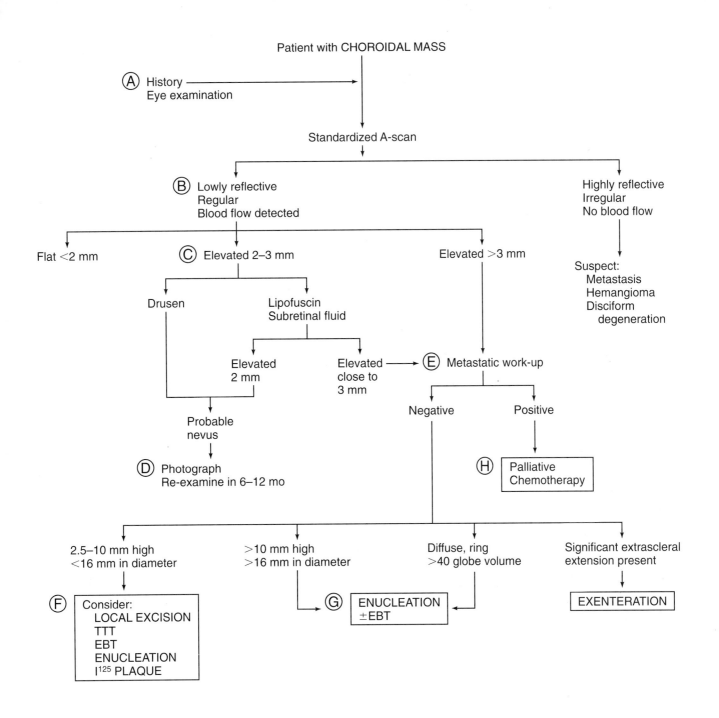

Patient with CHOROIDAL MASS

(A) History ——— Eye examination

Standardized A-scan

(B) Lowly reflective
Regular
Blood flow detected

Highly reflective
Irregular
No blood flow

Flat <2 mm

(C) Elevated 2–3 mm

Elevated >3 mm

Suspect:
Metastasis
Hemangioma
Disciform
degeneration

Drusen

Lipofuscin
Subretinal fluid

Elevated
2 mm

Elevated
close to
3 mm

(E) Metastatic work-up

Negative

Positive

Probable
nevus

(H) Palliative
Chemotherapy

(D) Photograph
Re-examine in 6–12 mo

2.5–10 mm high
<16 mm in diameter

>10 mm high
>16 mm in diameter

Diffuse, ring
>40 globe volume

Significant extrascleral
extension present

(F) Consider:
LOCAL EXCISION
TTT
EBT
ENUCLEATION
I¹²⁵ PLAQUE

(G) ENUCLEATION
±EBT

EXENTERATION

Gass IDM. Problems in the differential diagnosis of choroidal nevi and malignant melanomas: The XXXIII Edward Jackson Memorial Lecture. Am J Ophthalmol 1997; 83:299–323.

Grin JM, Grant-Kels JM, Grin CM, et al. Ocular melanomas and melanocytic lesions of the eye. J Am Acad Dermatol 1998; 38:716–730.

Shields CL, Shields JA, et al. Transpupillary thermotherapy for choroidal melanoma: Tumor control and visual results in 100 consecutive cases. Ophthalmology 1998; 105:581–590.

Zimmerman LE, McLean IW. An evaluation of enucleation in the management of uveal melanomas. Am J Ophthalmol 1979; 87:4741–4760.

VITREOUS OPACITIES

Lina M. Marouf, M.D.
Lanny Odin, M.D.
Bailey L. Lee, M.D.

A. Examination of the vitreous should be done using the slit lamp with the pupil dilated. This allows evaluation of the anterior third of the vitreous. High-power magnification provides information about the size, shape, and intensity of the vitreous cells when present. Use *indirect biomicroscopy* using 90-D or 78-D lenses, or contact lens *biomicroscopy* to visualize the posterior vitreous and retina. In cases of vitreitis, the location of the cells in the vitreous is important in classifying the type of inflammation. The vitreitis may be primary in origin, or it could be a sign of spillover from the anterior chamber or retina. Also perform indirect ophthalmoscopy with scleral depression to assess the peripheral retina and pars plana.

B. Patients with vitreous opacities may be asymptomatic, may complain of floaters, or may present with decreased vision. The change in vision may be secondary to dense vitreous opacities, cystoid macular edema, or associated retinal detachment. The presence of pain, photophobia, and eye redness should alert the physician to an inflammatory process. Floaters accompanied by photopsia indicate vitreoretinal traction as seen in vitreous detachment, retinal tears, and proliferative retinal diseases. A thorough ocular and medical history of trauma, surgery, or active medical problems could direct the analysis of the ocular disease.

C. A patient with vitreous degeneration most commonly presents with floaters. However, a patient may be asymptomatic. Increasing age, inflammation, or hemorrhage can result in liquefaction and syneresis of the vitreous. The vitreous fibers produce a shadowing effect on the retina that is perceived as floaters.

D. Asteroid hyalosis and synchysis scintillans are the two main entities associated with yellow crystalline opacities in the vitreous. Asteroid hyalosis are opacities composed of calcium-containing phospholipids and are found to be unilateral in 75% of patients. There has been an association with diabetes mellitus. When the retina detail is limited by dense asteroid hyalosis, fluorescein angiography may allow one to visualize the retina. Very rarely, vitrectomy may be required to remove the vitreous opacities to facilitate treatment of an underlying retinal pathologic condition. Synchysis scintillans or cholesterolosis occurs in eyes that have had repeated vitreous hemorrhages and is composed of cholesterol crystals. The opacities tend to settle inferiorly because these eyes often have a posterior vitreous detachment, in contrast to eyes with asteroid hyalosis.

E. Pigmented cells in the vitreous can be seen in conditions associated with the release of retinal pigment epithelium (RPE) cells into the vitreous or with vitreous hemorrhage as seen in posterior vitreous detachment, retinal, tears, and proliferative retinopathies. Proliferative retinal disease tends to be bilateral (except in retinal vascular occlusive disease). Examination of the fellow eye may help in establishing the diagnosis. In the absence of a known medical illness, a medical evaluation is indicated to rule out diabetes, hypertension, sickle cell disease, hyperviscosity syndrome, retinal embolization, and sarcoidosis. Posterior vitreous detachment resulting in vitreous hemorrhage is associated with a retinal tear in 80% of patients; therefore a thorough peripheral retinal examination is mandatory. When the vitreous hemorrhage precludes retinal visualization, ocular ultrasonography is warranted to rule out a retinal detachment. The presence of pigmented cells in the vitreous (Shafer's sign) indicates a retinal tear.

F. Tumor cells, such as retinoblastoma in children and malignant melanoma or large cell lymphoma, can produce vitreous seeding and masquerade as vitreitis. Intraocular large cell lymphoma occurs in patients in their sixties. It is bilateral in 80% of patients. The retina and choroid may also be involved by tumor cells, which have a yellow-white appearance. Amyloidosis of the vitreous produces a white stringy appearance of the vitreous fibrils that resembles a string of pearls. The diagnosis is established by the presence of the associated ocular findings.

G. Inflammation of the vitreous can present as vitreous cells, opacities, condensations, haze, cystoid macular edema (CME), or areas of vitreoretinal traction. The severity of the vitreous activity can be graded by assessing the amount of vitreous haze, the clarity of the optic nerve, retinal vessels, and nerve fiber layer reflex using a 20-D lens and indirect ophthalmoscopy.

H. Prior trauma or surgery to the eye can result in infectious endophthalmitis, lens-induced uveitis, or Irvine-Gass syndrome in the involved eye. The presence of bilateral iritis, vitreitis, and a yellow subretinal nodule after trauma is diagnostic of sympathetic ophthalmia. The clinical presentation, ocular findings, and course of the vitreitis should help in establishing the diagnosis.

I. Snowball opacities over the peripheral retina and pars plana occur in pars planitis, sarcoidosis, and Lyme disease. The medical history (e.g., tick bites, Lyme disease) and associated systemic findings such as erythema chronicum migrans (Lyme), erythema nodosum, and restrictive lung disease (sarcoidosis); laboratory tests such as VDRL, FTA-ABS, and Lyme titers; and chest film can help narrow the differential.

J. Vitreitis caused by posterior uveitis as seen in Vogt-Koyanagi-Harada syndrome or posterior scleritis can result in serous retinal detachment in the acute stage secondary to disruption of the outer blood retinal barrier. Chronic vitreitis and uveitis can lead to vitreous condensation, proliferative changes, and vitreous detachment, resulting in tractional or rhegmatogenous retinal detachment as seen in acute retinal necrosis, CMV retinitis, and pars planitis.

K. The diagnosis of several disorders associated with vasculitis is facilitated by multisystem involvement (e.g., Behçet's disease, Crohn's disease, Whipple's disease, sarcoidosis). Ocular involvement in sarcoidosis occurs in about 40% of patients. Usually, posterior segment disease is accompanied by granulomatous iridocyclitis. Posterior segment involvement includes snowball vitreous opacities, retinal vasculitis (termed candle-wax dripping), and optic nerve and choroidal granulomas. Toxoplasmosis presents as an area of focal retinitis seen as a "satellite" next to an old atrophic lesion. Consider syphilis in any patient with vitreitis because the clinical presentation may vary. Acute retinal necrosis syndrome classically presents with the triad of vasculitis, peripheral necrotizing retinitis, and vitreitis. Tuberculosis typically produces choroidal granulomas or iridocyclitis that is unresponsive to anti-inflammatory therapy. Pars planitis is characterized by bilateral ocular involvement, vitreitis, and snowball vitreous opacities with or without periphlebitis, peripheral neovascularization, and CME. It occurs in teenagers or young adults. Birdshot choroidopathy occurs in middle-aged patients, is bilateral, and clinically presents as multiple white spots in the choroid, vitreitis, CME, arteritis, and late optic atrophy. Color vision, electrooculographic, and electroretinographic abnormalities have been noted. Other laboratory tests that may confirm the diagnosis in some of the disease entities include chest film (sarcoid and tuberculosis); PPD skin testing (tuberculosis); ACE and serum lysozyme (sarcoidosis); MHA-TP, FTA-ABS, and VDRL (syphilis); serologic tests (toxoplasmosis); barium enema (Crohn's and Whipple's diseases); HLA typing (B_5, Behçet's, A29 birdshot choroidopathy).

L. Retinitis presents as an indistinct area of retinal thickening and whitening with overlying vitreitis. The most common cause in healthy individuals is toxoplasmic retinochoroiditis. In immunocompromised individuals, consider candidal retinitis, CMV, and septic retinitis. CMV retinitis produces a confluent hemorrhagic retinitis. Candidal retinochoroiditis lesions are multiple, are fluffy white, and may break into the vitreous to produce "fluff balls." Syphilis and tuberculosis can occur in both groups of patients. The medical work-up should include blood, urine, and catheter cultures.

M. Several entities have been found to present with vitreitis associated with white outer retinal or subretinal lesions. The white-yellow lesions in serpiginous choroidopathy involve the RPE-choroid complex. They begin in the peripapillary region, have a geographic appearance, and progress in a centripetal fashion. Serpiginous choroidopathy is a bilateral disease that can affect both sexes in the age group of 10–60 years. Multiple evanescent white dot syndrome is a self-limited ocular disease that affects young women, is unilateral, and is characterized by small discrete white dots occurring at the RPE level in the perifoveal region. The dots resolve, leaving RPE window defects. Accompanying vitreitis and periphlebitis may be present. Fluorescein angiography reveals early hyperfluorescence with late staining of the lesions. Posterior multifocal placoid pigment epitheliopathy is a bilateral disease characterized by large creamy-colored placoid lesions at the level of the RPE. The lesions involve the preequatorial region. Vitreitis and occasionally papillitis are present. The disease affects young people with good visual prognosis. Fluorescein angiography reveals early blockage and late staining of the lesions. Multifocal choroiditis, also called *pseudopresumed ocular histoplasmosis,* is a bilateral disease that usually affects women and is characterized by the presence of histoplasmosis-like "punched-out" lesions in the peripheral fundus. However, unlike in presumed ocular histoplasmosis syndrome, these patients present with significant iritis and vitreitis. In subretinal fibrosis and uveitis syndrome, a bilateral disease that affects young African-American women, irregular whitish lesions are seen in the subretinal space with accompanying vitreitis and iritis. Diffuse unilateral subacute neuroretinitis occurs in healthy individuals and is thought to result from a wandering nematode in the subretinal space. It is characterized by vitreitis, multiple evanescent gray-white outer retinal lesions, vasculitis, and papillitis. Several other parasitic infestations have also been reported to result in vitreitis with various ocular manifestations.

References

Bergren RL, Brown GC, Duker JS. Prevalence and association of asteroid hyalosis with systemic diseases. Am J Ophthalmol 1991; 111:289–293.

Hampton GR, Nelsen PT, Hay PB. Viewing through the asteroids. Ophthalmology 1981; 88:669–672.

Nussenblatt RB, Palestine AG, Chan CC, Roberge F. Standardization of vitreal inflammatory activity in intermediate and posterior uveitis. Ophthalmology 1985; 92:467–471.

Nussenblatt RB, Whitcup SM, Palestine AG. Uveitis: Fundamentals and clinical practice. 2nd ed. St Louis: Mosby, 1996.

Roy FH. Ocular differential diagnosis. Baltimore: Williams & Wilkins, 1997.

Patient with VITREOUS OPACITIES

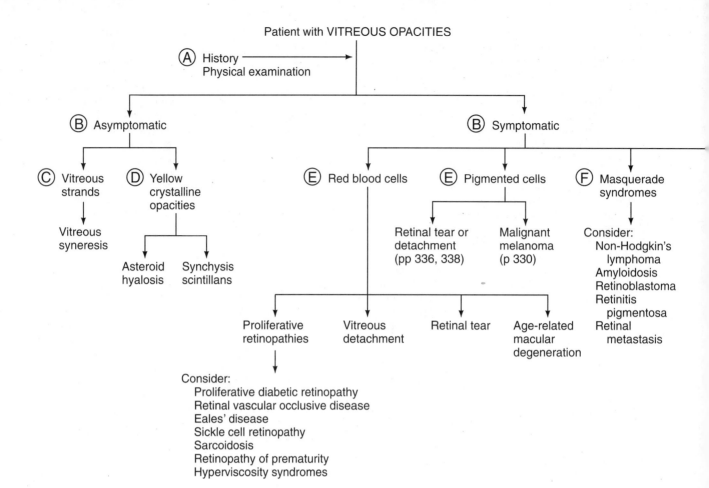

Consider:
    Proliferative diabetic retinopathy
    Retinal vascular occlusive disease
    Eales' disease
    Sickle cell retinopathy
    Sarcoidosis
    Retinopathy of prematurity
    Hyperviscosity syndromes

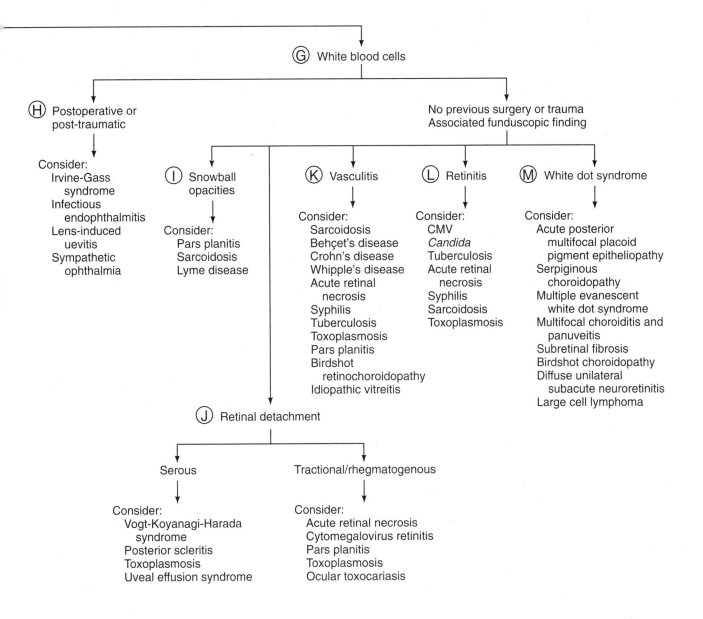

Ⓖ White blood cells

Ⓗ Postoperative or
post-traumatic

No previous surgery or trauma
Associated funduscopic finding

Consider:
  Irvine-Gass
    syndrome
  Infectious
    endophthalmitis
  Lens-induced
    uevitis
  Sympathetic
    ophthalmia

Ⓘ Snowball
opacities

Ⓚ Vasculitis

Ⓛ Retinitis

Ⓜ White dot syndrome

Consider:
  Pars planitis
  Sarcoidosis
  Lyme disease

Consider:
  Sarcoidosis
  Behçet's disease
  Crohn's disease
  Whipple's disease
  Acute retinal
    necrosis
  Syphilis
  Tuberculosis
  Toxoplasmosis
  Pars planitis
  Birdshot
    retinochoroidopathy
  Idiopathic vitreitis

Consider:
  CMV
  Candida
  Tuberculosis
  Acute retinal
    necrosis
  Syphilis
  Sarcoidosis
  Toxoplasmosis

Consider:
  Acute posterior
    multifocal placoid
    pigment epitheliopathy
  Serpiginous
    choroidopathy
  Multiple evanescent
    white dot syndrome
  Multifocal choroiditis and
    panuveitis
  Subretinal fibrosis
  Birdshot choroidopathy
  Diffuse unilateral
    subacute neuroretinitis
  Large cell lymphoma

Ⓙ Retinal detachment

Serous

Tractional/rhegmatogenous

Consider:
  Vogt-Koyanagi-Harada
    syndrome
  Posterior scleritis
  Toxoplasmosis
  Uveal effusion syndrome

Consider:
  Acute retinal necrosis
  Cytomegalovirus retinitis
  Pars planitis
  Toxoplasmosis
  Ocular toxocariasis

RETINAL HOLES AND TEARS

W.A.J. van Heuven, M.D.

Partial- or full-thickness holes in the retina are rarely present congenitally but usually develop later as a result of traction from the vitreous gel or tearing during ocular trauma. When a tear occurs, patients may have symptoms of retinal traction (seeing flashes of light) or may see floaters (a shower, cloud, or "spider web" of black or red spots), the latter usually indicating bleeding within the eye. Vitreous detachment (separation from retina), occurring either spontaneously in later adulthood or secondarily from vitreoretinal disorders (vasculopathy, inflammation, or trauma), usually is the cause of retinal tearing but may take place without causing retinal damage. In either case, flashes may occur. However, if no retinal damage is done, the floaters are often few, larger, and of specific shapes, representing some glial tissue from the disc on the posterior vitreous surface. In general, if the patient sees <10–12 floaters, one can assume a benign vitreous detachment and the eye examination can be scheduled during regular office hours. However, >12 floaters often indicates hemorrhage from a retinal tear and demands prompt attention.

A. Asymptomatic retinal holes are found incidentally during routine examination. Questioning yields no history of flashes or floaters.

B. The examination using the indirect ophthalmoscope and scleral depressor determines the type, size, and location of the holes, as well as the presence of subretinal fluid. Examination using the slit lamp and precorneal lens (contact lens gives best view) determines the presence of vitreous detachment.

C. Atrophic holes, such as those seen with high myopia and CMV, are caused by retinal atrophy and may not have obvious choroidal or vitreous components. The small round holes within lattice degeneration are similar, but the tears occurring at the edges of the lattice lesions are definitely tractional because of vitreoretinal adhesions, which tear the retina when the vitreous detaches.

D. As experience with AIDS and other immunosuppressed conditions accumulates, the treatment of retinal holes resulting from retinal necrosis continues to be controversial. Because retinal detachment in AIDS is so difficult to cure, prophylactic cryotherapy or laser therapy for retinal holes is often recommended. It may be necessary to treat widely around the holes to create chorioretinal adhesions in areas where the retina is still alive and able to scar.

E. The mere presence of retinal holes associated with myopia or lattice degeneration is not an indication for treatment. However, some ophthalmologists would treat prophylactically if the patient has a strong family history of retinal detachment from these causes and especially if the patient had a retinal detachment from such causes in the other eye. In addition, retinal tears located at the edge of lattice lesions should be considered as horseshoe-shaped tears and treated.

F. An operculated tear is a retinal tear caused by vitreous traction, which has torn a piece of retina completely away from its location, and no vitreoretinal traction remains on the remaining retina. The operculum is the piece of retina that is now completely located within the vitreous cavity on the surface of the detached vitreous gel. This is different from a horseshoe-shaped tear in which vitreoretinal traction persists at the base (flap) of the tear. Most rhegmatogenous (caused by a tear) retinal detachments do not occur unless three conditions are present simultaneously: a retinal hole, traction on the retina in the area of the hole, and liquid in the vitreous cavity overlying the hole. In operculated tears, traction is not present, so treatment is unnecessary.

G. If there is a significant amount of subretinal fluid around a tear, cryotherapy or laser treatment to create a chorioretinal adhesion is indicated to prevent liquid vitreous from going through the hole to detach the retina further. Clinically, a significant amount may be considered a rim of retinal detachment around a tear greater in diameter than the tear itself.

H. Many retinal surgeons treat all horseshoe-shaped retinal tears. However, if a careful history indicates no symptoms and if the tear shows evidence of having been present for a long time (demarcation line), the tear probably does not need to be treated, unless the patient plans to have limited access to physicians in the future or has a profession or sport in which eye trauma is common.

I. Dialysis (disinsertion) of the retina usually occurs inferiorly at the ora serrata as a result of trauma. If the dialysis is surrounded posteriorly by a chorioretinal scar, it is probably safe to leave it untreated. Not much is known about the natural history of asymptomatic dialysis, but it can cause retinal detachment, which is slowly progressive and often not noted until years after the injury. Most retinal surgeons treat asymptomatic as well as symptomatic dialysis with prophylactic cryotherapy.

J. Generally, symptomatic retinal tears tend to lead to retinal detachment, and asymptomatic tears are relatively benign. However, even symptomatic operculated holes may have a benign cause because there is no residual traction on the retina, unlike in horseshoe-shaped tears or tears associated with bridging vessels (see section F).

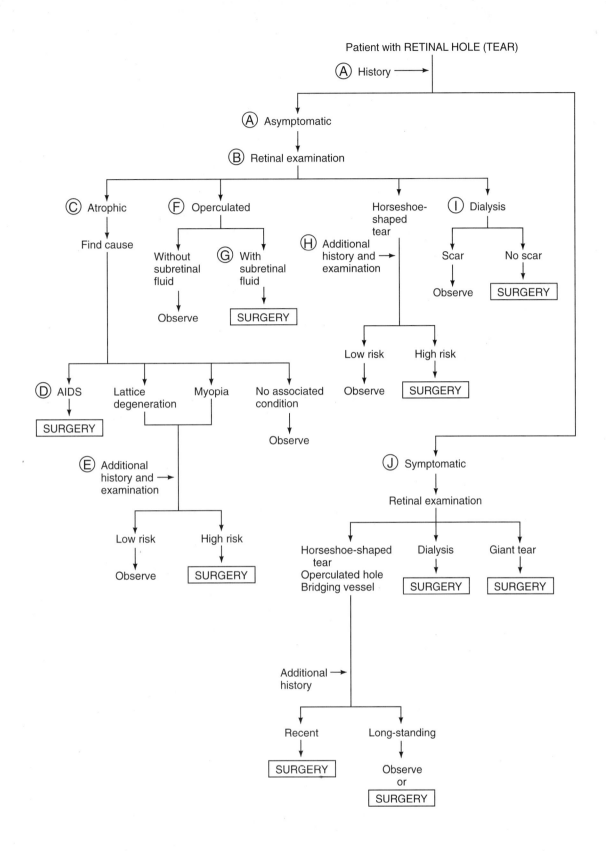

Patient with RETINAL HOLE (TEAR)

Ⓐ History →

Ⓐ Asymptomatic

Ⓑ Retinal examination

Ⓒ Atrophic

Find cause

Ⓕ Operculated

Without subretinal fluid

Observe

Ⓖ With subretinal fluid

SURGERY

Horseshoe-shaped tear

Ⓗ Additional history and examination →

Low risk

Observe

High risk

SURGERY

Ⓘ Dialysis

Scar

Observe

No scar

SURGERY

Ⓓ AIDS

SURGERY

Lattice degeneration

Myopia

No associated condition

Observe

Ⓔ Additional history and examination →

Low risk

Observe

High risk

SURGERY

Ⓙ Symptomatic

Retinal examination

Horseshoe-shaped tear
Operculated hole
Bridging vessel

Dialysis

SURGERY

Giant tear

SURGERY

Additional history →

Recent

SURGERY

Long-standing

Observe
or
SURGERY

References

Byer NE. The natural history of asymptomatic retinal breaks. Ophthalmology 1982; 89:1033–1039.

Byer NE. Long term natural history of lattice degeneration of the retina. Ophthalmology 1989; 9:1396–1401.

Folk JC, Bennett SR, Klugman MR, et al. Prophylactic treatment to the fellow eye of patients with phakic lattice retinal detachment. Retina 1990; 10:165–169.

Wilkinson CP, Rice TA. Michel's retinal detachment. 2nd ed. St Louis: Mosby, 1997.

RHEGMATOGENOUS RETINAL DETACHMENT

W.A.J. van Heuven, M.D.

Rhegmatogenous retinal detachment (RRD) is caused by a hole or tear in the retina. For such a hole to have caused the detachment, it must have been accompanied by the presence of liquid adjacent to the hole as well as traction on the retina in the area of the hole. Congenital, atrophic, or traumatic holes by themselves tend not to produce retinal detachment. The usual pathogenesis of RRD begins with a vitreous detachment, in which the vitreous gel either contracts or collapses and its surface separates from the retinal surface. Liquid from the vitreous gel then fills the space between the vitreous gel and the retina. As the vitreous separates from the retina, it occasionally tears the retina in an area of strong vitreoretinal adhesion. If the vitreous, as it separates, simply avulses a piece of retina, leaving no traction on the surrounding retina, the retinal hole usually does not cause retinal detachment. However, if the vitreous tears the retina and retains an adhesion to the edge of the tear (horseshoe-shaped retinal tear), traction in the area of the tear may cause retinal detachment to subsequently occur.

A. RRD is usually cured by closing the retinal hole; thus a thorough search for this hole or multiple holes is crucial. Binocular indirect ophthalmoscopy with scleral indentation, which brings the peripheral retina anterior to the equator into the examiner's view, is the best diagnostic method for finding retinal holes.

B. If the retinal holes are located in the upper two thirds of the eye, the injection of intravitreal gas can be used to close the hole by tamponade as part of the surgical cure. Because intraocular gas rises, proper positioning of the patient can help close superior holes. Closing inferior holes with the help of gas requires the patient to be upside down, which is not normally feasible.

C. Pneumatic retinopexy is the simplest surgical procedure for curing RRD. Approximately 40% of all retinal detachments can be managed with this technique, and 85% of selected cases can be successfully treated. The procedure consists of transconjunctival cryotherapy and intravitreal gas injection, followed by postoperative positioning of the patient. Specific indications are the presence of one break or a group of breaks located in the superior two thirds of the eye in a cooperative patient.

D. Complex RRDs, as defined here, are those associated with proliferative vitreoretinopathy (PVR), which consists of fibrosis in the vitreous cavity and on both surfaces of the retina to varying degrees, creating complex tractional forces on the retina and producing multiple fixed folds and retinal rigidity. This periretinal scarring makes surgical reattachment of the retina difficult, often requiring surgical dissection of the fibrosis from the surfaces of the retina.

E. Most RRDs, in which the retinal holes can be located, can be cured by scleral buckling techniques, which consist of temporary or permanent indentation of the globe to help approximate the pigment epithelium to the detached retina; the creation of chorioretinal adhesions around the retinal holes by cryopexy, diathermy, or laser; and at times, transchoroidal drainage of subretinal fluid and intravitreal injection of gas. The success rate in all retinal detachments, after one scleral buckling procedure, is about 85%, which can be increased to about 94% with revisions of the scleral buckle. Today, the sole reason for failure of scleral buckling procedures is the development of PVR.

F. In most cases of RRD, it should be possible to find the retinal hole. Inexperience of the examiner is probably the most common reason for failure to find the hole. Other reasons include opacities of the media, poor pupillary dilation, and a pale fundus, such as seen in albinism or high myopia. If no holes can be found using indirect ophthalmoscopy with scleral indentation, a more magnified view of the retina can be obtained using slit-lamp biomicroscopy with a three-mirror Goldman contact lens.

G. When an experienced examiner fails to find retinal holes after a diligent, the possibility that the retinal detachment is secondary must be considered (p 326). Typical characteristics of secondary detachments are that they do not extend to the ora serrata, are not associated with retinal folds, and do have shifting subretinal fluid, in addition to having an ocular cause, other than a hole, for the detachment. If secondary detachment is ruled out and the hole is still not found, a 360-degree scleral buckle can be used with 360 degrees of cryotherapy to create a circumferential chorioretinal adhesion over the buckle, which in most cases separates the peripheral retina from the posterior retina. Because most retinal holes occur between the equator and the ora serrata, the area of the holes will thus be separated from the posterior pole by the cryotherapy scar. Subretinal fluid drainage should also be done to reattach the retina in the operating room. Careful repeat examinations of the peripheral retina postoperatively may help locate the hole because the retina may again detach peripheral to the cryotherapy scar, initially in the area of the retinal hole. At that time, one can decide whether to revise the scleral buckling procedure to close the newly found retinal break.

H. Table 1 shows the classification of PVR. With increasing amounts of PVR, the curative operation increases in complexity. Without PVR, many different scleral buckling procedures alone will produce a cure. In mild PVR less than grade C2, scleral buckling must be combined with drainage of subretinal fluid and gas injection to maximize the postoperative period, during which the retina and the pigment epithelium remain apposed and the chorioretinal adhesion forms. In PVR greater than grade C2, vitrectomy surgery may be

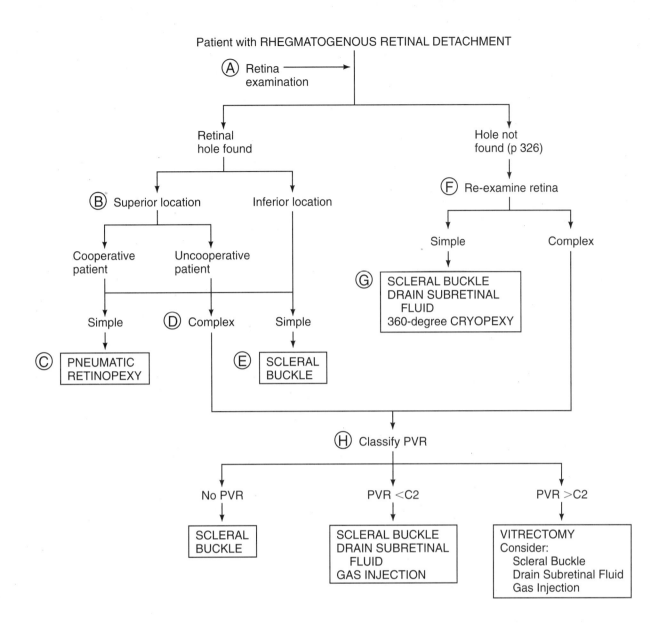

Patient with RHEGMATOGENOUS RETINAL DETACHMENT

(A) Retina examination

Retinal hole found

Hole not found (p 326)

(F) Re-examine retina

Simple

Complex

(G) SCLERAL BUCKLE
DRAIN SUBRETINAL FLUID
360-degree CRYOPEXY

(B) Superior location

Inferior location

Cooperative patient

Uncooperative patient

Simple

(D) Complex

Simple

(C) PNEUMATIC RETINOPEXY

(E) SCLERAL BUCKLE

(H) Classify PVR

No PVR

PVR <C2

PVR >C2

SCLERAL BUCKLE

SCLERAL BUCKLE
DRAIN SUBRETINAL FLUID
GAS INJECTION

VITRECTOMY
Consider:
    Scleral Buckle
    Drain Subretinal Fluid
    Gas Injection

needed to peel the periretinal fibrosis from the retina surfaces and permit the retina to settle back in its physiologic position. This can be combined with scleral buckling procedures, drainage of subretinal fluid, and injections of gases or oils.

References

Hilton CF, Kelly NE, Salzano TC, et al. Pneumatic retinopexy: A collaborative report of the first 100 cases. Ophthalmology 1987; 94:307–314.

Retina Society Terminology Committee. The classification of retinal detachment with proliferative vitreoretinopathy. Ophthalmology 1983; 90:121–125.

Ryan SI, ed. Retina. Vol 3. St Louis: Mosby, 1989.

Wilkinson CP, Rice TA. Michel's retinal detachment. 2nd ed. St Louis: Mosby, 1997.

TABLE 1   Classification of Proliferative Vitreoretinopathy

A. Vitreous haze and pigment
B. Wrinkling of inner retinal surface, rolled edge of retinal hole, vessel tortuosity
C. Full thickness, fixed retinal folds
    1. Same in one quadrant
    2. Same in two quadrants
    3. Same in three quadrants
D. Fixed retinal folds in four quadrants
    1. Wide funnel-shaped retinal detachment
    2. Narrow funnel-shaped retinal detachment
    3. Closed funnel-shaped retinal detachment

DIABETIC RETINOPATHY

W.A.J. van Heuven, M.D.

Diabetic retinopathy is one of the two leading causes of blindness in the Western world. In the United States it is the number one cause of new cases of blindness among people 20–74 years old. Generally, all of the changes of diabetic retinopathy are seen in both types of diabetes: type 1 insulin-dependent diabetes, juvenile diabetes (IDDM), and type 2 non–insulin-dependent adult-onset diabetes (NIDDM). However, there are significant differences in the way the eye disease presents and develops in these two types. In NIDDM the main reason for visual loss is neovascularization and bleeding. In NIDDM the main reason for visual loss is macular edema. Furthermore, in type 1 diabetes it takes several years for any retinopathy to develop, whereas in type 2 diabetes the retinopathy is often present at the time diabetes is diagnosed. In type 1, approximately 50% of patients have some retinopathy after 7 years of having diabetes, and 90% have retinopathy after about 20 years of having diabetes.

Systemic hypertension may be the strongest factor associated with progression of retinopathy. Furthermore, patients with severe proliferative retinopathy (PDR) are at a higher risk of stroke, myocardial infarction, and nephropathy. Whether good metabolic control of the diabetes can delay or prevent the development of diabetic retinopathy is still unknown, probably because good metabolic control is difficult to achieve, measure, and even define.

Some of the greatest changes in medicine in the last 10 years have been in the prevention of blindness from diabetes. Largely responsible for this improvement in eye care have been the three national collaborative studies supported by the National Institutes of Health (NIH): the Diabetic Retinopathy Study (DRS), which demonstrated the value of laser treatment for proliferative retinopathy; the Early Treatment Diabetic Retinopathy Study (ETDRS), which proved the value of earlier intervention with laser as well as the value of laser treatment for macular edema; and the Diabetic Retinopathy Vitrectomy Study (DRVS), which showed the value of early vitrectomy in some patients with severe retinopathy. The results of these studies currently form the basis for our rationale of treatment for diabetic retinopathy.

Any patient referred because of diabetes or anyone who has retinal changes suggestive of diabetes should have a thorough eye and physical examination. The eye examination should include gonioscopy to look for rubeosis of the iris and visual fields to rule out peripheral constriction from ischemic retinopathy or to rule out neurologic field defects from cerebrovascular disease. The physical examination is best done by an internist or endocrinologist to look specifically for systemic diabetic changes as well as to rule out systemic hypertension and other diseases that may mimic diabetes in the eye.

A. If a patient has good vision even with systemic diabetes and has no retinopathy or background retinopathy (BDR), take photographs of the entire fundus for documentation and future comparison and see the patient again 1 year later. In 5%–10% of these patients some retinopathy or increasing retinopathy develops within 1 year. In addition, if any severe systemic disease develops or the patient becomes pregnant during that year, it is wise for the ophthalmologist to be consulted again. BDR consists of microaneurysms, small round hemorrhages (blots and dots), and hard exudates.

B. Until recently, preproliferative retinopathy (PPDR) was defined as soft exudates (focal retinal edema in areas of recent capillary closure); venous beading (focal dilations of veins); intraretinal microvascular anomalies (IRMAs), which represent probably intraretinal neovascularization and are seen as irregular kinked nets of slightly dilated capillaries within the retina; and very severe BDR. It has been found, however, that some patients can have many soft exudates and almost no other retinopathy and that these exudates are not predictors of progression. Thus soft exudates are no longer considered proof of PPDR. Because BDR can be present for many years without apparent change, the category of PPDR was created, because such patients were seen to get PDR in a relatively short time. Thus identification of PPDR became a useful clinical tool for recommending the frequency of patient visits and for preparing the patient for future laser treatment. Because some IRMAs are difficult to differentiate from retinal neovascularization, fluorescein angiography is recommended. If patients are deemed reliable and can be expected to keep appointments, PPDR can simply be documented and observed every 4–6 months until higher-risk characteristics develop. However, in an unreliable patient or remote population, it may be wise to treat at least one eye with PPDR with panretinal photocoagulation.

C. Proliferative diabetic retinopathy is, by definition, preretinal proliferation of neovascularization at the disc (NVD) or elsewhere in the fundus (NVE). The DRS demonstrated that laser photocoagulation is beneficial at this stage. The DRS also identified high-risk characteristics for profound visual loss, which include NVD greater than one quarter of the disc area and vitreous or preretinal hemorrhage associated with NVD or with NVE. When these criteria are present, there is urgency in doing laser treatment soon, before further vitreous hemorrhage develops.

D. In a diabetic patient with decreased vision and clear media, the probable cause of vision loss is macular edema, although preretinal fibrosis and macular traction can also be causes. Slit-lamp biomicroscopy can differentiate these. The best view is obtained through a corneal contact lens, such as the Goldman posterior pole lens, which gives an excellent three-dimensional picture of the vitreous and retina. Angiography should also be done to confirm the diagnosis of macular edema, which will show late fluorescein leakage within the retina.

E. The determination of whether macular edema is clinically significant, which was defined by the ETDRS, is important in deciding whether to treat. The definition of clinically significant macular edema is as follows:
1. Thickening of the retina within 500 microns of the center of the macula
2. Hard exudates within 500 microns of the center of the macula, if associated with thickening of adjacent retina
3. A zone of retinal thickening 1 disc area or larger, a part of which is within 1 disc diameter of the center of the macula

The ETDRS demonstrated that laser treatment, according to its protocol, significantly reduced the risk of visual loss in clinically significant macular edema. Although definite proof is lacking, there is accumulating evidence that better hypoglycemic control, more precise blood pressure control, and the use of diuretics may decrease macular edema as well.

F. In eyes with opaque media, particularly vitreous hemorrhage and cataract, B-scan and quantitative A-scan ultrasonography are useful to determine the nature of vitreoretinal abnormalities in the posterior half of the eye. B-scan ultrasonography can provide good topographic information about the complex vitreoretinal relationships. Quantitative A-scan ultrasonography is helpful to differentiate retinal detachment from vitreous membranes. If the ultrasonography indicates vitreous traction on the macula or macular detachment, vitrectomy may be indicated.

G. If cataract is present and the lens opacities are sufficient to explain significantly decreased vision, cataract surgery is indicated. If ultrasonography shows the need for vitrectomy (macular detachment) and lens opacities are severe enough to interfere with vitreous surgery, cataract surgery should also be done, possibly in combination with vitrectomy. Both vitrectomy and cataract surgery tend to remove barriers between the posterior and anterior segments of the eye. Presumably, this permits neovascular factors produced by the ischemic retina to enter the anterior segment and produce neovascularization of the iris and angle, resulting in glaucoma. This scenario is especially likely if panretinal photocoagulation has not been previously done. Thus, if lensectomy and vitrectomy are contemplated for an eye that has not had laser treatment, panretinal photocoagulation should be done at the same time.

H. The DRVS demonstrated that early vitrectomy was better than vitrectomy after 1 year of vitreous hemorrhage in juvenile-onset diabetes. This benefit was not found in adult-onset diabetic vitreous hemorrhage. Thus, if more than trace vitreous hemorrhage occurs in a juvenile diabetic patient, vitrectomy is indicated unless it can be clearly demonstrated that the entire vitreous gel is detached from the posterior retinal surface. If vitreous hemorrhage occurs in a patient with adult-onset diabetes, biomicroscopy can be used to gauge the amount, mobility, and color of the hemorrhage, as well as the presence of vitreous detachment. If the amount of hemorrhage is little and the fundus can be seen through the hemorrhage, if the mobility of the blood is great, if the vitreous is detached from the posterior retina, and if the color is reddish, the vitreous hemorrhage can be observed and will probably clear spontaneously. However, if the vitreous hemorrhage is severe, relatively immobile, and yellow ochre in color or is associated with multiple vitreoretinal traction points, consider vitrectomy.

I. Many retinal ischemic conditions have features similar to those of diabetic retinopathy. These conditions include sickle cell disease and other hemoglobinopathies, hematologic diseases that cause small-vessel occlusions, collagen vascular diseases (lupus) that cause arteriolar occlusions, and talc retinopathy (which causes embolic phenomena in drug addicts). Many of these conditions show peripheral retinal occlusive phenomena with peripheral neovascularization, unlike the more central neovascularization of diabetes. Radiation retinopathy can mimic diabetic retinopathy precisely. The history indicates this as a possibility. Systemic hypertension and increased coagulability of the blood are common with diabetes. Thus patients may have a combination of hypertensive and diabetic retinopathy and may also have central or branch retinal vein occlusions together with diabetic retinopathy. Hypertensive retinopathy has many of the same features of diabetic retinopathy, except that the hemorrhages are in the nerve fiber layer and therefore are streaked rather than round, and microaneurysms occur only late in the disease. Vein occlusions also show many of the same features of diabetic retinopathy but are more prominently hemorrhagic, often with streak hemorrhages; are always associated with edema in the occluded areas; and have significant venous dilation, which is uniform, unlike the beading or sausagelike dilations in diabetic retinopathy.

References

Diabetic Retinopathy Study Research Group. Photocoagulation treatment of proliferative diabetic retinopathy: The second report of DRS findings. Ophthalmology 1978; 85:82–106.

Diabetic Retinopathy Study Research Group. Indications for photocoagulation treatment of diabetic retinopathy, DRS Report No. 14. Int Ophthalmol Clin 1987; 27:239–253.

Diabetic Retinopathy Vitrectomy Study Research Group. Early vitrectomy for severe proliferative diabetic retinopathy in eyes with useful vision. Results of a randomized trial, DRVS Report No. 3. Ophthalmology 1988; 95:1307–1320.

Early Treatment Diabetic Retinopathy Study Research Group. Photocoagulation for diabetic macular edema, ETDRS Report No. 1. Arch Ophthalmol 1985; 103:1796–1806.

Early Treatment Diabetic Retinopathy Study Research Group. Case reports to accompany ETDRS reports 3 and 4. Int Ophthalmol Clin 1987; 27:254–264.

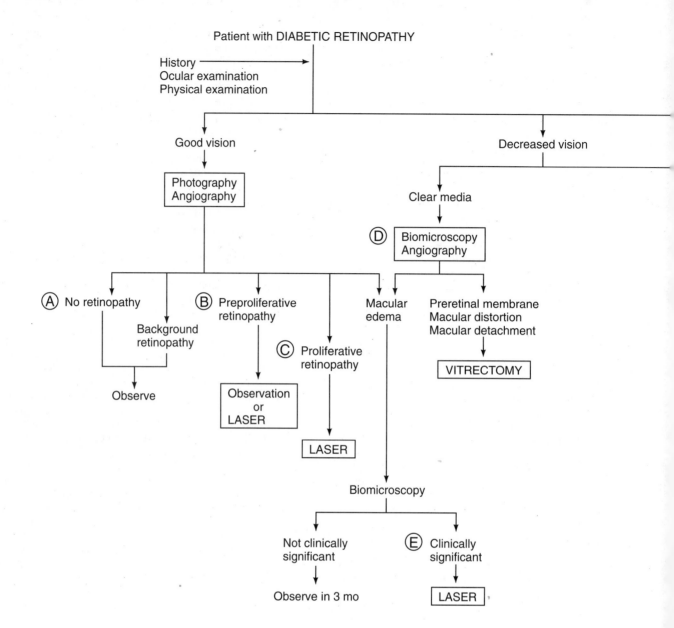

Patient with DIABETIC RETINOPATHY

History
Ocular examination
Physical examination

Good vision

Decreased vision

Photography
Angiography

Clear media

Ⓓ Biomicroscopy
Angiography

Ⓐ No retinopathy

Background
retinopathy

Ⓑ Preproliferative
retinopathy

Macular
edema

Preretinal membrane
Macular distortion
Macular detachment

Observe

Ⓒ Proliferative
retinopathy

VITRECTOMY

Observation
or
LASER

LASER

Biomicroscopy

Not clinically
significant

Ⓔ Clinically
significant

Observe in 3 mo

LASER

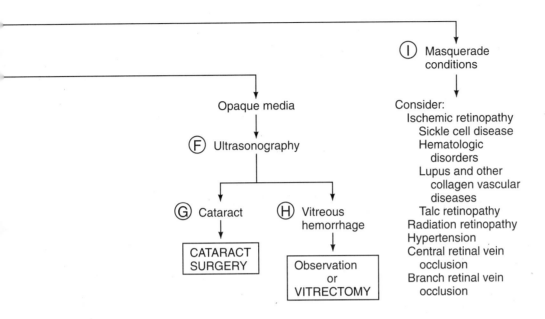

Opaque media

Ⓕ Ultrasonography

Ⓖ Cataract

Ⓗ Vitreous
hemorrhage

CATARACT
SURGERY

Observation
or
VITRECTOMY

Ⓘ Masquerade
conditions

Consider:
Ischemic retinopathy
Sickle cell disease
Hematologic
disorders
Lupus and other
collagen vascular
diseases
Talc retinopathy
Radiation retinopathy
Hypertension
Central retinal vein
occlusion
Branch retinal vein
occlusion

RETINAL DRUG TOXICITY

Bailey L. Lee, M.D.

A. A careful drug history must be taken in patients with suspected retinal drug toxicity, especially in patients whose medical history is incomplete or vague. Of course there will be those patients with an obvious history of drug use who are referred for evaluation, but even in those patients, the dosage and duration of the drug still needs to be documented.

B. Certain oral medications are well known for potential retinal toxicity. Chloroquine and hydroxychloroquine are used at higher dosages for the treatment of rheumatoid arthritis and systemic lupus erythematosus than for the treatment of malaria, and it is patients taking these higher dosages who are at risk for toxicity. For chloroquine, toxicity rarely occurs at a total cumulative dose of <300 g, but maintaining a daily dose of <250 mg may be more important. For hydroxychloroquine, toxicity rarely appears at dosages of ≤400 mg/day, but patients with many years of cumulative use may be at risk. These patients can develop macular pigmentary changes or bull's eye maculopathy. The phenothiazines thioridazine and chlorpromazine are believed to be concentrated within the melanin granules of the uvea and retinal pigment epithelium. Pigmentary retinopathy from chlorpromazine use is rare, whereas with thioridazine severe retinopathy can develop within weeks of taking dosages >800 mg/day. Clofazimine, used to treat *Mycobacterium avium* complex infections in AIDS patients, can cause a bull's eye-pattern of maculopathy. The antiestrogen drug tamoxifen, widely used for breast carcinoma, can lead to loss of central vision, macular edema, and superficial white refractile deposits in the inner layers of the retina with cumulative doses >90 g and also in cumulative doses as low as 15 g. Canthaxanthine is a carotinoid dye used as a tanning agent that can lead to deposits of golden-yellow crystal in the macular region, which usually does not affect the vision. Quinine toxicity typically occurs with doses >4 g and leads to atrophy of the inner layers of the retina. Used in the treatment of hypercholesterolemia, nicotinic acid can lead to cystoid macular edema without inflammation or leakage on fluorescein angiography. Digitalis and digoxin may cause blurred vision, color defects, and xanthopsia ("yellow vision") with normal-appearing fundus. Chronic ingestion of silver-containing compounds can lead to argyrosis, which can manifest itself as loss of normal choroidal markings, leopard-spot mottling, and a "dark" choroid on fluorescein angiography as result of deposition of silver in Bruch's membrane. Oral contraceptives can predispose patients to vascular occlusions.

C. Deferoxamine, whether administered intravenously or subcutaneously, can lead to a maculopathy with decreased vision, color vision abnormalities, nyctalopia, and ring scotoma. Vision may return after cessation of the drug. Intracarotid injection of cisplatinum and/or carmustine for the treatment of malignant gliomas of the brain can lead to either a clinical picture of retinal infarction or pigmentary retinopathy. Patients who have received chemotherapy intravenously for bone marrow transplantation have developed retinopathy even without radiation to the orbit or brain. A clinical picture similar to acute macular neuroretinopathy has developed after IV injections of sympathomimetics and iodine-contrast dye.

D. The anesthetic inhalation agent methoxyflurane, when administered to patients with renal dysfunction over a prolonged period, can lead to oxalosis or the deposition of oxalate crystals throughout the posterior pole. Inhalation of methamphetamine and cocaine may be associated with amaurosis fugax, retinal vasculitis, retinal hemorrhages, cotton-wool patches, and retinal artery occlusion. These manifestations are presumably caused by the rapid increase in systemic blood pressure. Carbon monoxide retinopathy presents as superficial retinal hemorrhages, disc edema, or retinal venous engorgement and tortuosity. This may represent hypoxic damage to the vascular endothelium.

E. Patients receiving subcutaneous interferon-α_2 for the treatment of systemic disorders (e.g., metastatic renal cell carcinoma, skin melanoma, Kaposi's sarcoma, hemangiomas of infancy) as well as for subretinal neovascular membranes can develop multiple cotton-wool patches and retinal hemorrhages. Deferoxamine administered subcutaneously can lead to a maculopathy with decreased vision, color vision abnormalities, nyctalopia, and ring scotoma.

F. Retinal toxicity can result from ocular medications or retained intraocular foreign bodies. Inadvertent injection of large doses of aminoglycosides into the anterior chamber after cataract surgery or even a previously considered safe dose of 200 μg for intravitreal injection of either amikacin or gentamicin in the treatment of endophthalmitis can lead to macular toxicity. Topical medications such as epinephrine, dipivefrin, and latanoprost used in the treatment of glaucoma have been noted to cause cystoid macular edema. After penetrating ocular injury, retained iron and copper can lead to siderosis and chalcosis, respectively.

G. Other local treatments away from the eye can also lead to retinal changes. Glycine is a substance used in irrigating fluid during transurethral resection of the prostate (TURP). Excessive systemic absorption can lead to transient visual loss lasting several hours with associated electroretinographic changes and a normal-appearing fundus. This may be because of glycine's role as an inhibitory neurotransmitter. A hemorrhagic maculopathy has been noted after subarachnoid and epidural injections, with the presumed mechanism being the sudden increase of the retinal venous pressure transmitted from elevated CSF pressure.

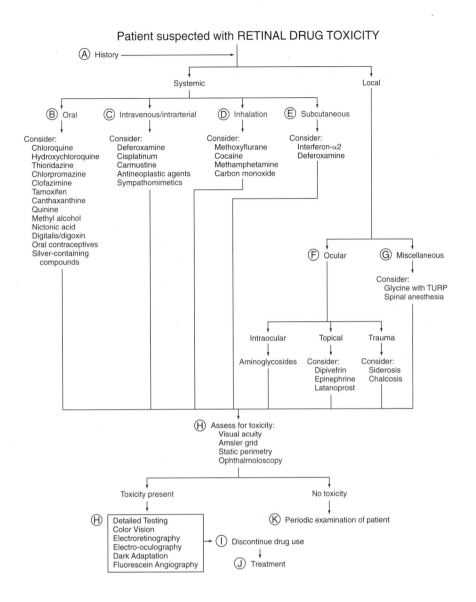

Patient suspected with RETINAL DRUG TOXICITY

(A) History

Systemic

(B) Oral

Consider:
Chloroquine
Hydroxychloroquine
Thioridazine
Chlorpromazine
Clofazimine
Tamoxifen
Canthaxanthine
Quinine
Methyl alcohol
Nictonic acid
Digitalis/digoxin
Oral contraceptives
Silver-containing
 compounds

(C) Intravenous/intrarterial

Consider:
Deferoxamine
Cisplatinum
Carmustine
Antineoplastic agents
Sympathomimetics

(D) Inhalation

Consider:
Methoxyflurane
Cocaine
Methamphetamine
Carbon monoxide

(E) Subcutaneous

Consider:
Interferon-α2
Deferoxamine

Local

(F) Ocular

(G) Miscellaneous

Consider:
Glycine with TURP
Spinal anesthesia

Intraocular

Aminoglycosides

Topical

Consider:
Dipivefrin
Epinephrine
Latanoprost

Trauma

Consider:
Siderosis
Chalcosis

(H) Assess for toxicity:
Visual acuity
Amsler grid
Static perimetry
Ophthalmoloscopy

Toxicity present

(H) Detailed Testing
Color Vision
Electroretinography
Electro-oculography
Dark Adaptation
Fluorescein Angiography

(I) Discontinue drug use

(J) Treatment

No toxicity

(K) Periodic examination of patient

H. Routine testing includes visual acuity, Amsler grid testing, and ophthalmoscopy on any patient taking or exposed to a drug that may cause retinal toxicity. Detailed studies, including color vision testing, electroretinography, electro-oculography, dark adaptation, and IV fluorescein angiography, may be helpful in some cases. Relative paracentral scotomas can be detected with a high degree of sensitivity using a red test object with static perimetry. Unfortunately, no single test is uniquely sensitive in detecting early retinal toxicity.

I. Visual function may improve with cessation of the drug at the earliest sign of retinopathy in the case of chloroquine or hydroxychloroquine. But even if these or other sight-threatening drugs are discontinued, visual defects may persist indefinitely or may progress.

J. Besides cessation of the suspected drug, there is no proven benefit of any therapy except the removal of the intraocular foreign body in the cases of siderosis and chalcosis.

K. Periodically examine patients taking high dosages of chloroquine, hydroxychloroquine, thioridazine, or other medication long term for the development of retinal toxicity.

References

Fraunfelder FT. Drug-induced ocular side effects and drug interaction. 3rd ed. Philadelphia: Lea & Febiger, 1989

Gass JDM. Stereoscopic atlas of macular diseases diagnosis and treatment. 4th ed. St Louis: Mosby, 1997: 775–808.

Grant WM. Toxicology of the eye: Effects on the eyes and visual system from chemicals, drugs, metals and minerals, plants, toxins and venoms: Also, systemic side effects from eye medications. 3rd ed. Springfield, IL: Thomas, 1986.

Swartz M. Other diseases: Drug toxicity and metabolic and nutritional conditions. In: Ryan SJ, ed. Retina. 2nd ed. Vol. 2. St Louis: Mosby, 1994: 1755–1766.

Weinberg DV, D'Amico DJ. Retinal toxicity of systemic drugs. In: Albert DM, Jakobiec FA, eds. Principles and practice of ophthalmology. Philadelphia: WB Saunders, 1994: 1042–1050.

UVEITIS

EXTERNAL OCULAR INFLAMMATION

David K. Scales, M.D.

External ocular inflammation encompasses the conjunctiva, episclera, and sclera. Conjunctival inflammatory evaluation and treatment is covered elsewhere (pp 58 and 62). The episclera is composed of Tenon's capsule and the vascular supply to the relatively avascular sclera. The sclera is the tough outer coat of the eye and is composed primarily of collagen. Inflammations of these tissues may look like conjunctivitis. Recognizing episcleritis and scleritis as distinct entities is important because these may be important harbingers of potentially lethal systemic diseases.

A. Inflamed vessels in episcleritis have a characteristic radial vascular pattern that differentiates it from the relatively more random pattern of inflamed vessels seen in conjunctivitis. Episcleritis may be associated with systemic disease in approximately one third of cases. Episcleritis is typically nonpainful but may have associated minor discomfort. Episcleritis usually presents as pink to red and may be sectoral or diffuse in distribution. The differentiation between episcleritis and scleritis is critical but may be difficult. Episcleral vessels characteristically blanch with phenylephrine eyedrops. Treatment of episcleritis in usually supportive with brief pulsed doses of topical steroids and systemic NSAIDs (indomethacin, 75 mg SR twice daily, or diflunisal, 500 mg orally two or three times daily).

B. Scleritis is associated with severe, potentially lethal diseases in up to 70% of cases. Scleritis is typically painful (deep ache or boring pain) and deep red or purple. Palpation of the globe through a closed lid shows tenderness in scleritis but not in episcleritis. Scleritis does not blanch with phenylephrine eyedrops. One hallmark of scleritis is the presence of scleral thickening revealed with a slit lamp using a narrow slit beam. Scleritis is treated with topical pulsed steroids and requires the use of systemic anti-inflammatory agents (NSAIDs, steroids, or immunosuppressives). Identification of the underlying diagnosis is key to successful management. Refer the patient to a uveitis specialist, internist, or rheumatologist if there is uncertainty about reaching a specific diagnostic conclusion.

C. Nodular and diffuse are the most common presentations of scleritis. Nodular is a relatively well-localized induration of the sclera and is less common than diffuse. Treatment is based on diagnosing and treating the associated systemic syndrome and controlling ocular inflammation with pulsed oral steroids. Scleritis that responds poorly to oral steroids may require the addition of immunosuppressive or steroid-sparing agents as well.

D. Necrotizing scleritis is often associated with rheumatoid arthritis (RA) and may be difficult to manage. It may require both aggressive medical treatment and surgical reinforcement of the necrotizing area. Fortunately, the area of thinned sclera rarely ruptures spontaneously but is at risk with trauma. The development of necrotizing scleritis in patients with RA places them at higher risk for developing lethal systemic vasculitis. If necrotizing scleritis fails to respond to treatment, undertake a diagnostic scleral biopsy with cultures to guide therapy.

References

de la Maza MS, Jabbur NS, Foster CS. An analysis of therapeutic decision for scleritis. Ophthalmology 1993; 100:1372-1376.

de la Maza MS, Jabbur NS, Foster CS. Severity of scleritis and episcleritis. Ophthalmology 1994; 101:389–396.

Foster CS, de la Maza MS. The sclera. New York: Springer-Verlag, 1994.

Foster CS, Forstot SL, Wilson LA. Mortality rate in rheumatoid arthritis patients developing necrotizing scleritis or peripheral ulcerative keratitis. Ophthalmology 1984; 91:1253–1263.

Tay-Kearney ML, Schwam BL, Lowder C, et al. Jabs clinical features and associated systemic diseases of HLA-B27 uveitis. Am J Ophthalmol 1996; 121:47–56.

Watson PG, Hayreh SS. Scleritis and episcleritis. Br J Ophthalmol 1976; 60:163.

Patient with EXTERNAL OCULAR INFLAMMATION

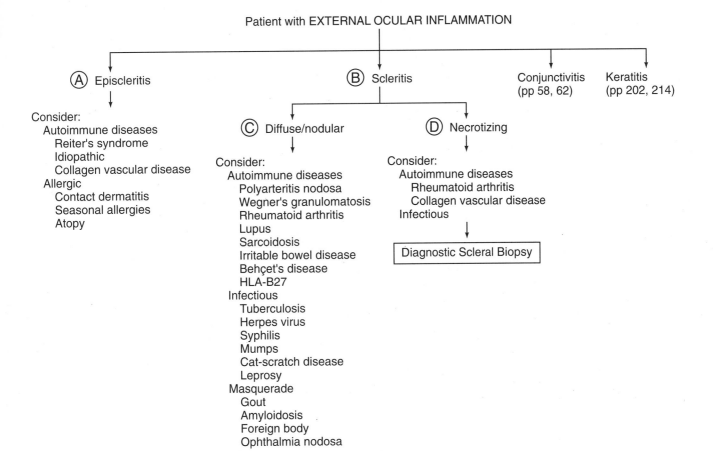

Ⓐ Episcleritis   Ⓑ Scleritis   Conjunctivitis (pp 58, 62)   Keratitis (pp 202, 214)

Consider:
  Autoimmune diseases
    Reiter's syndrome
    Idiopathic
    Collagen vascular disease
  Allergic
    Contact dermatitis
    Seasonal allergies
    Atopy

Ⓒ Diffuse/nodular   Ⓓ Necrotizing

Consider:
  Autoimmune diseases
    Polyarteritis nodosa
    Wegner's granulomatosis
    Rheumatoid arthritis
    Lupus
    Sarcoidosis
    Irritable bowel disease
    Behçet's disease
    HLA-B27
  Infectious
    Tuberculosis
    Herpes virus
    Syphilis
    Mumps
    Cat-scratch disease
    Leprosy
  Masquerade
    Gout
    Amyloidosis
    Foreign body
    Ophthalmia nodosa

Consider:
  Autoimmune diseases
    Rheumatoid arthritis
    Collagen vascular disease
  Infectious

Diagnostic Scleral Biopsy

349

ANTERIOR UVEITIS (IRIDOCYCLITIS)

David K. Scales, MD

Anterior uveitis (AU) encompasses acute, chronic, and recurrent forms of inflammation. The classical signs and symptoms of AU are pain, photophobia, limbal flush, and miotic pupil. In addition, blurred vision, keratic precipitates (KP) on the posterior surface of the cornea, a relative unilateral decrease in the intraocular pressure, and iris synechiae are often seen as well. Initially, iris synechiae can be broken by aggressive dilation; however, protracted efforts are usually unrewarding and make no functional visual difference. An AU-specific associated diagnosis can be made in approximately 50% of chronic or recurrent cases.

A. Because AU is often encountered with no associated disease, the first several episodes of typically presenting AU (mild anterior chamber reaction with good vision) can be treated without further investigation. Unresponsive, unusually severe, or acute presentations should prompt an evaluation for underlying disease. Topical steroids are pulsed hourly and tapered over several days to weeks depending on the severity of the AU. Adequate cycloplegia using Homatropine 5% or scopolamine 2% is maintained for the duration of treatment. Sudden withdrawal of therapy may result in a rebound or recurrence of inflammation that may be more difficult to manage than the initial presentation.

B. Diagnostic testing should be guided by a complete history, review of systems, and physical examination, but it should consist of at least a CBC, ESR, RPR, MHA-TP, ANA, and consideration of HLA-B27, IPPD with anergy testing, chest radiography, and rheumatologic consultation if indicated.

C. Recurrent AU presents in both acute and chronic forms. The acute form is usually present for <6 weeks and the chronic form for >6 weeks. Recurrent AU can be bilateral or alternating in presentation. Bilateral presentation should usually prompt systemic treatment (oral NSAID or steroid) in conjunction with topical or depot steroid injection (40 mg/ml triamcinolone).

D. Granulomatous forms of AU are differentiated from nongranulomatous forms by the presence of "mutton fat" KP (MFKP). These large greasy-looking KPs are usually located in the inferior one third of the cornea and may have associated relatively large cells floating in the anterior chamber. A highly localized pattern of MFKP with associated overlying corneal stromal edema should prompt an investigation into herpetic keratouveitis. Nongranulomatous KPs are usually smaller, and the anterior chamber cell is slightly smaller in appearance. The presence of small stellate-appearing KP evenly distributed across the cornea together with patchy iris transillumination defects, possible posterior subcapsular cataract, and small-angle vessels should prompt an investigation into Fuch's heterochromic iridocyclitis (HIC).

References

Foster CS, Barrett F. Cataract development and cataract surgery in patients with juvenile rheumatoid arthritis-associated iridocyclitis. Ophthalmology 1993; 100:809–817.

Kanski JJ. Juvenile arthritis and uveitis. Surv Ophthalmol 1990; 34:253–267.

Kanski JJ, Shun-Shin GA. Systemic uveitis syndromes in childhood: An analysis of 340 cases. Ophthalmology 1984; 91:1247–1252.

Opremcak EM. Uveitis, a clinical manual for ocular inflammation. New York: Springer-Verlag, 1995.

Rothova A, Veenedaal WG, Linssen A, et al. Clinical features of acute anterior uveitis. Am J Ophthalmol 1987; 103:137–145.

Wakefield D, Montanaro A, McClusky P. Acute anterior uveitis and HLA-B27. Surv Ophthalmol 1991; 36:223–232.

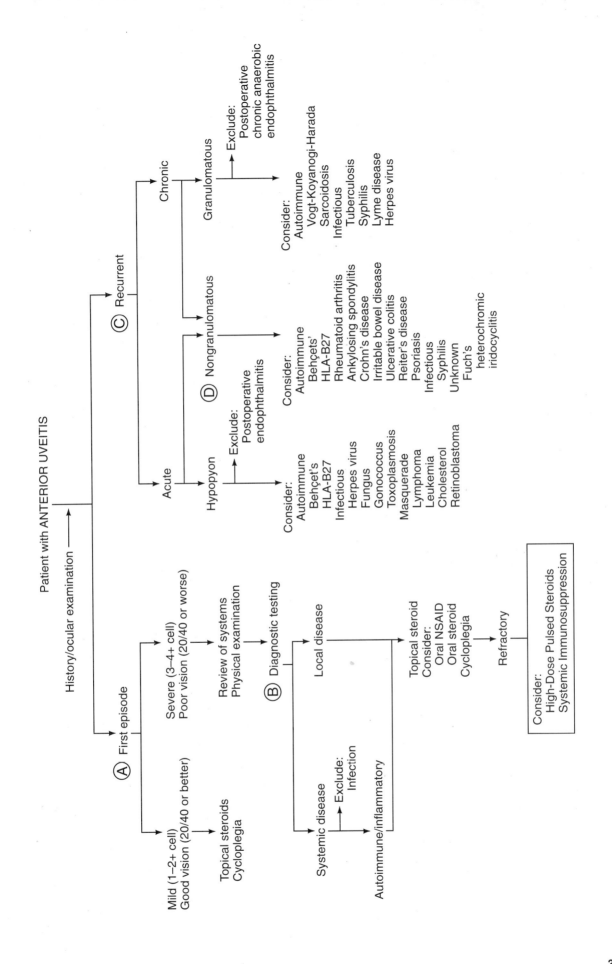

Patient with ANTERIOR UVEITIS

History/ocular examination

(A) First episode

Mild (1–2+ cell)
Good vision (20/40 or better)

Topical steroids
Cycloplegia

Severe (3–4+ cell)
Poor vision (20/40 or worse)

Review of systems
Physical examination

(B) Diagnostic testing

Systemic disease

Exclude:
Infection

Autoimmune/inflammatory

Local disease

Topical steroid
Consider:
Oral NSAID
Oral steroid
Cycloplegia

Refractory

Consider:
High-Dose Pulsed Steroids
Systemic Immunosuppression

(C) Recurrent

Acute

Chronic

Hypopyon

Exclude:
Postoperative
endophthalmitis

Consider:
Autoimmune
    Behçet's
    HLA-B27
Infectious
    Herpes virus
    Fungus
    Gonococcus
    Toxoplasmosis
Masquerade
    Lymphoma
    Leukemia
    Cholesterol
    Retinoblastoma

(D) Nongranulomatous

Consider:
Autoimmune
    Behçets'
    HLA-B27
    Rheumatoid arthritis
    Ankylosing spondylitis
    Crohn's disease
    Irritable bowel disease
    Ulcerative colitis
    Reiter's disease
    Psoriasis
Infectious
    Syphilis
Unknown
    Fuch's
    heterochromic
    iridocyclitis

Granulomatous

Exclude:
Postoperative
chronic anaerobic
endophthalmitis

Consider:
Autoimmune
    Vogt-Koyanogi-Harada
    Sarcoidosis
Infectious
    Tuberculosis
    Syphilis
    Lyme disease
    Herpes virus

INTERMEDIATE UVEITIS (PARS PLANITIS)

David K. Scales, M.D.

Patients with intermediate uveitis (IU) often complain of floaters and blurred vision. Less commonly, patients may have a vitreous hemorrhage or retinal detachment from pars plana neovascularization or peripheral retinal traction. Examination typically reveals a white-appearing eye with anterior vitreous cell. Further investigation may reveal anterior vitreous aggregates of cells (snowballs), inferior pars plana with exudate ("snowbanking"), and cystoid macular edema (CME) because these findings are associated with IU in 80% of patients. IU affects both eyes but may be asymmetric in presentation. Diagnostic testing should be guided by a complete history, review of systems, and physical examination, but it should consist of at least a CBC, ESR, RPR, MHA-TP, PPD with anergy screen, chest radiograph, and internal medicine/primary care consultation if indicated.

A. The vitreitis associated with IU is a rare cause of decreased vision. In patients with IU and decreased vision, evaluate and identify other possible causes of vitreitis and also rule out cystoid macular edema, using fluorescein angiography, as a consequence of vitreous inflammation. The presence of anterior vitreous cells alone (without decreased vision or other more serious vision-threatening conditions) is rarely an indication for treatment.

B. Although inflammation may be located primarily in either the anterior chamber (AC) or the anterior vitreous (IU), it is not uncommon in anterior uveitis (AU) for secondary inflammation to be present in the adjoining region (e.g., AU with "spillover" reaction in the anterior vitreous). The presence of this reactive cell in the anterior vitreous after resolved AU is not uncommon and does not indicate that the patient has IU.

C. Every patient with IU should receive a thorough examination with indirect ophthalmoscopy and scleral depression to identify the presence of important peripheral retinal and pars plana pathology, including snowbanking, neovascularization, retinal traction, or retinal detachment. The most common location for the exudative white mass is inferior on the pars plana. There may also be white deposits in the vitreous overlying the pars plana.

References

Foster CS. Medical treatment of intermediate uveitis. Dev Ophthalmol 1992; 23:156–157.

Henderly DE, Gentstler AJ, Smith RE, Rao NA. Changing patterns in uveitis. Am J Ophthalmol 1987; 103:131–136.

Jones NP. Fuch's heterochromic uveitis: An update. Surv Ophthalmol 1993; 37:253–272.

Kaplan HJ. Surgical treatment of intermediate uveitis. Dev Ophthalmol 1992; 23:185–189.

Margo CE, Hamed LM. Ocular syphilis. Surv Ophthalmol 1992; 37:203–220.

Nussenblatt RB, Whitcup SM, Palestine AG. Uveitis fundamentals and clinical practice. 2nd ed. St Louis: Mosby, 1996.

Opremcak EM. Uveitis a clinical manual for ocular inflammation. New York: Springer-Verlag, 1995.

Winterkorn JMS. Lyme disease: Neurologic and ophthalmic manifestations. Surv Ophthalmol 1990; 35:191–204.

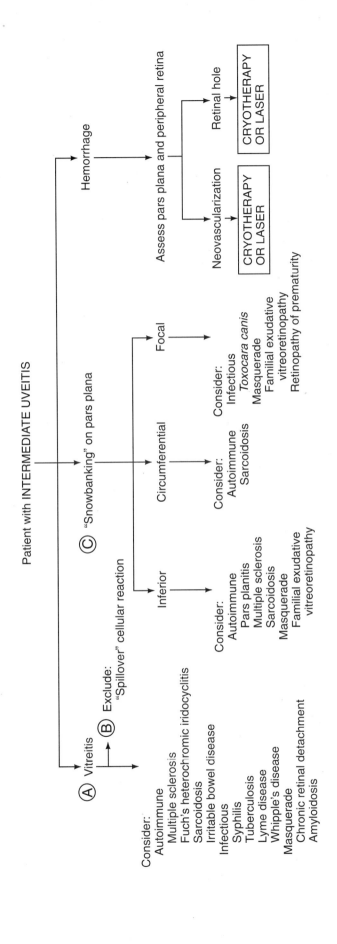

Patient with INTERMEDIATE UVEITIS

Ⓐ Vitreitis

Ⓑ Exclude:
"Spillover" cellular reaction

Consider:
Autoimmune
 Multiple sclerosis
 Fuch's heterochromic iridocyclitis
 Sarcoidosis
 Irritable bowel disease
Infectious
 Syphilis
 Tuberculosis
 Lyme disease
 Whipple's disease
Masquerade
 Chronic retinal detachment
 Amyloidosis

Ⓒ "Snowbanking" on pars plana

Inferior

Consider:
Autoimmune
 Pars planitis
 Multiple sclerosis
 Sarcoidosis
Masquerade
 Familial exudative
  vitreoretinopathy

Circumferential

Consider:
Autoimmune
 Sarcoidosis

Focal

Consider:
Infectious
 Toxocara canis
Masquerade
 Familial exudative
  vitreoretinopathy
Retinopathy of prematurity

Hemorrhage

Assess pars plana and peripheral retina

Neovascularization

CRYOTHERAPY
OR LASER

Retinal hole

CRYOTHERAPY
OR LASER

353

RETINITIS

David K. Scales, M.D.

Retinitis is a severe, often sight-threatening, form of posterior uveitis that is often associated with systemic disease. Retinitis may be primary (retinal inflammation or infection) or secondary (retina overlying a choroidal granuloma or resulting from ischemic vascular occlusion). Retinitis often has associated retinal hemorrhage, overlying vitreitis, vasculitis, and exudate. Most cases of retinitis are best evaluated with fluorescein angiography.

A. Retinitis may be single (classic "headlight in a fog" presentation for toxoplasmosis) or multifocal, occurring in several sites throughout the retina. A complete posterior pole examination, including contact lens examination to evaluate for associated vasculitis or choroiditis, is recommended. In general, unilateral and focal presentations are more often associated with infectious causes or local ocular inflammation than bilateral and multifocal presentations, which are more likely to be associated with systemic disease.

B. Although vitreitis may accompany many presentations of retinitis, its presence with certain patterns is significant. The triad of progressive, patchy, multifocal retinitis, arteritis, and vitreitis suggests acute retinal necrosis (ARN) caused by herpes virus in a healthy individual. It could also signify Behçet's syndrome in a patient with typical systemic findings. The appearance of intense retinitis associated with choroiditis (retinochoroiditis) and dense vitreitis suggests a diagnosis of toxoplasmosis but could also represent *Toxocara*, fungus, or nematode with the proper clinical and serologic findings. A rare nematode infection, where the worm is actually under or in the retina, is diffuse unilateral subacute neuroretinitis (DUSN), the early stages of which look like multifocal choroiditis and late stages look like retinitis pigmentosa in only one eye.

C. Infectious causes of retinitis are important to identify because they are potentially curable with appropriate antibiotic or antiviral agents. *Toxocara* may be either *T. canis* or *T. cati* and often presents as a solitary choroidal granuloma that forms after the worm dies. *Toxocara* presents in three forms: endophthalmitis, posterior pole granuloma, and asymptomatic peripheral granuloma. *Toxocara* is diagnosed by a positive serology from the blood or eye fluids.

D. Macular retinitis is a potentially blinding uveitis and requires rapid evaluation and treatment to preserve functional vision. The most common posterior retinitis is toxoplasmosis. The new area of retinitis is usually found in conjunction with an older chorioretinal scar (mother-daughter lesion). There is usually a significant vitreous reaction overlying the area of retinitis. A posi-

tive toxoplasmosis titer confirms infection, but in severe cases treatment must started pending results. The traditional treatment is sulfadiazine, pyrimethamine, and folinic acid. The difficulty in obtaining these medications, their significant side effects (thrombocytopenia and leukocytopenia), and their unclear role in treating children have prompted investigation into alternative strategies. New treatment regimens include trimethoprim-sulfamethoxazole DS orally twice daily for 6 weeks with added clindamycin, 300 mg orally four times a day for 3–4 weeks. Oral prednisone, 40–80 mg/day orally, can be added for severe vitreitis or sight-threatening lesions after 24–48 hours of systemic antibiotic treatment. Small peripheral lesions that do not interfere with vision may not require treatment.

E. Autoimmune causes for retinitis are commonly encountered. The retinitis accompanying Behçet's disease is essentially multifocal, vaso-occlusive, or ischemic in nature and can accompany other autoimmune diseases such as Wegener's granulomatosis, lupus erythematosus, and polyarteritis nodosa.

F. Retinitis presenting in immunocompromised individuals requires careful investigation for opportunistic infections, including CMV. CMV typically manifests as an advancing "brush fire" retinitis commonly associated with retinal hemorrhage. Syphilis is another infectious cause that should always be considered in retinitis and that may be associated with arteritis, choroiditis, optic neuritis, and occasionally, serous retinal detachments.

References

Chavis PS, Tabbara KF. Behçet's disease. Int Ophthalmol Clin 1995; 35:43–67.

De Laey JJ. Fluorescein angiography in posterior uveitis. Int Ophthalmol Clin 1995; 35:33–58.

Nussenblatt RB, Whitcup SM, Palestine AG. Uveitis fundamentals and clinical practice. 2nd ed. St Louis: Mosby, 1996.

Opremcak EM. Uveitis: A clinical manual for ocular inflammation. New York: Springer-Verlag, 1995.

Opremacak EM, Scales DK, Sharpe MR. Trimethoprim-sulfamethoxazole therapy for ocular toxoplasmosis. Ophthalmology 1992; 99:920–925.

Reed JB, Scales DK, Wong MT, et al. *Bartonella henselae* neuroretinitis in cat scratch disease. Ophthalmology 1998; 105:459–466.

Tabbara KF. Ocular toxoplasmosis: Toxoplasmic retinochoroiditis. Int Ophthalmol Clin 1995; 35:15–29.

Patient with RETINITIS

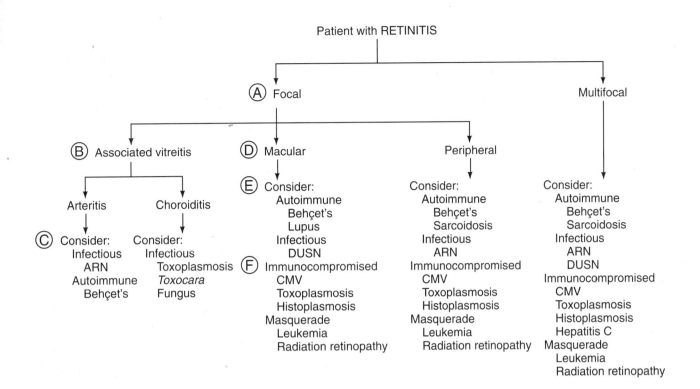

Ⓐ Focal   Multifocal

Ⓑ Associated vitreitis   Ⓓ Macular   Peripheral

Arteritis   Choroiditis

Ⓒ Consider: Consider:
Infectious   Infectious
ARN   Toxoplasmosis
Autoimmune *Toxocara*
Behçet's   Fungus

Ⓔ Consider:
   Autoimmune
      Behçet's
      Lupus
   Infectious
      DUSN
Ⓕ Immunocompromised
   CMV
   Toxoplasmosis
   Histoplasmosis
  Masquerade
   Leukemia
   Radiation retinopathy

Consider:
   Autoimmune
      Behçet's
      Sarcoidosis
   Infectious
      ARN
  Immunocompromised
   CMV
   Toxoplasmosis
   Histoplasmosis
  Masquerade
   Leukemia
   Radiation retinopathy

Consider:
   Autoimmune
      Behçet's
      Sarcoidosis
   Infectious
      ARN
      DUSN
  Immunocompromised
   CMV
   Toxoplasmosis
   Histoplasmosis
   Hepatitis C
  Masquerade
   Leukemia
   Radiation retinopathy

CHOROIDITIS

David K. Scales, M.D.
Brian B. Berger, M.D.

Choroiditis presents many diagnostic and therapeutic challenges. Because the choroid is sandwiched between retina and sclera, the choroid is secondarily affected by many primary retinal (i.e., toxoplasmic retinochoroiditis) and scleral (i.e., posterior scleritis) inflammations. Correspondingly, a primary choroiditis can secondarily affect both the retina and sclera (i.e., tuberculous choroidal granuloma with overlying retinitis, exudative retinal detachment, and adjacent scleritis). Choroiditis often may be asymptomatic or have metamorphopsia and decreased vision as presenting symptoms if the macula is involved. Included in this section are many of the so-called white dot syndromes.

A. A complete evaluation of choroiditis requires fluorescein angiography. The pattern of hyperfluorescence and leakage or staining is important in determining the correct diagnosis. Angiographic determination of focal, multifocal, geographic, and diffuse should be accomplished. A careful examination using both contact lens biomicroscopy and binocular indirect ophthalmoscopy is helpful in determining the presence of pigmentary changes or accompanying exudative retinal detachments.

B. Focal choroiditis is often infectious. Diagnostic evaluation is accomplished by a history, review of systems, and physical examination coupled with clinical suspicion in most cases because the relevant laboratory tests are often indeterminate. *Toxocara* and sarcoidosis require anti-inflammatory treatment (local or regional for *Toxocara* and systemic for sarcoidosis). Cysticercosis may require surgical removal of the cysts. Tuberculosis (TB) is often more difficult to diagnose and may be accompanied by other diseases. A history of "adequate" treatment for TB does not preclude TB-related uveitis (e.g., drug resistance, medication noncompliance). A positive PPD as the sole significant finding after exhaustive evaluation to exclude other possible causes in the correct clinical setting should suggest TB-related uveitis as the correct diagnosis. A positive response to a therapeutic trial of a triple drug regimen for a minimum of 2 months' duration confirms the diagnosis. Treatment after a successful therapeutic trial should be continued for 1 year. Consultation with an infectious disease specialist before starting triple drug therapy is recommended.

C. *Multifocal choroiditis* is a term that can be used to describe patients with multiple sites of choroidal and retinal pigment epithelial (RPE) inflammation. The lesions associated with multifocal choroiditis are usually scattered throughout the fundus and not localized to the posterior pole. Vogt-Koyonagi-Harada syndrome (VKH) and punctate inner choroidopathy (PIC) are presumably autoimmune diseases with typical clinical appearances but no other diagnostic criteria. VKH is a multifocal choroiditis that can become so effusive that the retinas can detach. It responds to steroids. Associated systemic signs are vitilligo, poliosis, a white streak of hair, dysacusia, and signs of meningeal irritation. PIC, as well as another similar syndrome (multifocal choroiditis and panuveitis) show multiple usually bilateral yellow-white lesions of the inner choroid and retina, mostly in the macular region, with occasional serous retinal detachment. No treatment is needed because the disease usually regresses spontaneously with good visual recovery. However, 40% of patients develop some subretinal neovascularization (SRNVM). The final picture resembles ocular histoplasmosis (POHS), but the histoplasmin skin test is negative. Presumed ocular histoplasmosis syndrome (POHS) classically presents as a multifocal chorioretinitis or scars without vitreitis. There are five potential findings in POHS (the first four are classically required for diagnosis): (1) "punched out" chorioretinal scars, (2) peripapillary pigmentary disturbance, (3) disciform macular scar, (4) no vitreitis, and (5) linear equatorial streaks. A subgroup of patients with multifocal choroiditis and panuveitis have serologic evidence of Epstein-Barr virus infection. The inflammation is usually bilateral and recurrent and may result in subretinal fibrosis.

D. Acute multifocal choroiditis may present as multiple gray-white subretinal spots throughout the fundus in specific syndrome patterns that have been termed the *white dot syndromes.* Several of these syndromes—multiple evanescent white dot syndrome (MEWDS), acute posterior multifocal placoid pigment epitheliopathy (APMPPE), and geographic helicoid peripapillary choroidopathy (GHPC)—tend to occur in people <60 years of age. MEWDS usually occurs in young women and is manifested by the acute onset of blurred vision in one eye. The lesions are small gray spots at the level of the retinal pigment epithelium and scattered throughout the posterior pole. The fovea has a granular appearance. The electroretinogram (ERG) and electro-oculogram (EOG) are abnormal. However, recovery of vision and of the electrophysiologic abnormalities is spontaneous within 2 months after the onset of symptoms. AMPPE usually causes the sudden onset of paracentral scotomas or blurred vision in both eyes. The acute lesions are yellow, measure 500–1000 microns, and are concentrated in the macula. Characteristically, they block choroidal fluorescence but show staining in the late phases of the fluorescein angiogram. During 1 or 2 months, the lesions spontaneously flatten and develop pigmentation. Most of the symptoms resolve, although paracentral scotomas may persist. Geographic helicoid peripapillary choroidopathy (GHPC) is a rare condition that occurs in a slightly older age group. Its appearance is similar to that of AMPPE, but it always begins at the optic nerve head and spreads in a serpentine manner. It tends to involve the macula, causing permanent loss of vision. In des-

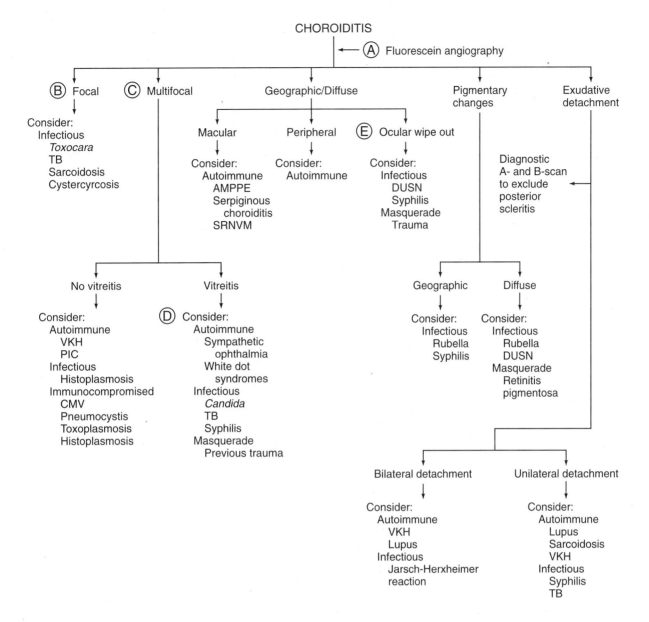

CHOROIDITIS

Ⓐ Fluorescein angiography

Ⓑ Focal

Consider:
Infectious
  Toxocara
  TB
  Sarcoidosis
  Cystercyrcosis

Ⓒ Multifocal

Geographic/Diffuse

Macular

Consider:
Autoimmune
  AMPPE
  Serpiginous
    choroiditis
  SRNVM

Peripheral

Consider:
Autoimmune

Ⓔ Ocular wipe out

Consider:
Infectious
  DUSN
  Syphilis
  Masquerade
  Trauma

Pigmentary changes

Exudative detachment

Diagnostic A- and B-scan to exclude posterior scleritis

No vitreitis

Consider:
Autoimmune
  VKH
  PIC
Infectious
  Histoplasmosis
Immunocompromised
  CMV
  Pneumocystis
  Toxoplasmosis
  Histoplasmosis

Vitreitis

Ⓓ Consider:
Autoimmune
  Sympathetic
    ophthalmia
  White dot
    syndromes
Infectious
  Candida
  TB
  Syphilis
Masquerade
  Previous trauma

Geographic

Consider:
Infectious
  Rubella
  Syphilis

Diffuse

Consider:
Infectious
  Rubella
  DUSN
  Masquerade
  Retinitis
  pigmentosa

Bilateral detachment

Consider:
Autoimmune
  VKH
  Lupus
Infectious
  Jarsch-Herxheimer
  reaction

Unilateral detachment

Consider:
Autoimmune
  Lupus
  Sarcoidosis
  VKH
Infectious
  Syphilis
  TB

perate cases, systemic corticosteroids, in conjunction with immunosuppressive agents, may be tried. Birdshot choroidopathy usually affects both eyes of Caucasian women in their fifties. The lesions are peripheral, creamy, subretinal infiltrates that tend to evolve into areas of atrophy and hyperpigmentation. The retinal arterioles become attenuated, and cystoid macular edema is a common cause of visual loss. The ERG and EOG become progressively more abnormal, and the result is often optic atrophy and blindness. From 80%–95% of patients are positive for the HLA-A 29 antigen. Corticosteroids and cyclosporine may prevent blindness.

E. Diffuse unilateral subacute neuroretinitis (DUSN) presents as a "unilateral wipe out syndrome" with transient white dots at the level of the RPE, hyperpigmentation, and optic atrophy. DUSN is caused by a motile nematode and can be treated, after identification of the worm, with laser photocoagulation (p 354).

References

Abu el-Asrar AM. Serpiginous (geographical) choroiditis. Ophthalmol Olin 1995; 35:87–91.

Nussenblatt RB, Whitcup SM, Palestine AG. Uveitis fundamentals and clinical practice. 2nd ed. St Louis: Mosby, 1996.

Opremcak EM. Uveitis a clinical manual for ocular inflammation. New York: Springer-Verlag, 1995.

Rao NA, Moorthy RS, Inomata H. Vogt-Koyanagi-Harada syndrome. Int Ophthalmol Clin 1995; 35:69–86.

Samy ON, D'Amico DJ. Infectious choroiditis in the acquired immune deficiency syndrome. Int Ophthalmol Clin 1996; 36:187–196.

Towler HM, Lightman S. Sympathetic ophthalmia. Int Ophthalmol Clin 1995; 35:31–42.

PANUVEITIS (DIFFUSE UVEITIS)

Brian B. Berger, M.D.
David K. Scales, M.D.

A. Panuveitis is inflammation of the entire eye. An important consideration in the evaluation of panuveitis is whether it is infectious. Bilateral panuveitis usually means that there is an underlying systemic disease, such as sarcoidosis, Vogt-Koyanagi-Harada syndrome (VKH), Behçet's syndrome, systemic candidiasis, or large-cell lymphoma. The review of systems should be oriented toward identifying systemic signs or symptoms of these diseases. For example, sarcoidosis can cause lymphadenopathy, shortness of breath, and skin changes. VKH is associated with dysacousia, meningism, poliosis, and alopecia. Behçet's syndrome includes aphthous ulcers of the oral and genital mucous membranes and polyarthritis. Panuveitis from *Candida* infection usually occurs in immunosuppressed patients, such as those who are undergoing chemotherapy for cancer, have had an organ transplantation, or have AIDS. It can also occur in patients who have had long-term antibiotic therapy or indwelling catheters or who have been IV drug abusers. Primary large-cell lymphoma of the retina and brain is sometimes associated with CNS symptoms. If the patient has had recent ocular surgery, suspect endophthalmitis.

B. Panuveitis that is chronic with granulomatous inflammation is usually not infectious. Granulomatous inflammation is characterized by "mutton fat" keratic precipitates on the corneal endothelium and iris nodules. Sympathetic ophthalmia is a bilateral uveitis that develops after an injury, either traumatic or surgical, that disrupts and exposes the uvea. Inflammation develops in the sympathizing eye after a latent period of at least 2 weeks but, more commonly, 4–8 weeks after injury to the exciting eye. It may also occur months or years later. In the sympathizing eye the inflammation may be mild and begin with a subacute iridocyclitis associated with small yellow lesions underlying the retina called *Dalen-Fuchs nodules*. Occasionally, systemic manifestations, identical to those seen in VKH, can develop. Sympathetic ophthalmia is extremely rare, but in an eye that is traumatized beyond hope for vision, enucleation within 2 weeks after the injury can prevent this disease. After sympathetic ophthalmia develops, treat with aggressive corticosteroids, immunosuppressive drugs, and enucleation of the exciting eye.

C. Sarcoidosis is the cause of 3% of all uveitis, and 20%–50% of patients with systemic sarcoidosis have uveitis. African-Americans are affected 10 times more often than whites. Sarcoidosis usually causes a bilateral chronic or recurrent iridocyclitis that can lead to secondary glaucoma, band keratopathy, and cataract. Less commonly, the posterior segment can be involved by choroiditis, retinal vasculitis that causes the characteristic "candlewax drippings" and snowball opacities in the vitreous, and optic nerve granulomas. Inflam-

mation of the posterior segment can lead to loss of vision through cystoid macular edema, retinal neovascularization with vitreous hemorrhage, and visual field defects. Of patients with ocular sarcoidosis, 80% have an abnormal chest radiograph. Angiotensin-converting enzyme (ACE) is usually elevated in the serum and aqueous humor. However, the diagnosis can be firmly established only by a tissue biopsy that shows a characteristic sarcoid granuloma. The ophthalmologist can make the diagnosis by performing a biopsy of conjunctival nodules or an enlarged salivary gland. Sarcoid uveitis is treated with corticosteroids, and most cases can be managed with a combination of topical and periocular therapy.

VKH consists of iridocyclitis, exudative retinal detachments, and uveoencephalitis. It is usually bilateral and is more common in pigmented races, especially Asians. Diagnosis may be difficult if only a few manifestations are present. If the posterior segment is involved, fluorescein angiography is usually diagnostic, with a pattern of diffuse punctate hyperfluorescence at the level of the choroid. Bilateral exudative retinal detachments are virtually pathognomonic of VKH, although this can occasionally be mimicked by hypertensive choroidopathy or severe AMPPE. The diagnosis is made on clinical grounds because no laboratory tests exist for this disease. VKH causes visual loss by recurrent retinal detachment, subretinal neovascularization leading to disciform scarring of the macula, and optic atrophy. Treat with high-dose systemic prednisone to resolve the serous retinal detachments as soon as possible. Tuberculosis is a rare cause of panuveitis.

D. Hypopyon panuveitis after surgery is endophthalmitis (p 276) until proven otherwise. When the patient has no history of surgery, consider Behçet's syndrome first.

E. *Candida* and rarely other fungi can cause panuveitis. Systemic and vitreous cultures are essential. If blood and urine cultures are negative, perform vitrectomy to visualize the retina and to obtain material for culture and cytologic examination. Cytologic examination may be diagnostic of primary large-cell lymphoma of the retina and brain. This condition is usually bilateral, occurring in people >60 years of age. It can mimic panuveitis. Further prompt evaluation, including MRI of the brain, lumbar puncture, and treatment by an oncologist, is indicated. A diagnosis of toxoplasmic panuveitis can usually be made once the retina is visualized after vitrectomy. *Candida* can often be cultured from the urine and blood. If systemic cultures are positive, treat the patient with amphotericin B with or without flucytosine (150 mg/kg/day) and remove the source of infection. Fluconazole is a newer drug that is effective orally (200 mg/day). If no evidence of

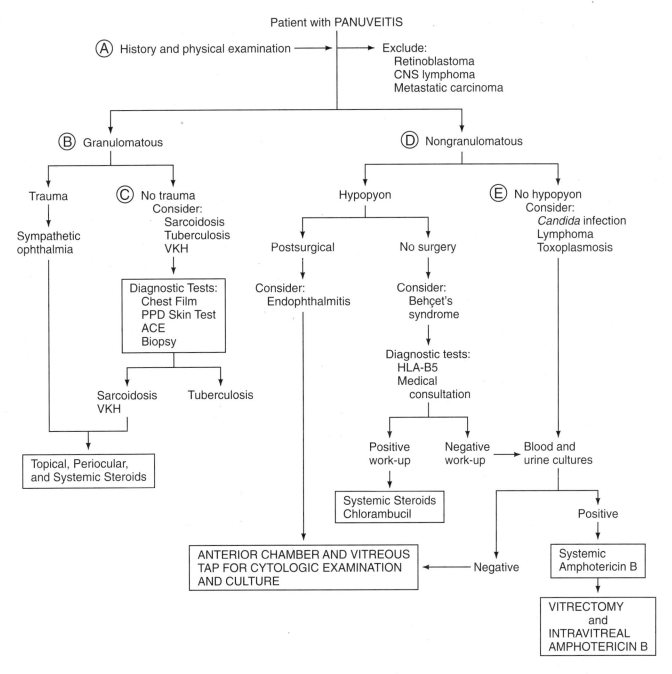

Patient with PANUVEITIS

Ⓐ History and physical examination ⟶ Exclude:
  Retinoblastoma
  CNS lymphoma
  Metastatic carcinoma

Ⓑ Granulomatous

Ⓓ Nongranulomatous

Trauma

Ⓒ No trauma
Consider:
  Sarcoidosis
  Tuberculosis
  VKH

Sympathetic
ophthalmia

Diagnostic Tests:
  Chest Film
  PPD Skin Test
  ACE
  Biopsy

Sarcoidosis
VKH

Tuberculosis

Topical, Periocular,
and Systemic Steroids

Hypopyon

Ⓔ No hypopyon
Consider:
  Candida infection
  Lymphoma
  Toxoplasmosis

Postsurgical

No surgery

Consider:
Endophthalmitis

Consider:
Behçet's
syndrome

Diagnostic tests:
  HLA-B5
  Medical
  consultation

Positive
work-up

Negative
work-up

Blood and
urine cultures

Systemic Steroids
Chlorambucil

Positive

ANTERIOR CHAMBER AND VITREOUS
TAP FOR CYTOLOGIC EXAMINATION
AND CULTURE

Negative

Systemic
Amphotericin B

VITRECTOMY
and
INTRAVITREAL
AMPHOTERICIN B

References

systemic infection is seen, systemic therapy is not necessary except to supplement the treatment of an overwhelming ocular infection. If the ocular infection is mild and systemic therapy is being given, the eye may simply be observed and often heals without further treatment. If the ocular infection is mild and systemic therapy is not being given, inject 5 mg of amphotericin B into the vitreous cavity. If the ocular infection is severe, vitrectomy with intraocular amphotericin B is recommended.

Chan CC, Li Q. Immunology of uveitis. Br J Ophthalmol 1998; 82:91–96.

Fraunfelder FW, Rosenbaum JT. Drug-induced uveitis. Incidence, prevention and treatment. Drug Safety 1997; 17:197–120.

McCluskey PJ, Wakefield D. Posterior uveitis in the acquired immunodeficiency syndrome. Int Ophthalmol Clin 1995; 35:1–14.

Moorthy RS, Inomata H, Rao NA. Vogt-Koyanagi-Harada syndrome. Surv Ophthalmol 1995; 39:265–292.

Nussenblatt RB, Whitcup SM, Palestine AG. Uveitis fundamentals and clinical practice. 2nd ed. St Louis: Mosby, 1996.

Opremcak EM. Uveitis: A clinical manual for ocular inflammation. New York: Springer-Verlag, 1995.

LOCAL OCULAR TREATMENT FOR UVEITIS

David K. Scales, M.D.

Determining the accurate diagnosis underlying uveitis is of absolute importance in the successful management, preservation of vision, and in some instances, preservation of the life in patients with ocular inflammation. No treatment of "uveitis" per se exists. Presentations of ocular inflammation have a specific underlying diagnosis that should be identified and then specifically addressed. Unfortunately, today we still cannot discover the specific underlying syndrome in every case of uveitis, and we are left with using a more general approach to its treatment. This decision tree is generic and does not supersede specific therapy more appropriately tailored to the patient's specific underlying diagnosis.

The goal of uveitis treatment is to preserve functional vision, prevent intraocular sequelae of media opacity or anatomic disruption, minimize potential medical complications from therapy, and prevent serious systemic complications of disease. These goals can best be accomplished when the correct diagnosis has been made.

A. Patients with normal vision and mild intraocular inflammation may not require treatment (i.e., intermediate uveitis [IU] with vitreitis alone, mild episcleritis, or Fuch's heterochromic iridocyclitis [HIC]). The decision to treat must be individualized for each patient's situation. One significant exception is patients with juvenile rheumatoid arthritis (JRA)-related anterior uveitis (AU) in which the eye does not appear inflamed externally but the sequelae of untreated internal inflammation are blinding. Patients with JRA-related AU require aggressive management despite "normal" vision.

B. Decreased vision requires a graduated response depending on the severity of the underlying inflammation. Thoroughly examine and treat patients with good vision to preserve the current visual function. Patients with poorer vision require the same thorough examination but a correspondingly more aggressive medical approach to recover and then maintain functional vision. If the decrease in vision is caused by media opacity, medical or surgical treatment of the opacity may be indicated. The execution of a successful surgical rehabilitation together with the perioperative management of uveitis patients is complex and requires specific expertise and careful planning. Patients for whom surgical rehabilitation is considered should have an evaluation by a uveitis or retina specialist if possible.

C. Hemorrhage as a cause of decreased vision in patients with uveitis is relatively common. A complete ocular examination, including ultrasound A- and/or B-scan imaging, should be accomplished to exclude vision- or sight-threatening complications that may require immediate action. Nonresorbing hemorrhages may require surgical removal after observation. Exudative retinal detachments are best managed medically but occasionally require scleral buckling and drainage of the subretinal fluid (if possible, some fluid should be obtained for culture and cytologic examination).

References

Hooper PL, Rao NA, Smith RE. Cataract extraction in uveitis patients. Surv Ophthalmol 1990; 35:230–144.

Jenning T, Rusin MM, Tessler HH, Cunha-Vaz JG. Posterior sub-Tenton's injections on corticosteroids in uveitis patients with cystoid macular edema. Jpn J Ophthalmol 1988; 32:385–391.

Kwon YH, Dreyer EB. Inflammatory glaucomas. Int Ophthalmol Clin 1996; 36:81–89.

Moorthy RS, Mermoud A, Baerveldt G, et al. Glaucoma associated with uveitis. Surv Ophthalmol 1997; 41:361–394.

Nozik RA. Periocular injection of steroids. Trans Acad Ophthal Otol 1976; 76:695–705.

Nussenblatt RB, Whitcup SM, Palestine AG. Uveitis fundamentals and clinical practice. 2nd ed. St Louis: Mosby, 1996.

Opremcak EM. Uveitis: a clinical manual for ocular inflammation. New York: Springer-Verlag, 1995.

Tabbara KF, Chavis PS. Cataract extraction in patients with chronic posterior uveitis. Int Ophthalmol Clin 1995; 35:121–131.

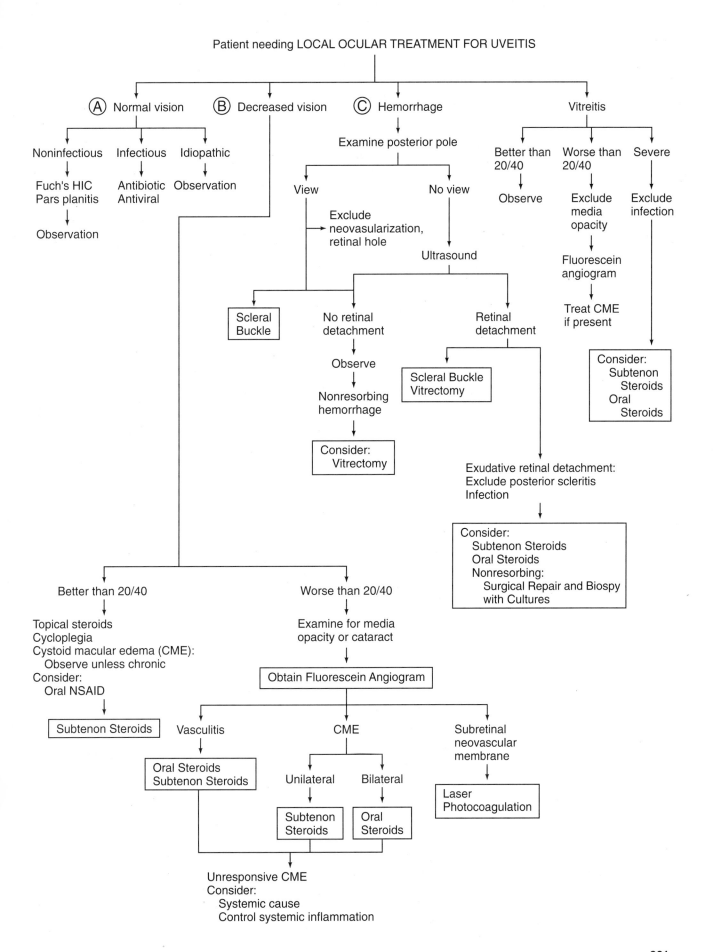

Patient needing LOCAL OCULAR TREATMENT FOR UVEITIS

A Normal vision

- Noninfectious
  - Fuch's HIC
  - Pars planitis
  - ↓
  - Observation
- Infectious
  - ↓
  - Antibiotic
  - Antiviral
- Idiopathic
  - ↓
  - Observation

B Decreased vision

C Hemorrhage

Examine posterior pole

- View
  - → Exclude neovasularization, retinal hole
    - Scleral Buckle
    - No retinal detachment
      - Observe
      - ↓
      - Nonresorbing hemorrhage
      - ↓
      - Consider: Vitrectomy
- No view
  - Ultrasound
    - Retinal detachment
      - Scleral Buckle Vitrectomy
      - ↓
      - Exudative retinal detachment: Exclude posterior scleritis Infection
        - ↓
        - Consider:
          Subtenon Steroids
          Oral Steroids
          Nonresorbing:
          Surgical Repair and Biospy with Cultures

Vitreitis

- Better than 20/40
  - Observe
- Worse than 20/40
  - Exclude media opacity
  - ↓
  - Fluorescein angiogram
  - ↓
  - Treat CME if present
- Severe
  - Exclude infection
  - ↓
  - Consider:
    Subtenon Steroids
    Oral Steroids

Better than 20/40

- Topical steroids
- Cycloplegia
- Cystoid macular edema (CME): Observe unless chronic
- Consider: Oral NSAID
  - ↓
  - Subtenon Steroids

Worse than 20/40

- Examine for media opacity or cataract
- ↓
- Obtain Fluorescein Angiogram

- Vasculitis
  - ↓
  - Oral Steroids
    Subtenon Steroids
- CME
  - Unilateral
    - Subtenon Steroids
  - Bilateral
    - Oral Steroids
- Subretinal neovascular membrane
  - ↓
  - Laser Photocoagulation

Unresponsive CME
Consider:
   Systemic cause
   Control systemic inflammation

SYSTEMIC TREATMENT FOR UVEITIS

David K. Scales, M.D.

Systemic treatment for uveitis serves as a foundation upon which the local ocular treatment rests. One of the most critical aspects of treating uveitis is to arrive at an accurate diagnosis and identify any associated systemic autoimmune, inflammatory, or infectious cause. Not only does identifying the correct systemic cause provide for the best possible outcome, but it also may prevent avoidable complications such as treatment of an infectious uveitis with steroids alone. Coordination of the systemic treatment of patients with ocular inflammation requires the active participation of both the treating ophthalmologist and the primary care physician for close monitoring of anti-inflammatory effectiveness and potential systemic side effects of treatment. In patients who require high-dose or prolonged use of systemic steroids or the use of immunosuppressant agents, comanagement with a suitable rheumatologist or hematologist-oncologist should be done.

A. The systemic disease underlying the ocular inflammation must be controlled as a priority. Uveitis from systemic disease cannot be managed successfully by local ocular treatment alone. After systemic disease is managed, the residual ocular inflammation can be suppressed. These two actions have to be performed simultaneously and in tandem.

B. Regularly observe patients with systemic disease and those at risk for ocular inflammation or with a history of uveitis.

C. After the systemic component of the patient's ocular inflammation has been satisfactorily addressed, many eyes will harbor some level of residual inflammation. Usually, local measures are sufficient to suppress this. If these are not sufficient, the systemic medication can be adjusted after the level of systemic control and potential treatment side effects are evaluated.

References

Hemady R, Tauber J, Foster CS. Immunosuppressive drugs in immune and inflammatory ocular disease. Surv Ophthalmol 1991; 35:369–385.

Nussenblatt RB, Whitcup SM, Palestine AG. Uveitis fundamentals and clinical practice. 2nd ed. St Louis: Mosby, 1996.

Opremcak EM. Uveitis a clinical manual for ocular inflammation. New York: Springer-Verlag, 1995.

Samily N, Foster CS. The role of nonsteroidal anti-inflammatory drugs in ocular inflammation. Int Ophthalmol Clin 1996; 36:195–206.

Scales DK. Immunomodulatory agents. In: Mauger TF, Craig EL, eds. Havener's ocular pharmacology. 6th ed. St Louis: Mosby, 1994: 355–364.

Tamesis RR, Rodriguez A, Christen WG, et al. Systemic drug toxicity trends in immunosuppressive therapy of immune and inflammatory ocular disease. Ophthalmology 1996; 103:768–775.

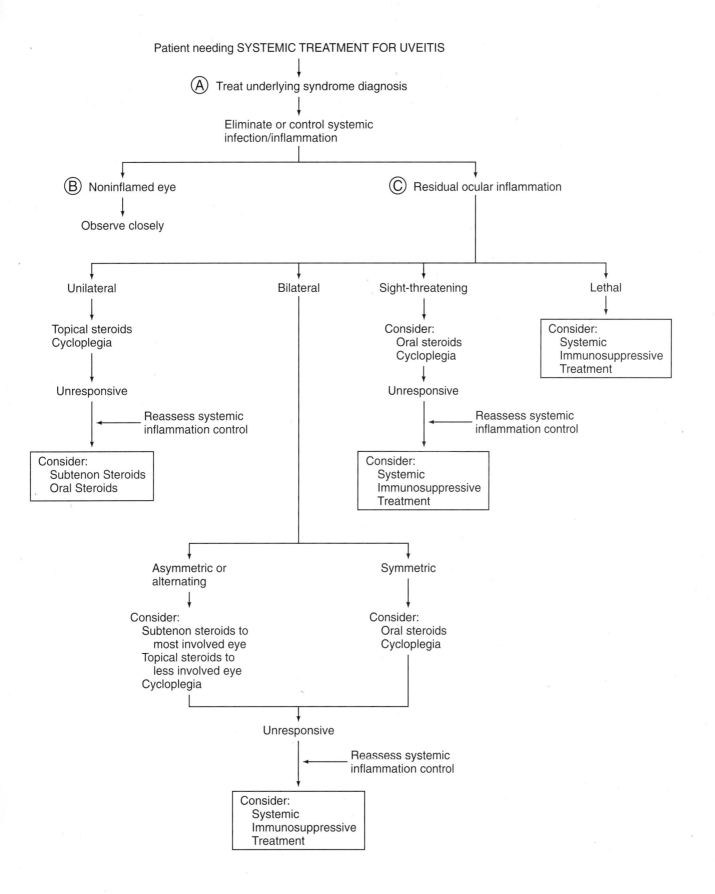

Patient needing SYSTEMIC TREATMENT FOR UVEITIS

Ⓐ Treat underlying syndrome diagnosis

Eliminate or control systemic
infection/inflammation

Ⓑ Noninflamed eye

Observe closely

Ⓒ Residual ocular inflammation

Unilateral

Topical steroids
Cycloplegia

Unresponsive

Reassess systemic
inflammation control

Consider:
  Subtenon Steroids
  Oral Steroids

Bilateral

Sight-threatening

Consider:
  Oral steroids
  Cycloplegia

Unresponsive

Reassess systemic
inflammation control

Consider:
  Systemic
  Immunosuppressive
  Treatment

Lethal

Consider:
  Systemic
  Immunosuppressive
  Treatment

Asymmetric or
alternating

Consider:
  Subtenon steroids to
    most involved eye
  Topical steroids to
    less involved eye
  Cycloplegia

Symmetric

Consider:
  Oral steroids
  Cycloplegia

Unresponsive

Reassess systemic
inflammation control

Consider:
  Systemic
  Immunosuppressive
  Treatment

NEURO-OPHTHALMIC DISORDERS

THE ABNORMAL PUPIL

Martha P. Schatz, M.D.
John E. Carter, M.D.
Susan M. Berry, M.D.

This chapter describes the observation of abnormal pupils in an awake and alert patient. The afferent pupillary defect to light stimulation, which is a clinical sign used in patients with visual loss, is not addressed here, nor are pupillary signs in a comatose patient. Associated signs of a third cranial nerve injury, such as ptosis and ocular muscle weakness, are described under acquired strabismus (pp 14 and 140).

A. A history and examination of the structure of the iris should exclude previous surgery of the iris or ocular trauma producing traumatic mydriasis or pupillary irregularity. The first step is to determine which pupil is abnormal. Observation of the pupil in bright and dim environments may be helpful. Anisocoria that is accentuated in dim light implicates the smaller pupil as having the defect. Anisocoria that is greater in bright light indicates that the larger pupil is abnormal. A unilateral tonic pupil, with its characteristic defect in both dilation and constriction, may be smaller in dim light but larger in bright light.

B. Light-near dissociation indicates a more intense constriction to a near stimulus than to light. There is rarely a situation in which the response to light is stronger than that to near stimulus as an isolated finding.

C. Bilateral light-near dissociation may indicate dorsal midbrain dysfunction (Parinaud's syndrome) or bilateral tonic pupils. Parinaud's syndrome always implies a lesion of the dorsal midbrain, either from an intrinsic process such as a neoplasm, infarct, vascular malformation, or demyelinating plaque or from an extrinsic lesion compressing the dorsal midbrain, most commonly a pinealoma.

D. In tonic pupils there are slow, "tonic" constrictions and dilations, segmental constriction, and spontaneous "vermiform movements" of the iris, which are best seen through the slit lamp.

E. Adie's tonic pupil syndrome is bilateral at the time of evaluation in a minority of cases and may be simultaneous in onset. However, each year, about 4% of patients with an Adie's tonic pupil develop a tonic pupil in the fellow eye. Sequential onset of tonic pupils, either by history or during observation of the patient, indicates Adie's tonic pupil syndrome. The list of pathologic processes that may cause bilateral tonic pupils is extensive, but all share the production of a peripheral polyneuropathy, which is responsible for the tonic pupils and which is a bilateral disorder.

F. Pharmacologic confirmation of a tonic pupil is achieved when 0.125% pilocarpine induces pupillary constriction in the mydriatic eye, indicating denervation hypersensitivity. Instill the drops in both eyes to provide a control before any manipulation of the eye, including tonometry and instillation of anesthetic drops. About 80% of tonic pupils react to dilute pilocarpine; thus the clinical findings are crucial in making the diagnosis of a tonic pupil. In unclear cases with mydriasis and failure to respond to diluted pilocarpine, 1% pilocarpine may be instilled. Failure to respond to 1% pilocarpine indicates a pharmacologically dilated pupil, usually caused by accidental exposure to atropinizing agents in health care workers or by ocular exposure to cocaine. Organophosphates produce mydriasis, and occasionally, individuals feign illness with the use of mydriatics. The pupillary response to pilocarpine is normal in mydriasis caused by injury to the third nerve. There may be a small response to dilute pilocarpine in third nerve palsy, again emphasizing the importance of the slit-lamp examination to distinguish mydriasis from a third nerve palsy and from a tonic pupil.

G. As in the mydriatic pupil, perform all pharmacologic studies of the miotic pupil before manipulating the cornea or instilling other drops. Testing with hydroxyamphetamine should not be done until 24–48 hours after cocaine testing.

H. Postganglionic Horner's syndrome (lesion distal to superior cervical ganglion) is only rarely caused by malignant lesions, whereas malignancy is responsible for up to 50% of cases when the lesion is preganglionic (lesion between C8-T1 and superior cervical ganglion). Associated CNS symptoms or signs identify the centrally located lesion, but processes in the apex of the chest, mediastinum, or neck account for most cases of Horner's syndrome.

I. Heterochromia iridis provides strong evidence of congenital Homer's syndrome, but a few cases of progressive heterochromia iridis in adults with acquired Homer's syndrome have been documented. The history, supplemented by earlier photos of the patient, should allow differentiation between these two conditions. Evaluate children without birth trauma for a possible cervical or mediastinal neuroblastoma.

J. The springing pupil is a benign syndrome with no associated symptoms or signs in which there is episodic mydriasis, usually in young women, associated with vague sensations in the eye and headache, as well as symptoms of defective accommodation. Migraine has also been described as producing episodic mydriasis.

K. Cluster headaches characteristically produce evidence of sympathetic paresis during the headache.

Patient with ABNORMAL PUPIL

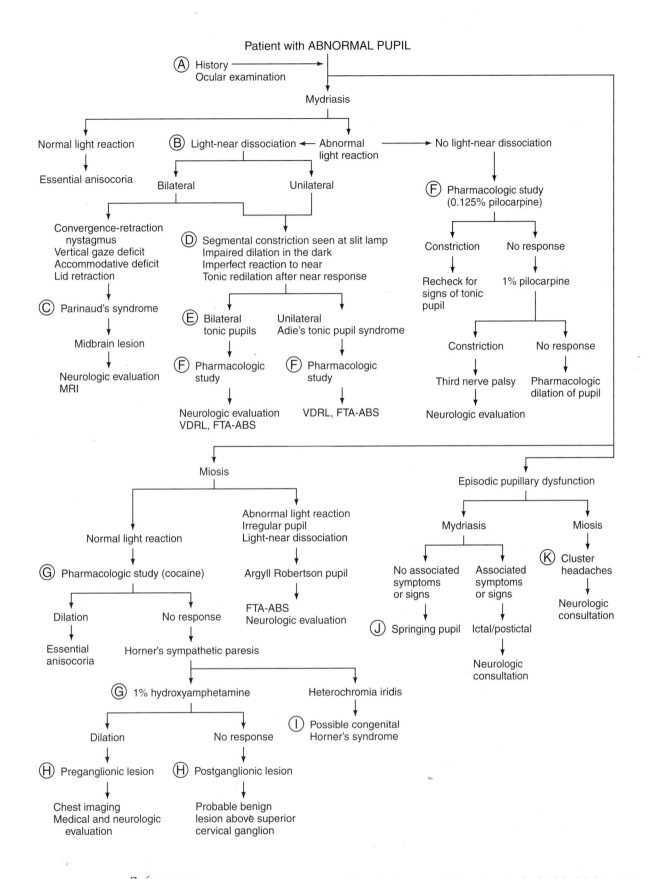

References

Burde RM, Savino PJ, Trobe JD. Clinical decisions in neuroophthalmology. 2nd ed. St Louis: Mosby, 1992.

Glaser JS. Neuro-ophthalmology. 2nd ed. Philadelphia: JB Lippincott, 1989.

Miller NR. Walsh and Hoyt's clinical neuro-ophthalmology. 4th ed. Vol. 2. Baltimore: Williams & Wilkins, 1985.

NYSTAGMUS

Martha Schatz, M.D.
John E. Carter, M.D.
Susan M. Berry, M.D.

Acquired nystagmus is most helpful diagnostically when it is present in the primary position. Any type of nystagmus discussed here may be caused by lesions in a variety of locations or may be congenital. In addition, drugs, especially anticonvulsants and psychoactive medications, may cause nystagmus in the primary position resulting in oscillopsia.

A. Three types of horizontal nystagmus maintain their horizontal character when the patient moves the eyes vertically: vestibular, periodic alternating nystagmus, and congenital nystagmus.

B. Congenital nystagmus has been described with a delayed onset for several years after birth. Pendular nystagmus in the primary position, which maintains its horizontal direction in vertical gaze, does not produce oscillopsia, and damps with convergence in a patient without other neurologic symptoms or signs, may still be congenital nystagmus even though it was not present for several years after birth.

C. Despite its name, ocular myoclonus is a nystagmus in that it is a steady, rhythmic oscillation of the eyes. It is a slow, coarse, vertical nystagmus and accompanies palatal myoclonus in which the palate or pharyngeal musculature exhibits the same rhythmic movement. Small lesions in the dentato-rubro-olivary pathway may produce only the palatal movement, whereas larger or bilateral lesions produce oculopalatal myoclonus. This is a delayed effect that may not develop for several months after the neurologic injury and does not necessarily mean that there is a new or progressive lesion.

D. Gaze-evoked nystagmus in the extremes of eccentric gaze is common. It is usually not sustained. Many drugs amplify gaze-evoked nystagmus. Gaze-evoked nystagmus to one side suggests a recovering gaze palsy from a lesion of the brainstem on the same side or a contralateral hemispheric lesion in the frontal lobe. However, significantly asymmetric gaze-evoked nystagmus may also be seen with ipsilateral brainstem lesions, especially cerebellopontine mass lesions. If eccentric gaze produces nystagmus in the abducting eye, there may have been an internuclear ophthalmoplegia that has recovered; slowing of adducting saccades in the fellow eye or saccadic dysmetria in the same eye confirms the diagnosis.

E. Upwards saccades, whether a single large amplitude movement or repetitive saccades induced by optokinetic stimulation, may produce co-contraction of all third nerve muscles and consequent convergence and retraction of the globe into the orbits. The repetitive phenomenon is convergence-retractory nystagmus when induced with optokinetic stimulation. This is one element of Parinaud's syndrome (lid retraction, light-near dissociation, and upward gaze palsy).

F. Superior oblique myokymia is identifiable by a history of intermittent vertical and torsional movement of one of the two images of the environment. It may be induced during the slit-lamp examination by various vertical eye movements. Spasmus nutans has a characteristic clinic profile of early onset, fine nystagmus, head bobbing, and resolution by age 3. Although it is usually benign, consideration must be given to intracranial mass lesions, especially if atypical features exist.

References

Burde RM, Savino PF, Trobe JD. Clinical decisions in neuro-ophthalmology. 2nd ed. St Louis: Mosby, 1992.

Glaser JS. Neuro-ophthalmology. 2nd ed. Hagerstown, MD: Harper & Row, 1989.

Miller NR. Walsh and Hoyt's clinical neuro-ophthalmology. Vol 2. Baltimore: Williams & Wilkins, 1985.

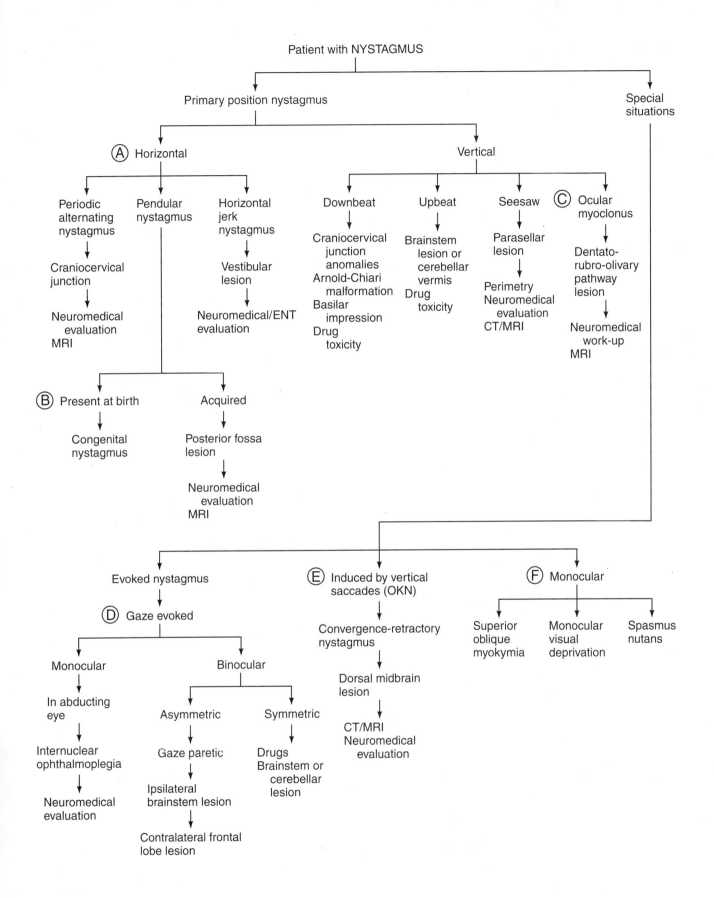

Patient with NYSTAGMUS

Primary position nystagmus — Special situations

(A) Horizontal — Vertical

Periodic alternating nystagmus — Pendular nystagmus — Horizontal jerk nystagmus

Periodic alternating nystagmus → Craniocervical junction → Neuromedical evaluation MRI

Horizontal jerk nystagmus → Vestibular lesion → Neuromedical/ENT evaluation

(B) Present at birth → Congenital nystagmus

Acquired → Posterior fossa lesion → Neuromedical evaluation MRI

Downbeat → Craniocervical junction anomalies Arnold-Chiari malformation Basilar impression Drug toxicity

Upbeat → Brainstem lesion or cerebellar vermis Drug toxicity

Seesaw → Parasellar lesion → Perimetry Neuromedical evaluation CT/MRI

(C) Ocular myoclonus → Dentato-rubro-olivary pathway lesion → Neuromedical work-up MRI

Evoked nystagmus
(D) Gaze evoked

Monocular → In abducting eye → Internuclear ophthalmoplegia → Neuromedical evaluation

Binocular
Asymmetric → Gaze paretic → Ipsilateral brainstem lesion → Contralateral frontal lobe lesion

Symmetric → Drugs Brainstem or cerebellar lesion

(E) Induced by vertical saccades (OKN) → Convergence-retractory nystagmus → Dorsal midbrain lesion → CT/MRI Neuromedical evaluation

(F) Monocular
Superior oblique myokymia
Monocular visual deprivation
Spasmus nutans

SWOLLEN DISC

Martha P. Schatz, M.D.
John E. Carter, M.D.

Occasional arbitrary distinctions are made in the terminology applied to swelling of the optic disc. Some use the term *disc swelling* descriptively and reserve the term *papilledema* for disc swelling caused by intracranial hypertension. Others use *papilledema* for any disc swelling but indicate passive disc swelling with intracranial hypertension by the term *choked disc.*

Disc swelling is produced by many processes. The most important question is whether the vision is affected. Impaired vision indicates that the swelling is unlikely to be passive, signifying that an active process is affecting the optic nerve. The character of the visual field (VF) defect is most helpful in determining the nature of the process. Diagnostic considerations are similar for unilateral and bilateral disc swelling with a cecocentral scotoma.

A. In any patient who presents with bilateral disc swelling, one must consider increased intracranial pressure (ICP) unless other parts of the clinical examination demonstrate otherwise (e.g., uveitis).

B. Optic neuropathy is diagnosed by the presence of an afferent pupillary defect, color vision deficit, and a neuropathic VF defect (i.e., altitudinal, arcuate, cecocentral, or constrictive). Non-neuropathic VF loss is that which does not have these features (i.e., macular).

C. Acute, bilateral blindness with disc swelling may be seen in patients with methanol poisoning. Bilateral optic neuritis is common in children and uncommon in adults. Unilateral, acute central scotoma with disc swelling in adults is most likely caused by central retinal vein occlusion (CRVO), which exhibits diffuse retinal hemorrhages. A more subacute onset over days indicates the presence of optic neuritis. Exclude chronic infectious processes such as lues, fungi, and tuberculosis; infiltrative processes such as leukemia and lymphoma; and chronic inflammatory processes such as sarcoid and collagen vascular disease before making a diagnosis of idiopathic demyelinating optic neuritis. A subacute onset over weeks suggests a compressive optic neuropathy. If the neuropathy is bilateral, consider optic nerve glioma or nerve sheath meningioma; unilateral optic nerve compression and disc swelling may be caused by these or any extrinsic mass lesion, including aneurysm.

D. Disc swelling and an altitudinal VF defect are highly suggestive of ischemia of the optic disc in the appropriate clinical situation. Most cases of anterior ischemic optic neuropathy (AION) are idiopathic, but temporal arteritis or giant cell arteritis (GCA) is treatable and must be excluded. Bilateral, simultaneous ischemic optic neuropathy is more often caused by temporal arteritis.

E. Monocular disc swelling with preserved vision may be seen with uveitis, in which case white blood cells should be present in the vitreous and anterior chamber. Disc swelling associated with prominent venous congestion is attributed to venous inflammation or papillophlebitis in younger patients or to "partial" central retinal vein occlusion, sometimes called *venous stasis retinopathy,* in older patients.

F. Unilateral disc swelling from intracranial hypertension is uncommon but usually becomes bilateral over weeks or months. Other symptoms may be used to determine the need to proceed to additional studies.

References

Burde RM, Savino PJ, Trobe JD. Clinical decisions in neuroophthalmology. 2nd ed. St Louis: Mosby, 1992.

Glaser JS. Neuro-ophthalmology. 2nd ed. Philadelphia: JB Lippincott, 1989.

Miller NR. Walsh and Hoyt's clinical neuro-ophthalmology. 4th ed. Vol. 1. Baltimore: Williams & Wilkins, 1982.

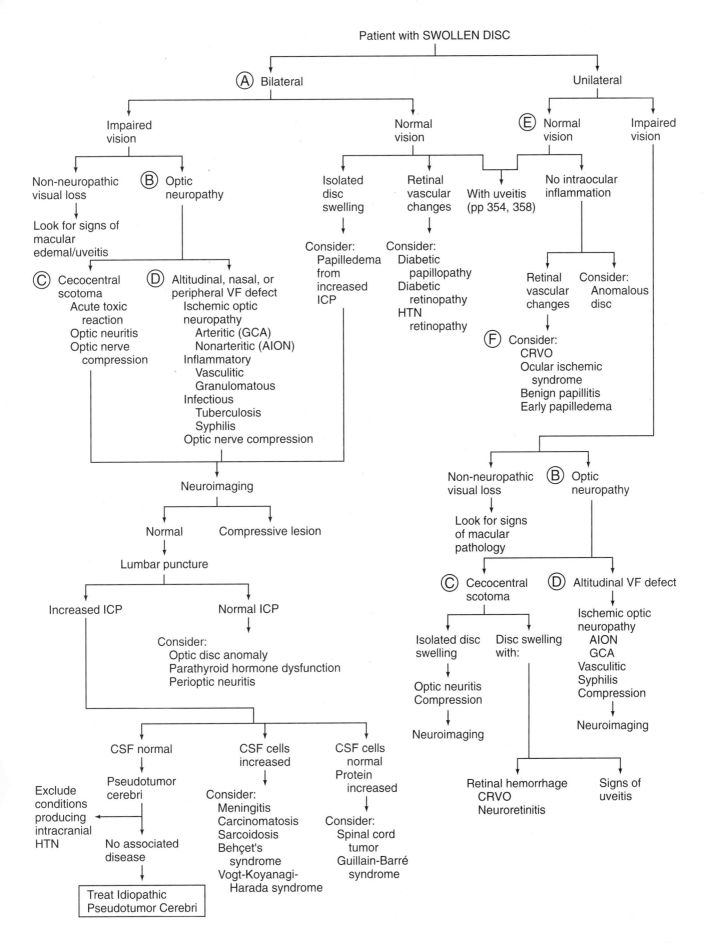

Patient with SWOLLEN DISC

Ⓐ Bilateral

- **Impaired vision**
  - **Non-neuropathic visual loss**
    - Look for signs of macular edemal/uveitis
  - **Ⓑ Optic neuropathy**
    - **Ⓒ Cecocentral scotoma**
      - Acute toxic reaction
      - Optic neuritis
      - Optic nerve compression
    - **Ⓓ Altitudinal, nasal, or peripheral VF defect**
      - Ischemic optic neuropathy
        - Arteritic (GCA)
        - Nonarteritic (AION)
      - Inflammatory
        - Vasculitic
        - Granulomatous
      - Infectious
        - Tuberculosis
        - Syphilis
      - Optic nerve compression

- **Normal vision**
  - **Isolated disc swelling**
    - Consider:
      - Papilledema from increased ICP
  - **Retinal vascular changes**
    - Consider:
      - Diabetic papillopathy
      - Diabetic retinopathy
      - HTN retinopathy

Unilateral

- **Ⓔ Normal vision**
  - **With uveitis** (pp 354, 358)
  - **No intraocular inflammation**
    - **Retinal vascular changes**
      - **Ⓕ Consider:**
        - CRVO
        - Ocular ischemic syndrome
        - Benign papillitis
        - Early papilledema
    - **Consider: Anomalous disc**
- **Impaired vision**

Neuroimaging
- **Normal**
  - Lumbar puncture
    - **Increased ICP**
    - **Normal ICP**
      - Consider:
        - Optic disc anomaly
        - Parathyroid hormone dysfunction
        - Perioptic neuritis
- **Compressive lesion**

- **CSF normal**
  - Pseudotumor cerebri
    - Exclude conditions producing intracranial HTN
    - No associated disease
      - Treat Idiopathic Pseudotumor Cerebri
- **CSF cells increased**
  - Consider:
    - Meningitis
    - Carcinomatosis
    - Sarcoidosis
    - Behçet's syndrome
    - Vogt-Koyanagi-Harada syndrome
- **CSF cells normal Protein increased**
  - Consider:
    - Spinal cord tumor
    - Guillain-Barré syndrome

- **Non-neuropathic visual loss**
  - Look for signs of macular pathology
- **Ⓑ Optic neuropathy**
  - **Ⓒ Cecocentral scotoma**
    - **Isolated disc swelling**
      - Optic neuritis
      - Compression
        - Neuroimaging
    - **Disc swelling with:**
      - Retinal hemorrhage
        - CRVO
        - Neuroretinitis
      - Signs of uveitis
  - **Ⓓ Altitudinal VF defect**
    - Ischemic optic neuropathy
      - AION
      - GCA
      - Vasculitic
      - Syphilis
      - Compression
        - Neuroimaging

OPTIC NEUROPATHY

John E. Carter, M.D.
Susan M. Berry, M.D.
Martha P. Schatz, M.D.
David K. Scales, M.D.

Optic neuropathy is diagnosed when complaints of decreased vision are accompanied by impaired color vision, afferent pupillary defect, and a visual field defect (or a combination thereof). Subjective abnormalities also include decreased color saturation and brightness in the involved eye. The appearance of the optic disc varies according to the duration of the process. Acute disease anteriorly produces disc swelling, but acute disease in the retrobulbar optic nerve may not change the appearance of the optic disc. Disease of the optic nerve of a more chronic nature usually produces atrophy, although compressive lesions may produce disc swelling for many months before atrophy develops.

A. Perform visual field testing in both eyes. Any defect that respects the vertical meridian indicates that the disease process is intracranial at the anterior chiasm and optic nerve junctions. Because most chiasmal lesions are caused by mass lesions, this distinction is critical in directing the diagnostic work-up.

B. The temporal profile of the visual loss is the most reliable indicator of the cause and permits tailoring of the examination and diagnostic studies toward the most likely diagnosis.

C. Bilateral, chronic, progressive optic atrophy is usually attributable to a hereditary optic atrophy, a nutritional or deficiency state, or exposure to environmental toxins or toxic medications. Visual field defects in those conditions are usually cecocentral. To be certain that these are not present may require examination of the parents or siblings as well as confirmation of historical data such as alcohol and tobacco abuse or dietary habits. If these conditions cannot be diagnosed, imaging studies are necessary to exclude mass lesions that simultaneously involve both optic nerves.

D. Young patients with acute or subacute visual loss and disc swelling most commonly have an inflammatory process involving the optic disc. Idiopathic optic neuritis is the most common, but history and laboratory studies should be used to exclude other more specific and more treatable inflammatory and infiltrative conditions.

E. The optic nerve head may be swollen with uveitis involving the posterior globe or with posterior episcleritis. Visual loss may or may not be present when the nerve is swollen in association with uveitis; when present, visual loss may be caused by inflammation of the nerve or by effects of the uveitis on the macula.

F. Visual loss with a very sudden onset is usually vascular in nature and in older patients indicates retinal vascular occlusion or, if disc swelling is present, ischemic optic neuropathy. Most ischemic optic neuropathy is related to either atherosclerosis of small arterioles, mechanical factors associated with small disc size, or a combination of these. However, temporal arteritis also causes ischemic optic neuropathy, and early treatment is important to prevent further visual loss. Symptoms that suggest temporal arteritis are progressive headache or head pains of recent onset, jaw claudication, nocturnal fevers or a recurrent fever of unknown origin, and polymyalgia rheumatica. Age >70 years and bilateral simultaneous ischemic optic neuropathy, especially with loss of most or all vision, also suggest temporal arteritis. The ESR is usually greatly elevated. A strong clinical diagnosis with significantly elevated ESR may be sufficient to make the diagnosis without a temporal artery biopsy.

G. Acute optic neuropathy with a normal optic disc indicates abnormality in the retrobulbar optic nerve. The diagnostic considerations are similar to those of patients with optic neuritis. Pituitary apoplexy (hemorrhage into a pituitary tumor) may cause acute visual loss bilaterally and is usually associated with severe headache and eye movement disturbances. An older patient with a history of cancer may have meningeal carcinomatosis, which involves the optic nerves bilaterally in a large percentage of patients.

H. A progressive optic atrophy in one eye is likely to indicate a compressive lesion, either neoplastic or aneurysmal.

References

Burde RM, Savino PJ, Trobe JD. Clinical decisions in neuro-ophthalmology. 2nd ed. St Louis: Mosby, 1992.
Glaser JS. Neuro-ophthalmology. 2nd ed. Philadelphia: JB Lippincott, 1989.
Miller NR. Walsh and Hoyt's clinical neuro-ophthalmology. 4th ed. Vol. 1. Baltimore: Williams & Wilkins, 1982.

Patient with OPTIC NEUROPATHY

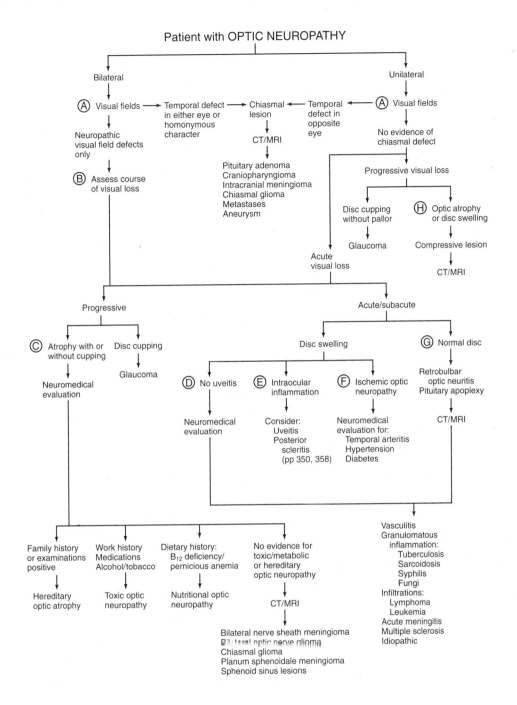

Bilateral
- Ⓐ Visual fields
  - Temporal defect in either eye or homonymous character → Chiasmal lesion → Temporal defect in opposite eye
    - CT/MRI
      - Pituitary adenoma
      - Craniopharyngioma
      - Intracranial meningioma
      - Chiasmal glioma
      - Metastases
      - Aneurysm
  - Neuropathic visual field defects only
    - Ⓑ Assess course of visual loss

Unilateral
- Ⓐ Visual fields
  - No evidence of chiasmal defect
    - Progressive visual loss
      - Disc cupping without pallor
        - Glaucoma
      - Ⓗ Optic atrophy or disc swelling
        - Compressive lesion
          - CT/MRI
    - Acute visual loss

Progressive
- Ⓒ Atrophy with or without cupping
  - Neuromedical evaluation
- Disc cupping
  - Glaucoma

Acute/subacute
- Disc swelling
  - Ⓓ No uveitis
    - Neuromedical evaluation
  - Ⓔ Intraocular inflammation
    - Consider:
      Uveitis
      Posterior scleritis
      (pp 350, 358)
  - Ⓕ Ischemic optic neuropathy
    - Neuromedical evaluation for:
      Temporal arteritis
      Hypertension
      Diabetes
- Ⓖ Normal disc
  - Retrobulbar optic neuritis
    Pituitary apoplexy
    - CT/MRI

- Family history or examinations positive
  - Hereditary optic atrophy
- Work history Medications Alcohol/tobacco
  - Toxic optic neuropathy
- Dietary history: B₁₂ deficiency/ pernicious anemia
  - Nutritional optic neuropathy
- No evidence for toxic/metabolic or hereditary optic neuropathy
  - CT/MRI
    - Bilateral nerve sheath meningioma
      Bilateral optic nerve glioma
      Chiasmal glioma
      Planum sphenoidale meningioma
      Sphenoid sinus lesions

- Vasculitis
- Granulomatous inflammation:
  Tuberculosis
  Sarcoidosis
  Syphilis
  Fungi
- Infiltrations:
  Lymphoma
  Leukemia
- Acute meningitis
- Multiple sclerosis
- Idiopathic

Patient with OPTIC NEUROPATHY WITH UVEITIS

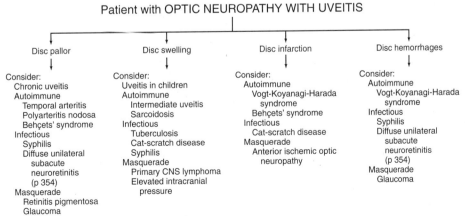

Disc pallor
Consider:
- Chronic uveitis
- Autoimmune
  - Temporal arteritis
  - Polyarteritis nodosa
  - Behçets' syndrome
- Infectious
  - Syphilis
  - Diffuse unilateral subacute neuroretinitis (p 354)
- Masquerade
  - Retinitis pigmentosa
  - Glaucoma

Disc swelling
Consider:
- Uveitis in children
- Autoimmune
  - Intermediate uveitis
  - Sarcoidosis
- Infectious
  - Tuberculosis
  - Cat-scratch disease
  - Syphilis
- Masquerade
  - Primary CNS lymphoma
  - Elevated intracranial pressure

Disc infarction
Consider:
- Autoimmune
  - Vogt-Koyanagi-Harada syndrome
  - Behçets' syndrome
- Infectious
  - Cat-scratch disease
- Masquerade
  - Anterior ischemic optic neuropathy

Disc hemorrhages
Consider:
- Autoimmune
  - Vogt-Koyanagi-Harada syndrome
- Infectious
  - Syphilis
  - Diffuse unilateral subacute neuroretinitis (p 354)
- Masquerade
  - Glaucoma

LOSS OF VISUAL FIELD

Johan Zwaan, M.D., Ph.D.

The interpretation of the loss of visual field (VF) is based on the anatomic organization of the retina and the visual pathways. Because lesions of different parts of the visual system can cause similar VF defects, interpretation of the VF is not always adequate to localize a lesion. Other clinical tests of pupillary reactions, color vision, ocular motility, perception of brightness, and light-stress recovery time may aid in refining the location of a lesion. Ophthalmoscopy is essential. MRI, CT scanning, or electrophysiologic testing is often necessary.

A. A central or paracentral VF defect can result from retinal or choroid disease or from a lesion in the optic nerve. The relation of the defect to the vertical and horizontal meridians of the VF is a helpful indication. Retinal lesions do not respect either of the meridians, whereas optic nerve lesions respect the nasal horizontal but not the vertical meridian. Ophthalmoscopy usually will aid in differentiating between the two. Age-related macular degeneration or other causes of macular scarring may cause central or paracentral scotomas. Consider optic neuritis or a mass lesion affecting the optic nerve. If the VF defect is bilateral and more or less symmetric, suspect optic neuropathies of hereditary (Leber's optic neuropathy), nutritional (vitamin B_{12} or folate lack, tobacco or alcohol amblyopia), or toxic (methanol, heavy metals) causes.

B. A cecocentral scotoma is a nerve fiber bundle (NFB) defect of the papillomacular bundle. It is, by definition, an extension of the blind spot.

C. The maculopapillary bundle consists of nerve fibers from the macula that enter the optic disc on the temporal side.

D. The nerve fibers from the nasal side of the retina are straight (nonarcuate) and enter the optic disc radially. A lesion of these fibers results in a temporal wedge-shaped VF defect. This type of a defect does not always respect the horizontal meridian.

E. Nerve fibers from the temporal peripheral retina arch around the maculopapillary bundle and the fovea on their way to the optic disc. This creates the superior and inferior arcuate NFB. This part of the VF is about 15 degrees away from the fixation point and is called *Bjerrum's area*. For unknown reasons, the superior and inferior temporal parts of the optic nerve are more sensitive to glaucoma. Therefore defects within Bjerrum's area are often an early indication of glaucomatous damage. Depending on the part of the arcuate NFB involved, different VF defects occur within Bjerrum's area.

F. The classical Bjerrum's scotoma has the shape of a scimitar and involves the entire arcuate NFB.

G. Seidel's scotoma is a comma-shaped extension of the blind spot. It indicates damage to the proximal part of the arcuate NFB.

H. Because the superior and inferior arcuate NFB do not cross the horizontal raphe of the retina, a defect of the distal part of the arcuate fibers will respect the horizontal meridian on the nasal side, leading to a nasal step.

I. Lesions of intermediate arcuate nerve fibers lead to isolated scotomas within Bjerrum's area, reminiscent of paracentral defects but more peripheral in the VF.

J. Altitudinal defects are larger than those from a nasal or temporal NFB defect alone. Those respecting the nasal horizontal meridian but not the temporal one are most likely caused by optic nerve or NFB defects. If they respect both parts of the horizontal meridian, the probable location for the lesion causing the defect is the calcarine cortex. Occipital cortex and retinal or optic disc lesions may cause altitudinal lesions. Uncommonly, contusions of the optic nerves or the chiasm or compression of their upper surfaces from above may cause altitudinal defects.

K. Embolism of the superior or inferior branch of the retinal artery is the most common cause of an altitudinal defect based on a retinal lesion. This generally occurs monocularly, but it is possible for emboli to affect both eyes. It is unusual for this to cause congruous lesions. Bilateral retinal detachments, rhegmatogenous or exudative, may also cause incongruous altitudinal defects.

L. A large nasal step may break through temporally, giving an altitudinal field defect. The defect will respect the horizontal meridian on the nasal side but not on the temporal side. This indicates an optic nerve lesion with the most likely causes being glaucoma or ischemic optic neuropathy.

M. The vascular supply of the optic disc is primarily from the posterior ciliary arteries. Occlusion may lead to altitudinal VF defects in one or both eyes. Usually, they will not be symmetric. Bilateral optic disc colobomas may cause altitudinal VF defects, and advanced glaucoma in both eyes can cause a large nasal step with temporal breakthrough in each eye.

N. Meningiomas originating from the olfactory groove usually grow backwards onto the planum sphenoidale and may compress the chiasma from above (suprachiasmatic meningioma). This may lead to inferior altitudinal VF defects. These tumors are often not recognized until significant and irreversible optic atrophy has occurred.

O. Bilateral and congruous altitudinal hemianopia, respecting both nasal and temporal horizontal raphe, is caused by lesions of the occipital lobe. If the calcarine branches of both posterior cerebral arteries are occluded, the brain tissue superior or inferior to the calcarine fissure may become infarcted. Similarly, inhibited circulation through the middle cerebral arteries may lead to infarction of the superior lips of the calcarine occipital cortex. A less likely cause is trauma to the area above the calcarine fissure, which results in an inferior congruous altitudinal VF defect. Because similar trauma from below most likely involves lacerations of the dural sinuses, therefore meaning the patient would not survive, superior altitudinal field defects from trauma are quite unusual.

P. Hemianopic VF defects split the point of fixation (macula) and respect the vertical meridian. In contrast, NFB defects originate from the blind spot (optic disc) and do not respect the vertical meridian.

Q. A junctional scotoma results when an optic nerve lesion of one eye impinges on the chiasm at the same side. Depending on its extent, the optic nerve lesion may cause a central or complete scotoma. The contralateral VF shows a superior quadrantanopic temporal defect or sometimes a hemianopic temporal defect because of involvement of the crossed nerve fibers in the chiasm.

R. Because of the decussation of nasal nerve fibers in the chiasm, both VFs are always affected by any lesion of the optic pathway behind the optic chiasm. Lesions at the chiasm may lead to binocular defects, but they are often asymmetric and almost always heteronymous.

S. Heteronymous hemianopia involves either both nasal or both temporal halves of the VF. Pituitary tumors will first affect the inferior part of the center portion of the chiasm, leading to bitemporal superior quadrantanopia. With further growth, the field defects expand to complete bitemporal hemianopia. Binasal hemianopia is rare. It is caused by compression of both lateral sides of the chiasm, usually secondary to aneurysmal or arteriosclerotic enlargement of both internal carotid arteries.

T. VF defects of the same side in both eyes (nasal hemianopia in one eye and temporal in the contralateral eye) are called *homonymous*. They are always caused by lesions behind the chiasm.

U. Congruity should be determined by performing central rather than peripheral VF tests. If the hemianopia affects the entire half of the VF, congruity cannot be determined. It can be tested only when the VF defect is incomplete. In general, the more congruous the hemi-anopia, the further posterior the causative lesion is located. The exceptions to this are lesions of the lateral geniculate body. Nerve fibers of corresponding areas from both eyes are not strongly associated in the optic tract, but they become organized in the lateral geniculate body. This is thought to lead to congruous VF defects. However, incomplete lesions in this area or preferential involvement of certain laminae with sparing of the other laminae may lead to incongruous defects.

V. Because of the loose association of corresponding areas in the optic tract, optic tract lesions cause highly incongruous VF defects.

W. The fibers of the middle part of the optic radiation, located in the temporal lobe, tend to be wider apart, and homologous fibers are not adjacent. This results in incongruous VF defects. The inferior fibers of the optic radiation swing anteriorly into the anterior tip of the temporal lobe, forming Meyer's loop. Superior fibers run back directly toward the optic radiation within the parietal lobe, separated from the inferior fibers. Hence anterior temporal lobe lesions cause (mid)peripheral superior quadrantanopia, known as "pie in the sky" scotomas. In more extensive temporal lobe lesions, the VF defects expand to hemianopia. Even then, the defects are denser superiorly.

X. The nerve fibers of the optic radiation become closer together and more homologously arranged in the parietal lobe and farther posterior. Superior and inferior fibers are still separated. Parietal lobe lesions tend to affect the superior fibers first, and the resulting VF defects tend to be congruous inferior quadrantanopia. If the lesions are larger, hemianopia follows with the defects being denser inferiorly.

Y. Occipital lobe lesions are the most congruous with one exception. Each eye has a temporal crescent of VF for which there is no counterpart in the contralateral eye. This crescent is represented in the occipital cortex along the most anterior part of the calcarine fissure. Thus a homonymous hemianopia with sparing of a temporal crescent localizes to the occipital cortex. The macula is represented at the tip of the occipital lobe. Lesions here result in a contralateral central hemianopia.

References

Burde RM, Savino PJ, Trobe JD. Clinical decisions in neuro-ophthalmology. 2nd ed. St Louis: Mosby, 1992.

Cogan OG. Neurology of the visual system. Springfield, IL: Charles C Thomas, 1966.

Trobe JD, Glaser JS. The visual fields manual. Gainesville, FL: Triad, 1983.

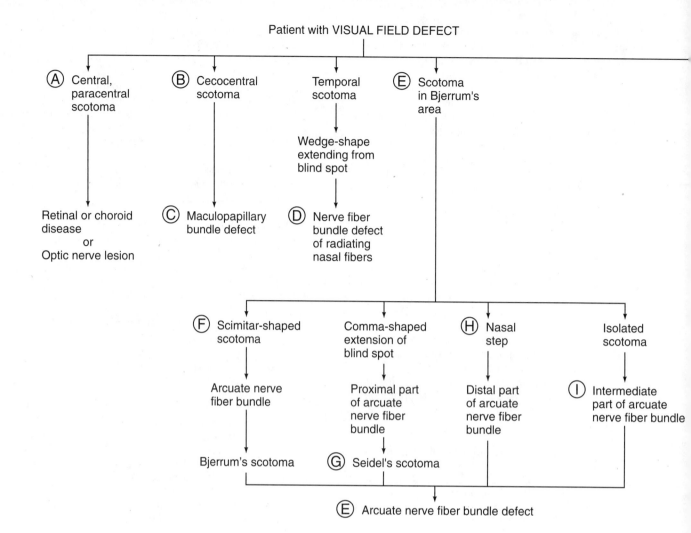

Patient with VISUAL FIELD DEFECT

(A) Central, paracentral scotoma

(B) Cecocentral scotoma

Temporal scotoma

(E) Scotoma in Bjerrum's area

Retinal or choroid disease
or
Optic nerve lesion

(C) Maculopapillary bundle defect

Wedge-shape extending from blind spot

(D) Nerve fiber bundle defect of radiating nasal fibers

(F) Scimitar-shaped scotoma

Comma-shaped extension of blind spot

(H) Nasal step

Isolated scotoma

Arcuate nerve fiber bundle

Proximal part of arcuate nerve fiber bundle

Distal part of arcuate nerve fiber bundle

(I) Intermediate part of arcuate nerve fiber bundle

Bjerrum's scotoma

(G) Seidel's scotoma

(E) Arcuate nerve fiber bundle defect

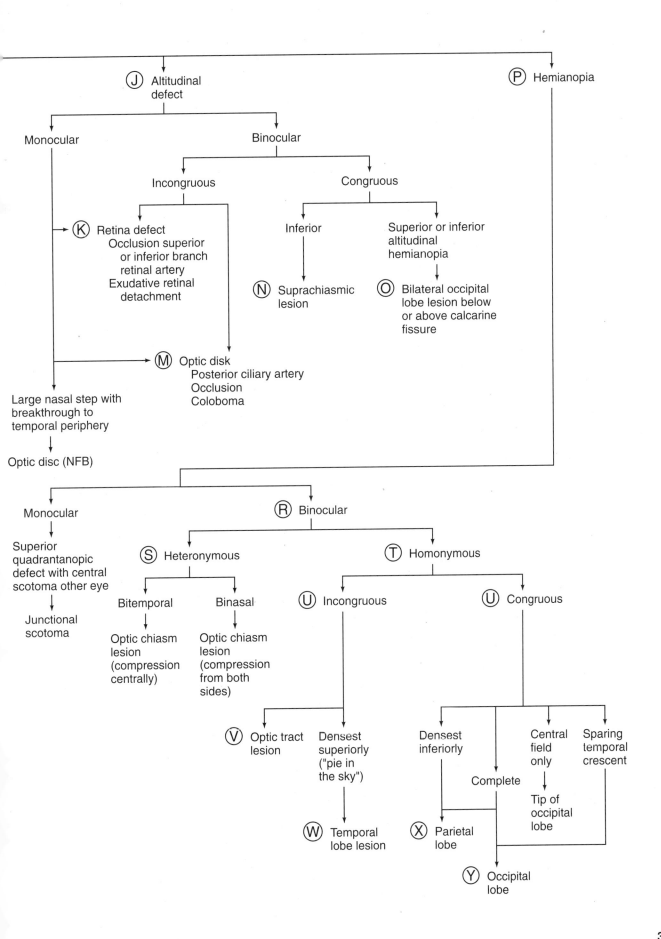

(J) Altitudinal defect

Monocular

Binocular

Incongruous

Congruous

(K) Retina defect
Occlusion superior
or inferior branch
retinal artery
Exudative retinal
detachment

Inferior

Superior or inferior
altitudinal
hemianopia

(N) Suprachiasmic
lesion

(O) Bilateral occipital
lobe lesion below
or above calcarine
fissure

(M) Optic disk
Posterior ciliary artery
Occlusion
Coloboma

Large nasal step with
breakthrough to
temporal periphery

Optic disc (NFB)

(P) Hemianopia

Monocular

(R) Binocular

Superior
quadrantanopic
defect with central
scotoma other eye

Junctional
scotoma

(S) Heteronymous

(T) Homonymous

Bitemporal

Binasal

(U) Incongruous

(U) Congruous

Optic chiasm
lesion
(compression
centrally)

Optic chiasm
lesion
(compression
from both
sides)

(V) Optic tract
lesion

Densest
superiorly
("pie in
the sky")

Densest
inferiorly

Central
field
only

Sparing
temporal
crescent

(W) Temporal
lobe lesion

Complete

Tip of
occipital
lobe

(X) Parietal
lobe

(Y) Occipital
lobe

Index

Lamellar keratectomy, 185
Lamellar keratoplasty, 226
Lanthony Desaturated Panel test, 8
Large-cell lymphoma, 358
Laser peripheral iridotomy (LPI), 236, 238
Laser transscleral cyclophotocoagulation, 252
LASIK keratorefractive surgery, 230
Latanoprost, 240, 244, 262, 263, 344
Lateral rectus (LR) muscle, 164, 166
Lateral rectus palsies, true, 144
Lattice degeneration, 336
Lattice dystrophy, 225, 228, 230
LCA; see Leber's congenital amaurosis
LCAT; see Lecithin cholesterol acetyltransferase deficiency
Le Fort fractures, 106, 107
Leber's congenital amaurosis (LCA), 178
Leber's idiopathic stellate retinopathy, 292
Leber's optic atrophy, 196
Leber's optic neuropathy, 374
Lecithin cholesterol acetyltransferase deficiency (LCAT), 224
Left hypertropia (LHT), 158
Leishmaniasis, 214, 217
Lens disorders, 267-287
    dislocated lenses, **272-275**
    opacities on lens surface, **268-271**
    pain after cataract surgery, **276-279**
    poor vision after cataract surgery, **280-283**
    shallow anterior chamber after cataract surgery, **284-287**
    subluxed lenses, **272-275**
Lens-cornea touch, 254, 255
Lensectomy, 190
Lenses
    dislocated, 86, **272-275,** 277
    subluxed, **272-275**
    surface of, opacities on, **268-271**
Lenticonus, anterior, 188
Lentiglobus, posterior, 22
Lentigo maligna, 54
Lenz's syndrome, 83
Leone tarsoconjunctival flap, 122
Leprosy, 214, 216, 231
Leptospirosis, 314
Leukemia, 32, 37, 68, 132, 196, 320
Leukocoria, **182-183,** 192, 194-195
Levobunolol, 206
Levodopa, 213
LGV; see Lymphogranuloma venereum
LHT; see Left hypertropia
Lid abnormalities, 32
Lid coloboma, 32
Lid lag, 114; see also Eyelid
Lidocaine hydrochloride (Xylocaine), 218, 277
Limbal conjunctival melanosis, 220
Limbal dermoids, 134, 185
Limited supraduction in children, surgery for, **164-165**
Lipid abnormalities, 13
Lipid layer of tear film, 44

Lipofuscinosis, neuronal ceroid, 291
Lipomas, 116
Lisch nodule, 76
Local anesthesia, 90-91
Local ocular treatment for uveitis, **360-361**
Long bone fractures, 66
Loss of visual field, 2-3, 4-5, **374-377**
Lower eyelid, reconstruction of, 124-125
Lower lid laxity, 48
Lowe's syndrome, 188, 268
Low-tension glaucoma, **246-247**
LP; see Lumbar puncture
LPI; see Laser peripheral iridotomy
LR muscle; see Lateral rectus muscle
Luetic retinopathy, 13
Lumbar puncture (LP), 28
Lupus choroidopathy, 101
Lupus erythematosus, 44, 66, 100, 101, 209, 217, 218, 314, 320, 341, 344, 354
Lyme disease, 214-215, 332
Lymphadenopathy, hilar, 104
Lymphangioma, 112, 132
Lymphocytic lymphoma, 320
Lymphocytic tumors, 112
Lymphogranuloma venereum (LGV), 215
Lymphoma, 32, 37, 44, 56, 88, 101, 102, 112, 314, 320, 358
Lymphoproliferative disorder, systemic, 132
Lysozyme level, 45

M

Macroaneurysm, 306, 316
Macrophthalmos, 86-87
Macropsia, 6
Macular bull's eye, 16, 101, 221, **290-291,** 310
Macular cherry-red spot, **294-295**
Macular degeneration, 2, 281, 296, 330, 374
Macular detachments, serous, 298
Macular disorders, 2
Macular dystrophy, 196, 228
Macular edema, 2, 78, 100, 105, 262, 280-281, 306, 332, 340-341, 352, 358
Macular epiretinal membranes, 314
Macular holes, 6
Macular hypoplasia, 16
Macular neuroretinitis, 292
Macular pucker, 18, 281
Macular retinitis, 354
Macular star, **292-293**
Maculopapillary bundle, 374
Maculopathy, 263, 281
Malabsorption syndromes, 13
Malar region, flattening of, 128
Malaria, 66, 214, 217, 344
Malignant glaucoma, 284
Malignant melanoma, 54, 56, **330-331**
Malingering, 18, 196
Malocclusion, 29
Mannitol, 256

Mannosidosis, 221
Map-dot-fingerprint dystrophy, 226
Marcus Gunn jaw winking syndrome, 116
Marcus Gunn pupil, 2, 66, 78, 106, 280
Marfan's syndrome, 22, 86, 216, 272
Marginal corneal ulcers, **208-209**
Marginal reflex distance, 116
Mast cell stabilizers, 203
Measles, 66
Medial canthal laxity, 118
Medial orbital wall fracture, 166
Medial rectus (MR) muscle, 164, 166
Medically uncontrolled primary open-angle glaucoma, surgery for, **252-253**
Medicamentosa, 202
Medications, glaucoma, **262-265**
Meesmann's dystrophy, 220, 226
Megacolon, aganglionic, 68
Megalocornea, 22, 86
Megalophthalmos, anterior, 86
Meibomitis, 36, 50-51
Meige's syndrome, 126
Melanin, 56, 72, 220
Melanocytic nevus, 54
Melanocytic tumors, 330
Melanocytoma, 76, 299
Melanocytosis, 308
Melanokeratosis, 226
Melanoma, 36, 54, 56, 76, 82, 299, 326, **330-331,** 344
Melanosis, 56, 68, 220
Membranous conjunctivitis, 59
Meningeal carcinomatosis, 372
Meningioma, 4, 302, 370, 374
Meningitis, 28, 58, 59, 102, 176
Meningococcal septicemia, 66
Meningococcus, 176
Mephenytoin, 16
Mercury, 218
Mestinon, 14
Metabolic disease, 13, 320
Metabolites, 86
Metachromatic leukodystrophy, 196, 221
Metamorphopsia, 6, 297
Metastatic carcinoma, 132, 314, 344
Methamphetamine, 344
Methanol, 246, 370
Methionine, 272
Methoxyflurane, 344
Methsuximide, 16
Methylmalonic aciduria, 291
Metipranolol, 262
MEWDS; see Multiple evanescent white dot syndrome
Meyer's loop, 375
MFKP; see Mutton fat keratic precipitates
Miconazole, 210
Microbial keratitis, 210
Microcornea, 82
Micronystagmus, 156
Micropannus, 216

Ocular cicatricial pemphigoid, 44, 230
Ocular compression from retrobulbar
 hemorrhage, 26
Ocular facial myokymia, 126
Ocular histoplasmosis, 296, 299, 333,
 356
Ocular hypotony, **260-261,** 326
Ocular inflammation, 26, 348-349
Ocular ischemia, 78, 248, 312, 314
Ocular micropsia, 6
Ocular motor apraxia, 179
Ocular motor nerve palsies, 14
Ocular myoclonus, 368
Ocular pain, 32-35
Ocular pemphigoid, 134
Ocular rosacea, 36
Ocular sarcoidosis, 358
Oculinum; see Botulinum A toxin
Oculocutaneous albinism (OCA), 16,
 68, 72, 178
Oculodermal syndromes, 330
Oculopalatal myoclonus, 368
Oculopharyngeal dystrophy, 116
Oculoplastics, 111-135
Oguchi's disease, 12
OID; see Orbital inflammatory disease
Olivopontocerebellar atrophy with
 retinal dystrophy (OPCA II), 291
Onchocerciasis, 112, 214, 217
ONH; see Optic nerve hypoplasia
Opacities, 268-271, 332-335
OPCA II; see Olivopontocerebellar
 atrophy with retinal dystrophy
Open-angle glaucoma, 101, 234,
 236-237, 244-245, 252-253, 262,
 263, **264-265**
Open-heart surgery, 66
Operculated retinal tear, 336
Ophthalmia, sympathetic, 358
Ophthalmia neonatorum, **176-177**
Ophthalmic artery occlusion, 320
Ophthalmic consultations, 97-109
 arthritis, **100-101**
 diabetes mellitus, **98-99**
 facial trauma, **106-107**
 head trauma, **106-107**
 HIV-positive patient, **102-103**
 sarcoidosis, **104-105**
 thyroid orbitopathy, **108-109**
Ophthalmic ultrasonography, 326
Ophthalmology, 1-95
 acquired hyperopia, **26-27**
 acquired increasing myopia, **22-25**
 acute conjunctivitis, **58-61**
 blepharitis, **50-51**
 chronic conjunctivitis, **62-65**
 decison making in; see Decision
  making in ophthalmology
 distorted vision, **6-7**
 dry eye, **44-47**
 epiphora, **48-49**
 eye pain, **32-35**
 eye trauma, **90-93**
 flashers and floaters, **18-21**
 headache, **28-31**
 hyphema, **78-79**
 hypopyon, **80-81**

Ophthalmology—cont'd
 increased transillumination of iris,
  72-75
 intraocular calcium density, **94-95**
 isolated diplopia, **14-15**
 itchy eye, **40-43**
 lesion of conjunctiva, **56-57**
 macrophthalmos, **86-87**
 microphthalmos, **82-85**
 nonpigmented lesion of eyelid,
  52-53
 painful orbital swelling, **88-89**
 pediatric; see Pediatric
  ophthalmology and strabismus
 photophobia, **16-17**
 pigment alterations of iris, **68-71**
 pigmented lesion of eyelid, **54-55**
 poor color vision, **8-11**
 poor night vision, **12-13**
 red eye, **36-39**
 subconjunctival hemorrhage, **66-67**
 transient visual loss, **4-5**
 tumor of iris, **76-77**
 visual loss, **2-3, 4-5**
Ophthalmopathy, 250
Ophthalmoplegia, 32
Ophthalmoscope, 91, 144, 326, 336
Optic atrophy, 29, 82, 101, 196, 372
Optic disc, 246, **370-371**
Optic nerve, 102, 105, 172, 236, 281,
 299
Optic nerve cupping, 247
Optic nerve disease, 91, 320
Optic nerve drusen, 94, 299
Optic nerve glioma, 370
Optic nerve granulomas, 333
Optic nerve hypoplasia (ONH), 178
Optic neuritis, 16, 32, 101, 102, 196,
 277, 370, 372, 374
Optic neuropathy, 29, 100, 101, 106,
 108, 320, 370, **372-373**
Optic pit, 298
Optociliary shunt vessels, 105
Oral contraceptives, 66, 344
Oral retinoids, 16
Orbicularis muscle, spasm of, 127
Orbital cellulitis, 59, 88, 132
Orbital edema, 128
Orbital fibrosis, 141
Orbital floor fracture, **128-129**
Orbital fractures, ocular compression
 from, 26
Orbital inflammatory disease (OID), 88,
 130, 132
Orbital lesions that press the posterior
 ocular wall anteriorly, 26
Orbital myositis, 32, 36
Orbital pseudotumor, 36
Orbital rim, displacement of portion of,
 128
Orbital swelling, painful, **88-89**
Orbital trauma, **128-129**
Orbital varix, 130, 250
Orbital wall fractures, 32
Orbitopathy, 108-109
Organophosphates, 366
Orofacial dystonia, 126

Oromandibular dystonia, 126
Oscillopsia, 368
Osmotic agents, 284
Osteoma, 94, 299
Outward rotation of everted eyelid
 margin, 119
Overaction
 of inferior oblique (OAIO), **146-147,**
  150, 168
 of superior oblique (OASO), 150,
  168
Overshoot, vitreous opacities that, 19

P

Paget's disease, 296
Pain, eye, 23, **32-35,** 36, 89, **276-279**
Painful orbital swelling, **88-89**
Palinopsia, 6, 14
PAN; see Periodic alternating
 nystagmus
Pancreatitis, 13, 314
Pannus, 216
Panretinal photocoagulation (PRP), 13,
 99, 230, 248, 312, 324, 341
Panuveitis, **358-359**
Pap smear, 59
Papillae, giant, 59
Papillary conjunctivitis, 36, 100
Papilledema, 4, 29, 94, 292, 302, 314,
 370
Papillitis, 16, 102, 292, 314, 333
Papilloma, squamous, 56
Papillomacular bundle, 374
Papillophlebitis, 370
Paracentral scotoma, 374
Parafoveal fixation, 140
Parafoveal telangiectasia, 306
Paralytic strabismus, 107
Paramethadione, 16
Paraproteinemia, 224
Parasellar area, tumors of, 32
Parasites, 66, 333
Parasympathetic nuclei in midbrain,
 lesions of, 26
Parasympathomimetic agents, 172,
 240, 244
Paresis of accommodation, 26
Paresthesias, 106
Parietal skull fracture, 28
Parinaud's oculoglandular
 conjunctivitis, 62
Parinaud's syndrome, 114, 366, 368
Parkinson's disease, 202
Paromomycin, 210
Parry-Romberg syndrome, 218
Pars plana vitrectomy, 6
Pars planitis, 19, 333, **352-353**
PAS; see Peripheral anterior synechiae
Patau's syndrome, 83
Patching, 78, **138-139,** 144, 152,
 254
Patent internal sclerostomy, 256
Pauciarticular disease, 101
PCF; see Pharyngoconjunctival fever
PDR; see Proliferative retinopathy
Pediatric cataracts, **188-189, 190-191**